Handbook of Youth Development

"This book will prove to be an invaluable resource for academics and all those working in a professional capacity with youth. Its positive, multi-disciplinary and cross-cultural content provides a deeply engaging theoretical and practical insight into the contemporary issues facing young people."

—Prof. Phillip Slee, Ph.D., *Professor in Human Development in the School of Education & Director, Student Wellbeing & Prevention of Violence (SWAPv) Research Centre, Flinders University, Australia*

"This collection grapples with the critical tensions between aspirations towards Positive Youth Development and the contemporary challenges facing young people in both formal and informal settings. It will help stakeholders, whether young people, youth workers, social development policymakers, educators or academic researchers, to consider a diversity of international contexts and disciplinary and technical approaches to promoting youth empowerment in the face of challenging political and institutional contexts. It is a valuable resource for exploring the varied policy and programmatic implications of intergenerational partnerships for the Sustainable Development Goals (SDGs) and investments in youth health and well-being, education, economic and professional advancement, civic and political participation, sports participation and digital engagement."

—Dr. Terri-Ann Gilbert-Roberts, Ph.D., *Research Manager, Social Policy Development, Commonwealth Secretariat & Founding Chair of the 50/50 Youth Research Cluster of the University of the West Indies*

"Sibnath Deb has a track record of bringing experts together to pool their knowledge about youth development. This volume, by a range of international experts, covers youth education, marginalisation, political involvement, employment, adversity, resilience, challenges and many other topics involving young people. It will become a valuable resource for educators, clinicians, policy makers, and clinicians."

—Prof. Kim Oates, *Emeritus Professor of Child and Adolescent health University of Sydney, Australia, Former President, International Society for Prevention of Child Abuse and Neglect (ISPCAN)*

"The editors bring together the voices of emerging and established scholars who cover a diverse range of topics from the well-established to more contemporary issues, such AI and COVID-19. This book will be of interest to specialists in the field seeking to update their knowledge, as well as newcomers seeking an introduction to the core topics and ideas in youth development. Insightful and analytic. I recommend this book to anyone interested in justice for young people, as it provides the tools by which it may be furthered."

—Prof. John Scott, Ph.D., *Head of School of Justice, Faculty of Creative Industries, Education and Social Justice, A Block, Kelvin Grove, Queensland University of Technology, Australia*

"I am happy to see the topics covered in the book. The book has important and relevant chapters that are important for the current times as well as the future. The topics on youth covered in the manuscript to name a few, range from expected topics such as youth development to the influence of COVID-19, and the impact of artificial intelligence. On the other hand, the book also addresses various aspects of the youth, such as sports, risky sexual behaviors, suicide, digital influence, and mental health. The book will surely be a significant valuable resource material for whoever is involved with youth affairs and youth development."

—Dr. Roopesh B. N., M.Phil., Ph.D., *Additional Professor, Consultant: Child N Adolescent Mental Health Unit, Adjunct Faculty: Department of Psychosocial Support in Disaster Management, Department of Clinical Psychology, National Institute of Mental Health and Neuroscience, Bengaluru, India*

"This handbook on youth development is a global resource. If the future of our world is contingent on the flowering of young people, it is incumbent upon us to read these chapters."

—Toni Nemia, M.S., *Executive Director, Centre for Child and Family Development, California Institute of Integral Studies, USA*

"This handbook edited by Sibnath Deb, an eminent scholar who have worked and published extensively on child rights and youth & Shayana Deb has five parts covering myriad issues ranging from positive youth development to challenges and issues faced by youth to models of intervention promoting youth development. There are several contributors to this handbook, both emerging and well-known in the field addressing core topics pertaining to youth development. This handbook deftly covers many areas pertaining to youth development and has much to offer for practitioners, policy makers, academicians, students and scholars working on youth development."

—Prof. Asha Banu Soletti, Ph.D., *Centre for Health and Mental Health, School of Social Work, Dean-Students' Affairs, Tata Institute of Social Sciences, Deonar, Mumbai-88, India*

"The *Handbook of Youth Development: Policies and Perspectives from India and Beyond* sets a standard for understanding in an exciting phase of life, youth development. The most salient aspect is that the reported research and literature covers almost all the aspects of youth development. The most comprehensive book I have seen on the topic in recent years. This should be must read for those who try to understand youth development. I highly recommend this book."

—Prof. Azizuddin Khan, Ph.D., *Psychophysiology Laboratory, Department of Humanities and Social Sciences, Indian Institute of Technology Bombay, Powai-400 076, Mumbai, Maharashtra, India*

"This Handbook provides a comprehensive and positive approach to youth development. It compiles valuable knowledge and experiences that highlight the importance of promoting well-being, health, quality of life, and academic-professional growth at this stage of life. It identifies the challenges and adversities that young people face and invites us to reflect on their active participation in communities in order to achieve the goals of the 2030 Agenda for Sustainable Development. It is required reading for academics, researchers, educators, and policymakers."

—Dr. Celina Korzeniowski, Ph.D., *Researcher at the National Scientific and Technical Research Council (CONICET), Argentina, Associate Professor at the School of Psychology, Aconcagua University, Mendoza, Argentina*

"*Handbook of Youth Development: Policies and Perspectives from India and Beyond*, a scientific research-based book demonstrates the complexity of adolescence in the 21st century in multicultural contexts. This innovative book by editors Sibnath Deb & Shayana Deb provides an up-to-date overview of cutting-edge international research and opens as a window to a variety of topics relevant to teenagers these days. This book is a must-read for teachers, teacher educators, school administrators, and school-based mental health professionals and parents."

—Prof. Nurit Kaplan Toren, *Senior Editor, Oxford Symposium in School-Based Family Counseling & Oranim Academic College of Education, University of Haifa, Israel*

Sibnath Deb · Shayana Deb
Editors

Handbook of Youth Development

Policies and Perspectives from India and Beyond

Springer

Editors
Sibnath Deb
Department of Applied Psychology
Pondicherry University (A Central University)
Puducherry, India

Shayana Deb
Faculty of Behavioural and Social Sciences
University of Groningen
Groningen, The Netherlands

ISBN 978-981-99-4968-7 ISBN 978-981-99-4969-4 (eBook)
https://doi.org/10.1007/978-981-99-4969-4

This Springer imprint is published by the registered company Springer Nature Singapore Pte Ltd.
The registered company address is: 152 Beach Road, #21-01/04 Gateway East, Singapore 189721, Singapore

Paper in this product is recyclable.

Foreword

It is axiomatic that adult health, mental health, and well-being rest on a foundation of youth development. Often youth development is seen as a trajectory where a challenge at one or another of the developmental stages leads to some later form of pathology. The *Handbook of Youth Development: Policies and Perspective from India and Beyond* looks at various facets of youth development that contribute to the experience of developing youth into becoming whole, functioning human beings. While the focus and many of the chapters are from an Indian context, the examples are relevant everywhere as the subtitle, "Policies and Perspective from India and Beyond," would suggest.

A survey of the sections of this rich anthology gives some indication of the course it follows: Positive Youth Development; Youth, Education, and Career; Youth, Adversities, and Challenges; The Role of Youth; Youth and Mental Health.

A selection of chapters attests to their diversity and their scope. They might be of interest to and useful to educators, health professionals, especially pediatricians, child psychiatrists, psychologists, social workers, and nurses. Indeed they may be relevant to all of us as self-understanding and self-awareness is an important aspect of coping with life.

The first chapter "Positive Youth Development Through Holistic Approach" by daughter and father, Shayana Deb & Sibnath Deb details the foundation for other chapters of the book. By holistic approach, they mean the quality upbringing of the child free from adversities. They note how physical, psychological, and social development influence child and youth development, and how child and youth development influence academic and career development, leadership development, moral development, and character building. This comprehensive approach with its emphasis on physical, psychological, and social factors echoes the significant work of George Engle's bio-psycho-social "new medical model" with was revolutionary when first published in 1977,[1] and has been widely acknowledged, but not always fully practiced or appreciated. I subsequently suggested that there was a need for a "new 'new' medical model", a bio-psycho-social-spiritual medical model.[2] The dominant medical model through much of the twentieth century has been a reductionistic biomedical model, which has been impressively successful, but has not fully recognized the psychosocial and economic determinants of disease and illness.

The chapters in this volume go beyond the traditional and even the new or new medical models to focus on human development, child and youth development. In rich and specific detail. While the ideal developmental pathway is free from adversities, youth and adults often encounter adversities, even disasters. This useful volume helps us imagine and plan for policies that foster resilience and community supports for life's challenges on the developmental path.

Allen R. Dyer, M.D., Ph.D.
Durham, CA, USA

Professor Emeritus of Psychiatry
and Behavioral Sciences
School of Medicine and Health
Sciences
The George Washington University
Washington, DC, USA

---

[1] In 1977, Engel published the seminal paper, "The Need for a New Medical Model: A Challenge for Biomedicine" [Science 196 (1977) 129–136]. He featured a **biopsychosocial** (BPS) model based on systems theory and on the hierarchical organization of organisms.

[2] Allen Dyer Published 1 April 2011. Southern Medical Journal My experiences as a cancer patient helped me understand the complexity of illness in ways which I could not fully appreciate as a physician trying to be attentive to my patients.

Preface

Youth development has become an important topic for discussion for global policy makers because of the size of the youth population and their potential for faster economic growth and possible contribution for social transformation and community development. Global estimates indicate that there are over 1.2 billion young people around the world, within the age group of 15 and 24 years, which accounts for approximately 16% of the global population. Statistical projections further suggest that India houses the world's biggest youth population, despite having a smaller population than China, according to a UN Study, followed by China in the second place (269 million youths), Indonesia (67 million), the USA (65 million), Pakistan (59 million), Nigeria (57 million), Brazil (51 million), and Bangladesh (48 million) (Source: https://economictimes.indiatimes.com/news/politics). It is expected that the demographic transition will eventuate in more than 60 countries, which are opening a window for a demographic dividend (UNFPA). Youth development in the present changing world necessitates a progressive procedure to empower the youth in facing their challenges and achieving their fullest potential, which is promoted through mentorship, career counseling in the educational institutions, organizing skill-based training programs, giving them the liberty to choose the carrier options based on their aptitude and interest and keeping the future job prospect into account and progressive policies for the youth holistic development. Youth leadership is an integral component of youth development and a potential career option, especially for those who exhibit leadership during their school and college days.

The concept of Positive Youth Development (PYD) received special attention from the researchers and academics especially those who are working with them in the last few decades. The broad objective of PYD is to utilize the potentials of youth by nurturing their internal abilities, providing a supportive and conductive environment and mentorship for optimal utilization of their inherent qualities, and producing responsible and productive citizens for community development and nation building.

Research and practice in areas concerning youths has underpinned the need for effective intervention programs that promote the strength of youths, instead of focusing only on the risk factors concerning them. Positive engagement of the youth in learning and social processes has drawn them away from high-risk and self-defeating behavior. Developing the youth requires focused planning, programming, interventions, monitoring, and evaluation, besides engaging them as partners in various developmental processes. In this regard, it is relevant to mention here that the Rajiv Gandhi National Institute of Youth Development (RGNIYD), an Institute of National Importance by Act of Parliament under the Ministry of Youth Affairs and Sports, Government of India published the first India Youth Development Index in 2010 highlighting the overall and state-wise status of youth respect to education, work, health, civic participation, political participation, and social inclusion and subsequently in 2017. The draft report of India YDI 2021 is ready in which one more domain is included i.e., safety and security of youth since a large number of youth experience violence and also get involved in risk behavior. This document is very much useful for the national policy makers as well as policy makers of every state to take appropriate measures for holistic development. In addition, it is an invaluable document for the young researchers and youth organizations working at the grass-root levels. The YDI should be developed by looking at the country-specific situation utilizing the reliable secondary source of data and sometime, if necessary, primary data also can be collected. New parameters can be considered from time to time considering the contemporary issues related to youth development. The present book is about Youth Development from a futuristic perspective. The main objective of the edited volume is to provide a clear picture about holistic youth development through education, games, sports, mental health support services, and mentorship. The book also presents risk behavior and way forward measures, role of institution-based family counseling, and status of youth with special reference to their role in the society and career options in the present situation in addition to providing a brief sketch about national and international policies and programs for youth development. The conceptualization of the idea behind the book is the outcome of intergenerational dialogue between father, daughter, and son during COVID-19 lockdown.

The volume contains 30 chapters under five broad parts.

Part I: Positive Youth Development

In this part, there are 10 chapters (Chaps. 1–10) discussing various aspects of positive youth development. For example, the first part is about positive youth development and this part has 10 chapters. Chapter 1 by Shayana Deb and Sibnath Deb discusses positive youth development through holistic approach with special reference to physical, psychological, social, academic, and professional development, as well as moral development and character building in addition to discussing theories concerning the PYD and its applications. The chapter also focuses on the role of family, educational institutions, peer group members, and virtual world, including social media, on children and youth. The factors which act as barriers for healthy growth and development of the youth have been emphasized in the chapter. This chapter also sheds light on the interconnection between child protection and youth development and suggests possible way forward measures. In Chap. 2, Peter Geiger and

Brian A. Gerrard describe how the application of School-Based Family Counseling (SBFC) in Higher Education can promote youth development. The use of a SBFC approach in Higher education is warranted because the evidence demonstrates that many youths struggle with family problems and college/vocational school problems that negatively affect academic performance. The chapter describes a pilot Higher Education SBFC project. A detailed case study illustrating the SBFC approach is provided. Literature has the power to mold the youth in the cognitive development of children and youth. Chapter 3, by Sudip Kumar Das, aspires to study how literature works in projecting a spectrum of values and insights to adolescent minds. Literature is known for enhancing academic and cognitive development among the budding youth and reading different genres enriches a young mind with refined aspects of social and emotional intricacies. This chapter also assesses canonical literary texts that are chiefly prescribed in the undergraduate and postgraduate curricula. Chapter 4 Nidup Dorji elaborates about the magnitude of youth population in Bhutan and their role in nation building. He further emphasizes on effective mentorship through educational institutions so that youth do not divert in negative directions. In Chapt. 5 Ruth Richardson discusses the barriers for youth development in the UK and presents the positive initiative taken by the government for the promotion of youth development in the UK.

Games and sports have a significant role in both physical and mental development of youth. In this regard, in Chap. 6, Shane Pill and Phillip T. Slee discuss the role of sports in shaping the outlook of youth to promote peace and harmony in the community. In particular, the authors stated that participation of youth in sports programs will fulfill their social and emotional needs such as having a sense of belongingness, a sense of mastery, a sense of "mattering" and so on. In Chap. 7, Anjali Gireesan and Sibnath Deb discuss the role of sports for developing a new culture for youth and highlight on the programs and initiatives at the national as well as at the international level, which have been brought into focus, to understand the emphasis being laid upon sports. Avinu Veronica Richa, Neivikuolie Khatsu & Amenu Richa in their Chap. 8 highlights the essence of Naga style wrestling or *Kene*—an indigenous sport of the Nagas and largely popular among the *Tenyimia* tribes like the Angami, Chakhesang, and Zeliang of Nagaland, and the Mao, Maram and Poumai Naga tribes of Manipur. Naga style wrestling or *Kene* is considered to be a sport which extends friendship amongst individuals, villages, and communities. This chapter makes the case that in the haste to professionalize traditional sports and games, the true spirit of the game for which it was laid down should not be lost. Chapter 9, by Sanjay Kumar, Shivendra Singh and Jaydeep Biswas discusses India's demographic dividend and its policy implications, especially emphasizing on more investment in health and education through proper coordination among allied Ministries of the Government of India. In Chap. 10 Sahen Gupta and K. Jayasankara Reddy elaborate the foundations of literature concerning confidence, resilience, and identity as cornerstones for positive youth development through sports. Further, the authors emphasize on positive youth development in terms of cognitive, social, and emotional development in addition to life skills to remain competent to face daily life challenges.

Part II: Youth, Education and Career

This part contains six chapters (Chaps. 11–16). In Chap. 11, Sabyasachi Mukhopadhyay and Amlan Chakraborty discuss the impact of Artificial Intelligence (AI) on youth and their career. Aleena Maria Sunny in her Chap. 12 gives a clear picture about teaching as a stimulating profession for youth. She also refers to the lack of young people in the teaching profession, in light of reports from various studies across the world. A brief overview about the changing roles a teacher has to play in the current setting is provided. The chapter also explores statistics on youth population in teaching across the world, as well as on the teacher attrition rates. The chapter ends with a few recommendations for policymakers and social scientists. In Chap. 13, Upasana Bagchi and K. Jayasankara Reddy illuminate upon the evolving scenario in the field of career decision-making among the youth and attempt to offer solutions to the challenges being faced by the youth.

Skill-based training is the need of the hour to achieve the mission of our government i.e., to become self-reliant and to transform India into digital India. Towards this end, RGNIYD organized a series of skill-based training programs during COVID-19 lockdown phase to enhance the knowledge and skills of young IT professionals. After the training program, feedback from the participants was collected by using a Google form. Analyzing the feedback Sibnath Deb, David Paul, Shayana Deb, Shikha Soni, and Emily Hernandez came out Chap. 14 discussing the efficacy of the online training. In particular, the objective of the chapter is to examine the participant's perceptions of the effectiveness of the Internet of Things (IoT) and automation online training. Similarly, Chap. 15 by Sukriti Pant, Bhuvana Manohari Nataraj and K. Jayasankara Reddy discusses the role of media literacy in combating the challenges posed by the usage of social media in addition to discussing various theories, frameworks, models, and components of media literacy. Further, the chapter highlights the impact of the various media literacy interventions on the youth. Chapter 16 examines the effectiveness of online professional and job oriented courses for youth by Sibnath Deb, Tusharika Mukherjee and David Paul.

Part III: Youth, Adversities and Challenges

There are eight chapters in Part III (Chaps. 17–24). Kaustuv Chakraborty in Chap. 17 illustrates how the global youth partakes in the challenge of adapting to a new and different culture and seeks to thrive in it and establish a renewed identity, all from the perspective of two young protagonists.

Young people across Canada are calling adults into action, particularly those in positions of power for addressing their issues like economic disparities, class inequalities, prejudicial thinking, and so on. They urge policy makers to become allies and to create more spaces for the voices of the youth to be heard. Chapter 18 by Jemma Llewellyn acts, not only as a direct answer to these calls to action, but also exemplifies practices of adult allyship in a community-university partnership project, in Ontario. Suicide, as well as self-harm among students and youth, are very high in India. Trina Banerjee and K. Jayasankara Reddy in their Chap. 19 emphasize on early detection and identification of vulnerability of risk behaviour of youth for prevention and enhancing their coping capacity. Intervention based on positive psychology is recommended to help youth in crisis management and also act as preventive and maintenance therapy through holistic mental health approach. The concepts of hope, forgiveness, self-compassion, gratitude, and resilience are suggested to incorporate into the intervention programs to build a better therapeutic system for youths dealing with suicidality. In Chap. 20 Prabhat Kumar Datta and Badri Narayan Kar present an overview of how the civil society actors, the young people, and the local government institutions responded to the COVID-19 pandemic in India, under the overall guidance of the state, to identify the challenges they have faced and what remains to be done to brave this kind of challenge in the future.

Chapter 21 by Tusharika Mukherjee discusses the digital transformation which brought about digital disruption for many youths, leading to the marginalization of those who lack the resources to adapt to the technological transition. Further, the chapter talks about building digital competence among youth so that they can take a greater advantage over automation. Durga P. Chhetri in Chap. 22 examines the progress in achieving the Sustainable Development Goals by 2030, especially in developing countries like India, and focuses primarily on the four important interrelated areas viz., poverty, education, gender equality, and employment for the attention of the policy makers for the overall development of the youth. Besides, this chapter also intends to offer information and analysis to the policymakers and stakeholders, which can help them gauge the progress made in addressing youth issues, assess policy gaps, and develop policy responses to achieve Agenda 2030, for sustainable development in India. Similarly in Chap. 23 Subhasis Bhadra discusses about inequalities experienced by marginalized youth resulting in systemic outcomes of several factors, namely, socio-economic deprivation, political upheavals, prejudices, and stereotypes associated with sex, gender, race, caste, and color, that compound the inabilities to cope with the challenges. Thereafter the author highlights the negative impact of oppressed social situations on career growth of youth and on their mental health. In Chap. 24, Pragati Dattatraya Ubale and T. V. Sekhar provide evidence of risk behavior of unmarried youth analyzing the 5th round of the National Family Health Survey (2019–2021).

Part IV: Role of Youth and Youth Development Index

This part consists of three chapters (Chaps. 25–27). For example, in Chap. 25, S. Lalitha focuses on youth participation in community development activities and the issues and concerns for youth participation. The importance of socio-economic and political contexts of the youth is also discussed in the chapter in addition to other factors that influence them in rendering their participation in community development. The strength-based approach in Social Work is suggested as a suitable intervention to work with youth and to enhance youth social capital for community development. Bishakha Majumdar, in Chap. 26, traces the recent trends in political participation of youth, globally and in India, the factors influencing political participation of youth, and the policy interventions that encourage political activism among the youth in a way that is constructive and beneficial for the new generations. It also suggests interventions that may encourage youth participation in politics, training them in political processes, and ensuring their active and informed participation in politics and policymaking. Chapter 27 by Gemma Wood discusses about the importance of bringing out Youth Development Index.

Part V: Youth and Mental Health

Part four comprises three chapters (Chaps. 28–30). Chapter 28 by Marianne Billington and Tom Billington highlights the conditions for the well-being of young people in contemporary Britain based on conversations between the two authors (daughter and father) that arose during family meals, walks, and coffees in their home city of Liverpool. The issues which emerged from the conversation and discussed in the chapter include culture, economics, gender, and politics and more specifically, issues relating to body image, humor, self-esteem, and the new standards and imperatives that are shaping and defining young people's identity and sense of wellbeing in the contemporary world. Chapter 29 by Tusharika Mukherjee, Sibnath Deb, Nudip Dorji, Shayana Deb, and Aleena Maria Sunny examines the role of resilience and hope in causing a substantial variance in the stress response to anticipation of crisis among Indians living in India and Germany during COVID-19. Resilience, hope, crisis apprehension, and the psychological response to the COVID-19 pandemic were measured among participants from India and Germany via an online survey. Finally, in Chap. 30 Sibnath Deb, Aleena Maria Sunny, Shinto Thomas, Shayana Deb, Fathima G. Ashra, V. S. Sujith and David Paul examine the importance of socio-demographic variables like age, gender, family environment, and relationship with parents and friends, in determining non-cognitive traits, such as flourishing and grit, during the tenure of doctoral research.

This edited volume will be beneficial for the young researchers and academics from social science disciplines viz., psychology, social work, public health, education, sociology, and sports science. It is also expected that NGOs working with children and youth, physical education institutes and teachers of the same institutions, policy makers, District Youth Officers of Nehru Yuva Kendra Sangathan (NYKS), and officers of National Service Scheme will find the volume comprehensive and useful. Every care is taken to produce an error free document. However, if there is any mistake or typographical errors, or errors in the citation of references, these are sincerely regretted.

Puducherry, India — Sibnath Deb
Groningen, The Netherlands — Shayana Deb

Acknowledgements

Conceptualization of a topic for bringing out an edited volume on an important issue by collecting chapters on diverse issues related to a topic requires a lot of thought, review of literature in addition to discussing it with other academics and researchers working in the same field. While conceptualizing the topic, the editors had discussion with a number of youth to understand their perspectives. The editors are grateful to all the youth with whom they discussed the volume for sharing their ideas and researchers whose articles were published in different journals which was a source of knowledge for the editors. The editors especially thank Ayushmaan Deb for his valuable inputs while editing the volume. In addition, the editors thank all the academics and researchers for exchanging their views by providing valuable inputs in shaping the outline of the volume. The significant contribution of all the contributors in this volume from across the world deserves high appreciation to come out with a comprehensive volume on youth development.

Sibnath Deb
Shayana Deb

About This Book

The book provides multiple perspectives of Youth Development from various disciplines. The book comprises of thirty chapters and reflects upon the rich experience of the researchers, academicians and youth activists of different countries. In addition to discussing various challenges faced by the youth, the book presents the best practices related to Youth Development. The book also discusses the status of the youth, with special reference to the perception of their role in the society, as well as their educational and career choices, in the present and rapidly altering world scenario. A wide range of contemporary and relevant issues relating to the holistic career growth of the youth and recognizing youth work as a profession, have been discussed in the volume. This edited volume shall be one of its kind, with a rare combination of bringing together a range of professions for the youth, in addition to traditional government jobs.

Given its comprehensive coverage, the book will be of interest to the youth, scholars, teachers, researchers and policy makers of population sciences, childhood and youth studies, development studies, psychology, sociology, social work, in addition to youth activists and NGOs working in the field.

Contents

Editors and Contributors

About the Editors

Sibnath Deb Ph.D., D.Sc., is a Professor of the Department of Applied Psychology at Pondicherry University (A Central University). He served the Rajiv Gandhi National Institute of Youth Development (An Institute of National Importance), Government of India, as Director from January 8, 2020, to June 30, 2023. He is also an Adjunct Professor at the School of Justice, Queensland University of Technology (QUT), Australia and Member Board of Directors, Institute for School-based Family Counselling, California, USA. From 2004 to 2008, he served the International Society for Prevention of Child Abuse and Neglect (ISPCAN) as a Council Member. He has produced 22 Ph.Ds., published 22 books (by Sage, Springer, Routledge, PEARSON, and so on), and more than 100 research articles. His research interests include child safety, students' mental health, youth development, adolescent reproductive health, family relationships and child protection. In recognition of his academic and research contribution, Prof. Deb has received many national and international awards, including "The Visitor's Award 2019" for his significant contribution to research from the Honourable President of India, Shri Ram Nath Kovind.

Shayana Deb holds a M.Sc. in Behavioural Science from the CHRIST (Deemed to be University), Bengaluru, India. Currently, she is doing a second Master's Degree in Youth Policy from the University of Groningen, The Netherlands. She did her undergraduate with a triple major, i.e., Biotechnology, Chemistry and Botany. She has a special interest in child protection and youth development. She volunteered in three research projects which developed her interest in child welfare and well-being and positive youth development.

Contributors

Nida Ansari College of Social and Applied Human Sciences, University of Guelph, Guelph, Canada

Fathima G. Ashra Department of Applied Psychology, Pondicherry University (A Central University), Puducherry, India

Upasana Bagchi Department of Psychology, CHRIST (Deemed to be University), Bengaluru, India

Trina Banerjee Department of Psychology, CHRIST (Deemed to Be University), Bengaluru, India

Subhasis Bhadra Department of Social Work, School of Social Sciences, Central University of Rajasthan, Bandarsindri, Kishangarh, Ajmer, Rajasthan, India

Marianne Billington University of Manchester, Manchester, UK

Tom Billington University of Sheffield, Sheffield, UK

Jaydeep Biswas Chief, Policy and Partnership, United Nations Population Fund (UNFPA), Lodi Estate, New Delhi, India

Amlan Chakrabarti A. K. Choudhury School of Information Technology, University of Calcutta, Salt Lake City, Kolkata, India

Kaustuv Chakraborti Department of English, Rajiv Gandhi National Institute of Youth Development, Sriperumbudur, Tamil Nadu, India

Durga P. Chhetri Department of Political Science, School of Social Sciences, Sikkim University, Gangtok, Sikkim, India

Sudip Kumar Das Faculty, Department of English, Rajiv Gandhi National Institute of Youth Development, Sriperumbudur, Tamil Nadu, India

Prabhat Kumar Datta Department of Political Science, University of Calcutta, Kolkata, India

Shayana Deb Department of Behavioral and Social Sciences, University of Groningen, Groningen, The Netherlands;
Department of Psychology, CHRIST (Deemed to Be University), Bengaluru, India

Sibnath Deb Department of Applied Psychology, Pondicherry University (A Central University), Puducherry, India;
Ministry of Youth Affairs and Sports (MYAS), Government of India (GOI), Pennalur, Sriperumbudur, India

Nidup Dorji Department of Public Health and Allied Health Sciences, Faculty of Nursing and Public Health, Khesar Gyalpo University of Medical Sciences of Bhutan, Thimphu, Bhutan

Peter Geiger Family Therapist, San Diego, CA, USA;
Consultant: Oxford Symposium in School-Based Family Counseling, San Diego, CA, USA

Brian Gerrard Institute for School-Based Family Counseling, San Diego, CA, USA

Anjali Gireesan Defence Research and Development Organisation (DRDO), Ministry of Defence, Government of India, New Delhi, India

Sahen Gupta Sport & High-Performance Psychologist/Lecturer in Applied Sport Psychology, University of Portsmouth, Portsmouth, UK;
School of Sport, Health & Exercise Sciences, University of Portsmouth, Portsmouth, UK

Emily J. Hernandez Rajiv Gandhi National Institute of Youth Development (RGNIYD), Ministry of Youth Affairs and Sports (MoYAS), Government of India (GoI), Sriperumbudur, Tamil Nadu, India

Badri Narayan Kar Department of Political Science, University of Calcutta, Kolkata, India

Neivikuolie Khatsu Nagaland Olympic Association, Office Complex, Kohima, Nagaland, India

Sanjay Kumar Population Dynamics and Research Specialist, United Nations Population Fund (UNFPA), Lodi Estate, New Delhi, India

S. Lalitha Department of Social Work, RGNIYD, Sriperumbudur, India

Jemma Llewellyn College of Arts, University of Guelph, Guelph, Canada

Bishakha Majumdar Organizational Behavior and Human Resource Management, Indian Institute of Management Visakhapatnam, Visakhapatnam, India

Tusharika Mukherjee Work and Organizational Psychologist, Münster, Germany;
Associated with Justus-Liebig University, Giessen, Germany

Sabyasachi Mukhopadhyay Centre for Computational and Data Sciences, IIT Kharagpur, Kharagpur, India

Bhuvana Manohari Nataraj Department of Psychology, CHRIST (Deemed to be University), Bengaluru, India

Sukriti Pant Via News Didi, Jalandhar, India

David Paul Rajiv Gandhi National Institute of Youth Development (RGNIYD), Ministry of Youth Affairs and Sports (MoYAS), Government of India (GoI), Sriperumbudur, Tamil Nadu, India;
Department of Applied Psychology, Pondicherry University (A Central University), Puducherry, India

Shane Pill Flinders University, Adelaide, SA, Australia

K. Jayasankara Reddy Department of Psychology, CHRIST (Deemed to be University), Bengaluru, India

Amenu Richa North East Initiative Development Agency (NEIDA), Kohima, Nagaland, India

Avinu Veronica Richa Rajiv Gandhi National Institute of Youth Development (RGNIYD), Sriperumbudur, Tamil Nadu, India

Ruth Richardson University of Derby, Derby, UK

T. V. Sekher International Institute of Population Sciences, Mumbai, India

Shivendra Singh Data Analyst, United Nations Population Fund (UNFPA), Lodi Estate, New Delhi, India

Phillip T. Slee Flinders University, Adelaide, SA, Australia

Shikha Soni Rajiv Gandhi National Institute of Youth Development (RGNIYD), Ministry of Youth Affairs and Sports (MoYAS), Government of India (GoI), Sriperumbudur, Tamil Nadu, India

V. S. Sujith Department of Applied Psychology, Pondicherry University (A Central University), Puducherry, India

Aleena Maria Sunny Department of Psychology, St. George's College, Weybridge, UK;
PGCE Teacher Trainee at, UCL Institute of Education, London, UK

Shinto Thomas Teacher of Psychology, St. George's College, Weybrigde, UK

Pragati Dattatraya Ubale International Institute of Population Sciences, Mumbai, India

Gemma Wood Numbers and People Synergy, Canberra, Australia

Part I
Positive Youth Development

Chapter 1
Positive Youth Development Through Holistic Approach

Shayana Deb and Sibnath Deb

Abstract Youth development has become a poignant topic of discussion due to the sheer size of this population. Therefore, policy makers of most countries are focusing on youth development by introducing suitable policies and programs, with an objective to utilize their full potential for community development. Youth can play a very important role in social and community development, as well as in climate change, as they are very creative, innovative, energetic, and dynamic. For nation building the role of youth is very crucial. During the last few decades, researchers and academics have been focusing on positive youth development (PYD) for optimal utilization of their potential and for producing responsible and productive citizens for community development and nation building. Mentorship through educational institutions, for imparting value education and imbibing a spirit of nationalism, would be rewarding. This chapter discusses positive youth development through holistic approach with special reference to physical, psychological, social, academic, and professional development, as well as moral development and character building. The chapter also focuses on the role of family, educational institutions, peer group members, and virtual world, including social media, on children and youth, in addition to discussing factors which act as barriers to healthy growth and development of the youth. This chapter also sheds light on the interconnection between child protection and youth development and suggests possible way forward measures in addition to providing a brief overview of policies and programs for youth development.

Keywords Child · Youth · Positive development · Physical development · Psychological development · Social development · Academic and career development · Moral development

---

S. Deb (✉)
Department of Behavioral and Social Sciences, University of Groningen, Groningen - 9712 CP, The Netherlands
e-mail: shayanadeb65380@gmail.com

S. Deb
Department of Applied Psychology, Pondicherry University (A Central University), Puducherry 605 104, India

S. Deb and S. Deb (eds.), *Handbook of Youth Development*,
https://doi.org/10.1007/978-981-99-4969-4_1

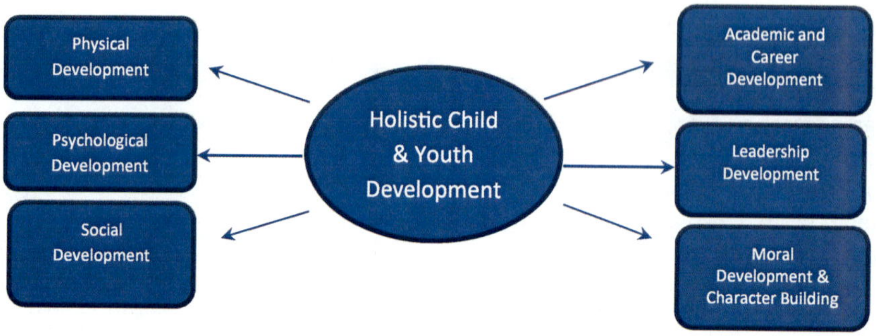

Fig. 1.1 Holistic child and youth development

Introduction

The root of holistic and healthy youth development lies in the quality upbringing of a child, free from all adversities. This goes back to the period prior to childbirth. Nutritional status of a mother during pregnancy, age of conceiving a child, health care facilities for a pregnant mother, mothers' educational background and life styles, as well as other support facilities, play a very important role in the healthy upbringing of a child, which impacts their entire life. Therefore, basic care for the potential mothers, as well as basic care and support facilities to every child after delivery and during the formative years, are crucial to healthy physical growth and enjoy childhood with parents' love and affection. Nevertheless, adversities in different forms on account of internal and external factors are barriers for a large number of children for their healthy childhood development. This chapter discusses positive youth development through holistic approach with special reference to physical, psychological, social, academic, and professional development, as well as moral development and character building in addition to focusing on the role of family, educational institutions, peer group members, and virtual world, including social media, on children and youth. The following diagram provides a clear idea about holistic child and youth development (Fig. 1.1).

Physical Development

Healthy physical development of a child and youth keeps them active, productive, and energetic, in addition to staying away from sickness. Proper physical development largely depends upon adequate nutrition, timely medical care in case of health problems, and physical activities, in terms of games and sports, yoga, and/or pranayama. Generally, during childhood, every child gets maximum pleasure, joy, and happiness through games and sports. Unfortunately, most of the children and youth of the current generation do not get such opportunities, because of urbanization and lack of space for playgroups in the educational institutes. On and above, hectic pressure for study i.e., time table of the educational institute, does not allow children to find time from their daily routine to spend time on the playground. Educational institutes stress more on teaching and less on extra-curricular activities, although educational policy of most of the countries directs educational institutes to give special emphasis on physical activities and experiential learning. In reality, learning is mostly classroom based mostly in the developing countries like India. At the same time, most of the parents and teachers want their children to remain occupied in their studies only resulting in poor physical development. Another interesting feature is that a large number of rural children and youth suffer from malnutrition, mostly caused by poverty, while urban children and youth suffer from obesity because of special preference for fast food. Too much dependence on mobile phones is another contributing factor for poor physical development of children and youth.

The Indian school education system is textbook-oriented, focusing on memorization of lessons, and demands long hours of systematic study every day. The elaborate study routines, which are expected by high school students, spanning from the morning till late evening hours, leaving little time for socialization and recreation. A number of studies highlighted that "mental health problems among children and adolescents are frequent in India as well" (Basu et al., 2020; Madasu et al., 2019; Mohapatra et al., 2014).

Academic stress during childhood and youth is found to be associated with retarded physical growth and physical fitness. A large number of children and youth remain so busy in studies throughout the year that they get no time for physical or recreational activities. Findings disclosed that the impact of academic stress is also far-reaching. For example, one study reported that "high levels of academic stress have led to poor outcomes in the areas of exercise, nutrition, substance use, and self-care (Weidner et al., 1996). Furthermore, academic stress is found to be a risk factor for psychopathology. Another study observed that "fourth, fifth, and sixth-grade girls who have higher levels of academic stress are more likely to experience feelings of depression" (Wenz-Gross & Siperstein, 1997). Many adolescents in India are referred to hospital psychiatric units for school-related distress—exhibiting symptoms of depression, high anxiety, frequent school refusal, phobia, physical complaints, irritability, weeping spells, and decreased interest in school work (Basu et al., 2020; Madasu et al., 2019; Verma et al., 2002).

Because of academic stress, failure in examinations and other challenges, every day, 41 Indian students commit suicide (Crime in India, 2020), raising questions regarding the effects of the school system on the well-being of young people. Suicide among students has increased from 10,335 in 2019 to 14,825 in 2020. That is why psychiatrists have expressed their concern at the emergence of education as a serious source of stress for school-going children, causing high incidence of deaths by suicide (D'Mello, 1997).

In order to ensure physical fitness, the Ministry of Youth Affairs and Sports, Government of India, has come out with a program called "FIT INDIA". The basic concept of this program is that every individual should go for at least half an hour to one hour of physical exercise in any form every day to remain physically fit. In the

New Education Policy 2020, much emphasis is given to extra-curricular activities and choice-based education with multiple exit options keeping the overall welfare and well-being of the children and youth. Hopefully, above initiatives will improve the situation in near future so far as health of children and youth are concerned.

Psychological Development

Psychological and/or emotional development of a child and youth primarily depends upon the family environment. If a child is born in a family where both the parents are caring and provide basic support facilities, including love and affection to the child and the intra-parental relationship is positive, it will have a positive impact on the mental health of a child and the youth. Parents' educational and cultural background, outlook, profession, lifestyles, and values in life have also a significant impact on the psychological and emotional development of a child. On the contrary, children born and brought up in a disturbed family environment suffer from adjustment problems, temper tantrum, inferiority complex, loss of interest and motivation in studies, anxiety, depression, and suicidal ideation (Artz et al., 2014). Children victims of intimate partner violence are vulnerable to lifelong negative outcomes and in turn, the negative consequences are reflected in the society in terms of involvement of those children in socially undesirable activities (Artz et al., 2014).

Adversities in early childhood and in the youth phase have been found to be associated with distorted mind-set of children as well as youth, and they become vulnerable to academic backwardness, social isolation, social deviance, and risk behavior (Björkenstam et al., 2017; Logan-Greene et al., 2017; Roberts et al., 2018). Evidence also demonstrates that childhood adversities have a positive association with later life mental health challenges, like depression and anxiety. For example, one study carried out in Sweden covering 478,141 individuals reported that cumulative childhood adversity is associated with early adulthood depression, in terms of a clinical diagnosis and antidepressant medication (Björkenstam et al., 2017). The same study highlighted that parental psychiatric disorders are particularly associated with depression.

One Indian study observed that "about half of the school students experienced moderate levels of anxiety while 13.2% suffered from high levels of anxiety during the COVID-19 pandemic. The study also disclosed that more than one-third (34.8%) and one-fourth (27.5%) of students were suffering from moderate and high levels of depression, respectively" (Deb et al., 2022). Another study carried out in Germany reported that "two-thirds of the children and adolescents were highly burdened by the COVID-19 pandemic. They experienced significantly lower health-related quality of life (HRQoL) (40.2% vs. 15.3%), more mental health problems (17.8% vs. 9.9%), and higher anxiety levels (24.1% vs. 14.9%) than before the pandemic. Children with low socio-economic status, migration background, and limited living space were affected significantly more" (Ravens-Sieberer et al., 2022).

Social Development

Relationships with different social agents make a significant difference in the life of an individual, as well as in the success of their career. As we maintain good relationships with parents, we need to maintain good interpersonal relationships with peer group members, extended family members, teachers, elderly people, and significant others. In turn, it would ensure a strong social network and an individual will remain likely to get social support at times of crisis. Therefore, during the development phase, parents should take their children to social gatherings and encourage them to mingle with others and maintain social relationships, in addition to taking part in different social, cultural, spiritual, and other outgoing activities. This initiative by parents will make a child and youth more social and proactive in life.

Emotional intelligence has a very important role for an individual to maintain harmonious relationships with different social agents. In simple words, emotional intelligence means regulating one's own emotions and understanding the emotion of others. In other words, "emotional intelligence or emotional quotient is the ability to understand, use, and manage your own emotions in positive ways to relieve stress, communicate effectively, empathize with others, overcome challenges, and defuse conflict" (Source: https://www.helpguide.org/articles/mental-health/emotional-intelligence). It assists an individual build stronger relationships, succeed at school and work, and achieve career and personal goals. It also helps an individual at every step of their life, while dealing with challenges effectively in social and community life. Therefore, youth should apply this concept in their life to be well-adjusted in social life and to overcome stress caused by various factors.

There are four dimensions of emotional intelligence and they include:

1. **Self-management**—You're able to control impulsive feelings and behaviors, manage your emotions in healthy ways, take initiative, follow through on commitments, and adapt to changing circumstances.
2. **Self-awareness**—You recognize your own emotions and how they affect your thoughts and behavior. You know your strengths and weaknesses, and have self-confidence.
3. **Social awareness**—You have empathy. You can understand the emotions, needs, and concerns of other people, the ability to pick up on emotional cues, feel comfortable socially, and recognize the power dynamics in a group or an organization.
4. **Relationship management**—You know how to develop and maintain good relationships, communicate clearly, inspire and influence others, work well in a team, and manage conflict (Source: https://www.helpguide.org/articles/mental-health/emotional-intelligence).

Academic and Career Development

Every child should get the opportunity for education. Education helps in cognitive development and rational thinking, as well as intellectual development. For better academic and career development, a child requires quality education, proper guidance, and values in life, in addition to a supportive family environment. The career path of a child needs to be decided based on the aptitude and interest of a child, considering the market demand of a particular subject. In this regard, the role of a career counselor or psychologist is very important. They can help in choosing the right career path, by examining the aptitude and interest of a child. With the changing global scenario, with respect to the development and diversification of education, children and the youth have multiple options to choose for career progression. Children and youth should be informed about all possible options and opportunities within the country and at the global level. In this regard, student support services of the educational institutes need to play a vital role.

It has been observed that parents with low levels of education i.e., non-graduates, pressure their children more for better academic performance than the parents with graduation and post-graduation backgrounds. In developing countries like India, education is highly correlated with better job prospects and enhanced quality of life. That is why parents wish their children to perform well in studies for leading a quality of life and in turn, it also ensures support for parents during their old age. The findings of a secondary data based study covering low and middle income countries confirmed the association between indicators of poverty and the risk of common mental disorders (Patel & Kleinman, 2003). One study observed low academic anxiety among adolescents from high socio-economic classes—which may be partly attributed to their secured future at least in material aspects. The prevalence of anxiety disorders tends to decrease with higher socio-economic status (Sadock & Sadock, 2000). Another study has also reported that social disadvantage is associated with increased stress among students (Goodman et al., 2005).

In a study, Deb et al. (2015) observed that nearly two-thirds (63.5%) of the students reported stress due to academic pressure while about two-thirds (66%) reported getting more pressure from their parents for better academic performance. The degree of parental pressure experienced differed significantly across the educational levels of the parents, mother's occupation, number of private tutors, and academic performance. In particular, children of fathers possessing a lower education level (non-graduates) were found to be more likely to perceive pressure for better academic performance. Further, the study disclosed that about one-thirds (32.6%) of the students were symptomatic of psychiatric caseness and 81.6% reported examination-related anxiety.

Close mentorship and/or careful guidance meted out to children and youth are highly beneficial to generate interest among them in studies and guide them in the right direction as per their aptitude and interest, for successful career progression. In this regard, a study found that a close mentoring initiative program benefited the high school students to express and discuss their research and their social and emotional concerns (Qua et al., 2020).

Limited research has been undertaken to examine the causal and contributory factors for motivating underprivileged youth in academic and career development. In a longitudinal study carried out in California, covering Black and Latino youth from lower social strata found that "youth's beliefs about their ability to engage politically (i.e., socio-political efficacy) predict motivations for post-secondary plans (e.g., encouragement; pressure from parents/family), is subsequently related to engagement in academic and career activities, albeit in different directions" (Uriostegui et al., 2021). Further, the authors suggested that "to continue fostering positive youth development, critical consciousness programming will need to integrate how youth understand their role in changing social inequality in relation to their perception of and interactions with parents and mentors" (Uriostegui et al., 2021).

A large number of children and youth suffer from different forms of disorders and disabilities, which do not draw the attention of the institutional authorities, mostly due to lack of knowledge and understanding about the issue and lack of specialized support service facilities. However, this issue requires the attention of the administrators of academic institutes, so that the potential of children and youth with disorders or disabilities can be utilized to the maximal level, by providing need-based support services at an early age. In this regard, Nguyen et al. (2020) carried out a meta-analysis study titled "understanding the essential components and experiences of youth with autism spectrum disorders in peer mentorship programs during the transition to adulthood: A qualitative meta-ethnography" and found that "peer mentors played an essential role to facilitate the positive experiences that mentees had with program components, including interactions with peer groups. Successful peer mentorship programs created a safe environment for mentees to practice skills and helped mentees gain confidence to expand their roles to take leadership in their learning".

Moral Development and Character Building

Moral development of a child and youth plays an important role in their social and personal life. It gives a special identity to an individual. Moral development as well as rational thinking helps an individual to distinguish between right and wrong. It is mostly developed among children through socialization in the family and observing the behavior and lifestyles of the parents. The role of schools, peer group members, family culture, neighborhood, and religious institutions greatly influence the moral development of children and youth in terms of cognitive changes, emotions, and even neurodevelopment. Moral development is a continuous process across a lifetime. Daily life experiences and real life challenges also influence the morality of an individual.

In addition, a positive mind-set, patience, and tolerance add additional value to a young person to interpret any situation judiciously and/or from the right perspective. Broadly, there are four qualities of moral development and they include moral reasoning, conscience, empathy, and self-control.

Character building of children and youth is the beginning of becoming a responsible citizen and contributing toward nation building. Values like humanity, sincerity, hard work, honesty, integrity, and positivity are some of the defining qualities of human beings. All these qualities are to be inculcated among children and youth through educational institutions and teachers should be mentors in this regard. A good character helps an individual to win over others by their pleasing personality, behaviors, and manners. A person with good character always remains loyal to the institutions and plays a responsible role in social life. It is very important for a child and youth to become a good human being first, whose presence will make a positive difference in the community.

Children and youth should be exposed to various social issues concerning humankind so that they can identify them with the issues and think of finding viable solutions. Close connection with the community would insist children and youth to take a leading role in introducing transformational changes in the community, to improve the overall quality of life of common people.

Swami Vivekananda's mantra for the youth is evergreen. He stated: *"Until you can trust yourself, you cannot trust Allah or God."* If we are not able to see God in other humans and ourselves, then where can we find divinity? This is the best example of the moral development of a child and youth.

Digital Literacy Among Children and Youth

In today's technology-driven society, children and youth should be oriented with digital literacy to meet the academic expectations of the institutes and to gather academic related information from the websites from time to time, for career progression. During the last two years when educational institutions were closed on account of COVID-19, children and youth from the rural areas could not progress much in terms of learning, due to lack of computer facilities and/or non-availability of android phones and lack of digital literacy. According to UNICEF's (2020) report on the access to digital education during the COVID-19 pandemic, 1.3 billion children aged between 3 and 17 years presently do not have access to the internet, forming 66% of the school-going population. Sambuli and Magnoli (2019) reported that thousands of youths in the developing nations do not have access to connectivity or digital literacy, exposing them to what is called the 'digital divide'.

To avoid a similar situation, every educational institution should be provided adequate computer and internet facilities and rural youths need to be oriented on digital literacy, so that they can move ahead with urban children and youth in their career growth.

Leadership Development

Every child is born with some qualities. It should be identified by the parents and teachers by observing their performance and role in day to day life. At the same time, educational institutes should organize extra-curricular activities like debate and discussion on contemporary issues, extempore contests, essay competitions, creative writing competitions, assignments on different issues, project presentations, science exhibitions, as well as games and sports. Every student should be encouraged to participate in all those activities as per their interest, which will in turn bring out their creative and in-born talent. Children's creativity has been manifested during childhood and parents as well as teachers should encourage them in the same direction, considering the circumstances and social situation. Students should also be encouraged to take part in community-based development activities like cleanliness drives, social awareness related to the environment, factors related to climate change, social myths and misconceptions concerning health and nutrition, and so on. In the process of engagement in community development activities, the leadership role of the children and youth ought to be visible in their behavior and some of them might get interested in those activities and play the role of a leader to bring a social change.

Since children and youth are the future of the nation and from them, some will come to politics, special leadership development programs may be organized in every educational institute for children and youth. Leadership development programs focusing on issues like personality development, counseling skills, especially how to become an active listener, becoming empathetic, conflict resolution, peace-building, life skills, communication skills, disseminating information about various welfare schemes and legislative measures on contemporary issues, and demonstration of understanding about an issue through lectures and so on will be highly beneficial for children and the youth. Youth can take the lead role in various activities of knowledge dissemination among peer group members about best practices, cleanliness drives, literacy campaigns, climate change, myths and misconceptions, providing support to poor people, rehabilitation of street children, health and hygiene, etc.

Educational institutes are the platforms to produce future leaders through value-based education and the involvement of students in different community-based activities in generating special interest among students in serving the community. The National Service Scheme (NSS) of the Ministry of Youth Affairs and Sports, Government of India attracts a large number of school, college, and university students in community development activities and in the long run, aligns some students toward politics and leads the community as a leader. Inculcating spirituality among students to act as responsible leaders through mentoring has been found to be beneficial (Nolan-Arañez, 2020). For formulation of various policies for the welfare of children and youth, youth participation and its positive implications has been acknowledged by the policy makers. However, limited research documented the effectiveness of youth participation in policy formulation and their implementations. Nevertheless, the issue requires more investigation (Villa-Torres & Svanemyr, 2015).

Interestingly, narcissism is found to be associated with child leadership. Brummelman et al. (2021) reported that "children with higher narcissism levels more often emerged as leaders in classrooms. When given a leadership role in the task, children with higher narcissism levels perceived themselves as better leaders, but their actual leadership functioning did not differ significantly from that of other leaders. Finally, the authors concluded based on analysis of data from primary research stating that children with relatively high narcissism levels tend to emerge as leaders, even though they may not excel as leaders".

For success in any service or activity, perseverance is mandatory. A lot of people perceive various initiatives from time to time emotionally and are unable to continue their activities, resulting in failure to achieve the objectives. Similarly, youth engagement in community development activities requires continuity, which is missing in case of some youths. In this regard, Christens et al. (2022) undertook a study titled "Persistence of a youth organizing initiative: cultivating and sustaining a leadership development ecosystem". Analyses of interviews with 19 adolescent and young adult participants revealed that engagement often began before high school and continued long afterward, with more established older leaders playing a variety of roles to engage younger participants and support their development as leaders. The outcome of the study suggested that practical strategies should be thought of, which can enhance the sustainability of these initiatives among students, for witnessing the positive impacts of youth leadership on social justice.

In a secondary study on school-based positive youth development, Curran and Wexler (2017) observed the benefits of peer mentorship, which enhances social confidence and healthy behaviors. However, the authors suggested that "peer mentorship activities should be actively facilitated by an adult supervisor to ensure positive communication and trust between the mentor and mentee".

Child Protection for Faster Economic Growth and Healthy Society

Protection of the rights of the children, including safety of the children from all adversities, yields a number of benefits as highlighted in the conceptual mode (Fig. 1.2). The conceptual model shows what measures need to be taken at the individual, family, and community levels, as well as the State and National levels, and its subsequent impact on building competent youth, which will lead to higher quality of life, less health expenses and better life span. Holistic youth development is not possible until we ensure child protection.

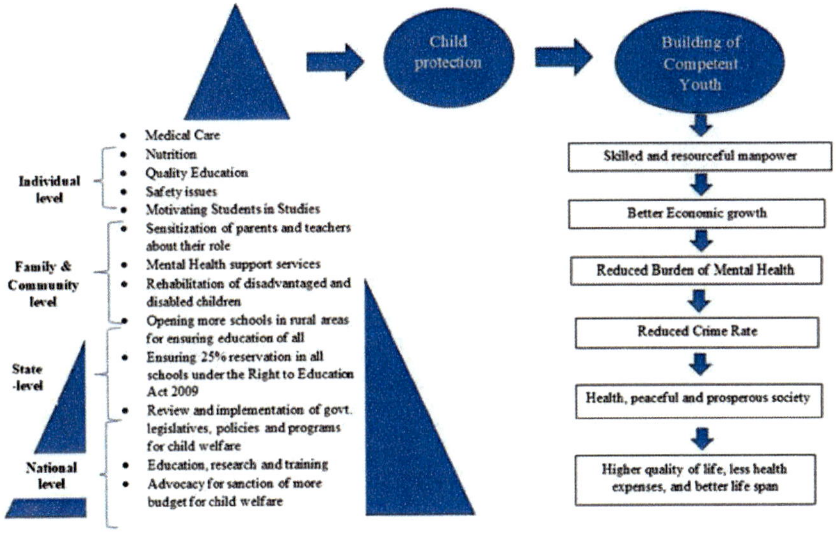

Fig. 1.2 A conceptual model for faster economic growth and healthy society through child protection and youth development (*Source* Deb, 2017)

Positive Youth Development

During the last few decades, researchers and academics have been focusing on positive youth development (PYD) for optimal utilization of their potential and for producing responsible and productive citizens for community development and nation building. PYD is all about inculcating the practice of developing or nurturing internal abilities among the youth population by providing a creative and supportive environment through appropriate mentorship and encouragement so that they can believe in their potential and make positive changes in the society by influencing the world around them. Positive youth development awareness programs fortify youth's sense of character, faith, self-adequacy, and self-esteem as well as their social, behavioral, and emotional competence. PYD programs engage young people in purposeful, productive, and valuable ways while recognizing and enhancing their strengths. These programs enhance positive results by providing a variety of opportunities, fostering positive relationships, and giving the appropriate amount of support that is needed to develop young people's assets and prevent risky behaviors in future. Several research studies have demonstrated that youngsters who are encircled by several opportunities for positive experiences have less chances of engaging themselves into risky and unusual behavior and ultimately are proven to show a successful transition into adulthood (Alberts et al., 2006; Lerner et al., 2012; Roth & Brooks-Gunn, 2000). Cultural diversity and prior experiences can effectively influence a positive development among the young minds. For example, youth living in the United States of America, represent many different background foundations, cultural norms, and lifestyles. The issues faced by these youth are also diverse in nature. PYD can assist and benefit the youth service providers and public health professionals by identifying different circumstances to understand and address the needs of the youth in a better way. PYD improves the feelings of having a sense of belongingness, helps in establishing a positive relationship with peers, strengthens companionship, and also helps in identifying an individual's culture in a society. Increased resiliency and risk reduction can be fostered by utilizing PYD norms and practices with youth and communities of different nationalities, cultures, and specific needs with respect to learning and behavior (Catalano et al., 2004).

PYD proves that fundamental psychosocial conditions are important determinants of youth prosperity (Lerner et al., 2009). Positive youth development depends on the social developmental framework hypothesis, which proposes that youngsters have assets that can be created, supported, and developed (Lerner et al., 2009). A significant PYD asset is the social setting where youths reside like the family, school, and local area associations. Lerner et al. (2009) depicted PYD as a model that promotes the "5Cs". It's a nationally known youth commitment model that deals with not "fixing" behavioral issues, but rather builds and nurtures a child's beliefs and their ways of behaving, perceiving things, and abilities. The outcome ought to be a healthy and positive childhood phase which in turn promotes a fruitful adulthood. The 5cs of positive youth development include:

- **Competence**: It is the capacity and expertise to manage the difficulties, undertakings, and stresses throughout everyday life.
- **Confidence**: It is a positive thought or belief in one's own value and viability. **Connection**: It portrays positive relationships with others, including relatives, friends, and society.
- **Character**: Furthermore, character defines principles of conduct that promote day to day social functioning in various types of social settings.
- **Caring**: Last but not the least, caring emphasizes on showing sympathy and having empathy for others living in the society.

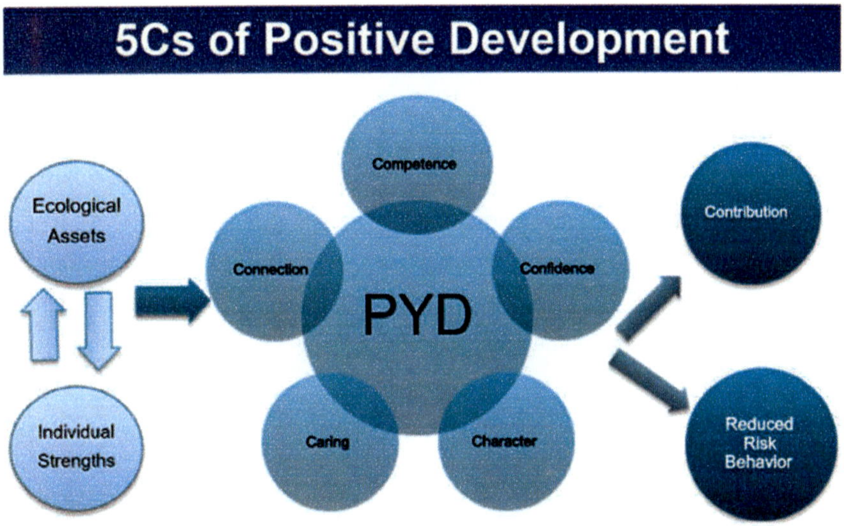

Source: Institute for Applied Research in Youth Development, Tufts University. Medford, Massachusetts.

Over the last many years, most researchers have focused on investigating and deciding psychological wellness utilizing different types of mental health problems (Vaillant, 2012). Up to this point, not many studies connect the 5Cs of PYD. Psychological wellness has been compared to studies about mental health issues. In the positive youth development field, a lot of exploration consideration has been spent on examinations that look at the psychometric properties of the 5Cs of PYD (Chen et al., 2018; Dvorsky et al., 2019), positive improvement corresponding to positive and negative psychological wellness (Holsen et al., 2017; Zhu & Shek, 2020), the improvement of instruments to be adjusted into nearby settings, and the viability of mediations utilizing a positive improvement approach (Ciocanel et al., 2017; Smith et al., 2018). Regardless of these different scopes of examination, the exact relationship between positive youth development, the 5Cs specifically, and mental health is yet to be analyzed.

Socializing has numerous positive implications, such as presenting youth to positive social norms like school commitment, helping peers, donating money, and volunteering for a good cause. For example, the social development model developed by Catalano and Hawkins (1996), asserts that youngsters who experience formatively suitable opportunities for dynamic association in their families, schools, and communities, and are most likely to have positive bonds and attachment with others that reduce or inhibit problematic behavior (Catalano et al., 2003). According to the authors (1996), the following salient factors are vital for prevention:

Community Protective Factors

- Opportunities for prosocial community involvement
- Rewards for prosocial community involvement

School Protective Factors

- Opportunities for prosocial school involvement
- Rewards for prosocial school involvement

Family Protective Factors

- Opportunities for prosocial family involvement
- Rewards for prosocial family involvement
- Family attachment

Peer and Individual Protective Factors

- Religiosity
- Belief in a moral order
- Social Skills
- Prosocial Peer Attachment
- Resilient Temperament

Besides there are a number of examples of positive youth development where researchers got positive results in multicultural set-ups and they include:

- Inside societies of the United States, Local American youth with a high sense of social identity and confidence showed lower levels of liquor and drug use (Zimmerman & Arunkumar, 1947).
- Vietnamese-American youth displayed a more prominent association with their culture and community when they took part in a youth development program that improved their interpersonal skills and boosted their self-confidence (McConachie et al., 2000).
- Youth in Panama, Costa Rica, and Guatemala who had PYD encounters, like associations with peers, educators, and their families, were better at making choices in regard to substance abuse than those with less positive encounters and relationships (DiClemente et al., 2004).
- Youth in Hong Kong who underwent positive youth development awareness programs were encouraged to make contributions to their communities through service-learning activities, and parents and teachers were empowered to serve in supportive roles (Kliewer & Murrelle, 2007).

Factors Influencing Healthy Child and Youth Development

All children in the developing countries are not fortunate to enjoy basic care and support facilities for their healthy growth and development. A good number of children experience a variety of adversities, which adversely affect their healthy growth and development. The factors which adversely affect the healthy growth and development of children and youth include pregnancy before marriage, unwanted pregnancy, preference for male child, dependence of parents on substances, mental health challenges of either of the parents, family violence, common childhood disorders, poor knowledge among the parents about child rights and the quality of the upbringing of children, poverty, lack of social support, abuse of children, girl child marriage, special and/or unique characteristics of children, high expectations of parents from their wards, not listening to the children and youth, lack of educational and medical facilities, and so on (Fig. 1.3). If children enjoy their basic rights, they will grow with positive mental health along with quality education and in turn will be able to contribute to nation building. At the same time, the children who will be deprived from their basic rights i.e., deprivation from nutrition, medical care, education, safety, and experience adversities will affect their healthy growth and development and in turn, they will remain unskilled and vulnerable to exploitation.

In addition, parenting styles and behavior have significant impacts on the healthy growth and development of Children and Youth. As is known, the role of parents is very important for imparting values among children and youth and for their career growth and development. In particular, parenting styles and parental behaviors have significant impacts on personality and emotional development of children and youth. Broadly, there are four types of parenting styles viz., authoritative, authoritarian, permissive (Baumrind, 2013), and uninvolved. Among these four, authoritative parenting style is found to be effective in the quality upbringing of children and

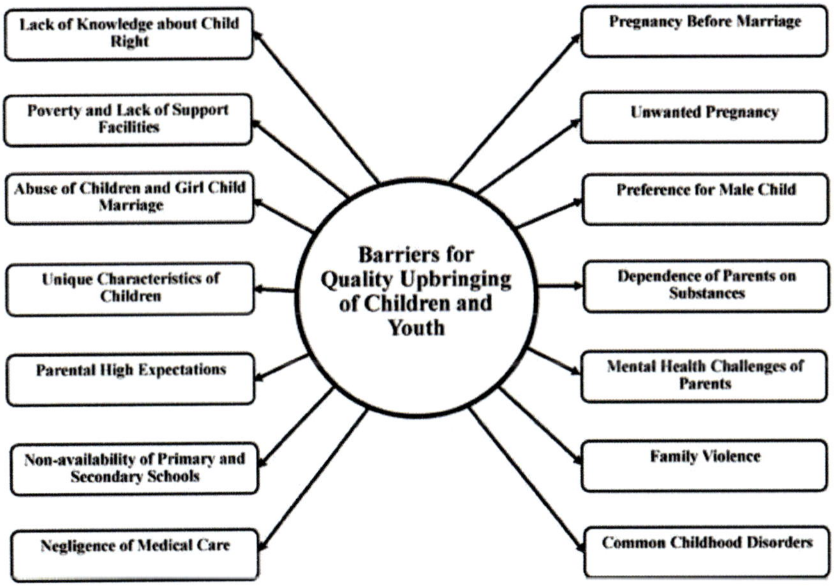

Fig. 1.3 Factors influencing early childhood care, safety and overall well-being of children and youth. *Source* Deb et al. (2022)

youth. Parents following this are highly responsive and they clearly tell their children about their expectations. They are also very supportive and extend support to their child when needed. As compared to authoritative parenting, authoritarian parents lack responsiveness. They are very demanding (Baumrind et al., 2010). Further, they do not rely on their child and their regarding their career and family decision-making processes. They also discourage open discussions with their child about any issue (Gonzalez et al., 2002).

On the other hand, permissive parenting style refers to engaging in child care and parents of this category do not have high expectations from their child. They discuss various issues with their child, even family-related decision-making processes. They allow their child to think differently instead of setting rules for their child. Parents of the uninvolved parenting style category are indifferent about their child's welfare. They also do not extend support to their child in times of crisis (Baumrind et al., 2010). Parents of this category are low in responsiveness and low on demands.

Similarly, parenting behavior such as parental warmth and support, inductive reasoning, and parent–child communication facilitate positive child and youth adjustment and in turn, children and youth feel emotionally secure, happy and become more confident and resilient. Evidence indicates that the socio-economic background of the family and living environment determines the parenting behaviors while guiding their children (Conger et al., 2000). Previous studies demonstrated that children and youth who are exposed to social and community violence tend to indulge in such violent activities while some suffer from anxiety and depression (Ceballo et al., 2003).

Role of Socialization Process During Childhood

Socialization during early childhood plays an important role in every child's life. Socialization refers to behaving in a society following the cultural beliefs, norms, and practices. It helps a child respond to social demands in an appropriate manner. In later life, they are able to behave in a responsible manner, and as adults, they can control their impulses. Family is the place where a child gets orientation on the socialization process, by observing the behavior and lifestyles of parents. This is called informal training. Therefore, parents are the role model for children in terms of behavior, manners, punctuality, honesty, styles of interaction with different social agents, and so on. If a child comes across a parent who leads a disciplined and honest life, is responsible and well-mannered, the child will automatically follow his father or mother and stand out to be a good human being. On the contrary, if a child is brought up between parents who are manipulative in nature, misbehave with others, and do not value and respect others, they are going to follow such parents and subsequently, will be regarded as problematic children.

Therefore, parents should be very careful about their behavior, manners, and lifestyles. Honesty, integrity, humanity, and a positive outlook are very important characteristics of individuals. If a child finds all the characteristics in some of their family members, it will greatly influence them and they will consider them as role models (Deb et al., 2020).

Educational institutions impart formal training to children on the socialization process through participation in various group activities and discipline them to perform every activity systematically. Through group activities, children and youth are able to show their adjustment capacity, tolerance, and acceptability of other views and opinions, as well as social norms and rationality. The outcome of the socialization process within the family and institutions is developing good manners, good habits, and developing a good outlook toward life, in addition to developing good qualities like respecting others and their views, acceptance, adjusting in different situations in life, learning to cooperate, tolerate and respond to different situations in appropriate manner and develop a positive attitude toward interpreting any situation positively, which, in turn, helps a child to remain psychologically happy and lead a well-adjusted life (Deb et al., 2020).

Role of School in Child Growth and Development

The role of school and teachers, like family, is equally important to shape the future of every child and transform them into responsible citizens. The values of school, positive schooling environment, teaching styles, and pedagogy adopted by the teachers and teachers' positive gestures inside and outside the classroom toward students create an encouraging environment for children to study with interest and perform well, in addition to taking part in various cultural and extra-curricular activities. While dealing with the students, a teacher should always remember that no two children are identical in any respect and accordingly, they should deal with them. A teacher should pay special attention to children who are backward and try to clarify their confusions, if any, so that they can proceed in completing his/her studies.

In the process of participation in various activities of the school and higher learning institutes, the potential of a child and youth, in terms of leadership qualities, emerges and in the long run, they play the role of a leader in the community.

Disciplining children when they make a mistake is necessary. But, it should be done in a manner which will not hurt them. At the same time, they will understand their mistake, accept them and correct them.

Role of Peers and Other Social Agents in the Socialization Process of Children and Youth

Developing friendship with peer group members in the educational institutions and in the community is a common practice for every child as they can play with them, spend leisure time and finally get a lot of happiness out of it. In the process of interaction with the peer group members, children and youth also learn a lot from each other. However, there is a possibility to be misguided by some peer group members and get involved in socially undesirable activities, including risk behavior. At the same time, the role of significant others in the community like political/community leaders, extended family members, and elderly persons has an important role to create a positive environment in the community, by organizing cultural programs and games, and sports in which children and youth can take part and develop a sense of belongingness.

Role of Social Media, Mobile, and Internet in the Life of Children and Youth

Information technology, including social media, has become a part and parcel of life for everyone. Now one cannot think of moving from one place to another without a mobile phone as it has multiple facilities and we can connect to anyone easily. Without mobile phones, most people feel helpless and even some suffer from anxiety. Social media consumes a good amount of time from our life as we engage in social media (viz., WhatsApp, Facebook, and Instagram) for long hours every day. In today's society, every grown up child and youth has a mobile and it has become a status symbol and the brand of the mobile is a topic of reference. Sometimes, wrong information uploaded on social media misguides the children and youth and divert their mind from studies to other issues. It also compels people, including children and youth, to form opinions about various issues based on social media information, which is dangerous for a healthy society. Children and youth should be sensitized about the misuse of social media and pay more attention to their studies.

The Influence of the Virtual World on Children and Youth

The advantages of the virtual world are enormous in terms of gaining knowledge, career development, social networking and civic engagement, entertainment, as well as accessibility to health-related valuable information (Burgess & Green, 2018; UNESCO-UNEVOC, 2020).

It is relevant to mention here that the online mode of education and virtual facilities has benefitted a large number of youth pursuing higher education who could not pursue higher education earlier due to various reasons. In addition, online education has empowered youth to access remote resources, best lectures of resource persons from other parts of the world and learn at a comfortable pace. Further, youth are taking advantage of the internet to gain various professional skills such as video editing, website design, cooking, and so on. According to the 2020 IGPP Report (IGPP, 2020), over 70% of youth use the internet for studies and learning new skills along with accessing social media and playing games. According to The World Youth Report (United Nations, 2020 July), "*young people that have Internet access may have opportunities to extend their social networks, strengthen their knowledge base, and identify financing opportunities to support venture creation and development.*" (p. 73). Social media has been found to provide youth with information that helps them to form their identity in addition to providing valuable social services like suicide prevention through tele-counseling and online reporting of child abuse and neglect cases, across the society as it has no boundaries (Chan & Ngai, 2019). The role of digital mental health interventions was found to be very beneficial during the COVID-19 Pandemic, with the youth as one of the main stakeholders. The Government of India also launched the program Manodarpan, which constitutes a website and helplines were also launched to provide mental health assistance during the pandemic (PIB, 2020 July 21).

On the other hand, the virtual world has multiple side effects and they include cognitive decline (Firth et al., 2019; Uncapher & Wagner, 2018; Zhou et al., 2019), mental health challenges due to disconnection with close ones, resulting in lack of emotional attachment and support (Jelenchick et al., 2013), too much dependence on virtual world (Balhara et al., 2018) and vulnerability to cybercrimes (Aboujaoude et al., 2015; Anderson & Jiang, 2018). Evidence indicates that frequent internet users tend to lack emotional and social skills and also tend to be lonely in real life (Engelberg & Sjöberg, 2004). Figure 1.4 depicts the contributions of the virtual world on children and youth and its potential threats.

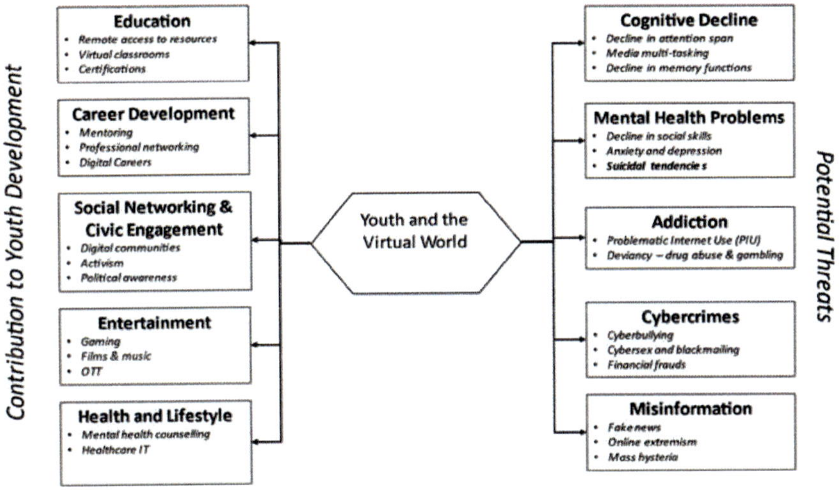

Fig. 1.4 Virtual world and influences on the youth. *Source* Deb et al. (2022). Youth Development in India: Future Generations in a Changing World, London, Routledge

Policies and Programs for Youth Development: International and National Scenario

Globally various youth development policies and programs have been taken by various national and international organizations. In this section, a brief sketch of those policies and programs has been provided including policies and programs taken by the government of India.

Youth Development: International Scenario

i. Commonwealth Youth Development Program

The Commonwealth Youth Program (CYP) aims to work with young people aged between 15 and 29 years in all the 54 Commonwealth member countries and its head office is being stationed in London. The Commonwealth Youth Ministers Meeting decides the activities of CYP. Broadly, it focuses on

- Enterprise/vocational training and microcredit
- Youth participation in decision-making and youth policy
- Professionalization and training for youth workers
- Citizenship, peace-building, and human rights education
- HIV/AIDS awareness and counseling
- Information and Communications Technology
- Democracy (through Commonwealth election observer missions)
- Youth mainstreaming
- Youth Development Index.

In order to encourage youth in development and social work, the Commonwealth Youth Awards for Excellence is given to youth every year for their outstanding activities in the fields of environment protection, education, health and well-being, skill-based training, sports, protection of human rights and so on.

II. International Initiatives for Youth Development

The United Nations (UN) has taken several initiatives for the promotion of youth development globally which in turn helped many member states, particularly the developing nations to focus on their youth population. Some of the agencies of UN for youth related activities are as follows:

1. **UN Department of Economic and Social Affairs Division (DESA)**: The World Program of Action for Youth was set up by DESA with the aim of increasing their understanding about the global situation of the youth. This has played an important role in strengthening the National Youth policies of their member states. They also provide youth the opportunity to partake in the country's official delegations to the UN.

2. **UN Centre for Human Settlements (UCHS)**: Particular emphasis is given to the livelihood aspects of the youth, specifically for the disadvantaged and underprivileged youth who stay in slums and unplanned settlements. It also provides financial support to many developing countries through the UN-Habitat Urban Youth Fund. Poverty reduction and employment generation are also included in their objectives.
3. **United Nations Development Program (UNDP)**: Program provides an array of initiatives: both short and long in nature. Equality, national ownership and leadership, volunteerism, knowledge sharing, and working by, with and for young people are a few among their guiding principles. UNDP being the first to explicitly state their commitment to the youth, expect economic empowerment of the youth, their civic participation in political processes, and engagement in resilience building
4. **United Nations Environment Program (UNEP)**: Promotion of environmental awareness among youth has been taken up as a global agenda. Through regular conferences, information exchange, and capacity building programs, the intention is to cultivate an environmental consciousness youth population across the world.
5. **United Nations Population Fund (UNPF)**: Empowerment of youth is done first by understanding their conditions, and then by bringing together governments through advocacy for more investment in young people. They also provide support to sustainable organizations which are led by young people with the intention of promoting human rights as a priority.
6. **Voice of the youth (VOF) by UNICEF**: Online platform for young people to share their thoughts and opinions as well as understand the issues affecting the world in terms of youth population. The topics may vary from education to violence to conflict to disaster management to human rights. This has various online subsidiaries: Cross-cultural interactions are entertained through 'Voice of Youth Connect', information is gathered through 'Voice of Youth Citizens', and skill training is provided through 'Voice of Youth Maps'.
7. **International Labor Organization (ILO)**: Dedicated to enhancing working opportunities and conditions for young men and women across the world. ILO actively associates with various alliances at various sectors of different countries and is involved in the development of youth employment policies and programs. It has a crucial role to play in the UN Secretary General's Youth Employment Network.
8. **Food and Agriculture Organization of United Nations (FAO)**: FAO has a new strategic objective that has considered youth as their priority. The Feeding Minds, Fighting Hunger Portal, and Education for Rural People (ERP) are some of their education resources provided to children and young adults across the world. Specific needs of vulnerable youth in the rural parts of developing countries, FAO has developed the Junior Farmers Field and Life School Program (JFFLS) that is intense to work toward long term food security.
9. **United Nations Volunteer (UNV)**: UNV has a long history of working for youth across the world. As per reports, "by 2011 23% of UN volunteers and 62% of

UN online volunteers were under the age of 30" (National Youth Policy, 2017). Through youth volunteerism and partnerships, the United Nations agencies ascribe that best to work for and with youth.

10. **The World Program of Action Youth (WPAY)**: it is an initiative that provides a framework for policy building and guidelines for action plans that can be taken up by national or international agencies to work toward improving the conditions of young people. They aim to ensure constructive participation of youth by improving the quality and quantity of opportunities available for them. Hunger and poverty, drug abuse, juvenile delinquency, and armed conflicts are some of the priority areas identified by them.

The Government of India Initiatives for Youth Development

Although all the Ministries of the Government of India have some programs focusing on the welfare and well-being of youth, the Ministry of Youth Affairs and Sports is exclusively engaged in holistic youth development through its various schemes and programs. Let us discuss the National Youth Policy 2014 and 2021 (draft) in brief.

National Youth Policy 2014 (NYP 2014), Ministry of Youth Affairs and Sports, the Government of India

The NYP 2014 was implemented with the mission to empower the youth of the country to achieve their full potential and make them productive and responsible citizens so that they can contribute to the economic prosperity of the nation. Installing social values and motivating them for volunteering was another objective of NYP 2014. The policy document encompasses five well-defined objectives, eleven priority areas, and policy interventions in each priority area. The priority areas include: Education; Employment and Skill Development; Entrepreneurship; Health and healthy lifestyle; Sports; Promotion of Social values; Community engagement; Participation in politics and governance; Youth engagement; Inclusion; and Social Justice (National Youth Policy 2014). Along these lines, the National Policy for Skill Development and Entrepreneurship 2015 laid great emphasis and defined skill development of the youth as a joint responsibility of all stakeholders. The conceptualization behind NYP 2014 was in line with the vision of 'Skill India' which aimed at enabling the youth in the country to attain their full potential as a lifelong process. With the growth of individuals comes the growth of the country and is found to be one of the most sustainable ideas (Deb et al., 2021).

National Youth Policy 2021 (NYP 2021, Draft), Ministry of Youth Affairs and Sports, the Government of India

The NYP 2021 develops a ten-year road map for youth development which is aligned with the SDGs and serves to 'unlock the potential of the youth to advance India' and target to achieve the broad objective by 2030. In particular, the NYP 2021 wishes to take measures for youth development in five most important priority areas and they include education, employment and entrepreneurship, youth leadership and development, health, fitness and sports, and social justice. Social inclusion approach is emphasized in designing, planning, and implementation of all schemes and programs for youth development.

The National Education Policy 2020, Ministry of Education, the Government of India

This National Education Policy 2020 is the landmark development after independence to facilitate flexible, interest and aptitude oriented multi-disciplinary education for children. It emphasizes experiential learning in addition to classroom teaching. Pedagogy is given special emphasis in the NEP 2020 stating that education should be inquiry-driven, discovery-oriented, learner-centered, discussion-based, and enjoyable.

The NEP 2020 provides an opportunity to reform at all levels of education from school to higher education in addition to focusing on strengthening teacher training, reforming the existing examination system, early childhood care and restructuring the regulatory framework of education, and to create a new system that is aligned with the aspirational goals of twenty-first century education, including SDG4, while building upon India's traditions and value systems. The NEP 2020 states that.

> The teacher must be at the center of the fundamental reforms in the education system. The new education policy must help re-establish teachers, at all levels, as the most respected and essential members of our society, because they truly shape our next generation of citizens. It must do everything to empower teachers and help them to do their job as effectively as possible. The new education policy must help recruit the very best and brightest to enter the teaching profession at all levels, by ensuring livelihood, respect, dignity, and autonomy, while also instilling in the system basic methods of quality control and accountability. The new education policy must provide to all students, irrespective of their place of residence, a quality education system, with a particular focus on historically marginalized, disadvantaged, and underrepresented groups. Education is the best tool for achieving economic and social mobility, inclusion, and equality. Initiatives must be in place to ensure that all students from such groups, despite inherent obstacles, are provided various targeted opportunities to enter and excel in the educational system (The New Education Policy, 2020).

The Integrated Child Protection Scheme (ICPS), Ministry of Women and Child Development, the Government of India

ICPS is a centrally sponsored scheme with the objective to build a protective environment for children in difficult circumstances, as well as other vulnerable children, through Government and Civil Society Partnership. This scheme brings all related schemes concerning child protection under one umbrella and emphasizes on safety of the children in addition to introducing a data management system for effective implementation of all the programs and for close monitoring so that need-based corrective measures can be taken from time to time.

National Institute of Rural Development and Panchayati Raj (NIRD & PR), Ministry of Rural Development, the Government of India

An education institution under the Ministry of Rural Development that offers programs in over seven brought social science disciplines such as social justice, local governance, public policy, rural management science and technology, and sustainable development to name a few. The institution is known to provide support services for the rural youth through their eminent research and capacity building programs.

Schemes and Programs of the Ministry of Youth Affairs and Sports, the Government of India for Youth

The Ministry of Youth Affairs and Sports, Government of India has taken several initiatives for catering the needs of the youth of diverse categories. Some of them are as follows:

(i) **Rajiv Gandhi National Institute of Youth Development (RGNIYD), Ministry of Youth Affairs and Sports, Government of India**: The RGNIYD—an institute of national importance was established in 1993 with the objective to impart skill-based training programs to the youth of the country. In 2014, it introduced six Master's Degree programs in the field of social sciences. Further, in 2021, the institute introduced six new job oriented courses and they include Master's Degree in Data Science, Artificial Intelligence and Machine Learning, Cyber Security, Mathematics, English, and Sociology. The institute proposes to introduce two more courses on Child Rights and Protection and Cloud Computing in the next year. Apart from the post graduate programs, the institution also offers Ph.D. programs and also engages in research in youth development. The institute is actively engaged in skill-based training programs and 15 day orientation programs for the District Youth Officers of the Nehru Yuva Kendra Sanghatan (NYKS). Frequently it organizes training programs for NSS volunteers across the country. Most of the training programs are organized in partnership with other higher learning institutes and industries. The Whistling Wood International, Mumbai an affiliating institute of RGNIYD is engaged in running creative and film related courses. The extension activities of the institute give emphasis on occupational rehabilitation of marginalized youth. The institute publishes the India Youth Development Index every five years which provides the status of youth across the states with respect to six domains like education, employment, health, civic participation, political participation, and safety.

(ii) **Nehru Yuva Kendra Sangathan (NYKS)**: It is one of the largest programs with nearly 8.5 million members for mobilization of youth and youth club members for community development activities in addition to focusing personality development of youth. The Tribal Youth Exchange Program, the Adolescent Health and Development Programme, the Promotion of Folk Art and Culture, and the National Integration Camps are some of the outstanding programs of NYKS.

(iii) **National Service Scheme (NSS)**: NSS is another large scale institute-based activity which encourages school, college, and university students to take part in social service. This program is based on the ideologies of Mahatma Gandhi which encourages voluntary community services among the youth. The NSS volunteers are given the opportunity to learn through their field experience while working with real life issues of the citizens of a country. This includes issues related to awareness generation about social issues, cleanliness drives, tree plantation, women empowerment, disaster management, and so on.

(iv) **National Program for Youth and Adolescence Development (NPYAD)**: This scheme provides financial assistance to 5 major objectives focusing on youth and adolescence development, which are personality development, national integration, promotion of adventures, adolescence empowerment, adolescent empowerment, and resource development.

(v) **National Young Leaders Programs (NYLP)**: The primary aim is to encourage the leadership skills of theyouth and utilize it for nation building. Its components are: Neighborhood Youth Parliament (educating through debates and discussions at a village or community level), Youth for Development Program (promoting dignity of labor through volunteerism), National Youth Leaders award (rewarding youth for their outstanding performance in their respective areas), National Youth Advisory Council (involving youth leaders and stakeholders in important decision-making processes) and National Youth Development Fund (mobilizing financial resources for Youth Development).

In order to recognize and motivate youth in social development work, the Ministry of Youth Affairs and Sports, Government of India and UN Volunteers give awards to youth every year for their exemplary work in the community. Every year National

Youth Festival is organized in India in different parts of the country to create a platform for exchanging knowledge and experience of youth.

Some of the Skill Development Programs for Youth Under Different Ministries of the Government of India

(i) **Mahatma Gandhi National Rural Employment Guarantee Act (MGNREGA), Ministry of Rural Development, Government of India: This Act provides** employment opportunities to unskilled workers through promotion of self-reliance. As can be inferred from the given table from the standing committee report on the seven years of performance of MGNREGA, the program has succeeded in providing jobs for people in rural areas where participation of women, SC/ST, and other marginalized societies has been ensured.

(ii) **Deen Dayal Upadhyaya Grameen Kaushalya Yojna (DDU-GKY), Ministry of Rural Development, The Government of India**: The broad objective of this program is to improve employability skills of youth from poor socio-economic background. It is a part of the Skill India Campaign that has initiated several renowned programs such as Make in India, Digital India, and Stand-up India campaigns.

(iii) **Deen Dayal Antayodaya Yojana (DDAY), Ministry of Rural Development, The Government of India**: The program that was initially known as National Rural Livelihood Mission (NRLM) aims at providing an institutional platform for youth from poor socio-economic background that offers easy access to financial services which can be converted to sustainable livelihood options. Some of the key objectives of the program are: (1) creation of a productive workforce, (2) strengthening and diversifying livelihoods, (3) skill training and placement support (4) rural entrepreneurship development. Mahila Kisan Sashaktikaran Pariyojana (MKSP) that empowers women in agriculture and Start-up Village Entrepreneurship Program (SVEP) which motivates and promotes start-up Enterprises for the youth are other programs coming under this program.

(iv) **Prime Minister's Employment Generation Program (PMEGP), Ministry of Micro, Small and Medium Enterprises, The Government of India**: This program aims at promoting opportunity through micro-enterprises for unemployed youth interested in the non-farming sector. The program is interested in investing in both urban and rural areas. The Khadi and Village Industries Commission (KVIC) has been reported to have achieved more than 100% of its target under the PMEGP program during 2016–17.

(v) **Enterprise and Skill Development, Ministry of Micro, Small and Medium Enterprises, The Government of India**: Along with the focus on entrepreneurial skills, specific skills relating to electronics and food processing are particularly encouraged in this program. The program also includes Entrepreneurship Development Programs (EDP), Entrepreneurial Skill Development Program (ESDP), Management Development Program (MDP), Industrial Motivation Campaign (IMC), and Vocational Education Training (VET).

(vi) **Pradhan Mantri Kaushal Vikas Yojana (PMKVY), Ministry of Skill Development and Entrepreneurship, The Government of India**: This is a skill certification scheme that trains in industry relevant skills and aptitude that can increase the probability of youth having a better livelihood. Fees for both training and assessment are completely taken care of by the government and are implemented through the Ministry of Skill Development and Entrepreneurship. Several states are to assess the impact of PMKVY training on youth skill development by providing encouraging reports.

Conclusion and Way Forward

Holistic development of the youth is the outcome of child safety and protection of child rights. Providing basic care and support facilities to all children and protecting them from all adversities and creating a safe community environment through sensitization of larger society will ensure positive youth development and thereby responsible future citizens. Further, quality and need-based education in addition to skill-based training and involvement of children and youth in physical and extra-curricular activities will make them physically and mentally strong, more productive, and a resource toward nation building. However, the issues and challenges faced by the children and youth require attention of the administrators of the educational institutions.

In this regard, the New Education Policy (NEP, 2020) of the Government of India is a paradigm shift for meaningful upbringing of children and youth through multidisciplinary aptitude and interest oriented education. Every educational institute is in the process of implementing it, which will ensure the utilization of the full potential of every child and youth. Along with emphasis on aptitude and interest oriented education, creativity, extra-curricular activities, and experiential learning will get special attention of the educational administrators for the benefit of the students. Certain issues require attention of the authorities of the Ministry of Education and other ministries and they include,

- For imparting quality education, qualified and experienced teachers should be appointed and they should be sensitized to adopt appropriate pedagogy to make the teaching–learning process more interesting.
- Emphasis should be given on experiential learning by engaging students in project work and other creative activities.
- Every educational institute should arrange skill-based training programs and workshops for improving the communication skills and personality development of the students.

- Mental health of the children and youth needs special attention. Therefore, every educational institute should appoint trained school counselors or psychologists to address the mental health needs of the students in a scientific manner i.e., based on evidence. In order to address serious mental challenges, school counselors should involve parents (Pedrelli et al., 2015). In addition, institute-based family counseling programs should be initiated to address the challenges faced by children and youth at the familial level.
- Institute authorities should come out with a proper plan of action to engage students in community development activities periodically without disturbing the regular teaching–learning process.
- At the community level, local community leaders should mobilize the community for addressing the local issues by themselves in which youth can be encouraged to participate. For example, in Rwanda, every Sunday, all the community members get together to clean their locality and it is practiced diligently.
- For effective implementation of various youth development related schemes and programs under different ministries, close monitoring is required by appointing efficient and capable personnel at the top. Periodic evaluation of programs by the third party would help to understand the shortcomings and challenges in implementation and taking corrective measures.

References

Aboujaoude, E., Savage, M., Starcevic, V., & Salame, W. (2015). Cyberbullying: Review of an old problem gone viral. *Journal of Adolescent Health, 57*, 10–18. https://doi.org/10.1016/j.jadohealth.2015.04.011

Alberts, A. E., Christiansen, E. D., Chase, P., Naudeau, S., Phelps, E., & Lerner, R. M. (2006). Qualitative and quantitative assessments of thriving and contribution in early adolescence: Findings from the 4-H Study of Positive Youth Development. *Journal of Youth Development, 1*(2), 20–32.

Anderson, M., & Jiang, J. (2018, May 31). Teens, social media & technology. *Pew Research Center Internet and Technology*. Retrieved from https://www.pewresearch.org/internet/2018/05/31/teens-social-media-technology-2018/

Artz, S., Jackson, M. A., Rossiter, K. R., Nijdam-Jones, A., Géczy, I., & Porteous, S. (2014). A comprehensive review of the literature on the impact of exposure to intimate partner violence on children and youth

Balhara, Y. P. S., Mahapatra, A., Sharma, P., & Bhargava, R. (2018). Problematic internet use among students in South-East Asia: Current state of evidence. *Indian Journal of Public Health, 62*(3), 197.

Baumrind, D. (2013). Authoritative parenting revisited: History and current status

Baumrind, D., Larzelere, R. E., & Owens, E. B. (2010). Effects of preschool parents' power assertive patterns and practices on adolescent development. *Parenting: Science and Practice, 10*(3), 157–201.

Basu, S., & Banerjee, B. (2020). Impact of environmental factors on mental health of children and adolescents: A systematic review. *Children and Youth Services Review, 119*, 105515.

Burgess, J., & Green, J. (2018). *YouTube: Online video and participatory culture*. Wiley.

Björkenstam, E., Vinnerljung, B., & Hjern, A. (2017). Impact of childhood adversities on depression in early adulthood: A longitudinal cohort study of 478,141 individuals in Sweden. *Journal of Affective Disorders, 223*, 95–100.

Brummelman, E., Nevicka, B., & O'Brien, J. M. (2021). Narcissism and leadership in children. *Psychological Science, 32*(3), 354–363.

Catalano, R. F., & Hawkins, J. D. (1996). The social development model: A theory of antisocial behavior. In J. D. Hawkins (Ed.), *Delinquency and crime: Current theories* (pp. 149–197). Cambridge University.

Catalano, R. F., Mazza, J. J., Harachi, T. W., Abbott, R. D., Haggerty, K. P., & Fleming, C. B. (2003). Raising healthy children through enhancing social development in elementary school: Results after 1.5 years. *Journal of School Psychology, 41*(2), 143–164.

Catalano, R. F., Berglund, M. L., Ryan, J. A. M., Lonczak, H. S., & Hawkins, J. D. (2004). Positive youth development in the United States: Research findings on evaluations of positive youth development programs. *Annals of the American Academy of Political and Social Science, 591*, 98–124.

Ceballo, R., Ramirez, C., Hearn, K. D., & Maltese, K. L. (2003). Community violence and children's psychological well-being: Does parental monitoring matter? *Journal of Clinical Child and Adolescent Psychology, 32*(4), 586–592.

Chan, C., & Ngai, S. S. Y. (2019). Utilizing social media for social work: Insights from clients in online youth services. *Journal of Social Work Practice, 33*(2), 157–172.

Christens, B. D., Morgan, K. Y., Cosio, M., Dolan, T., & Aguayo, R. (2022). Persistence of a youth organizing initiative: Cultivating and sustaining a leadership development ecosystem. *Journal of Community Psychology, 50*(5), 2491–2507.

Chen, B. B., Wiium, N., & Dimitrova, R. (2018). Factor structure of positive youth development: Contributions of exploratory structural equation modeling. *Personality and Individual Differences, 124*, 12–15.

Ciocanel, O., Power, K., Eriksen, A., & Gillings, K. (2017). Effectiveness of positive youth development interventions: A meta-analysis of randomized controlled trials. *Journal of Youth and Adolescence, 46*(3), 483–504.

Conger, K. J., Rueter, M. A., & Conger, R. D. (2000). The role of economic pressure in the lives of parents and their adolescents: The family stress model. In *Negotiating adolescence in times of social change* (pp. 201–223)

Crime in India (2020). National Crime Records Bureau. Retrieved from http://ncrb.nic.in/cii2020/cii-2020/figure%20at%20a%20glance.pdf

Curran, T., & Wexler, L. (2017). School-based positive youth development: A systematic review of the literature. *Journal of School Health, 87*(1), 71–80.

Deb, S., Strodl, E., & Sun, H. (2015). Academic stress, parental pressure, anxiety and mental health among Indian high school students. *International Journal of Psychology and Behavioral Science, 5*(1), 26–34.

Deb, S. (2017). Child protetion: The key for better growth statistics and hormany in the nation. Delivered Prof. Anima sen memorial special lecture in the Indian Science Congress held in Shri Venkaterswara University, Triputi during January 3–7, 2017

Deb, S., Kar, S., Deb, S., Biswas, S., Dar, A. A., & Mukherjee, T. (2022). A cross-sectional study on mental health of school students during the COVID-19 pandemic in India. *Data, 7*(7), 99.

Deb, S., Majumdar, B., & Sunny, A. M. (2021). *Youth development in India: Future generations in a changing world*. Routledge India

Deb, S., Bhadra, S., Sunny, A. M. & Sahay, S. (2000). *Childhood to adolescence: Issues and concerns*. New Delhi, PEARSON.

D'Mello, P. (1997). Forcing kids to be counterproductive. In *The Tribune* (p. 17)

DiClemente, C. C., Schlundt, D., & Gemmell, L. (2004). Readiness and stages of change in addiction treatment. *American Journal on Addictions, 13*(2), 103–119.

Dvorsky, M. R., Kofler, M. J., Burns, G. L., Luebbe, A. M., Garner, A. A., Jarrett, M. A., & Becker, S. P. (2019). Factor structure and criterion validity of the five Cs model of positive youth development in a multi-university sample of college students. *Journal of Youth and Adolescence, 48*(3), 537–553.

Engelberg, E., & Sjöberg, L. (2004). Internet use, social skills, and adjustment. *Cyberpsychology and Behavior, 7*(1), 41–47.

Firth, J., Torous, J., Stubbs, B., Firth, J. A., Steiner, G. Z., Smith, L., & Sarris, J. (2019). The "online brain": How the Internet may be changing our cognition. *World Psychiatry, 18*(2), 119–129.

Goodman, E., Ewen, B. S., Dolan, L. M., Schafer-Kalkhoff, T., & Adler, N. A. (2005). Social disadvantage and adolescent stress. *Journal of Adolescent Health, 37*(6), 494–492.

Gonzalez, A. R., Holbein, M. F. D., & Quilter, S. (2002). High school students' goal orientations and their relationship to perceived parenting styles. *Contemporary Educational Psychology, 27*(3), 450–470.

Holsen, I., Geldhof, J., Larsen, T., & Aardal, E. (2017). The five Cs of positive youth development in Norway: Assessment and associations with positive and negative outcomes. *International Journal of Behavioral Development, 41*(5), 559–569.

IGPP (2020). Patterns of internet usage among youths in India. Institute for Governance, Polices & Politics & Social Media Matters & Youth Online Learning Organisation, New Delhi. Retrieved from https://www.socialmediamatters.in/patterns-of-internet-usage-among-youths-in-india

Jelenchick, L. A., Eickhoff, J. C., & Moreno, M. A. (2013). Facebook depression? Social networking site use and depression in older adolescents. *Journal of Adolescent Health, 52*(1), 128–130.

Kliewer, W., & Murrelle, L. (2007). Risk and protective factors for adolescent substance use: Findings from a study in selected Central American countries. *Journal of Adolescent Health, 40*(5), 448–455.

Lerner, R. M., Bowers, E. P., Geldhof, G. J., Gestsdóttir, S., & DeSouza, L. (2012). Promoting positive youth development in the face of contextual changes and challenges: The roles of individual strengths and ecological assets. *New Directions for Youth Development, 2012*(135), 119–128.

Lerner, J. V., Phelps, E., Forman, Y., & Bowers, E. P. (2009). *Positive youth development*. Wiley.

Logan-Greene, P., Tennyson, R. L., Nurius, P. S., & Borja, S. (2017, December). Adverse childhood experiences, coping resources, and mental health problems among court-involved youth. In *Child & youth care forum* (Vol. 46, No. 6, pp. 923–946). Springer US

Madasu, S., Malhotra, S., Kant, S., Sagar, R., Mishra, A. K., Misra, P., & Ahamed, F. (2019). Anxiety disorders among adolescents in a rural area of Northern India using screen for child anxiety-related emotional disorders tool: A community-based study. *Indian Journal of Community Medicine: Official Publication of Indian Association of Preventive and Social Medicine, 44*(4), 317.

McConachie, H., Huq, S., Munir, S., Ferdous, S., Zaman, S., & Khan, N. Z. (2000). A randomized controlled trial of alternative modes of service provision to young children with cerebral palsy in Bangladesh. *The Journal of Pediatrics, 137*(6), 769–776.

Mohapatra, S., Agarwal, V., Sitholey, P., & Arya, A. (2014). A clinical study of anxiety disorders in children and adolescents from North Indian children and adolescents clinic. *Asian Journal of Psychiatry, 8*, 84–88.

Nguyen, L., Jack, S., Ketelaar, M., Di Rezze, B., Soper, A. K., & Gorter, J. W. (2020). Understanding the essential components and experiences of youth with autism spectrum disorders in peer mentorship programmes during the transition to adulthood: A qualitative meta-ethnography. *Child: Care, Health and Development, 46*(6), 667–681.

Nolan-Arañez, S. I. (2020). The intersectionality of leadership and spiritual development through mentoring. *New Directions for Student Leadership, 2020*(166), 97–110.

Patel, V., & Kleinman, A. (2003). Poverty and common ental disorders in developing countries. *Bulletin of the World Health Organization, 81*(8), 609–615.

Pedrelli, P., Nyer, M., Yeung, A., Zulauf, C., & Wilens, T. (2015). College students: Mental health problems and treatment considerations. *Academic Psychiatry, 39*(5), 503–511.

PIB (2020, July 21). Union HRD Minister launches MANODARPAN initiative of Ministry of HRD to provide psychosocial support to students for their mental health and well-being.

Press Releases. Retrieved from https://www.education.gov.in/sites/upload_files/mhrd/files/Manodarpan-merged_0.pdf

Qua, K., Pinkard, O., Kundracik, E. C., Ramirez-Bergeron, D., & Berger, N. A. (2020). Near peer mentors to address socio-emotional issues among underrepresented minority high school students in research intensive STEM programs: Perceptions of students and mentors. *Journal of STEM Outreach, 3*(1).

Ravens-Sieberer, U., Kaman, A., Erhart, M., Devine, J., Schlack, R., & Otto, C. (2022). Impact of the COVID-19 pandemic on quality of life and mental health in children and adolescents in Germany. *European Child and Adolescent Psychiatry, 31*(6), 879–889.

Roberts, Y. H., English, D., Thompson, R., & White, C. R. (2018). The impact of childhood stressful life events on health and behavior in at-risk youth. *Children and Youth Services Review, 85*, 117–126.

Sadock, B. J., & Sadock, V. A. (Eds.) (2000). *Kaplan & Sadock's comprehensive textbook of psychiatry* (7th ed., Vols. 1–2). Lippincott Williams & Wilkins Publishers

Sambuli, N., & Magnoli, S. (2019, April). What is digital equality? An interview with Nanjira Sambuli. In *World economic forum*

Smith, E. P., Osgood, D. W., Oh, Y., & Caldwell, L. C. (2018). Promoting afterschool quality and positive youth development: Cluster randomized trial of the PAX good behavior game. *Prevention Science, 19*(2), 159–173.

The New Education Policy (2020). Ministry of Education, Government of India

UNESCO-UNEVOC (2020). *Virtual Conference on Skills for a Resilient Youth: Virtual Conference Report. UNESCO-UNEVOC TVeT Forum, 6–14 July 2020. Skills Development, Commonwealth of Learning.* Retrieved from https://unevoc.unesco.org/home/Virtual+conference+on+skills+for+a+resilient+youth

UNICEF. (2020). *How many children and young people have internet access at home? Estimating digital connectivity during the COVID-19 pandemic.* UNICEF

United Nations (2020, July). The World Youth Report: Youth Social Entrepreneurship and the 2030 Agenda. Retrieved from https://www.un.org/development/desa/youth/wp-content/uploads/sites/21/2020/07/2020-World-Youth-Report-FULL-FINAL.pdf

Uncapher, M. R., & Wagner, A. D. (2018). Minds and brains of media multitaskers: Current findings and future directions. *Proceedings of the National Academy of Sciences, 115*(40), 9889–9896. Retrieved from https://www.pnas.org/content/pnas/115/40/9889.full.pdf?

Uriostegui, M., Roy, A. L., & Li-Grining, C. P. (2021). What drives you? Black and Latinx youth's critical consciousness, motivations, and academic and career activities. *Journal of Youth and Adolescence, 50*(1), 58–74.

Vaillant, G. E. (2012). Positive mental health: Is there a cross-cultural definition? *World Psychiatry, 11*(2), 93–99.

Verma, S., Sharma, D., & Larson, R. W. (2002). School stress in India: Effects on time and daily emotions. *International Journal of Behavioral Development, 26*(6), 500–508.

Villa-Torres, L., & Svanemyr, J. (2015). Ensuring youth's right to participation and promotion of youth leadership in the development of sexual and reproductive health policies and programs. *Journal of Adolescent Health, 56*(1), S51–S57.

Weidner, G., Kohlmann, C. W., Dotzauer, E., & Burns, L. R. (1996). The effects of academic stress on health behaviors in young adults. *Anxiety, Stress, and Coping: An International Journal, 9*, 123–133.

Wenz-Gross, M., & Siperstein, G. N. (1997). Importance of social support in the adjustment of children with learning problems. *Exceptional Children, 63*, 183–193.

Zhu, X., & Shek, D. T. (2020). Impact of a positive youth development program on junior high school students in mainland China: A pioneer study. *Children and Youth Services Review, 114*, 105022.

Zhou, F., Montag, C., Sariyska, R., Lachmann, B., Reuter, M., Weber, B., & Becker, B. (2019). Orbitofrontal gray matter deficits as markers of Internet gaming disorder: Converging evidence from a cross-sectional and prospective longitudinal design. *Addiction Biology, 24*(1), 100–109.

Zimmerman, M. A., & Arunkumar, R. (1994). Resiliency research: Implications for schools and policy. *Social Policy Report, 8*(4), 1–20.

Shayana Deb obtained M.Sc in Behavioural Science from the CHRIST (Deemed to be University), Bengaluru, India. Currently she is pursuing second Master Degree on Youth Policy at the University of Groningen, The Netherlands. She did her undergraduate with a triple major i.e., Biotechnology, Chemistry and Botany. She attended a number of online courses on different subjects based on her areas of academic interest. She has a special interest in child protection and youth development. On a voluntary basis, she worked in two research projects which created interest in her on child welfare and well-being issues and positive development of adolescence and youth. She has published three articles, eight book chapters and one conference proceedings as co-author. Recently she co-authored two books and they include (i) Social Psychology: Theories and Applications and (ii) Community Psychology: Emerging Issues and Challenges (in press, Routledge).

Prof. Sibnath Deb Ph.D. & DSc, is Professor of the Department of Applied Psychology, Pondicherry University (A Central University), Puducherry, India. Prior to that, Prof. Deb served the Rajiv Gandhi National Institute of Youth Development (An Institute of National Importance), Ministry of Youth Affairs and Sports, Government of India as Director for three and half years (January 8, 2020 to June 30, 2023). Professor Deb was also acting as Director (I/C), Directorate of Distance Education, and Dean (I/C), School of Law, Pondicherry University. He also taught at the University of Calcutta. In 1994, Professor Deb did an intensive course on 'HIV/AIDS and Qualitative Research' from the University of Western Australia. From April 2009 to August 2009, Professor Deb visited the School of Public Health, Queensland University of Technology (QUT), Brisbane, Australia, as Visiting Faculty. Currently, he is also Adjunct Professor at the School of Justice, QUT, Australia. During 2004–2008, he served the International Society for the Prevention of Child Abuse and Neglect (ISPCAN) as Council Member. In brief, he has 32 years of teaching, research and administrative experience and has produced 22 Ph.Ds. in addition to publishing more than 100 research articles/book chapters in the leading national and international journals. Professor Deb has written 10 books and edited 11 books. Some of his latest published books are (a) Child Safety, Welfare and Well-being: Issues and Challenges (2nd Edition, 2022, Springer Nature, Singapore); (b) School-based Family Counseling For Crisis and Disaster (2023, Routledge, California); (c) Health and Wellbeing: Challenges, Strategies and Future Trends (2022, Springer Nature, Singapore); (d) Youth Development in India: Future Generations in a Changing World (2021), Routledge. Professor Deb has received three national and three international awards in recognition of his contribution in the field of psychology including "Visitor's Award-2019" from the Hon'ble President of India Shri Ram Nath Kovind. His current areas of research interest include family dynamics, parenting styles, child safety, students' mental health, adolescent reproductive health and applied social psychology

Chapter 2
The Promotion of Youth Development in Higher Education Through School-Based Family Counseling

Peter Geiger and Brian Gerrard

Abstract This chapter describes how the application of school-based family counseling (SBFC) in Higher Education can promote youth development. The use of a SBFC approach in Higher education is warranted because the evidence demonstrates that many youths struggle with both family problems and college/vocational school problems that negatively affect academic performance. The chapter describes a pilot Higher Education SBFC project. A detailed case study illustrating the SBFC approach is provided. Challenges to developing a SBFC youth development approach are discussed and different solutions recommended.

Keywords Youth development · Higher education · Promotion · School-based family counseling

Introduction: The Strengths of School-Based Family Counseling

School-based Family Counseling (SBFC) is an integrated systems approach to helping children and youth succeed academically and personally through the linking of school-focused and family focused mental health approaches (Gerrard & Soriano, 2019). SBFC has nine strengths: interdisciplinary focus; educational focus; family and school focus; systems orientation; parent partnership; multicultural sensitivity; child advocacy; promotion of school transformation; and evidence-based support.

SBFC is an interdisciplinary metamodel (see Fig. 2.1) in that it may be practiced by any of the mental health professions: psychology, psychiatry, psychiatric nursing,

P. Geiger (✉)
Family Therapist, San Diego, CA, USA
e-mail: ptrgeiger@aol.com

Consultant: Oxford Symposium in School-Based Family Counseling, San Diego, CA, USA

B. Gerrard
Institute for School-Based Family Counseling, San Diego, CA, USA
e-mail: gerrardb@usfca.edu

S. Deb and S. Deb (eds.), *Handbook of Youth Development*,
https://doi.org/10.1007/978-981-99-4969-4_2

social work, counseling, marital and family therapy. In addition, and crucially, many SBFC psycho-educational and counseling interventions may be made by educators. SBFC interventions include counseling, psychotherapy, and psychoeducation strategies. The term SBFC practitioner is used to indicate that the SBFC approach is not specific to any particular mental health discipline. In this regard, SBFC bears a similarity to the way family counseling/therapy developed outside the traditional mental health disciplines and then became incorporated into all of them.

SBFC has an educational focus with an emphasis on promoting the academic success of the student. This educational emphasis is appealing to teachers as well as parents and guardians because it avoids the message "you need therapy", which many families find stigmatizing, and the goal—adaptation to life challenges (Geiger, 2017;

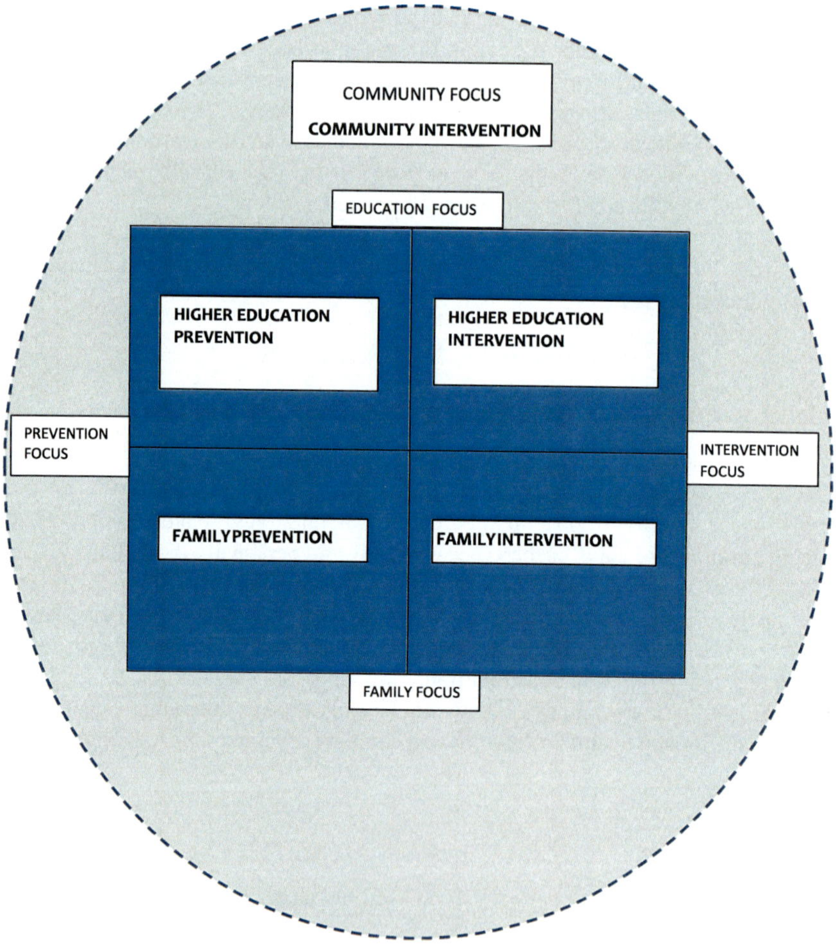

Fig. 2.1 The SBFC meta-model applied to higher education

Ivey et al., 2005)—is experienced as more client-centered and less pathologizing than many traditional mental health approaches. There is research demonstrating that when parents are referred to community mental health clinics for therapy because their child or youth is struggling at school because of "family problems", many families refuse to go. In many cultures, there is a stigma around seeking therapy. Seeing a mental health practitioner means that you are "crazy" or have poor mental health (American Psychiatric Association, n.d.; Glied & Cuellar, 2003). SBFC avoids this stigmatizing effect by framing the meetings between the SBFC practitioner and the family as having a primary goal of promoting the educational success of the child or youth. Furthermore, the SBFC practitioner is acutely aware that families are valuable resources for empowering children and youth and that a reason for collaborating with families is not just to address problems in the family, but also to mobilize family strengths. Conversely, the SBFC practitioner is also aware that schools can have both positive and negative effects on students and that a SBFC approach also involves making changes at the school level. For example, bullying is common in schools. School transformation is considered as important as family transformation.

The combined family and school focus is a hallmark of SBFC. Both play an important role in child and youth development. Children and youth spend a significant portion of their lives in educational institutions (primary, secondary, and tertiary) and in families. A core premise of SBFC is that students who are struggling academically can best be helped by mental health interventions that influence both family and school. The term "school" here is used to refer to any educational institution at the primary, secondary, or tertiary (also referred to as higher education) levels. Even at the university level, the term school is widely used to refer to how departments are organized around disciplines: e.g. School of Engineering, School of Education, School of Medicine, etc.

SBFC uses a systems approach to understand the multiple relationships in which students are embedded: family of origin, extended family, families of choice, couple relationships, peer relationships, the school community, the classroom, teacher-student relationships, and the broader community. Because of the strong focus on the importance of family, SBFC emphasizes family systems theory, in addition to broader systems theories such as Bronfenbrenner's ecological systems theory.

SBFC emphasizes the importance of approaching the student's parents/guardians as partners with the SBFC practitioner. This collaborative approach in which parents/guardians are treated respectfully as resources and sources of wisdom is fundamental to the SBFC approach. Even in situations where family members are in conflict (e.g. marital conflict between parents) causing a negative impact on the student, often there are other family members (e.g. grandparents, uncles and aunts, siblings) who can be a source of strength and empowerment to the student.

Because of the importance it places on family SBFC is a multiculturally sensitive approach. Unlike many Americentric and Eurocentric approaches to mental health that emphasize individualism and independence from family, the SBFC approach emphasizes interdependence with family. Although the client system in SBFC involves the child/youth, the family, the school, and the community, the

SBFC practitioner is primarily an advocate for the child/youth because they are more vulnerable.

Research using randomized control groups shows moderate evidence-based support for SBFC with children and youth at the primary and secondary education levels (Apisitwasana, et al., 2018; Conduct Problems Prevention Research Group, 2007; Crozier et al., 2010; Eddy et al., 2000; Flay et al., 2004; Kratochwill et al., 2004, 2009; Lochman & Wells, 2004). In addition, there are a large number of correlational and descriptive studies in the mental health literature supportive of a SBFC approach (Gerrard, 2008).

The Need for SBFC in Higher Education

Worldwide there are over 220 million students in higher education and the majority of these are youth (UNESCO Institute for Statistics, 2022) (see Fig. 2.2).

Is there a need for a SBFC approach at the Higher education level? This is a reasonable question given the developmental needs of older youth to separate from their families of origin and develop enough independence to cope with the challenges of navigating higher education and developing careers and families of their own. In addition, Higher education typically involves large classes at universities and vocational schools where traditional school interventions like classroom meetings and guidance groups are rare.

The literature is supportive of applying SBFC at the Higher education level. The evidence consists of numerous studies indicating that a significant percentage of youth in different countries experience relationship problems at the family and/or Higher educational level that interfere with their ability to learn or graduate. In addition, there is research demonstrating that family support and Higher education support play a critical role in promoting student well-being that contributes to academic success.

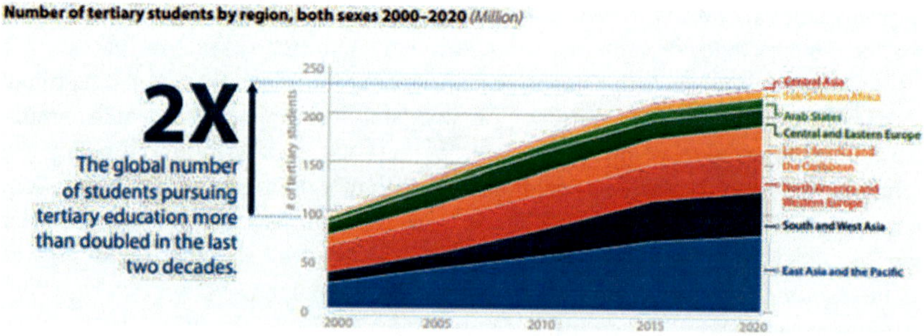

Fig. 2.2 Number of higher education students worldwide 2020–2022 (reprinted from UNESCO Institute of Statistics: Higher Education Statistics at a Glance)

Research on How Family Problems Affect Youth Academic Behavior

Hargrove et al. (2006) have pointed out that the concerns that college students bring to college counseling centers are mainly family related. A common problem experienced by students, especially students from a minority culture, is the socialization in higher education into values that conflict with the parents' values. The intergenerational conflict that results can have a negative effect on students' mental health and academic behavior (Castillo et al., 2012; Lee & Liu, 2001; Lee et al., 2005; Su et al., 2005).

> Scholars have suggested that, by late adolescence, when many children of immigrant parents are in college, parent–child cultural value differences accentuate the typical intergenerational conflict (Lee & Liu, 2001; Lee et al., 2000). Because the university culture is composed of U.S. values and beliefs (Castillo, Conoley, & Brossart, 2004), many Asian American college students may feel pressured to assimilate to the university culture in order to be successful in college. However, adoption of White American beliefs and behaviors, such as individualism, independence, and assertiveness, can lead to conflict with parents who may expect the maintenance of Asian cultural values, such as collectivism, filial piety, and humility (Kim et al., 1999).

A study by Hunt et al. (2017) reported a lower grade point average among college students who experienced more interparental conflict, especially female students and those living away from home. Research by van Ingen et al. (2015) on "helicopter" parents found that this style of parental overprotectiveness had negative effects on college students contributing to poor peer relationships and low self-efficacy. Little (2004) has described how 25%-35% of college students in the USA who come from divorced families experience family stress that affects their studies. Deng et al. (2022) found that family stress contributed more to Pakistani college student stress than did academic stress. Perera (2012) made the following comments giving a perspective on the role of family in higher education in India:

> While deeply investigating major problems faced by the students as personal, social, psychological, economic, and education problems, it could be clearly identified that the root causes of many problems were based on their family backgrounds. It was also revealed that 1/5th of students have to face various types of family problems frequently. Some prominent family problems identified are "economic difficulties", "broken families/single parent families", "fathers' addiction to drugs/alcohol", "parental conflicts", and "illnesses". However, most of the students' problems were directly related with economic background of their families. (p. 2).

Krumrei-Mancuso et al. (2010) report that 87% of college students in their multi-site sample came for counseling for personal (not academic) problems, including family problems. Other researchers have noted the correlation between the quality of student-parent relationship and college grades (Fass & Tubman, 2002; Schwanz et al., 2014). Schnyders and Lane (2018) summarize the importance of family relationships, and relationships in general, for college youth:

> Among college students, relationship quality with family, peers, and romantic partners is an important component of well-being (Lane & Fink, 2015). Relationship problems are a

> primary concern among college students seeking counseling (Mistler et al., 2012). Other common presenting concerns among college student clients—namely, eating disorders, suicidality, and abuse—may also be related to relational factors (Gallagher, 2007). (p. 239)

Research on How Higher Education Problems Affect Youth Academic Behavior

At some higher education institutions, when students have mental health challenges, they have difficulty getting help because of an academic culture of silence and stigma around the need for mental health support (Siegel & Keeler, 2020). Often professors are not viewed as individuals that students can seek help from when they are experiencing emotional problems. Siegel & Keeler (2018) make the following in comments:

> When the group discussion turned to disclosure to professors, many participants noted they did not want their professors to know about their experiences with depression: "I would be horrified if my professors ever knew. Like, seriously I would definitely not want my professors to know at all." A reason students' put forth for not wanting professors to know about their experiences with depression was a fear of being stigmatized as a result. As described by one participant, "I'm definitely afraid of being written off if I bring it up. There is so much pressure to be taken seriously and I feel like that would hinder people's ability to think of me seriously." Another student explained, "I think there is still a stereotype where depression equals laziness." (p. 216).

A similar study by Sabaner and Arnold (2021) gives further examples:

> In contrast, however, Ceebee had a professor who "rejected" her request to take the day off after a Black man was killed by the police in her hometown, which caused her to feel "drained" for the rest of the week. Daniel's negative experiences with his math professor caused him to isolate further. He said, "It's frustrating that [professors] don't necessarily care about your success. They kind of just care that you can eventually get out of their hair, and they can move on with their day and get their paycheck." His social isolation was exacerbated further by his professor's apathy: "It's really weird being in this void of "Do people around me really care about my success and all that? Do I mean something, or am I just a person existing? Am I just a number on your attendance? Am I a name on your sheet? Is that all I am, or am I actually a person?" (p. 26)

A survey of Australian college students by Stallman and Hurst (2016) found the following sources of stress prevalent (the percentage of students affected are shown in parentheses): academic coursework demands (95.6%), friendships (59.8%), family (57.8%), romantic relationships (56%), university environment (50.6%), parental expectations (46%), relationship breakdown (36.3%). Five of the top sources of stress are relational. However, academic course demands were the top stressor.

A challenge that many minority students encounter in universities where the majority of students, faculty, and staff belong to the majority group (e.g. white) is discrimination. They experience the university environment as inhospitable. Consequently, there is low minority student retention, i.e. failure to graduate (McClain & Perry, 2017). In addition, minority youth at universities are often negatively impacted by microaggressions (Nadal et al., 2014). One study indicated that 18% of college undergraduates have experienced bullying (MacDonald, 2010), and it is estimated that 100,000 students drop out of college each year because of bullying (Cardin, 2014).

Research on How Family Support Facilitates Youth Academic Behavior

Jones et al. (2018) reported the following observations regarding the importance of family support to youth:

> Students rely on family for emotional support (Budescu & Silverman, 2016). Research has demonstrated that family support offers emotional adjustment (Larose & Boivin, 1998), which in turn leads to greater academic dedication and efficacy (Budescu & Silverman, 2016) as well as reduced test anxiety (Song et al., 2015). Although emerging adulthood is characterized by increased autonomy (Goldscheider & Davanzo, 1986), maintaining strong ties to one's family is important for adjustment to college (Wintre & Yaffe, 2000). In fact, individuals who remain emotionally close to their families find it easier to adjust to a new social environment and display increased help-seeking behavior (Holt, 2014).

Schnyders and Lane (2018) make a similar point: "… our findings suggest that parent relationships may be a salient protective factor from perceiving the early emerging adult years as a time of instability" (p.249). Studies by Fass and Tubman (2002) and Schwanz et al. (2014) suggest that positive college student-parent relationships are associated with higher grades.

Research on How Higher Education Support Facilitates Youth Academic Behavior

Jones et al. (2018) make the following observations about the importance of peer support to youth in Higher educational institutions:

> Given that many college students live away from home, they often rely on other students for support (Thompson, 2008). Peers who understand the pressure of higher education may be more equipped to provide empathy relating to academics and financial stressors (Larose & Boivin, 1998). For example, students in Thompson and Mazer's (2009) study indicated that peers were often more successful than instructors at explaining or clarifying class content and that venting to peers was the most useful form of academic support that they received.

Several studies indicate that faculty support is important for student retention (Kalkbrenner et al., 2021; Sabaner & Arnold, 2021; Siegel & Keeler, 2020). Siegel and Keeler (2020) give the following example:

> One student, who did speak to professors, noted a relatively positive response: "Eventually, it got to a point where it was affecting my work and I had to tell some of my professors. They were very supportive, so I feel very fortunate." (p. 216).

Sabaner and Arnold (2021) provide this example:

> Professors played a large role in either alleviating or exacerbating academic stress and other difficult situations. Tristan's professors were immensely helpful in easing his battle with depression and helping him succeed academically: "I had professors that cared, I had instructors that listened and worked with me.... They helped me go around the issues that I was having in my life to get to the destination of my grade." Ceebee's African American Studies teacher, the only Black professor she had during her first semester, helped her be more comfortable as a Black woman at a PWI and served as a mentor throughout the semester.

Deng et al. (2022) recommend that higher education institutions help students with depression by facilitating organizational changes that improve the social climate in the educational institution:

> According to the findings of this study, high levels of depressive symptoms among college students should be brought to the attention of relevant departments. To prevent college student depression, relevant departments should improve the study and life environment for students, try to reduce the generation of negative life events, provide adequate social support for students, and improve their cognitive and coping capacities to improve their mental qualities...The administration of the school should work to create a good and safe atmosphere. Furthermore, teachers should assume responsibility for assisting and guiding sad pupils, since this will aid in their learning and performance. (p. 9).

The above references provide examples of how educators (in addition to mental health professionals) can make prevention, psychoeducation, and counseling interventions that benefit college youth.

Summary

There is a remarkable similarity between the challenges, and the resources, present in families and schools at the elementary/secondary level and at the higher education level. The need for a SBFC approach at the higher education level is indicated by the numerous studies indicating the strong positive, as well as negative, impact families can have on youth. A further indication for the need for an SBFC approach in higher education is the traditional absence of family counseling/therapy training for mental health professionals in Student Affairs and Counseling training programs.

College counseling is helpful for dealing with academic stress (Choi & Miller, 2014; Lockard et al., 2012; Turner & Berry, 2000; Nafziger et al., 1999). However, Student Affairs and College Counseling programs typically do not provide training in family counseling/therapy. This means that many college mental health professionals lack the training to help students with family problems. Mental health professionals who lack training in family counseling/therapy and refer college students and their families to community mental health clinics are in the same position as school mental health professionals who make similar referrals. The referred families often refuse to go because of the stigma associated with "therapy" (Choi & Miller, 2014; Corrigan et al., 2014; Nafziger et al., 1999).

It is important to note that several researchers on college counseling have recommended that parent intervention is important in counseling college youth (Castillo et al., 2012; Chang et al., 2018; Deng et al., 2022; van Ingen et al., 2015). Deng et al. (2022) in describing the need for intervention to help depressed youth in higher education in Pakistan emphasize: "Furthermore, these findings support the importance of the home environment as a source of depression risk factors among university students, implying that family-based treatments and improvements are critical in reducing depression among university students" (p. 9). Chang et al. (2018) found a significant correlation between family support and college student suicidality, and made the following observations:

> Relatedly, our findings also indicate the importance of working with family members to foster and maintain a positive support system for the student. For example, parents might be trained to look for and identify early signs of suicide risk (e.g., anxiety, dysphoria, and suicide ideation) in students (Power et al., 2009). Thus, parents can serve as a first line of defense in efforts to prevent or reduce the risk of suicide in students and to help students get the professional help needed when family support is simply not enough. Alternatively, our findings also point to the importance of having family counselors work with the family system to help promote and sustain positive and supportive environments for students that may be at risk of suicide. At the very least, when it comes to potentially reducing suicide risk in students, our findings indicate that in addition to having hope, having a supportive family is also likely to make a difference (p. 128).

Several college mental health professionals have recommended the use of family therapy in college counseling centers (Alishio, 1993; Jackson, 2009; Haber & Merck, 2010; Dumont, 2021. Katharine Jackson (2009), associate professor and staff psychologist at Suffolk University Counseling Center, advocates for the use of family therapy in college counseling centers:

> This reflective paper is written on the premise that now, more than ever, family therapy is an appropriate and useful modality to consider utilizing in working with college students. And parents of students, instead of being demonized as overinvolved or too demanding, can thus be seen as potential allies who can offer important insight into family history and clinical concerns. It is not unusual for so-called "hovering" parents to also be harboring their own personal problems that need to be acknowledged and attended to in some way by counselors. Sensitivity to the nuances of family dynamics and the "launching" phase of the family life-cycle (Blacker, 1999; McGoldrick, 1999) is important in grasping the full context of students presenting problems. Thus, this writer advocates for a family therapy perspective in working as a psychologist at a university counseling center.

Some college mental health professionals have also recommended the use of couples therapy (a fundamental part of family therapy) for college students (Gibbons & Shurts, 2010; Henry et al., 2013; Toth et al., 2002).

There is a lack of outcome studies on family therapy by college counselors with students. A randomized control group study by Chen et al. (2021) compared the effects of a traditional medication-based treatment with a systematic family therapy treatment with depressed college students and found that the family therapy significantly reduced student depression and increased their social adaptability. One reason for this lack of research appears to be that college counselors are not trained in family therapy and use an individual development model rather than a family systems developmental model for understanding youth development (Alishio, 1993).

How SBFC Can Be Applied in Higher Education

The need for mental and behavioral health development, and professional services assistive to such development, occurs at any age and in any context. This writing concerns itself with the context of tertiary and vocational education, in settings as disparate as the prestigious graduate school "ivory tower", and the "hands-on" technical or community college, or apprenticeship.

The roots of our metamodel are Adlerian. The metamodel (see Fig. 2.1) further draws from systems and family systems theory, as well as from developmental and life-cycle theory. Because it is a metamodel, it is able to inform the work of practitioners trained in diverse models of counseling, therapy, and social work, including cognitive-behavioral therapy, solutions-focused therapy, and contemporary psychodynamics, including self-psychology.

Our metamodel arose out of a 30-plus year experiment in what we called "school-based family counseling"; as the literature around SBFC (sometimes SBFC&T—"and therapy") grew, so did our realization that the model is simply too widely applicable, and too effective to be restricted only to the setting of schools in primary and secondary education.

The "-based" in school-based family counseling refers to the fact that it is in the educational setting that the symptoms become apparent, when the environmental demands (Geiger, 2017; Ivey et al., 2005) posed by the tasks of being a school student become too burdensome. It mostly falls to the school staff to raise the alarm, and seek to ameliorate the situation, and treatment is greatly facilitated by having a mental health professional trained in family counseling/therapy on-site at the school.

When we conducted a limited pilot study of the model in the tertiary education setting, an undergraduate college in the United States, we found the model absolutely and completely applicable to the older students in tertiary education.

We, therefore, propose a developmental amendment to the taxonomy of the SBFC metamodel:

> SBFC–1: School-based family counseling in the kindergarten/primary/elementary school setting
>
> SBFC–2: School-based family counseling in the middle/secondary/high school setting
>
> SBFC–3: School-based family counseling in the university/tertiary/technical-vocational school setting

See Table 2.1 for a comparison of mental health strategies that can be used at the different SBFC levels.

SBFC–1 arose out of a need to address children's mental health needs within the school setting. From its early origins, SBFC theory (Adler; Friesen; Gerrard) focused on, and met demands associated with children of elementary school age and up to

Table 2.1 Comparison of SBFC 1,2,3 on prevention/intervention levels and mental health strategies

Prevention/ intervention		**SBFC-1**	**SBFC-2**	**SBFC-33**
		Primary	**Secondary**	**Tertiary**
Level	Mental Health Strategies	**Education**	**Education**	**Education**
School intervention	Individual counseling/ therapy	+	+	+
	Group counseling/therapy	+	+	+
	Crisis intervention	+	+	+
	Teacher consultation	+	+	+
	Educational administrator consultation	+	+	+
School prevention	Classroom meetings	++	++	+
	Guidance groups	++	++	
	Whole school intervention	+	+	+
	Classroom management	++	++	+
	Student support groups	+	+	++
Family intervention	Conjoint family counseling/therapy	+	+	+
	Family counseling/therapy with individuals	+	+	++
	Parent consultation			
	Couple counseling (Family of Origin)	++	+	+
	Couple counseling (Student and Partner)		+	++
Family prevention	Parent education training	++	++	+
	Parent support groups	+	+	
Community intervention	Crisis intervention (e.g. Disasters)	+	+	+
	Advocacy for students, families, schools	+	+	+
Community prevention	Educational resources (e.g. Guest Speakers on anti-racism)	+	+	+
	School outreach to community	+	+	+

Note + = Important intervention at this level
++ = Especially Important intervention at this level

high school age. SBFC–1 and SBFC–2 are now practiced very widely, and a sizable body of literature is available. However the practice of SBFC–3 is not so widespread.

We believe a number of macro-systemic factors have contributed to the failure of SBFC–3, thus far, to gain a wider acceptance in schools and colleges of tertiary and vocational education. To begin with, the culture in many localities follows a medico-political model, in which the "child" becomes an "adult" at age 18 or thereabouts. Policymakers—as well as many SBFC theorists and practitioners—rightly deem children to be especially vulnerable and at risk, hence the strong tradition of SBFC in elementary schools. "Adults" on the other hand are seen as capable, for example, of seeking counseling/therapy of their own volition.

Furthermore, staff at primary and secondary schools often have regular contact with parents, and are more aware of family problems, and the need for family-level intervention to combat a young student's developmental challenge, than tertiary educators.

Even so, many colleges in the developed world now offer some kind of counseling or psychological services to tertiary students. However in our experience, it is a minority (albeit growing) of these college counseling centers that are staffed by clinicians fully trained in family therapy and systems theory, and this has for over a decade been a concern to us. We are therefore pleased to record here that our review of the literature suggests a sea-change.

The evidential data unmistakably point policymakers, SBFC theorists, and practitioners to regard post-high-school students—whether in a university (graduate or undergraduate) or in a vocational or technical college, or an apprenticeship setting—as a population every bit as likely to benefit from SBFC programs as are minor children: many youths struggle with both family problems and university problems in a conjunction that negatively affects academic performance.

A Pilot Project in SBFC-3

We had the good fortune to institute a very small, very short-lived pilot SBFC–3 program for undergraduates under the auspices of a college academic advisor who instinctively recognized the benefits. Our observations do not constitute an academic study; yet they are persuasive. Our conclusions are presented here not in lieu of a study, but as anecdotal support for and rationale behind our recommendation to education policymakers.

Four students were referred to our pilot program. The referral criterion was evidence of academic distress in the guise of inability to meet demands posed by course assignments, and potential for academic failure. Treatment was successfully completed with only one of the four referred students, following an intervention by the provost, who took the position that if the experimental program failed it might damage the chances of the referred students, while if it succeeded it would be impossible/impracticable to extend and augment it.

- Student A. male client whose parents' recent divorce was of enormous worry to him (handful of sessions)
- Student B. female client, also a child of divorce, whose hitherto undiagnosed information-processing learning difference was causing her to fail all her written assignments (handful of sessions)
- Student C. male client, a child of divorced immigrant parents, with profound intergenerational acculturation issues (treatment successfully completed)
- Student D. male client, an immigrant and also a child of divorce, with more profound characterological issues (1 session)

A detailed family and educational intake revealed, in each case, a severe stressor in one of two areas:

1. *Family.* All four cases had divorced parents; these students were preoccupied with what was, had been, or might be going on at home, and beset with divided loyalties to troubled parents.
2. *Educational and characterological preparation.* Each of these students was in some way unprepared for college; history-taking and a phenomenological assessment revealed that Student B had a significant learning difference that should or might have led to her being held back at the end of the year and refused an advance to the next grade level repeatedly during her primary and secondary schooling. In the cases of students A and C, the burden of the divorced or antagonistic parents' developmental challenges and associated familial scripts affected the development of self-efficacy in the transition to adulthood and college, leading to considerable doubts about why they were even in tertiary education, and to what purpose. These doubts were altogether more marked in student D, and resulted in behavioral difficulties in the classroom.

The four students were, in each case, intelligent and personable, and the university's admissions process had either not flagged the developmental deficits, or had chosen to wave the student onward, much in the manner as had Student B's primary and secondary school teachers.

The Developmental Challenge

We draw from the (neo-Piagetian) Developmental Counseling and Therapy (DCT) model of Dr. Allen E. Ivey. DCT holds that our development into higher and more complex cognitive-emotional functioning arrives only in response to environmental challenges (Ivey et al., 2005). Society often has difficulty with developmental outliers, such as Student B, who should or might have been held back at the end of the academic year in her primary and secondary school. Affording special, tailored tuition to such students is often expensive (in all the meanings of the word), and many academic-achievement laggards manage to catch up in a subsequent year all by themselves and with no discernible intervention having been made. Thus school personnel may experience strong temptation to advance the laggard student to the next grade, including interpersonal pressures (see below). But if, by the time the young adult in this developmental outlier category has entered the vocational school or university setting, the developmental deficits persist, they will become all too obvious in a way that causes profound upset to both students and educators. It is then necessary and appropriate for both education institutions and young adults that a proactive approach be taken to address the long delayed problem.

It will immediately be apparent to readers that the developmental/family-of-origin problems encountered in these first-year university students (median age 19–20) are analogous to those found in school students aged 9–10; in many cases, our literature review suggests, the overlay of young adult dating/partner-search issues will compound and be compounded by the longer-standing problems. We agree therefore with Mistler et al. (2012), even though, in the pilot study, only Student C was dating, and the dating relationship was not a prime focus of treatment.

While divorcing or antagonistic parents is prima facie a family issue, each student in our pilot study was in some way characterologically held back by their parents' own developmental challenges. Taking a phenomenological approach to the evidence presented by Student B, who should or might have been held back to repeat grades, the clinician hears ideation of the following nature:

- "I can't hold her back: her mother, who's on the school board, would be embarrassed and upset" (teacher)
- "My parents let me know in no uncertain terms that I was NOT going to repeat a grade" (Student B)
- "To be honest, we wanted to graduate her out of here as soon as possible, not least to get the mother off our backs" (principal)

All three of these comments encode important evidence, necessary for complete case conceptualization, of the family dynamic and parents' developmental insufficiencies. In this case, they suggest a narcissistic family structure demanding that a certain "face" be displayed, come what may. The greater the narcissistic challenges of the parents, the less able are they to provide adequately for their child's narcissistic developmental needs, and the more challenging is the emotional field surrounding the child.

In this connection, we draw attention to Twenge et al. (2008), whose cross-temporal meta-analysis found that.

> …narcissism levels have risen over the generations in 85 samples of American college students who completed the 40-item forced-choice Narcissistic Personality Inventory (NPI) between 1979 and 2006 (total n516,475). Mean narcissism scores were significantly correlated with the year of data collection when weighted by sample size (b 5.53, po.001). Since 1982, NPI scores have increased by 0.33 standard deviation. Thus, almost two-thirds of recent college students are above the mean 1979–1985 narcissism score, a 30% increase. The results complement previous studies finding increases in other individualistic traits such as assertiveness, agency, self-esteem, and extraversion. (p. 875)

Having taught in US colleges during this period, we too have observed the same: whether at undergraduate or at graduate level, each year's new intake of students seems less prepared than its predecessor for the developmental challenges of adulthood and tertiary education. This may or may not be the case in other localities around the globe.

Case Example

Joshua presents as a lanky, athletic, well-spoken, and polite young man; his parents immigrated from eastern Africa. Joshua is enrolled in a BA program to study economics. The SBFC–3 clinician, who is Caucasian, chooses a brief psychodynamic therapy model, predicated on the fact that treatment must come to a hard stop at the end of the semester. The primary intervention, *Mirroring*, is taken from self-psychology following Geiger (2017). Mirroring builds "self-structure", thereby allowing for identity cohesion and the ability to rise to challenges in decision-making.

Joshua's family consists of a much older father, now divorced from his mother and remarried; his mother, who lives by herself not far from the father; a younger sister in a boarding school in their home country; and Joshua's steady girlfriend.

Most people glancing at Joshua cannot see that he is not "African American" but *African*. Joshua spins tales of his family's life in their home country, where they were personages of significant prestige. Between the expectations of his ancestors, his powerful, at times punitive older father, his girlfriend, his buddies on the basketball court, the college's academic advisor who referred him to the pilot SBRC–3 program, the White cop who pulls him over and gives him a ticket, and his African American neighbors and friends, Joshua finds himself, so the clinician assesses, pulled in a variety of directions. In Eriksonian lifecycle terms, his struggle is between *identity* and *role confusion*. In self-psychology terms, the Mirroring he received from his parents was lopsided and *conditioned*, leading to a self-structure insufficient to meet them, in terms of Ivey's et al. (2005) DCT, developmental challenge presented by this life stage and its inherent transitions.

Although we have earlier noted that several researchers on college counseling have emphasized the importance of parent intervention, the possibility did not present itself in the case of Joshua. The SBFC–3 clinician is nevertheless able to contextualize and conceptualize the therapeutic conversation as *family therapy with only one family member present in the consulting room* (Gerrard, 2019). Holding the SBFC frame allows the clinician to connect empathically with all family members, and all the generations participating in the difficult and painful process of immigration and acculturation. As Joshua brought into the therapeutic conversation conflicts with, in turn, his father, his mother, and his girlfriend (who is *not* from their country), the SBFC–3 clinician each time "held space" for the other family member, using techniques like "If your mother were a part of our conversation here, I wonder if she would say/think/feel…?"

Course of Treatment (13 Sessions)

The clinician begins with a structured intake, "dreaming" himself (following Ogden, 2005, and Borges, 1970, p. 13) into Joshua's experience and history. Joshua projects vivid pictures into the clinician's countertransference of the family's almost royal lifestyle in Africa, of the respect due to his older, punitive, somatizing father, almost as from a subject to his king, and of his sense of moral duty to continue in their aristocratic tradition; and, as the clinician Mirrors back enthusiastically, Joshua responds well, and becomes able to show more of himself.

The SBFC–3 therapist is immediately struck by Joshua's almost complete lack of enthusiasm for the academic path into which he is enrolled. In the first sessions, the clinician *feels himself into* (Geiger, 2017) a transference presentation suggestive of a child anxious to forestall any criticism by demonstrating his first-class understanding of events. The clinician accesses waves of sadness around Joshua's experience of his "misguidedly abusive" father, and these are processed along with the powerful mutual desire for love between son and father. The mutual *dreaming* allows Joshua to access his own metaphor of "dad's torn vessel inside between culture and personality". Creating and understanding metaphors are manifestations of the *Dialectic-Systemic* style of cognitive-emotional functioning (Geiger, 2017; Ivey et al., 2005), and pave the way for Joshua to discriminate between the "legislative" aspect of the father–son relationship, and the empathic, loving aspect; the clinician takes these developments in Joshua's self-narrative as further evidence that adaptive developmental augmentation is taking place.

The conversation next turns to Joshua's mother, who believes God commands that he should not live with his girlfriend. Joshua is at a loss: since the divorce, his default stance has been to make sure he "keeps others happy", which he is now utterly unable to do. He "feels worse", yet accepts the clinician's framing that this is because he is now feeling feelings long defended against. The clinician accordingly makes space to talk about sad feelings and "hating crying". The clinician also sets homework: Joshua is to write a letter to his father, about whom he says: *I love him and also hate him,* and for whom their culture demands "first love and loyalty".

Around the half-way mark, both of the semester and of the treatment, a new thread weaves its way into the conversation, evidencing enhanced self-structure and identity cohesion. Joshua for the first time openly entertains the idea of abandoning his studies in economics in a series of *what if...* conversations. While Joshua has little interest in economics, he has a great deal of interest in and enthusiasm for sport, fitness, and athleticism: can he make himself a future in this area—and what are the implications for his place in the college—and would this conform to the expectations of his father, and the ancestral traditions and obligations?

At this time too the clinician notices changes in Joshua's demeanor. At the outset, his transferential stance vis-à-vis the clinician was unusually respectful and deferential, having a quality of "one-down-ness" that, according to the clinician's "working hypothesis" (Geiger, 2017), emanates from his relationship with his powerful, "misguided" father. Gradual at first, the changes are now unmistakable as Joshua enters into an enthusiastic, open-eyed, direct-gazing conversation about *what might be possible* for him in terms of a career path.

In the last week of the therapy, Joshua requests a meeting with the college's academic advisor to review and revise his courses to include anatomy and kinesiology. The academic advisor allows the changes only after consulting with the SBFC–3 clinician. Five years later Joshua seeks out the clinician and sends a grateful message: after his graduation, and having married his girlfriend and started their family, he is successfully and happily working in his own fitness business.

Challenges and Solutions

This section discusses some challenges in developing an SBFC-3 approach in higher education and solutions that might be applied.

Challenge: An Absence of Mental Health Professionals in the Tertiary Institution

The tertiary educator as SBFC–3 front-line clinician

We are aware that our readership includes Tertiary educators whose school or college—and therefore whose students or apprentices—do not have access to clinicians formally trained in the SBFC–3 metamodel or in any model of counseling, therapy, or social work. And we have earlier discussed that "many SBFC psycho-educational and counseling interventions may be made by educators" who are not trained in the same way as the licensed or credentialed mental health clinician, the literature records several examples cited above.

We are also aware of the tension, in the past two decades, within the teaching profession, between, on the one hand, those teachers who like a strict division between the developmental tasks allocated to the home and to the school, and who do not wish to do any of the behaviors done by the SBFC clinician, and those who are content to recognize that, in the world we live in today, it is the teachers who are, inescapably, the "front-line" SBFC professionals. It is they who first notice the student's distress and/or underperformance, and who are charged with first response and triage. We, therefore, welcome the work and findings of Deng et al. (2022) cited above, that "teachers should assume responsibility for assisting and guiding sad pupils". For the purposes of this writing, then, we will assume that the Tertiary educator *is* content with performing this important function.

Reflecting on the case of Joshua, we offer the following "primer" to the Tertiary educator interested in assisting student development:

1. *Look for what isn't there, and be curious about it.* This is no longer about criticizing, coaching, or encouraging. Approach the student instead with curiosity,

attempting to *dream* (Borges, 1970; Ogden, 2005) and/or *feel yourself into* (Geiger, 2017) an understanding of the phenomena, and the differences. Can you spot what the student is not thinking, not assuming, not feeling, not noticing, that the more successful students do appear to be thinking, assuming, feeling, and noticing?

2. *See if you can figure out if the student is "leading" with her or his Doing Style or Feeling-Sensing Style* (Geiger, 2017), and if the student's "predominant" Style (Geiger, 2017; Ivey et al., 2005) is in some way hampering or hindering the student. We recently had a graduate student who simply couldn't turn in a paper. The student's *frame of reference* was that a paper "should" be a mechanical regurgitation of the writings of authorities; discovering this, we suggested that the student, whose inclination is more to Feeling-Sensing, write what he wanted and what was true, and *interesting* for him, and then compare his writing with the authorities and, drawing attention to any divergences or discrepancies, draw conclusions; delighted and augmented, he wrote an excellent paper and earned a coveted A grade.
3. *When you notice a frame of reference that isn't serving the student, be curious about how and from whom the student learned it.* Joshua's frame of reference was the aristocratic tradition of his father's African family; while our graduate student's "paper = regurgitation" ideation came from his parents' sense of academic inferiority and powerlessness.
4. *Be mindful of, and sensitive to any cultural idiosyncrasies in the students' family.* Our parents bequeath us their *family scripts*, thereby serving as our principal role models in all aspects of our approach to life. Our development and differentiation occur as we *adapt* and *modify* the scripts. As *Joshua* shows us, we can both honor the old scripts and write ourselves an augmented version.

Of course, it goes without saying that, where these more gentle counseling methods prove insufficient to help the student, and in more serious presentations involving depression, mania, suicidality, or psychosis, the educator should make a referral and seek additional help for the student.

Challenge: Higher Education Mental Health Professionals May Lack Training in Family Therapy

This challenge can be addressed in two ways: (1) by the higher education mental health professional undertaking additional training in family therapy (e.g. by taking a certificate program in family therapy) and by becoming familiar with the SBFC and family therapy literature; (2) by the tertiary institution having on staff a marital and family therapist. For example, the Counseling and Psychological Services program at San Francisco State University in California, USA has on staff an interdisciplinary team of 6 marital and family therapists, 4 psychologists, and 3 social workers (San Francisco State University: Counseling and Psychological Services, 2022).

Challenge: Mental Health "Turf' Issues

It is a sad truth that "turf" issues are common among the mental health professions and there are numerous instances where one mental health profession has attempted to restrict the practice of another mental health profession. Carter et al. (2017) provide examples of this for psychiatry, counseling psychology, social work, marital and family therapy, and school-based family counseling. This attitude of "my mental health discipline is superior to yours" can have destructive effects on clients.

Carter et al. (2017) describe 10 strategies for reducing inter-professional conflict between SBFC practitioners and members of other mental health disciplines. Here are five examples:

> *Strategy #1*: *Do not attack other disciplines.*
>
> While it may be true that SBFC is a superior approach in many respects, describing other mental health disciplines as "narrower" or "insufficient" will make your colleagues more likely to view your proposed SBFC program unfavorably.
>
> *Strategy #2*: *Use discipline-inclusive language.*
>
> Emphasize that SBFC is a metamodel that is used by all mental health approaches. Use inclusive language such as "SBFC professional" rather than "SBFC counselor/therapist".
>
> *Strategy #3*: *Be familiar with the SBFC literature within other disciplines.*
>
> You can do this by reading SBFC literature reviews (such as Gerrard, 2011). Building bridges with members of other mental health guilds is extremely important. Point out that SBFC is a metamodel already being used within their profession. Emphasize that an SBFC program is not intended as a replacement for what they do, but is an approach that can make their mental health guild's practices more effective.
>
> *Strategy #4*: *Make friends with the opposition.*
>
> This is the Nelson Mandela strategy of "If you want to make peace with your enemy, you have to work with your enemy. Then he becomes your partner". This strategy may take time, and involves looking for opportunities to build a friendship. It may also involve sitting down with a professional colleague who disagrees with you and/or feels threatened by an SBFC program. Showing empathy for this colleague may plant the seeds of collaboration (p.10).
>
> *Strategy #5*: *Gather evidence-based support for the program.*
>
> This is important in getting funding for the SBFC program, as well as help persuade wavering and doubting colleagues to green-light the program (p.10).

Challenge: The Parents/Guardians Are not Available for Family Counseling

This is a common SBFC challenge at primary, secondary, and (as discussed above), particularly at tertiary levels. There may be several reasons for the parents/guardians being unavailable:

1. The higher education student does not want the SBFC–3 practitioner to contact the parents/guardians. One reason for this is that the SBFC–3 practitioner has not developed sufficient trust with the student and more time is needed to develop rapport.

2. The SBFC practitioner has made an insufficiently skilled effort to contact the parents/guardians.
3. The parents/guardians live in the locality of the educational institution but are not able to come for counseling because they are working. This can be sometimes handled by the SBFC–3 practitioner adopting a more flexible meeting schedule, including scheduling phone-only consultations with the parents.
4. The parents/guardians live too far away to attend a counseling session. The use of phone-only consultations, or, where practicable, a Zoom meeting or other video call can overcome this difficulty.
5. The parents/guardians refuse to participate in counseling despite being invited by the student and the SBFC-3 practitioner. In this situation, the clinician can use a (above discussed) family therapy approach called family therapy with individuals (Gerrard, 2019). Alternatively, there may be another family member who is willing to participate in counseling and who is in a position to have a positive influence on the parents/guardians (for example, an aunt, uncle, grandparent, or close family friend).

Challenge: The Higher Education Mental Health Professional Has an Individualistic Approach to Youth Development

In countries like the USA and Canada individualism, personal assertiveness, and the rights of the individual over those of the group, are highly valued. This can lead to higher education mental health professionals emphasizing the independence of college students from their families of origin. However, this Americentric individualistic approach may be culturally inappropriate for students who come from cultural backgrounds that emphasize family cohesion, family loyalty, and interdependence. This issue is summarized by Chadda and Deb (2013):

> Unlike the Western society, which puts emphasis on 'individualism', the Indian society is 'collectivistic' in that it promotes interdependence and cooperation, with the family forming the focal point of the social structure….Application of Western psychotherapy, primarily focused on dynamic models, ego structure, and individuals, therefore, becomes difficult in the Indian collectivist context (p. 300).

The solution we recommend is for mental health professionals to develop multicultural sensitivity, not just for how they relate to individual clients, but for the clients' families as well.

Challenge: The Higher Education Institution Cannot Afford a Mental Health Student Services Program

Our response to this challenge is: "Can your higher education institution afford *not* to have a mental health student services program, particularly one that can help students with family problems?" Student retention is a widespread problem in higher education. Many of the students who drop out do so because of family and relationship problems that an SBFC mental health professional could address. There is therefore a fiscal reason for developing a SBFC-3 program. Institutions of higher education also have an "in loco parentis" responsibility for the oversight of the youth who are their students. That is to say, there is a moral imperative that higher education institutions should take steps to ensure they protect their students from mental health challenges, and from failure due to those challenges.

Conclusion

We have attempted to outline in this chapter a blueprint for promoting youth development through SBFC applied to higher education. Although there is evidence-based support for the application of SBFC to primary and secondary education, more evidence-based support for what we call SBFC-3 has yet to be developed building on the research of Chen et al. (2021). Nevertheless, there is strong support in the mental health literature, particularly the college counseling literature, for bringing a family systems approach to higher education mental health intervention. There are over 200 million youth worldwide studying in higher education. A significant percentage of these students could benefit from SBFC programs that reduce family conflicts, strengthen family support, and promote academic success twinned with culturally consonant completion of life-stage-appropriate developmental tasks.

References

American Psychiatric Association (n.d.). Stigma, prejudice and discrimination against people with mental illness. Retrieved from https://www.psychiatry.org/patients-families/stigma-and-discrimination

Alishio, K. (1993). Applying trans-generational family theory and therapy to college student psychotherapy. *Journal of College Student Psychotherapy, 6*(3–4), 97–116. https://doi.org/10.1300/J035v06n03_06

Apisitwasana, Perngparn, U., & Cottler, L. (2018). Effectiveness of school and family-based interventions to prevent gaming addiction among grades 4–5 students in Bangkok, Thailand. *Psychology Research and Behavior Management*, 11, 103–115. https://doi.org/10.2147/PRBM.S145868

Blacker, L. (1999). The launching phase of the life cycle. In B. Carter & M. McGoldrick (Eds.), *The expanded family life cycle: Individual, family, and social perspectives* (3rd ed., pp. 287–306). Allyn & Bacon.

Borges, J. L. (1970). Preface. *Dr Brodie's report*, N.T. DiGiovanni, transl. (p. 11–4). Penguin, 1976

Budescu, M., & Silverman, L. (2016). Kinship support and academic efficacy among college students: A cross-sectional examination. *Journal of Child and Family Studies*, 25, 1789–1801. https://doi.org/10.1007/s10826-016-0359-z

Chang, E., Chang, O., Martos, T., & Sallay, V. (2018). Loss of hope and suicide risk in Hungarian college students: How the presence of perceived family support makes a positive difference. *The Family Journal, 26*(1), 119–126. https://doi.org/10.1177/1066480718756595

Cardin, K. (26 January 2014). Bullying in college: Silent yet prevalent. *Usatoday.com*. N.p., n.d. Web. https://www.usatoday.com/story/news/nation/2013/10/18/college-bullying-silent-yet-prevalent/3008677/

Carter, M., Garner, W., Geiger, P., Gerrard, B., & Soriano, M. (2017). Reducing inter-professional barriers affecting school-based family counseling. *International Journal for School-Based Family Counseling, 4*, 1–16. https://www.schoolbasedfamilycounseling.com/_files/ugd/e85353_49e5740a79744c8c90b9f6016a9c2441.pdf

Castillo, L., Zahn, M., & Cano, M. (2012). Predictors of familial acculturative stress in Asian American college students. *Journal of College Counseling, 15*(1), 52–64. https://doi.org/10.1002/j.2161-1882.2012.00005.x

Chadda, R., & Deb, K. (2013). Indian family systems, collectivistic society and psychotherapy. *Indian Journal of Psychiatry, 55*, S299-309. https://doi.org/10.4103/0019-5545.105555

Chen, Q., Zhao, W., Li, Q., & Sagi, H. (2021). The influence of family therapy on psychological stress and social adaptability of depressed patients. *Work, 1*, 613–624. https://doi.org/10.3233/wor-213503

Choi, N., & Miller, M. (2014). AAPI college students' willingness to seek counseling: The role of culture, stigma, and attitudes. *Journal of Counseling Psychology., 61*, 340–351. https://doi.org/10.1037/cou0000027

Conduct Problems Prevention Research Group. (2007). Fast track randomized controlled trial to prevent externalizing psychiatric disorders: Findings from grades 3 to 9. *Journal of the American Academy of Child and Adolescent Psychiatry, 46*(10), 1250–1262. https://doi.org/10.1097/chi.0b013e31813e5d39

Corrigan, P., Druss, B., & Perlick, D. (2014). The impact of mental illness stigma on seeking and participating in mental health care. *Psychological Science in the Public Interest, 15*(2), 37–70

Crozier, M., Rokutani, L., Russett, J., Godwin, E., & Banks G. (2010). A multisite program evaluation of families and schools together (FAST): Continued evidence of a successful multifamily community-based prevention program. *The School Community Journal, 20*(1), 187–207; ERIC: EJ891838

Deng, Y., Cherian, J., Khan, N, Kumari, K., Sial, M., Comite, U., Gavurova, B., Popp, J. (2022). Family and academic stress and their impact on students' depression level and academic performance. *Frontiers of Psychiatry, 13*, 869337. https://doi.org/10.3389/fpsyt.2022.869337

Dumont, D. (2021). Facing adulthood: Helicopter parenting as a function of the family projection process. *Journal of College Student Psychotherapy, 35*(1), 1–14. https://doi.org/10.1080/87568225.2019.1601049

Eddy, J., Reid, J., & Fetrow, R. (2000). An elementary school-based prevention program targeting modifiable antecedents of youth delinquency and violence: Linking the interests of families and teachers (LIFT). *Journal of Emotional and Behavioral Disorders, 8*(3), 165–176.

Fass, M. E., & Tubman, J. G. (2002). The influence of parental and peer attachment on college students' academic achievement. *Psychology in the Schools, 39*(5), 561–574. https://doi.org/10.1002/pits.10050

Flay, B., Graumlich S., Segawa, E., Burns, J., Amuwo, S., Bell, C., Campbell, R., Cowell, J., Cooksey, J., Dancy, B., Hedeker, D., Jagers, R., Levy, S., Paikoff, R.,Punwani, I, & Weisberg, R. (2004). Effects of 2 prevention programs on high-risk behaviors among African American youth: A randomized trial. *Archives of Pediatrics and Adolescent Medicine, 158*(4), 377–384. https://doi.org/10.1001/archpedi.158.4.377

Gallagher, R. P. (2007). National survey of counseling center directors, 2006 (Monograph Series No. 8P). Retrieved from University of Pittsburgh website: http://d-scholarship.pitt.edu/28167/1/2006_survey.pdf

Geiger, P. B. (2017). *Intentional intervention in counseling and therapy: Goals and process in client engagement*. Routledge.

Gerrard, B. (2008). School-based family counseling: Overview, trends, and recommendations for future research. *International Journal for School-Based Family Counseling, 1*, 1–30.

Gerrard, B. (2019). How to do family counseling with individuals. In B. Gerrard, M. Carter, & D. Ribera (Eds.), *School-based family counseling: An interdisciplinary practitioner's guide.* Routledge.

Gerrard, B., & Soriano, M. (2019). School-based family counseling: The revolutionary paradigm. In B. Gerrard, M. Carter, & D. Ribera (Eds.), *School-based family counseling: An interdisciplinary practitioner's guide.* Routledge.

Gibbons, M., & Shurts, W. (2010). Combining career and couples counseling for college students: A narrative approach. *Journal of College Counseling., 13*(2), 169–181.

Glied, S., & Cuellar, A. E. (2003). Trends and issues in child and adolescent mental health. *Health Affairs, 22*, 5. https://doi.org/10.1377/hlthaff.22.5.39

Goldscheider, F. K., & Davanzo, J. (1986). Semiautonomy and leaving home in early adulthood. *Social Forces, 65*(1), 187–201. https://doi.org/10.2307/2578942

Haber, R., & Merck, R. (2010). Intruder or resource? The family's influence in college counseling centers. *Journal of College Student Psychotherapy, 24*(3), 162–180. https://doi.org/10.1080/87568225.2010.486286

Hargrove, D. S., McDaniel, S. H., Malone, E., & Christiansen, M. D. (2006). Family problems. In P. A. Grayson & P. W. Meilman (Eds.), *College mental health practice* (pp. 79–93). Routledge.

Henry, W. J., Mitcham, M. A., & Henry, L. M. (2013). Conflict resolution strategies adopted from parenting coordination: Assisting high-conflict coparenting students. *Journal of College Counseling, 16*(2), 176–190. https://doi.org/10.1002/j.2161-1882.2013.00035.x

Holt, J. (2014). Help seeking and social competence mediate the parental attachment–college student adjustment relation. *Personal Relationships, 21*(4), 640–654. https://doi.org/10.1111/pere.12055

Hunt, J., Krueger, L., Lacy, E., & Limberg, D. (2017). The Relationship between interparental conflict and self-reported grade point average among college students. *Journal of College Counseling, 20*(3), 237–249. https://doi.org/10.1002/jocc.12072

Ivey, A. E., Ivey, M. B., Myers, J. E., & Sweeney, T. J. (2005). *Developmental counseling and therapy: Promoting wellness over the lifespan.* Lahaska Press, Houghton Mifflin.

Jackson, K. (2009). The use of family therapy within a university counseling center. *Journal of College Student Psychotherapy, 23*(4), 253–261. https://doi.org/10.1080/87568220903163983

Jones, P., Park, S., & Lefevo, G. (2018). Contemporary college student anxiety: The role of academic distress, financial stress, and support. *Journal of College Counseling, 21*(3), 252–264. https://doi.org/10.1002/jocc.12107

Kalkbrenner, M. T., Jolley, A. L., & Hays, D. G. (2021). Faculty views on college student mental health: Implications for retention and student success. *Journal of College Student Retention: Research, Theory and Practice, 23*(3), 636–658. https://doi.org/10.1177/1521025119867639

Kim, B. S. K., Atkinson, D. R., & Yang, P. H. (1999). The Asian values scale: Development, factor analysis, validation, and reliability. *Journal of Counseling Psychology, 46*(3), 342–352. https://doi.org/10.1037/0022-0167.46.3.342

Kratochwill, T., McDonald, L., Levin, J., Scalia, P., & Coover, G. (2009). Families and schools together: An experimental study of multi-family support groups for children at risk. *Journal of School Psychology, 47*, 245–265. https://doi.org/10.1016/j.jsp.2009.03.001

Kratochwill, T., McDonald, L., Levin, J., Bear-Tibbetts, H., & Demaray, M. (2004). Families and schools together: An experimental analysis of a parent mediated multi-family group program for American Indian children. *Journal of School Psychology, 42*(5), 359–383.

Krumrei-Mancuso, E., Newton, F., & Kim, E. (2010). A multi-institution look at college students seeking counseling: Nature and severity of concerns. *Pepperdine University, All Faculty Open Access Publications.* Paper 156. https://digitalcommons.pepperdine.edu/faculty_pubs/156

Larose, S., & Boivin, M. (1998). Attachment to parents, social support expectations, and socioemotional adjustment during the high school-college transition. *Journal of Research on Adolescence, 8*(1), 1–27. https://doi.org/10.1207/s15327795jra0801_1

Lee, R. M., Choe, J., Kim, G., & Ngo, V. (2000). Construction of the Asian American family conflicts scale. *Journal of Counseling Psychology, 47*(2), 211–222. https://doi.org/10.1037/0022-0167.47.2.211

Lee, R. M., & Liu, H.-T.T. (2001). Coping with intergenerational family conflict: Comparison of Asian American, Hispanic, and European American college students. *Journal of Counseling Psychology, 48*(4), 410–419. https://doi.org/10.1037/0022-0167.48.4.410

Lee, R. M., Su, J., & Yoshida, E. (2005). Coping with intergenerational family conflict among Asian American college students. *Journal of Counseling Psychology, 52*(3), 389–399. https://doi.org/10.1037/0022-0167.52.3.389

Little, J. (2004). The collision: College students, family problems and university Life. *The Vermont Connection, 25*(1). https://scholarworks.uvm.edu/tvc/vol25/iss1/7

Lochman, J., & Wells, K. (2004). The coping power program for preadolescent aggressive boys and their parents: Outcome effects at the 1-year follow-up. *Journal of Consulting and Clinical Psychology, 72*(4), 571–578.

Lockard, A. J., Hayes, J. A., McAleavey, A. A., & Locke, B. D. (2012). Change in academic distress: Examining differences between a clinical and nonclinical sample of college students. *Journal of College Counseling, 15*(3), 233–246. https://doi.org/10.1002/j.2161-1882.2012.00018.x

MacDonald, C. (26 March, 2010). Cyberbullying among college students: Prevalence and demographic Differences. N.p., Web. https://doi.org/10.1016/j.sbspro.2010.12.436

McClain, K., & Perry, A. (2017). Where did they go: Retention rates for students of color at predominantly white institutions. *College Student Affairs Leadership, 4*(1) Article 3. https://scholarworks.gvsu.edu/csal/vol4/iss1/3

McGoldrick, M. (1999). History, genograms, and the family life cycle: Freud in context. In B. Carter & M. McGoldrick (Eds.), *The expanded family life cycle: Individual, family, and social perspectives* (3rd ed., pp. 47–68). Allyn & Bacon.

Mistler, B., Reetz, D., Krylowicz, B., & Barr, V. (2012). The association for university and college counseling center directors annual survey. In *Association for university and college counseling center directors*. Retrieved from. https://www.researchgate.net/publication/275970421_Integration_of_College_Counseling_and_Health_Services_A_Phenomenological_Study

Nadal, K. L., Wong, Y., Griffin, K. E., Davidoff, K., & Sriken, J. (2014). The adverse impact of racial microaggressions on college students' self-esteem. *Journal of College Student Development, 55*(5), 461–474. https://doi.org/10.1353/csd.2014.0051

Nafziger, M., Couillard, G., & Smith, T. (1999). Research: evaluating therapy outcome at a university counseling center with the college adjustment scales. *Journal of College Counseling, 2*. https://doi.org/10.1002/j.2161-1882.1999.tb00137.x

Ogden, T. H. (2005). On psychoanalytic supervision. *The International Journal of Psychoanalysis, 86*, 1265–80

Perera, R. (2012). Family relations and the problems of university students. In *First International Research Conference on Humanities and Social Sciences – IRCHS*. At University of Sri Jayewardenepura

Power, L., Morgan, S., Byrne, S., Boylan, C., Carthy, A., Crowley, S. … Guerin, S. (2009). A pilot study evaluating a support programme for parents of young people with suicidal behaviour. *Child and Adolescent Psychiatry and Mental Health, 3*, 20.

Sabaner, C., & Arnold, K. (2021). Mental health in the transition to college: Experiences of six low-income, high-achieving students. *Journal of College Counseling, 24*(1), 18–35. https://doi.org/10.1002/jocc.12174

San Francisco State University: Counseling & Psychological Services (2022, October 2). Retrieved from https://psyservs.sfsu.edu/content/counseling-psychological-services-faculty-and-staff

Schnyders, C. M., & Lane, J. A. (2018). Gender, parent and peer relationships, and identification with emerging adulthood among college students. *Journal of College Counseling, 21*(3), 239–251. https://doi.org/10.1002/jocc.12106

Schwanz, K., Palm, L., Hill-Chapman, C., & Broughton, S. (2014). College students' perceptions of relations with parents and academic performance. *American Journal of Educational Research.*, *2*(1), 13–17. https://doi.org/10.12691/education-2-1-3

Siegel, J., & Keeler, A. (2020). Storm, stress, silence: A focus group examination of mental health culture and challenges among graduate students currently or previously experiencing depression. *Journal of College Counseling, 23*(3), 207–220. https://doi.org/10.1002/jocc.12166

Song, J., Bong, M., Lee, K., & Kim, S.-I. (2015). Longitudinal investigation into the role of perceived social support in adolescents' academic motivation and achievement. *Journal of Educational Psychology, 107*(3), 821–841. https://doi.org/10.1037/edu0000016

Stallman, H., & Hurst, C. (2016). The university stress scale: Measuring domains and extent of stress in university students. *Australian Psychologist, 51*(2), 128–134. https://doi.org/10.1111/ap.12127

Su, J., Lee, R. M., & Vang, S. (2005). Intergenerational family conflict and coping among Hmong American college students. *Journal of Counseling Psychology, 52*(4), 482–489. https://doi.org/10.1037/0022-0167.52.4.482

Thompson, B. (2008). How college freshmen communicate student academic support: A grounded theory study. *Communication Education, 57*(1), 123–144. https://doi.org/10.1080/03634520701576147

Thompson, B., & Mazer, J. (2009). College student ratings of student academic support: Frequency, importance, and modes of communication. *Communication Education, 58*(3), 433–458. https://doi.org/10.1080/03634520902930440

Toth, P., Harnishfeger, B., & Shea, A. (2002). Finding the silver lining: Counseling a couple in conflict. *Journal of College Student Psychotherapy., 16*(3–4), 269–285. https://doi.org/10.1300/J035v16n03_07

Turner, A. L., & Berry, T. R. (2000). Counseling center contributions to student retention and graduation: A longitudinal assessment. *Journal of College Student Development, 41*(6), 627–636.

Twenge, J. M., Konrath, S., Foster, J. D., Campbell, W. K., & Bushman, B. J. (2008). Egos inflating over time: A cross-temporal meta-analysis of the Narcissistic Personality Inventory. *Journal of Personality, 76*(4), 875–902. https://doi.org/10.1111/j.1467-6494.2008.00507.x

van Ingen, D., Freiheit, S., Steinfeldt, J., Moore, L., Wimer, D., Knutt, A., Scapinello, S., & Roberts, A. (2015). Helicopter parenting: The effect of an overbearing caregiving style on peer attachment and self-efficacy. *Journal of College Counseling, 18*(1), 7–20. https://doi.org/10.1002/j.2161-1882.2015.00065.x

Wintre, M. G., & Yaffe, M. (2000). First-year students' adjustment to university life as a function of relationships with parents. *Journal of Adolescent Research, 15*(1), 9–37. https://doi.org/10.1177/0743558400151002

Prof. Peter Geiger is an educator and writer and marriage and family therapist licensed in California. Between 2006 and 2013 he taught in the counseling psychology graduate program of the University of San Francisco. His book *Intentional Intervention in Counseling and Therapy: goals and process in client engagement* was published by Routledge in July 2017. Based on Geiger's teaching and research and motivated by his desire to improve outcomes for clients of counselors and therapists, *Intentional Intervention* has generated international acclaim. Geiger is in private practice in San Francisco and consults with pre licensed and licensed clinicians on case conceptualization and countertransference. He supervises clinical practicum students at California Institute of Integral Studies and pre-licensed clinicians at the Marina Counseling Center and the Center for Mindful Psychotherapy. Geiger is a consultant to and Fellow of the Oxford Symposium in School-Based

Family Counseling, and member of the Symposium's Disastershock Global Response Team. A keen observer of current affairs, Geiger has been a prolific writer of letters to the Financial Times newspaper, with twenty three published.

Dr. Brian A. Gerrard has a Ph.D. in Sociology from the University of New South Wales, Sydney, Australia, and a PhD in Counseling Psychology, from the University of Toronto. He holds teaching awards from two universities. He has extensive experience teaching a wide variety of Master's and Doctoral level courses in counselor education. Dr. Gerrard is Emeritus Faculty Member of the University of San Francisco where he developed the masters Marital and Family Therapy (MFT) program and for 14 years served as MFT Coordinator. His orientation emphasizes an integration of family systems and problem-solving approaches. He has been Chair of the USF Counseling Psychology Department three times. Currently, he is Member of the Board, Western Institute for Social Research: Center for Child and Family Development. The center, co-founded by Dr. Gerrard, has for years managed the largest longest running School-Based Family Counseling program of its type in the USA. Its Mission Possible program has served more than 30,000 children and families in over 70 Bay area Schools. Dr. Gerrard is also Chair of the Institute for School-Based Family Counseling and Symposium Director for the Oxford Symposium in School-Based Family Counseling. Currently, Dr. Gerrard is Chief Administrative Officer and Core Faculty Member in the Western Institute for Social Research in Berkeley, California. He is Senior Editor of the book *School-Based Family Counseling: An interdisciplinary Practitioner's Guide* (Routledge, 2019).

Chapter 3
Literature as a Moral Tool for Youth: A Select Study of Canonical Texts

Sudip Kumar Das

Abstract The paper aims to study how literature imparts a spectrum of values and insights to adolescent minds. Literature is known for academic and cognitive development in budding youths and reading through different genres benefits a young mind with refined aspects of social and emotional intricacies. This article is designed with an assessment of canonical literary texts chiefly prescribed in the undergraduate and postgraduate curricula. It will deal with an appraisal of select novels in terms of inculcating ethics and integrity that play a pivotal role in holistic development. Apart from the pressing value system, literature induces utilitarian features such as an intuitive approach, and problem-solving skills that increase empathy and enhance the sensibility of any individual who is involved in the task of reading and analyzing any work of literary merit. This chapter will consider canonical texts from different ages of literary productions and will attempt to analyze how they aid in inculcating essential values in the individuals reading them.

Keywords Value · Soft skills · Youth · Morality · Literary canons

Introduction

Definitions and terminologies exist to facilitate us in conceptualizing a word or idea comprehensively but often we find difficulty in elucidating an intricate notion holistically. Morality is one such abstract value that has undergone argument and deliberation to assimilate it into a broad spectrum. It has emerged as a concept of personal law or behavioral yardstick for every individual in a society, which will make society function smoother without the intervention of actual law and order. Morality works as a guide in our daily actions forcing us to stick to the codes of society for personal happiness as well as abstaining from lawlessness. We often associate morality with happiness and think whatever makes an individual happy without

S. K. Das (✉)
Faculty, Department of English, Rajiv Gandhi National Institute of Youth Development, Sriperumbudur, Tamil Nadu, India
e-mail: sudipdas448@gmail.com

S. Deb and S. Deb (eds.), *Handbook of Youth Development*,
https://doi.org/10.1007/978-981-99-4969-4_3

harming others is morally righteous and good. But happiness is a subjective matter, our actions are determined by our desires and requirements which are susceptible to good and bad.

In every language, children's literature very delicately creates a perception of 'good' and 'bad' through fables, parables, fairy tales, allegories, and legends folk-tales. Of late, this exclusive genre of literature is scrutinized on gender, sexuality, and politics study but the prime goal was to build a moral sensibility through a habit of reading during formative years. Children's literature does not necessarily indulge in the niceties of ethics nevertheless transitional literature also known as youth literature focuses on problems of adolescent life and its emerging principles. Youth literature delineates themes like the quest for identity and psychological and physical changes. The corpus of youth literature bridges the adult literary world through its representation of mature scruples and the nuanced human psyche. Bridge literature is that stepping stone that prudently glides young minds into a classical literary sphere.

Literature, Morality and Youth

A taste of classical literature in the early stages of life presents different perspectives on an experience and inculcates a deep understanding of an unfamiliar world through the lens of fictional characters. The literary experience helps to execute things judiciously in real life and aids in cognitive development. Our social surroundings in early-stage shape our outlook toward foreign cultures, religions, and races which are not always accommodating and inclusive in nature. We as human beings become overtly critical of an imported ideology, language, or people. This limitation can be eradicated by rigorous study of different branches like anthropology, philosophy, and history. But reading literature is the only process to provide us with an experience of living fictive lives, positing different arguments and evaluating the same challenges from multiple aspects. This distinction is no less a critical practice; it allows us a glance at the flip side of the problem.

From its inception literature serves a greater role in human life than merely conveying stories, entertainment, and romances; it disseminates certain truths and philosophy. This philosophy often contains some universal message or value without which literature loses its significance. Knowledge can be gained by occupying a point of view of another self in imagination. Through this imaginative participation, we expand our moral wisdom and practical knowledge.

Even within the concourse of fictional events, a literary work cannot be estranged from any ethical standpoint. A literary work is a tapestry of cultural fibers deeply rooted in the circumstance of the writer. The writer cannot produce anything completely different remaining within the traditional society. The question of morality in literature and its pragmatic usage is arguable concerning our perception of literature. Theorists of cognitive aspects believe in literature's ability to create a mock individual experience; a challenge where readers have to undergo moral struggle and come to a moral resolution through multiple attempts. This imaginary mental drill of fierce ethical skirmishes and precarious situations aids to polish moral propositions.

Literature's primary prerogative is to bring out the essential truth without any overt didactic approach. The moral consciousness should not be a burden on the work but rather attuned to the texture of a particular work. W. H Hudson's remark surmises this aptly:

> The ethics must be wrought into the texture of a story, the philosophy must be held in solution the novelist (for that matter the artist) must never for a moment be lost in the propagandist or preacher.

The present chapter aims to look into three British fiction, two American fiction and one Russian novel which have undergone a lot of studies and critical evaluation. The literature will unravel the concept of morality laid down by literary stalwarts in different countries and times of history. This work addresses morality in general, and how it plays across human lives and situations. The novels are taken up from diverse authors, cultures, and literature, it displays a person's disposition to ethics. The moral ambiguity, complexity, and amoral heroes are taken into study in respect of their values without delving deep into the nuances of the philosophy of morality.

Selected British Fiction Through the Lens of Morality

Henry Fielding's novels are the major works that tried to moderate the excessive morality of British fiction through his mode of satirical response to the contemporary standard set by a writer like Samuel Richardson. It is imperative to take Richardson's name because his impetus in Fielding's novel writing is undeniable. The first prominent work *Shamela* was written criticizing the overtly sensational *Pamela* for its representation of the protagonist as a paragon of virtue. In *Shamela*, unlike Pamela, the heroine is a prurient woman who proceeds to lure her master for monetary profit. His works contain moral undertones which run in all his novels but there are incongruences. Chastity and marriage are the most deliberated topics which he addressed with a moralistic tool of existing societal norms. He is harshly critical of the sexual and financial motifs involved in a marriage and his condemnation remains the same across his different novels even though there are deviations and idealism in his approach to virtuousness. *Joseph Andrews* is a continuation of Fielding's scathing attack against Richardson through his presentation of the eponymous character Joseph who is the brother of Pamela. Joseph and his girlfriend Fanny are unrealistically virtuous and he almost mechanically resists all the sexual mores of Lady Booby and Mrs Slipslop for his commitment to Fanny. To establish as an epitome of principles and impeccability, Fielding gives an expressive account of Joseph as "outwardly a pretty fellow, his morals remained entirely uncorrupted, though he was at the same time smarter and gentler than any of the beaus in town, either in or out of livery" (Fielding 13). Lady Booby relentlessly tries to seduce Joseph but her subsequent failure prompts her to mock his excessive virtue. But he stands for his moral position which might seem amusing as men are often portrayed to succumb easily to sexual provocation. Joseph advances to a rational argument when his virtue is ridiculed just because a woman is trying to be flippantly voluptuous: "I can't see why her having no virtue should be a reason against my having any; or why, because I am a man, or because I am poor, my virtue must be subservient to her pleasures" (Fielding 28). 'To treat male chastity with the seriousness with which Richardson treated female chastity is to treat it comically, but the very fact that such treatment inevitably turns out to be comic is a comment on the moral confusion implied in Richardson's position' (Daiches 713). Fielding has reinforced their chastity in the romantic relationship and the prolonged fixation with physical purity has also been compensated in the end with a happy marriage. Fielding has allowed the moral aspect to flow through the parson, Adams from a religious outlook. Parson Adams and Joseph are often unyielding in their faith and believe that humankind is marked by their action, charity, and love. 'Parson Adams mistakes the real world because he lives in the world of Christian values which everybody else professes to live in but which in fact everybody else ignores' (Daiches 715). Faith in Christianity is Parson's unwavering weathervane that directs his actions even after the world treats him unfairly for his beliefs.

Jane Austen's works are often read in a light-hearted manner where young women indulge a great time in procuring good husbands; the range of emotions, the role of society in standard matrimony, and the character's levity are all part of that sojourn. But unlike Samuel Richardson's propagandist morality, she gently floats the dilemma between social norms and the individual's spontaneity, 'moral seriousness', and conventional standards of duty through lucid narrative and measured humor. David Daiches has remarked:

> The greatest of all the novelists of manners of this or any other period, and one who raised the whole genre to new level of art, was Jane Austen (1775–1815). With no exhibitionist critical apparatus, such as Fielding's theory of the comic epic, no pretentiously announced moral purpose such as Richardson kept repeating, and indeed with no apparent awareness that she was doing more than essaying some novels in an established social mode, this unpretentious daughter of a Hampshire rector, with her quietly penetrating vision of man as a social animal, her ironic awareness of the tensions between spontaneity and convention and between the claims of personal morality and those of social and economic propriety, her polished and controlled wit, and beneath all her steady moral apprehension of nature of human relationship, produced some of the greatest novels in English… (Daiches 743–44)

F. R. Leavis's critical reflection on novel and morality is interwoven and follows certain ideas such as 'form in fiction, 'moral fable', 'moral enactment', and 'moral exploration'. He points out the moral interest novelists exhibit intervenes with their form in fiction. In his book *The Great Tradition*, he took Jane Austen's reference who puts plots in the novel 'deliberately and calculatedly' and 'the principle of development in her work is an intense moral interest of her own in life that is in the first place a preoccupation with certain problems that life compels on her as personal ones' (Leavis 116).

In *Northanger Abbey (1818)*, a naïve young girl Catherine ventures out of her place where she encounters new people and society. Her jocund demeanor and simplicity fail to gauge friends and partner as the man she chooses is an egoist and immoral.

He leaves her at the sight of a better prospect to her dismay. She later falls in love with Henry Tilney but had to face resistance from General Tilney as he was more concerned with the value and wealth Catherine would bring to the family name. Jane Austen through this simple portrayal of life shows the dinginess of life. Life is dull and the dullness makes it real, far from the rouge of French romantic novels. Respect and appreciation in love are prerequisites that her lovers shower in abundance. Through the characters' life and approach, the readers can choose a definite moral path to live in appreciation or discontentment. We see our moral reflection in the mundane life and attitudes of characters. Austen's deep understanding helps us to plunge into our minds through everyday events.

Charles Dickens's one of the major novels, *Great Expectation* displays 'the relation between gentility and morality' and is based on the Victorian era with the booming industrialization and development in England. But the plot focuses chiefly on the young protagonist Pip's beginning in society. The novel is a bildungsroman where the growth of the central character Pip is followed and his development into new relationships, friendships, and society. The portrayal of the characters and events is much more mature and flawless to complement the 'central moral vision' of the novel. Pip befriends Herbert Pocket who aspires to be a merchant despite the adverse present condition and his friendship is a cherished treasure for Pip. His kindness and generosity toward Pip to make him fit into the London-based lifestyle show his openness and sense of morality which is free from any pecuniary status. Herbert took it as his moral responsibility to make Pip prepare for the upper-class society, the decorum of table manners. As he starts to accept the questionable source of his success in the world, Pip's ability for love is shown throughout the book. It is brutally made apparent to Pip that he feels mortified and that he is aware of his vanity and elitism. In his journey to becoming a gentleman, Pip tries to forget his initial years, especially his association with the convict but both of them had a realization. The convict understands that attaining refinement is the greatest reward and Pip's appreciation of the convict as his benefactor is where Dickens's mastery lies. The moral shift is from respect for oneself to social commitment. This idea of moral change or advancement is predicated on the writer's positivism.

Moral transformation or change of heart is a recurrent theme in *Great Expectation*, Pip's character is an embodiment of this conversion because he used to have a hard, ingrateful attitude but he realizes his vanity with shame. He transforms from a proud snob to a person with humility and gratitude. Estella's change is quite similar but it is not described in the narrative. Miss Havisham also transforms. Although Miss Havisham teaches her self-made student a lesson, it is clear from their argument that she has been indoctrinating her with a lovelessness that she desperately needs. The novel displays numerous facets of nature and morals.

Depiction of Human Values and Ethics in Select American Fiction

A text with moral lessons often seems to be didactic in nature and devoid of any literary essence for the soul. But Harper Lee's *To Kill a Mockingbird* is one of the most significant works of the abolitionist movement in America which showed solidarity with black people. Lee has asserted an empathetic attitude through the character of Atticus Finch who is an advocate and believes in the unprejudiced treatment of people. He agrees to defend a fellow black man, Tom Robinson who is accused of a false rape charge by a white woman, Mayella Ewell. The decision of defending Tom's case itself makes him a 'nigger-lover' in his community that profusely attracts animosity and hateful slurs. His compassionate outlook toward black people essentially brings in the question of empathy as an attribute of professionalism. Finch's daughter Scout and son, Jem too imbue with the same empathetic attitude as their father for which they had to encounter community prejudices and the underlying racism. The character of Atticus Finch embodies humane qualities which permeate the inclusive, egalitarian approach of the children. His moral conscience manifests in the remark to Scout that "You'll get along a lot better with all kinds of folks. You never really understand a person until you consider things from his point of view-" that is "-until you climb into his skin and walk around in it" (Lee 33).

Boo Radley, who is a recluse has been shunned by the community and lives alone in isolation. Scout tries to befriend him as she realizes society's cruel motifs and Boo's traumatic past made her sympathetic and understanding toward his behavioral anomaly. Boo has voluntarily withdrawn himself from the hatred and biasedness as he does not want to associate with mean bigoted people. Jem who had an edgy relationship with Atticus also realized his father's constant predicament to prove Tom's innocence. Finch's striving to give justice irrespective of all the odds made Jem understand the determination it takes to stand with a belief you strongly adhere to. His expression of admiration toward Atticus is a testament to his inner conflict. The character of Maudie is significantly central in resistance to the condescending attitude against black people who constantly extended her support to Atticus and his family, her moral principle is not insubstantial. She emboldens Scout to be firm in her decisions without getting compromised for her integrity.

Narrative criticism has often pointed out the problematics of empathy in professional character portrayal as it entails partiality. The nature of prejudice might not be innocuous and often lead to haze the judgment due to personal follies. In *To Kill a Mockingbird*, critical reading would re-examine the mode of empathy which is complex and less shifted toward professional objectivity. The ethical value system instilled by the protagonist in his children and young readers per se is focused. Finch's postulation on compassion is not superficial and he wants to impart that in children's consciences:

> … it's not fair for you and Jem, I know that, but sometimes we have to make the best of things, and the way we conduct ourselves when the chips are down—well, all I can say is,

when you and Jem are grown, maybe you'll look back on this with some compassion and some feeling that I didn't let you down (Lee 120).

He has full respect for people's entitlement to their personal opinion but has a deeper conviction in his integrity which is not supposed to be determined by a 'majority rule'.

Ernest Hemingway's *The Old Man and the Sea* is a classic novella that talks about human perseverance, and mankind's place in nature. According to Hemingway, dignity is attained by perseverance in the face of hardship and the capacity to slog through discomfort and tiredness. Santiago is an old fisherman who was not having enough luck in fishing. The fact that Santiago is an angler who depends on catching fish for a living in no way lessens his profound admiration for nature and his amazing awareness of his surroundings. His identification as a fisherman plays a significant role in his innate humility. He goes fishing one day and catches a marlin. But he gets dragged out into the water after struggling to kill the marlin. The marlin grows close to Santiago and he refers to it as his "brother". Santiago becomes stronger by thinking about the things he enjoys and is passionate about, like Manolin, a young fisherman. After three days of combat, Santiago successfully kills the marlin. Santiago faces several challenges to capture a large fish, but when he does, sharks that prey on marlins steal it from him. Santiago respects his rival marlin rather than despises it. The only distinction he can make between humans and fish is that they are not as intellectual as we who kill them; albeit they are more honorable and more competent. In his struggle, he respects the fish. Both the marlin and he has strong qualities. Santiago is aware that amid the unspoiled beauty of nature, every life is equal. The ocean doesn't have any favorites. The honorable fisherman recognizes his big fraternity with everyone around him rather than establishing himself as a master of the animals.

Santiago is out of the ordinary in his community because of his beliefs and personal rules of conduct. Santiago distinguishes himself from the realist fishermen driven by profit by his devotion to his trade which goes beyond worries of financial profit or existence. He contrasts with Cuba's shift to neo-capitalism and the transformation of fishing from a local tradition to an organization. He continues to be committed to a line of work that, in his eyes, represents an even more holistic approach to life and is a necessary component of evolution, in the never-ending cycle that unites all living things as brothers because they are all hunters. He thinks that even though he did it to sustain himself and others, killing the fish could have been sinful. Santiago decides to set aside his feeling of existential guilt and leave the discussion of sin to those who are more suited to do so. He consoles himself stating this is how nature works, he was born to be a fisherman, just as the fish was born to be a fish, to make sense of his activities. The spirit of the human force is encapsulated in the lines that human beings can be destroyed but cannot be defeated.

Morality and Crime in Dostoevsky's Novel

Morality is the simple perception of good and bad behavior. Man's goals for power and recognition inevitably lead to his downfall because of his dreams, passions, and wants. It forces someone to give up their moral principles. He sacrifices his moral principles to obtain anything. In such cases, one's morality is called under doubt. Following socially established norms is a key component of morality. However, there are divergent viewpoints on this situation. Morality is subjective and may mean different things to different people. Some ideas have been shaped by assumptions and biases in law and religion. Everyone has a responsibility to uphold morality since it was developed by people for people and they work to make it legal. Righteousness demonstrates appropriate behavior.

Fyodor Dostoevsky's *Crime and Punishment* is not only a difficult and unsettling novel but it also addresses a number of difficult moral dilemmas. Dostoevsky with sheer skill and artistry has intertwined social and political aspects which lead to a common man's resort to committing the crime of murder. Raskolnikov's murderous story is told in Crime and Punishment, which is set in St. Petersburg. Despite being a work of crime fiction, the author fails to create any suspense because there is no suspense created about the identity of the criminal. It is entirely focused on Raskolnikov, his idealized universe, and the psychological consciousness of what was going through his mind prior to the crime and after the crime. Raskolnikov is portrayed by Dostoevsky as a young, attractive intellectual who is fascinated with a variety of popular views about figures like Napoleon, Hegel, and Nietzsche and applies them without completely understanding them. He broke the law by forming such views without fully developing them. Such unrealistic ideas ultimately bring him great anguish.

It demonstrates how an intelligent young man affected by nihilistic views commits a crime and becomes unwell. After killing a pawnbroker his horrible thoughts and isolation drove him to break down, but he eventually found relief by admitting his wrongdoing and receiving redemption. His utilitarian beliefs persuade him that killing the woman will not be a loss for society at large and that her only motivation is to hurt the underprivileged clients she receives. "'The old woman is of no consequence,' he thought, hotly and incoherently. 'The old woman was a mistake perhaps, but she is not what matters! The old woman was only an illness.... I was in a hurry to overstep.... I didn't kill a human being, but a principle! I killed the principle, but I didn't overstep, I stopped on this side.... I was only capable of killing" (Dostoevsky 389). But even though he thinks the sense of remorse or guilt will not touch him, the statement proves he is troubled in his conscience. The author tries to look into the matter of what motivates an ordinary man to commit a crime. It gave rise to a series of questions which include the cause of resorting to an extreme crime and the consequent impact on his actions. The remainder of the book discusses his desperation, sorrow, and grief as well as how he overcame them with Sonia's help and ultimately found redemption. Dostoevsky demonstrates how Raskolnikov finds atonement as a result of his repentance and adoption of Christian principles. It explains the psychological anguish and moral ambiguity Raskolnikov experiences all through the work. The book features a wide range of people with both favorable and negative characteristics. Raskolnikov occupies a middle position because, as his name implies, he is "double," possessing both good and evil. He is portrayed as having both flaws and merits.

Raskolnikov is not a character devoid of morality, he is haunted by his conscience. In the end, he chooses the path of righteousness and resurrects himself with Christian principles. Dostoevsky inspires him to believe in Christian love and morality.

Role of Literature in Inculcating Human Values

Literature imparts a moral cognizance in our behavioral pattern, which is an essential part of humane qualities, judiciousness, and logical aptitude. The perception of the moral value of one's character and the moral quality of one's deliberate and ingrained behavior is referred to as moral awareness. Through constant value judgments, we create our moral consciousness, and that entails reasonable inference from moral norms. Moral conscience typically includes the awareness of obligations, rights, attributes, character flaws, benefits, and drawbacks. The cognitive components run parallel with moral judgments. Literature is a significant medium that deals with life and the universe, the complexities of the mind. It is highly unlikely that literature would be "art for art's sake" and refrain from revealing any moral values.

Literary works are expected to reveal imaginative power and imitative aspects but through these aspects, literary values are also revealed. Literary value is a concept, which formed as the conventional body gets shaped by certain traditions, beliefs, and ideas. A fundamental rewriting of the canonical works would represent a denial of the literary body rather than just altering what our society values. The contemporary criticism of canon contends for the feasibility of a different range of canon while maintaining the literature's fundamental role in culture. In the justification of canon which adopts the stance of ideals presented in the canonical works are the basic principles that characterize our civilizations. These values can be found independent of any literary canon and the impact of it on a person and community can be gauged from a distance. Nevertheless, the question of literature charting the way for the life of any individual, problems that exist in human life irrespective of literary activity, cannot be supported in any meaningful way. We can only argue how literature evaluates the objectives established by literary convention. Literary works are molded through the creative faculty of individuals who are open to pluralistic discourses and often the conditions shy away from practical simulations. Literature is more than just a way to communicate pre-existing ideals or a reaction to fundamental challenges. It is a mode of defining and developing fundamental issues as well as ideals.

Conclusion

Our perception of literature—moral and aesthetic value—is determined by the kind of literature we consume as readers. Fictions of different genres will evoke various emotional receptivity and fiction in general will provide a deep understanding of human relations and conflicts. Even though these works have a specific goal and sensible decisions, there is not much to ponder about and grow in them. The substitute literature is often very inconsequential that shows straightforward decisions and immediate objectives. But such a simple inference would be shallow and elusive of the nuances. Certain themes go well beyond the immediate circumstances, for example, legal and ethical rights, and regard for the kind of cosmos we live in.

We should be concerned about how literature affects our moral development. Apart from fulfilling the modest purpose of education, literature deals with learning. The moral component of education and its quasi-characteristics should be considered. Our moral awareness is greatly enriched by literary fiction. A literary work's worth is determined by how much it adds to the entire moral life. It conveys enduring and commonplace views toward life as well as ideas, sentiments, and emotions.

References

Adiguzel, F. B., & Ayaz, P. (2020). Values in youth literature: The case of bridge books. *African Educational Research Journal., 8*(3), 551–559.

Austen, Jane (n.a). *Northanger Abbey*. Planet eBook

Barton, J. (2004). Being Atticus Finch: The professional role of empathy in to Kill a Mockingbird. *Harvard Law Review, 117*(1682–1702), 2022. https://doi.org/10.2307/4093264.Accessed7Oct

Bloom, H. (Ed.). (2010). *Viva modern critical interpretations: Fyodor Dostoevsky's crime and punishment*. Viva Books. Print.

Daiches, D. (1994). *A critical history of english literature* (Vol. 2 Revised Edition). Mandarin Paperbacks.

Dickens, C. (n.a). *Great expectation*. Rupa Publication India. Print.

Dostoevsky, F., & Garnett, T. B. C. (2018). *Crime and punishment* (p. 250). Dreamscape Media

Dostoevsky, F. (n.a). *Crime and punishment*. Planet eBook

Fielding, H. (2013). *Joesph Andrews*. Rupa Publication India, Print.

Frank, J. (1866). Introduction. In *Crime and punishment*. By Fyodor Dostoevsky. Trans. Constance Garnett. Bantam classics, v-xxiii. Print.

Hemingway, E. (1994). *The old man and the sea*. Penguin Random House, Print.

Hudson, W. H. (2000). *An outline history of english literature*. Surjeet Publication, Reprint.

Leavis, F. R. (1976). Basic concepts of Leavis' Novel criticism. In: *Leavis' criticism of poetry and the novel* (pp. 116–117). Heinermann

Leavis, F. R. (2011). *The great tradition*. Faber and Faber. Ebook.

Lee, H. (2002). To kill a mockingbird. In *Perennial classics* (1st ed.). Harper Collins, Print

Mehar, S. (2010). Fyodor Dostoevsky crime and punishment. Rama Brothers India PVT. Ltd., Print

Parmar, P. C. (n.a). *Temptation of crime facets of crime and morality in Fyodor Dostoevsky's crime and punishment and Aravind Adiga's the white tiger*. Department of English, Kadi Sarva Vishwavidyalaya. http://hdl.handle.net/10603/202897

Shukla, R. *Moral consciousness in the English Novel with special reference to the major Novels of Jane Austen and Charles Dickens*. Department of English, Chhatrapati Sahuji Maharaj University. http://hdl.handle.net/10603/222501

Strem, G. G. (1957). The moral world of Dostoevsky. *Russian Review, 16*(3), 15–26

Mr. Sudip Kumar Das completed his Postgraduate degree from Pondicherry University in 2015 with First Class. He did his Undergraduate degree from The University of Burdwan. Currently, he is pursuing a D.Phil. degree from the University of Allahabad. He is also working as a teaching faculty in the Department of English, Rajiv Gandhi National Institute of Youth Development. His research topic is on Partition Literature which incorporates regional literary works and western thinkers. He has chapters in two Edited Books on the theme of Partition Trauma and Literature and Culture. He has published articles in two reputed journals and presented papers at multiple National and International Conferences. His research interest includes Partition studies, Gender studies, Canadian Literature, Indian Writing and British Poetry. He keeps an interest in Creative writing and Subaltern studies.

Chapter 4
Developing Bhutan: Nurturing Youth

Nidup Dorji

Abstract Nurturing youths is a critical investment for a better tomorrow. Bhutan has the youngest population with nearly 60% under 25 years of age. This represents a positive force in contributing toward Bhutan's development. Bhutan abreast collectivism with greater family and community participation. However, with economic modernization and infringement of individualistic ideologies, the value of interdependence may be at threat with vulnerable youths at greater risk of harm and violence. The revelation of rising drug use among Bhutanese youth (84%) and students (43%) remains a huge concern for its family system and society. Social problems that lay hidden when triggered by external events such as modernization and urbanization are not exhaustible especially when youths are exposed to fast changing outside world filled with attractions and distractions. Besides, lack of social and parental support and family breakups do not provide protection or serve as inspiration to youths but rather contribute to a higher prevalence of addiction. It is not that children today are born with a greater propensity to cause problems, but the change in the environment and upbringing needs critical attention. Therefore, the objective of the Chapter is to reach out to multiple approaches to harm and risk reduction among the youths, which need to be rooted in the wisdom that all living beings own basic goodness. The approach also merits attending to their needs and care, keeping them occupied within multiple environments—homes, schools, institutions, and communities. The solution is not in avoidance but in reaching out to youths. Certainly, the 'mud' with the Bhutanese youth is not that thick for now. Therefore, education can be used as a flame to ignite curiosity and explore better. Besides, nurturing the immeasurable values of loving-kindness, compassion, and equanimity to create a compassionate society is possible for a spiritually rich acclaimed Bhutan.

Keywords Youth · Interdependence · Mindfulness · Sacred outlook · Values · Adverse childhood experiences · Bhutan

---

N. Dorji (✉)
Department of Public Health and Allied Health Sciences, Faculty of Nursing and Public Health, Khesar Gyalpo University of Medical Sciences of Bhutan, Thimphu, Bhutan
e-mail: nidupdorji.dorji@gmail.com

S. Deb and S. Deb (eds.), *Handbook of Youth Development*,
https://doi.org/10.1007/978-981-99-4969-4_4

Introduction

Youth represents the future of any nation state. They are the main agents of change and progress and have a greater effect on socio-economic development. The future of the world is even more promising with young generations more creative, innovative, hardworking, and to a greater extent aware of their future. For this, family is regarded as a building block of society for playing a critical role for the growth and development of children and youth who contribute to social development. Family is crucial in one's life and they shape the person's characteristics, values, and sound health. Children first learn how to manage their emotions, interact with others, communicate, and instill the values of citizenship and belonging in the society and family. Nevertheless, research indicated a steady rise in the number of divorces across the globe and the single parent household has increased that could have bearing consequences on children. They include the risk of developing behavioral disorders, poor performance in school, substance abuse, and greater risk of psychiatric pathologies and difficulty in relationships in later adult life. In contrast, depending on the degree of conflictive separation, findings from some studies have not supported the notion that children coming from single parents perform poorly in school. Empirically, drugs and drinking are more common and teenage pregnancies rapidly increasing. Wanting what everyone else does, measuring success in life through how much one has, lack of feeling important unless one has, pressure to be perfect, and living under poverty that contributes to social, behavioral, and educational problems are the common features of the twenty-first century. There is a need of emphasis to understand how the youth and children of the twenty-first century face issues differently from that of the previous generations. As much as modernity has greater influence on youth and children, this chapter is believed to blend modern approaches of empowering youth and children and reconnection with the fundamental truths of 'basic goodness', impermanence, interdependence, and the criticality of developing sacred outlook to one's life and surrounding for the better future of Bhutan.

Investing in Children and Youth

Investing in children and youth and their development is an opportunity to unite social and economic goals now and in the future. It is one of the crucial remedies any country may offer to the problems and challenges brought in by rapid socio-economic developments and demographic environmental changes. Working for positive youth development can strengthen self-awareness and regulations; self-efficacy at the social, emotional, spiritual, cognitive, and behavioral competence levels, and believes in their future. However, such development and progress would require networks of supportive adults and their facilitation. In the face of unavoidable changes, children and youth must acquire greater thinking, social, coping with emotions and stress, political skills, and self-assurance. Investment in children and youth today would therefore reduce future adults' welfare issues (Canoy et al., 2006). Considerable research findings have emphasized the significance of massive mainstream early investment in children and youth to avoid the development of problematic groups of children. Prevention is better than cure and continues to be significant to this day and age. Therefore, the need to shift social investment strategies from cure to prevention is critical.

Reconnection with Basic Goodness

Not necessarily influenced by Western psychology commonly based on Freud's psychodynamic model that is grounded on the model of causation apparently moving towards blame, Buddhist psychology is informed by personal responsibility. In Buddhism, looking into the blame game whether it is internal or external as the stimulus of distress is not significant. Instead, it asks us first to be present with our experience and observe our reaction to that experience, then look inside to uncover its source. It demands the realization of personal responsibility to any outcome and enables us to move away from blame.

The experience of basic goodness is universal and does not belong to any one culture or tradition. There is nothing religious talking about it. However, living in the time of uncertainty it feels hard to see and uncover the goodness vested in each one of us. Unless the ground of goodness is discovered in our own lives, it is difficult to hope to improve the lives of others. Basic goodness is being authentic, which is heavily challenged with the advent of globalization and modernization where talking about the mind is a much neglected area. We all experience glimpses of goodness all the time, but we simply fail to acknowledge them. Perhaps, modern education, technology, and life encourage competition, speed efficiency, and productivity discourses that fuels stress, especially among the young people and farther them away from seeing their basic goodness. Although the mind is not an entity but free from concepts, it is significantly related with all kinds of extreme emotions. A Bhutanese born Tibetan Lama, His Eminence Dzongsar Jamyang Khyentse remarked "Without the workable mind, perception of adversities and feeling of suffering will continue to bother people especially the young. We can't change any human behavior until we learn to deal with our mind." (https://www.youtube.com/watch?v=KsP9IUv6cHM&t=452s). Reconnecting to basic goodness will be challenging without familiarizing with one's mind.

Empower Youth to Be Leader

We are tempted to think that modernity, its advancement towards higher altitudes of technology, and scientific temper have made youth more self-important, and ignorant of the real issues that society faces. Temptations such as drug addiction, smoking, drinking, sexual relationship followed by violence in the family, neighborhood, and communities, money, personal relationships, and intense competition create more anxiety among the youths fueling more social and mental health problems including stress and depression. The persistent crises that the world faces also disengage youths at the extreme margins of society influencing the loss of hope for their future. The provision of an enabling environment for the youth to prosper, a platform to exercise their rights, regain hope, and a sense of community to engage as a responsible social actor, policies and programs that are youth friendly remain critical. Hence, the starting point is to recognize and consider youth as a solution, not as a problem, and fully potentiate them in social change through empowerment (Singh, 2018). Empowering youth is a human resource development tool and a process designed to assist in the development of productive individuals. Empowerment enables children and youth to solve their own problems and contribute to the development of their community. Youth-led empowerment actions offer learning opportunities and create spaces for young people to participate in the community movements (Soe, 2020). In a study by Schwartz and Suyemoto (2013), youth community organization programs and empowerment were found to influence a wide range of youth development outcomes, including knowledge, skills, civic engagement, and change in the positive outlook of self and others. Young people are often seen as one of the victims of social problems in the community, weak education system, political instability, and poverty. Young people from such backgrounds tend to have lower quality education, which in turn contributes to higher levels of communal stress bringing in the burden to the future generations (Schwartz & Suyemoto, 2013). Our job is not to tell the children what to be, but to show them the possibilities of being a good human.

Appreciate Independence and Understand Interdependence

Perhaps the only country in the world to pursue happiness as a central policy goal, and guided by the philosophy of Buddhism that believes in dependent co-origination, Bhutan has valued the significance of interdependence. This is evident in Bhutan where the developmental activities are guided by the philosophy of "Gross National Happiness" and strict wildlife and environmental conservation policy of forest coverage to remain not less than 60 percent at all times. The value of realizing the significance of interdependence is healthy and its inculcation among the youth is even more imperative.

Individualism or independence is more frequently observed in European American culture in contrast to interdependence and collectivism more frequently observed in the East Asian cultural context (Ogihara & Uchida, 2014). Although individualism brings benefits such as enjoying free choices and a stronger sense of self-sufficiency, it also urges people to pursue personal achievements, thereby creating competition between the individuals and bringing in the feeling of being lonely and selfish. It is a pity to observe that some birth families fail to consistently provide support to the young, which forces them to become independent living. With such developments, the focus on fostering connections falls and gives rise to a new focus often characterized by self-sufficiency. Such a premature transition could be harsh and shocking, especially to youth. Empirically, with the individualistic ideologies creeping into the Bhutanese society, especially among the urban dwellers, the traditional belief of extended family system and collectivism that remained as a protective factor may be at threat.

"Reap What You Sow—Karma" and Impermanence

Karma is a Sanskrit word meaning 'action' or 'doing' which is closely related with Hinduism, Jainism, and Sikhism, and is heavily used in Buddhism. Karma believes that every action including behavior, speech, and thought continuously produces reactions that influence the future of the individual (Lee et al., 2017). Even among the nonreligious individuals, the idea of karma is resonated with the belief in some sort of forces at work as what goes around comes around. Science is no different, as it believes in the association of 'cause-condition and effect'. In fact, entailing certain symmetry in nature, Newton's third law states that for every action there is equal and opposite reaction, which means that action cannot be wasted but leaves a lasting imprint that the consequences of it will have to be reaped anyhow. People can forget but karma will never. As is enshrined in the teaching of Gautama Buddha 'You are your own master and you make your own future.' The classic proverb 'You reap what you sow' implies that the future consequences are inevitably shaped by present action(s) and hence the need to watch our doings. As much as we are the maker of happiness, we are also the maker of our own problems and suffering. Not wishing to have a problem is as easy as not engaging with the causes of it. Many of us fail to understand this simple cause-effect relationship in a world full of attractions and distractions. On the other hand, one of the chronic practices even more so in today's time is believing in permanency. The process of change and impermanence is an integral part of existence. Deeper awareness and appreciation of this fact can lead to happiness that every being wishes to have. However, the mere intellectual understanding of impermanence is inadequate. It requires existential understanding through the expansion of consciousness and attention to these processes (Dwivedi, 2006). How much do we have time to contemplate on impermanence? If we seriously contemplate impermanence, there is nothing inherent in nature except aggregation, which does not last forever. Realizing in life about simple facts such as all born will die can curtail wrong intentions and the wrong doings. Our actions become impure when the inner poison of ignorance, aversion, and greed contaminates one's mind. Our ignorance stops us from seeing our potential to lighten the darkness. In ignorance, we busy ourselves doing non-virtuous activities. We do almost everything as if we will live forever. Wars, famine, exploitations, separation, and disharmony, are not the results of smartness and farsightedness but the results of the action of exercising our own ignorance.

Strengthen Mindfulness and Lessen Mental Health

Globally, mental and substance use disorders are the leading cause of disability among children and youth and is a significant contributor to disease burden among these groups (Erskine et al., 2015) with far reaching effects on social, economic, and health. Mindfulness interventions are increasingly becoming popular among the world population. Mindfulness is the state of consciousness including the incorporation of purposeful awareness and attention, as well as non-judgmental reactions to the present moment (Huang et al., 2021). Mindful-based interventions are also found to reduce the consumption of several substances including alcohol and cigarettes, via a reduction in craving and increased mindfulness (Chiesa & Serretti, 2014). Considerable empirical studies have shown positive influence of mindfulness on social and emotional competence (Klingbeil et al., 2017), academic performance (Caballero et al., 2019), at the same time reduction in the behavioral problems (Van de Weijer-Bergsma et al., 2012). Mindfulness practices can deliver lasting improvements in self-awareness and contribute to emotional stability (Thompson & Gauntlett-Gilbert, 2008). Although the practice of mindfulness depends on life events such as adverse childhood experiences (ACEs), mindfulness practices are also found to have numerous positive effects on life outcomes including mental health and educational achievement (Huang et al., 2021). In a world filled with attractions and distractions, the negative effect of distractions on recognition, recall, and social presence was revealed in the study by Oh et al. (2019). For the Bhutanese, where the teachings of Gautama Buddha are still prevalent, monastic leaders and communities play a greater role to strengthen and reach out the true teachings of Buddha, blend to fit in the modern Bhutanese lifestyle heavily influenced the ideologies of the affluent societies.

Prevent Adverse and Promote Positive Childhood Experiences

A growing body of research identifies that multiple ACEs are the major risk factors for several negative health outcomes (Kajeepeta et al., 2015). Increase in ACEs increases the risk of age-related health problems and the effects of ACEs such as childhood maltreatment can be long lasting (Dorji et al., 2020). As per Springer et al. (2007), ACEs particularly physical abuse predicted the worst physical and mental health outcomes decades after the occurrence of the event. Individual with a history of emotional neglect and sexual abuse while still a child are more likely to develop more than one lifetime affective disorders such as depression and social phobia (Spinhoven et al., 2010). According to a systematic review (Fliege et al., 2009), the most recurrently found associations between adolescent or adult self-harm behavior are rooted in childhood experiences of emotional neglect, physical (such as sexual) or psychological abuses. Engaging in more risky behavior is further exacerbated by more adverse experiences encountered in childhood and consequently suffers from poor health (Ramiro et al., 2010). Ramiro et al. (2010) claimed that suicide ideation and attempts significantly increased with four or more ACEs. ACEs also increase health-risk behaviors such as smoking, drug, and alcohol use (Norman et al., 2012). Although eradication of ACEs is aspirational, screening for the history of ACEs can help both the client and the care provider to understand more about the underlying causes of it and its influence on health conditions. This would in turn facilitate better-informed care and treatment options (Hughes et al., 2017).

On the other hand, positive childhood experiences (PCEs), which are the experiences of building a sense of belongingness and connection in childhood, are found to have numerous positive effects on life. Although, less is known about how PCEs provide protection and counter the negative impacts of ACEs, research into psychology have demonstrated that exposure to advantageous childhood experiences can improve future social experiences, and healthy relationships, predict better productivity and responsibility in adulthood (Narayan et al., 2018). This is because exposure to positive experiences and supportive relationships could help children build resilience to withstand adverse experiences and mitigate its negative consequences (Sege & Harper Browne, 2017). PCEs have shown dose–response associations with depression and poor mental health outcomes. Compared to none to two PCEs, those reporting six to seven PCEs had 72% lower odds of reporting depression and poor mental health outcomes (Bethell et al., 2019). Regardless of the importance of PCEs and ACEs and its impact on multiple health conditions and wellbeing, nothing is available about the prevalence of ACEs and PCEs among young people in Bhutan, and its influence on their health, wellbeing, and quality as of today. However, existing evidence suggests the positive influence of PCEs as much as ACEs, and its negative influence on multiple dimensions of life, deserve promotion and prevention, respectively. It is because both ACEs and PCEs are attainable.

Human Values Education and Human (Youth) Outcomes

Understanding human values is a never-ending process. Although there is no one universal consensus definition of value, Schwartz (1994, p. 21) summarized the most widely shared conception of values in social psychology as "Values are desirable trans situational goals, varying in importance, that serve as guiding principles in the life of a person or other social entity". This definition is obvious that values motivate action and give direction. Values are standards or principles considered critical in life. They come from within, the boundless qualities such as loving-kindness, compassion, rejoice, and equanimity, can be reinforced further by practicing generosity, punctuality, patience, diligence, concentration, and wisdom. They are the foundation of human existence (Radha, 2016). Values make a difference, influence behavior and therefore serve as criteria for selecting action.

Depending on the context of its use, the meaning of value differs. All values have cognitive, affective, and directional aspects (Rokeach, 2008) and are not necessarily concrete rules of conduct. As educational institutions are the sacred places where learners build in their characters and career, a quality education, which includes imparting of value education with the highest intellectual excellence that helps the learners emerge as leaders in their chosen field. Hence, true education must be human-making, implying that all education must stem from value-based education (Shobha & Kala, 2015). True education must be based on the knowledge of the whole human being and that such knowledge cannot be attained without loving-kindness, compassion, rejoice, and equanimity. A nation of people with a strong character is indeed a greater nation.

Human beings are the ones that give value and meaning to the world. As education is a process of all-round development of an individual, physically, intellectually, emotionally, socially, morally, and spiritually, teachers are not only expected to facilitate in the gaining of knowledge but also inculcate values and bring in the transformation of inner being through the process of inner development (Gul, 2017). Therefore, in building the character of human beings, values are desirable to become a part of the character building and guide for self-development.

Although change is inevitable, there is a growing concern about the erosion of values because of modern education that gradually undermines the values and its significance, especially among the youth today. In addition, society is becoming more materialistic and values appear to be pushed into the far background. Therefore, the promotion of human values in the society depends on the promotion of good qualities among the individuals. Value-based education is a solution to empower youth and restore the values that are apparently dwindling. With the fast changing technology, socio-economic development, ecology, and environment, value education is of unique importance that the educational institutions including the family system will have greater stress on human values and concern for others (Shobha & Kala, 2015). While the value system of people is genetically predetermined, significant parts of values are established in the early years from parents, teachers, friends and others. Almost in every culture, children are taught to be honest and truthful but never to be little honest or little truthful. Although values are relatively stable and enduring, the number of values could change with more people growing up and getting exposed to other value systems.

The contemporary world demands greater intercommunication and unanimity. Consequently, there is an urgent need for cultivating values of mutual cooperation and harmony, which can be best fostered through education at home and formal schooling. In fact, the quest for excellence stresses the need for value education at all levels of human training. Since teachers' actions convey more than their words, an ordinary teacher can bring about extraordinary transformation in the society. Teachers need to understand, appreciate, and uphold life sustained moral values. Indeed, teachers are supposedly the watchdog of the society for being the role model for their students and the society. A value-based, spiritual, ethical, and a need based education is crucial for sustainable human development and social growth in the current world where materialism and capitalistic ideas dominate (Gul, 2017).

Develop Sacred or Positive Outlook

In Bhutan, most Bhutanese would dare not urinate on a prayer flag. This is a great value of viewing the surroundings sacred. Both spiritual belief and environmental practices which can be at odds in the reductionist paradigm are aligned in the service of environmental conservation in Bhutan (Allison, 2017). Presently about 71% of the landmass are under forest coverage, which is more than the constitutional mandate of 60% (Devkota et al., 2022) for ages to come. Furthermore, the centuries old Bhutan's Buddhist heritage and the following Buddhist philosophy of 'Middle-path' have promoted the preservation of nature, understanding the sanctity of life and abstention from killing of living creatures greatly contributing to the prevention of biodiversity degradation. For a small nation like Bhutan, the sacrosanctity outlook must continue to be transferred and valued for generations to come. Connection to land and water is vital in Australian Aboriginal culture. Nicholas Lucas Ticum, a Maya priest and a researcher, told the Permanent Forum on Indigenous Issues that "The earth does not belong to human beings. Human beings belong to the earth". He further called for the care of the planet by building sustainable development alliances and strategies and on scientific and research community to 'recognize the spiritual dimensions of human beings, the connection and interconnectedness of all the elements of the universe and scientific pluralism" (United Nations Meetings Coverage & Press Release, 2009). The sacrosanctity outlook to surroundings is crucial to enable beings to harmonize their living with Mother Nature more and combat the mass-scale environmental destruction that the blue planet earth currently faces. Youth-led climate activists such as Greta Thunberg is an indication that there are young who are empowered to make a positive and lasting difference and ensure a sustainable and healthy future for earth that continues to support life in it. Thus, life sustenance will only continue if and only if, humans with selfish desires wear sacred lenses and change their outlook. Developing a positive outlook to life is critical for every human to save the future.

Buddhist psychology is based on the notion that human beings are fundamentally good and that their most basic qualities are positive, open, intelligent, and warm (Trungpa, 2005). According to Trungpa (2005), a great deal of chaos in the world is mostly deep rooted in people lacking to appreciate themselves. Having never developed loving-kindness, empathy, and gentleness towards themselves lead to projecting outside inharmonious and confusion. Instead of appreciating our lives, we often take our existence for granted or we find it depressing and arduous. People threaten to attempt or complete suicide because they do not get what they think deserves out of their life. It is when we do not punish or condemn ourselves, relax more, and appreciate our body and mind, we begin to come closer to the fundamental notion of basic goodness in ourselves. Developing tenderness towards ourselves allows us to see our problems and our potentials accurately. Seeing this allows us to feel that we need not have to ignore our problems or amplify our potential. Such kind of gentleness toward self and appreciation are important that provide the ground for helping others and ourselves. Therefore, in the context of Bhutanese, not daring to urinate on the prayer flags is a notoriously precious value worth an investment among the youth for developing sacrosanctity and the sacred outlook. It is only through the sacred outlook towards one's surroundings that an individual would learn to harmonize in living together. Not having a sacred outlook fuels selfish motives and limits farsightedness.

Conclusion

For the future, there is no greater investment than on youths. Empowerment and investing in children and youth is an opportunity, a crucial remedy to combat problems and challenges brought in by rapid socio-economic development, modernization, urbanization, and environmental changes. Reconnection with the basic goodness entrusted upon every individual deserves revitalization in the changing world. As nothing is inherent in nature, the understanding and appreciation of interdependence and co-habitation outweigh the benefits brought in by individualism. Understanding and deeper awareness that nothing lasts forever and being mindful are the long-term investment for a better future. Let the knowing 'what goes around comes around' or 'you reap what you sow' be not in words, but in individual realization. This would in turn mitigate adverse life experiences such as ACEs and promote positive experiences for instance PCEs. Value-based education in the institutions and family are critical for positive human outcomes. Developing a positive and sacred outlook toward surroundings is the basis for harmonious living, happiness, and better wellbeing.

References

Allison, E. (2017). Spirits and Nature: The intertwining of sacred cosmologies and environmental conservation in Bhutan. *Journal for the Study of Religion, Nature & Culture, 11*(2)

Bethell, C., Jones, J., Gombojav, N., Linkenbach, J., & Sege, R. (2019). Positive childhood experiences and adult mental and relational health in a statewide sample: Associations across adverse childhood experiences levels. *JAMA Pediatrics, 173*(11), e193007. https://doi.org/10.1001/jamapediatrics.2019.3007

Caballero, C., Scherer, E., West, M. R., Mrazek, M. D., Gabrieli, C. F., & Gabrieli, J. D. (2019). Greater mindfulness is associated with better academic achievement in middle school. *Mind, Brain, and Education, 13*(3), 157–166.

Canoy, M., Carvalho, G., Hammarlund, C., Hubert, A., Lerais, F., & Melich, A. (2006). Investing in Youth: from childhood to adulthood. *Bureau of European Policy Advisers (BEPA), 11*

Chiesa, A., & Serretti, A. (2014). Are mindfulness-based interventions effective for substance use disorders? A systematic review of the evidence. *Substance Use & Misuse, 49*(5), 492–512. https://doi.org/10.3109/10826084.2013.770027

Devkota, D., Miller, D. C., Wang, S. W., & Brooks, J. S. (2022). Biodiversity conservation funding in Bhutan: Thematic, temporal, and spatial trends over four decades. *Conservation Science and Practice*, e12757

Dorji, N., Dunne, M., & Deb, S. (2020). Adverse childhood experiences: Association with physical and mental health conditions among older adults in Bhutan. *Public Health, 182*, 173–178. https://doi.org/10.1016/j.puhe.2020.02.013

Dwivedi, K. N. (2006). An Eastern perspective on change. *Clinical Child Psychology and Psychiatry, 11*(2), 205–212. https://doi.org/10.1177/1359104506061445

Erskine, H. E., Moffitt, T. E., Copeland, W. E., Costello, E. J., Ferrari, A. J., Patton, G., & Scott, J. G. (2015). A heavy burden on young minds: The global burden of mental and substance use disorders in children and youth. *Psychological Medicine, 45*(7), 1551–1563. https://doi.org/10.1017/s0033291714002888

Fliege, H., Lee, J.-R., Grimm, A., & Klapp, B. F. (2009). Risk factors and correlates of deliberate self-harm behavior: A systematic review. *Journal of Psychosomatic Research, 66*(6), 477–493.

Gul, S. B. A. (2017). Teacher and value education: An exploratory study. *Online Submission, 37*.

Huang, C., Yang, M., Geng, Y., Chen, Y., Cheung, S. P., Deng, G., & Zhuo, G. (2021). Adverse childhood experiences and mindfulness in Chinese college students during the COVID-19 pandemic. *Front Psychiatry, 12*, 619128. https://doi.org/10.3389/fpsyt.2021.619128

Hughes, K., Bellis, M. A., Hardcastle, K. A., Sethi, D., Butchart, A., Mikton, C., & Dunne, M. P. (2017). The effect of multiple adverse childhood experiences on health: A systematic review and meta-analysis. *The Lancet Public Health, 2*(8), e356–e366.

Kajeepeta, S., Gelaye, B., Jackson, C. L., & Williams, M. A. (2015). Adverse childhood experiences are associated with adult sleep disorders: A systematic review. *Sleep Medicine, 16*(3), 320–330.

Klingbeil, D. A., Renshaw, T. L., Willenbrink, J. B., Copek, R. A., Chan, K. T., Haddock, A., & Clifton, J. (2017). Mindfulness-based interventions with youth: A comprehensive meta-analysis of group-design studies. *Journal of School Psychology, 63*, 77–103.

Lee, K. C. G., Oh, A., Zhao, Q., Wu, F.-Y., Chen, S., Diaz, T., & Ong, C. K. (2017). Buddhist counseling: Implications for mental health professionals. *Spirituality in Clinical Practice, 4*(2), 113.

Narayan, A. J., Rivera, L. M., Bernstein, R. E., Harris, W. W., & Lieberman, A. F. (2018). Positive childhood experiences predict less psychopathology and stress in pregnant women with childhood adversity: A pilot study of the benevolent childhood experiences (BCEs) scale. *Child Abuse and Neglect, 78*, 19–30.

Norman, R. E., Byambaa, M., De, R., Butchart, A., Scott, J., & Vos, T. (2012). The long-term health consequences of child physical abuse, emotional abuse, and neglect: A systematic review and meta-analysis. *PLoS Medicine, 9*(11), e1001349.

Ogihara, Y., & Uchida, Y. (2014). Does individualism bring happiness? Negative effects of individualism on interpersonal relationships and happiness. *Frontiers in Psychology, 5*. https://doi.org/10.3389/fpsyg.2014.00135

Oh, C., Herrera, F., & Bailenson, J. (2019). The effects of immersion and real-world distractions on virtual social interactions. *Cyberpsychology, Behavior, and Social Networking, 22*(6), 365–372.

Radha, P. (2016). *Role of Teachers in Imparting Value Education.* Paper presented at the National Conference on "Value Education Through Teacher Education"

Ramiro, L. S., Madrid, B. J., & Brown, D. W. (2010). Adverse childhood experiences (ACE) and health-risk behaviors among adults in a developing country setting. *Child Abuse and Neglect, 34*(11), 842–855. https://doi.org/10.1016/j.chiabu.2010.02.012

Rokeach, M. (2008). *Understanding human values.* Simon and Schuster

Schwartz, S. H. (1994). Are there universal aspects in the structure and contents of human values? *Journal of Social Issues, 50*(4), 19–45.

Schwartz, S., & Suyemoto, K. (2013). Creating change from the inside: Youth development within a youth community organizing program. *Journal of Community Psychology, 41*(3), 341–358.

Sege, R. D., & Harper Browne, C. (2017). Responding to ACEs with HOPE: Health outcomes from positive experiences. *Academic Pediatric, 17*(7s), S79–S85. https://doi.org/10.1016/j.acap.2017.03.007

Shobha, S., & Kala, N. (2015). Value education towards empowerment of youth-A holistic approach. *Procedia - Social and Behavioral Sciences, 172*, 192–199. https://doi.org/10.1016/j.sbspro.2015.01.354

Singh, A. K. (2018). Empowering youth through Buddhist education. *The Journal of International Association of Buddhist Universities (JIABU), 11*(3), 298–310.

Soe, T. M. (2020). The significance and impacts of a youth-led empowerment program and youth-led community development interventions in Myanmar

Spinhoven, P., Elzinga, B. M., Hovens, J. G., Roelofs, K., Zitman, F. G., van Oppen, P., & Penninx, B. W. (2010). The specificity of childhood adversities and negative life events across the life span to anxiety and depressive disorders. *Journal of Affective Disorders, 126*(1–2), 103–112.

Springer, K. W., Sheridan, J., Kuo, D., & Carnes, M. (2007). Long-term physical and mental health consequences of childhood physical abuse: Results from a large population-based sample of men and women. *Child Abuse and Neglect, 31*(5), 517–530.

Thompson, M., & Gauntlett-Gilbert, J. (2008). Mindfulness with children and adolescents: Effective clinical application. *Clinical Child Psychology and Psychiatry, 13*(3), 395–407. https://doi.org/10.1177/1359104508090603

Trungpa, C. (2005). *The sanity we are born with: A Buddhist approach to psychology*. Shambhala Publications

United Nations Meetings Coverage and Press Release. (2009). The earth does not belong to human beings; Human beings belong to the earth [Press release]. Retrieved from https://press.un.org/en/2009/hr4988.doc.htm#:~:text=Lucas%20Ticum%20said%2C%20adding%20that,generations%20of%20mankind%2C%20he%20said

Van de Weijer-Bergsma, E., Formsma, A. R., de Bruin, E. I., & Bögels, S. M. (2012). The effectiveness of mindfulness training on behavioral problems and attentional functioning in adolescents with ADHD. *Journal of Child and Family Studies, 21*(5), 775–787.

Dr. Nidup Dorji is an Assistant Professor and Dean of Public Health and Allied Health Sciences at the Faculty of Nursing and Public Health (FNPH), Khesar Gyalpo University of Medical Sciences of Bhutan (KGUMSB). After obtaining his Doctor of Philosophy in Public Health from Queensland University of Technology, Australia, he rigorously worked in the area of psychological well being, happiness, and quality of life among older adults in Bhutan. He also obtained his Postdoctoral Fellowship from University of Quebec at Montreal (UQAM), Canada. He has published book chapters and scientific articles in the national and international peer-reviewed journals as first and second author through independent research undertakings and collaborations. Dr Dorji is currently teaching international public health, epidemiology and biostatistics, environmental health, sexual and reproductive health including HIV/AIDS, and health research at FNPH. Besides his interest to study more about happiness, quality of life, elderly health, life skills education, end-of-life care and spirituality, he also developed his patience to research more about adverse and positive childhood experiences and their influence on health and wellbeing.

Chapter 5
Youth Development: International Perspectives

Ruth Richardson

Abstract The decimation and the negative impact on the extent of youth provisions in England over the last ten years have been widely documented. There are grave concerns about the implications for young people of the destruction of youth work. Additionally, there is mounting evidence that young people are currently facing unprecedented challenges. The time is ripe to provide support to young people and therefore, arguably, for youth work to serve as a much more secure provision. This chapter provides an overview of the historical development of youth work in the United Kingdom and the contests of defining youth work. The drive toward quantitative data collection and the impact agenda is evaluated. This chapter goes on to present a strand of youth work, called Global Youth Work, that was developed in England before the series of budget cuts and redundancies inundated youth work services. In describing the framework of 'Connect, Challenge, Change' which is related to Global Youth Work, this chapter outlines how England might foster positive international partnerships and revive an appreciation for the importance of the methodology of youth work. This chapter asserts that England needs to engage much more with youth work. Additionally, that Global Youth Work could be an effective tool for England in reinvigorating and reimagining youth work.

Keywords Youth development · Economic · Social · Political · United Kingdom

Introduction

From the Albemarle Report published in 1960, recommendations for the delivery of youth services began to be implemented across England. It has been suggested that this may have been the beginning of the youth service in the United Kingdom (UK) and that this approach to youth work became an international model that was

'Between the cracks' and over time: Youth Work approaches in England.

R. Richardson (✉)
University of Derby, 2 Boden Street, Derby DE23 8GX, UK
e-mail: r.richardson@derby.ac.uk

S. Deb and S. Deb (eds.), *Handbook of Youth Development*,
https://doi.org/10.1007/978-981-99-4969-4_5

emulated by many other countries across the world (Nicholls, 2011). However, some critiques of the Albemarle Report suggest that youth work had been taking place extensively prior to the publication of the Albermarle Report and additionally that the report appeared to be centered on a largely deficit-based model (Muirhead, 2020). Increasingly, a significant critique is made of deficit approaches where working with young people views them from the onset as inherently flawed and requiring help (De St Croix, 2018; Muirhead, 2020).

The economic, social, and political climate in the UK has been tumultuous in recent years and youth work has in no way escaped the challenges that this has presented. Arguably, youth work in the UK was decimated in 2010 when government-led austerity measures were implemented and resulted in numerous youth provisions closing including the statutory youth services (YMCA, 2020). Youth work practitioners from across the UK have endeavored to ensure that young people have continued to be supported and that the methodological approach to youth work is maintained (UNISON, 2016). Additional recent concerns regarding the state of youth work in the UK query if competitiveness for funding has negatively affected more localized, grassroots initiatives and pushed youth work projects into an outcome driven approach (De St Croix, 2018). Furthermore, there are concerns that argue that youth work is only taking place at larger, national scales in response to societal frenzies about topics, usually criminal in nature, such as Anti-Social Behavior (ASB) and young people being associated with drug dealing and knife crime (Legane, 2018).

Consequently, from seemingly enthralling beginnings, what youth work there is now in the UK can be queried and considered problematic. Despite this, it should be acknowledged that numerous infrastructure organizations such as the Federation of Detached Youth Workers, In Defence of Youth Work, the Institute for Youth Work (IYW), the National Youth Agency (NYA), and UK Youth all lobby to raise awareness of the importance of the youth work sector. Universities alongside the auspices of the Professional Association of Lecturers in Youth and Community Work (PALYCW) successfully train youth workers every year to the nationally recognized level six and above in line with the Joint Negotiating Committee (JNC) standard for Youth Work (NYA, n.d.).

Youth work in the UK has undergone seismic changes to the sector and many youth workers have been left feeling burnt-out and jaded (Wonder Foundation, n.d.). Despite this, young people in the UK, like young people all over the world, have never needed support through the unique methodology of youth work more (UK Youth, 2021). Young people in England are proven to be disproportionately experiencing issues related to racism, mental health, the cost-of-living crisis, and limited employment opportunities (Children's Commissioner, 2021).

Exploring how the conception of youth work in the UK has developed can assist in a better understanding of how youth work best functions under differing circumstances and pressures (Davies, 2008). An appreciation for how youth work is defined and how various definitions have evolved may help expose where the practice of youth work has become misaligned and no longer serving its original purpose.

Around 2005 a collective of organizations from across England worked together on a youth project underpinned by a shared interest and passion for youth work, especially a certain strand called Global Youth Work (Development Education Association, 2009). A project, called Global Youth Action (GYA), worked with young people from a variety of backgrounds including Pakistani, Bangladeshi and Malaysian heritage, growing up in post-industrial towns in northern England as well as predominantly white British heritage GYA groups from the Midlands and the Southwest of England. In addition, a youth group made up of largely refugee and asylum seeker young people in West London participated. Through this national GYW project, a theoretical framework was created and entitled 'Connect, Challenge, Change' (Development Education Association, 2010). The key components to the 'Connect, Challenge, Change' (3Cs) framework were generated through core parts of generic youth work practice such as youth led, reflective practice, and critical thinking skills.

Within this 3Cs framework, 'Connect' encourages youth workers to get to know their youth groups much better. Through this initial stage, the youth worker is encouraged to find out what topics the young people are most interested in. Approaches here can relate to consensus decision making to encourage the groups to collectively agree on a singular topic which they will focus on throughout the framework process. Following 'Connect' the young people enter the 'Challenge' phase of the learning journey where they debate their collectively chosen topic. Importantly, within 'Challenge', the young people view the topic from multiple perspectives. Once these two stages have taken place the youth groups are supported to consider what action they might like to take. It is here that 'Personal, Local, National and Global (PLNG)' ideas are drawn upon in order to encourage the young people to consider the various approaches that they can take to participate in positive social change (National Occupational Standards, 2008).

Global Youth Work (GYW) and the Connect, Challenge, Change (3Cs) approach is rooted in good youth work practice where young people are central (Davies, 2008; NYA, 2020; Smith, 2013). The GYW approach to youth work is adaptable and would be effective for youth engagement in a diverse range of settings. Importantly, the 3Cs approache encourages young people to be active, engaged, and critically minded about the world around them. The youth worker walks alongside the young people as they participate in the 3Cs learning journey together. There is a "long-standing youth work assumption that adults will seek respectful relationships with young people rather than dominate them or patronize them as not yet quite complete" (Davies, 2008, p. 6).

Despite the numerous challenges that face youth work today, such as a lack of funding and infrastructure, it could be beneficial to reconnect with the core of the methodological approach of youth work, maybe by engaging with GYW, and particularly in England. It could be argued that now is the critical time to increase sharing of good practice on the international stage, such as through international partner projects, conferences, and research, coupled with generating greater awareness of the 3Cs framework.

Youth work in England occupies a unique space. There are ongoing and increasing concerns regarding the lack of top-down appreciation of what constitutes youth work (De St Croix, 2018). In the contemporary, internationally connected world, there is a lot that England could learn regarding youth work from other countries. In many Commonwealth countries, the high percentage of youthful populations has propelled youth work into a much more prestigious role, especially within the State apparatus (Commonwealth Secretariat, 2017). In fact, more than 60% of the Commonwealth's population is aged under thirty (BBC News, 2022). The 3Cs framework that was developed as part of GYW could be utilized elsewhere. Through increased reciprocity and international partnerships, youth work should grow for the benefit of all. It is also hoped that the English Government might once again embrace youth work approaches.

The remainder of this chapter will explore this discussion in greater depth. Initially, perspectives on the history of youth work in the UK will be presented. An appreciation of how and where youth work approaches began is important for considering 'what next' for youth work, particularly in England. Indeed, an understanding of the history of youth work in the UK results in a greater appreciation for why, even in 2022, many still struggle to define it. Following an exploration of the past, there will be a brief overview of the current status of youth work. The framework of the 3Cs will be presented in more depth. The chapter will end with an exploration of the benefits and scope of international youth work partnerships in relation to GYW. Finally, the author queries whether there is scope for international partnerships relating to GYW and to potentially prompt these discussions.

Background to Youth Work in the UK

Some perspectives suggest that the Albemarle Report published in 1960 was the beginning of youth work in the UK (Nicholls, 2011). However, there are critiques that argue that there were a multitude of iterations representing youth work in existence prior to 1960. It is useful to explore these earlier youth work approaches in order to have a practical appreciation of how youth work in England operates today. As far back as the eighteenth century there were activities taking place that are purported to be the beginnings of youth work. During these times, Sunday schools proliferated. Sunday schools were largely linked to Christian churches (Smith, 2013). During the eighteenth century, the idea of Ragged Schools also emerged. Ragged Schools often had a local focus and endeavored to meet the holistic needs of children in very deprived areas (Smith, 2019). Although there were set objectives within Ragged School settings, there were also informal approaches to engagement that were employed, and it is these which may constitute the beginnings of what is now called youth work. A critical feature of Ragged Schools was that they would often take place in any space that could be made available for free, and which were accessible to the young people that they served such as covered railway arches. Unlike the Sunday Schools, the Ragged Schools were non-denominational and primarily advocated to serve the emotional, physical, social, and economic needs of the young people. Smith (2019) argues that:

Ragged Schools movement grew out of recognition that charity, denominational and Sunday schools were not providing for significant numbers of children in inner-city areas (p. 2).

Through these two examples, it is evident that informal education and approaches to engaging with young people within their own settings were beginning to take place in England even as far back as the eighteenth century. In addition, there were significant initiatives to emerge that had a clear impact upon the development of youth work. Most notably, in 1844, the youth organization entitled the Young Men's Christian Association (YMCA) began in London (YMCA, 2020). The initial inception of the YMCA was directed at young men, aimed largely at engaging in bible reading and the promotion of Christianity (YMCA, 2020). However, this type of community engagement was entirely in keeping with the cultural traditions of that time. 'Lads Clubs' were emerging at the end of the nineteenth century and often these provisions had a religious element too. Following the initial opportunities for predominantly boys and men, girl's clubs started in the late nineteenth century (Smith, 2013). The YMCA and Lads Clubs aided the development of youth work by designating specific spaces to meet the needs of young people at that time.

Additionally, at the end of the 1890s the term 'youth' started to emerge as a social category utilized in the popular press. Often, the framing of young people was that they were both a source of issues such as crime as well as a key group encountering unprecedented issues, such as unemployment (Smith, 2013). More radical forms of youth work began to emerge during these times. Whilst many of the early examples of youth work stemmed from Christian-based activities, there started to be an emergence in the nineteenth century of youth workers motivated by social and political factors rather than religion. Smith (2013) points out that whilst some youth work schemes were derived from conservative views, others sought radical social change. These historical contributions illustrate a recognition of the importance of social and political dimensions to work with young people. Often this work had a strong emphasis on fellowship and social justice. Consequently, even in these early inceptions of youth work, there were clear tensions between differing motivations and approaches. Davies (2008) suggests that these early signs of youth work were embedded within what is often referred to as 'popular' education movements and that the root of youth work was in "working-class activism based on self-help and self-organization" (p. 5). The suggestion here is that acknowledging the significance of 'class' was instrumental in the historical development of youth work in the UK. Class has continued to become a more contentious issue (Richmond, 2008). Economic inequality has got progressively worse in the UK and continues to be a significant issue today (The Equality Trust, 2019). However, very few contemporary youth projects will mention addressing class issues specifically in their strategic plans.

At the start of the twentieth century, the UK saw the emergence of the Scouts (2023), followed shortly by the Guides (World Association of Girl Guides and Girl Scouts, n.d.). The Scouts were the first large-scale youth movement in England (Smith, 2013). However, there were Brigades groups across the country precursing the establishment of the Scouts. In fact, Baden Powell, the founder of the Scouts, expressed concerns that the Brigades were too evangelical and regimented (Smith,

2013). It is argued that scouting is a democratic, voluntary movement that strives to not be static. Many of the concurrent themes of youth work relate to this conception of youth work as a 'movement' (UK Youth, 2020).

Following the First World War (1914–1918), there was support toward specific funding and State involvement in youth work (Davies, 2008). The first booklet with youth work in the title: 'Methods in Youth Work' was published in 1931 (Smith, 2013). Davies (2008) suggests that, at this time, the ideal goal of youth work was largely to encourage youth leaders rather than a broader goal of exploring citizenship for all young people. However, with the onset of the Second World War (1939–1945), the burgeoning of an organized youth service began to focus on how to best deal with the situations arising in wartime England. At around this time, the concept of young people gathering in safe spaces, such as open access youth clubs, and detached youth work started to take form and were regarded as youth work.

Key clauses were inserted into the Education Act in 1944, which required Local Authorities in the UK to secure leisure-time occupation and facilities for recreation for young people (Davies, 2008). Consequently, the UK emerged from the Second World War with a 'Service of Youth' formally designated by the State, which was required to be delivered locally and in connection with voluntary organizations.

As a consequence of these developments, it begins to become clear why there is so much disquiet at the idea that youth work in the UK began with the publication of the Albemarle Report in 1960. Davies (2008) argues that the Albemarle Report was written as a result of an independent review of the youth services that were already in existence. However, Smith (2013) goes on to support the idea that "with the publication of the Albemarle Report followed something of a golden age for youth work in England and Wales" (p. 21). The Albemarle Report declares that young people should have the right to free association, access training and be safely challenged. Words such as commitment, association, recreation, counsel, and self-determination appear in relation to the concept of youth work. The Albemarle Report placed a very high value on the active participation of young people and young people's peer relationships, which should both remain an important feature of modern youth work (Davies, 2008). This Report in 1960 was the trigger for a significant expenditure on youth centers, an expansion of training, and the development of project work, including detached youth work (Smith, 2013).

At the same time of the publication of the Albemarle Report, the importance of the professionalization of youth work entered the dialectic. This debate regarding professionalization of youth work has arguably raged since this time. As can be appreciated from the history of youth work, the voluntary sector and volunteers have always been instrumental. Davies (2008) queries whether the voluntary sector would survive a professionalizing onslaught of the youth work sector and vice versa. Not least because, if professionalism was equated to a qualification (and gaining a qualification is almost universally at a price) then there is a certainly that people from poorer backgrounds or people desiring to switch professions would not be able to join the youth work workforce.

In the 1970s, the UK youth workers were benefiting from a youthful boost to the population. The number of young people had grown substantially in what is often now referred to as the baby boomer generation. Beyond this post-war population growth, the trend has consistently been lower birth rates and decreasing numbers of young people. In the UK, the post 1970s period also witnessed the growth of home entertainment for example through TV. Consequently, there began to be fewer young people and many of those young people were being drawn into different media. This is contrary to the social and economic barriers that previous older generations could have experienced.

The 1980s and 1990s revealed increasing pressure for resources from organizations delivering services for young people. It was during this time that the national consensus appeared to deem work such as criminal justice, teaching, and social work as more necessitated as well as more professional. As a consequence, youth work activities began to move away from being embedded in the places that young people met to targeting and responding to specific issues. Policy and practice moved away from open access youth provisions towards activities working with specific groups of young people that could be deemed to be 'at risk' (Davies, 2013; Smith, 2013; UNISON, 2016). Youth workers were being told that their work needed to prioritise young people who would be considered to be at social margins such as unemployed young people or those young people at risk of being involved in crime (Davies, 2008). During this time, it is possible to observe how State involvement fundamentally altered youth work objectives from youth led to more top-down. "The role of youth work within State-sponsored services was, in effect, downgraded and increasingly marginalized" (Smith, 2013, p. 26). This may have been in response to social narratives about youth crime and a pervasive belief that there needed to be a national response to at-risk, so-called problematic groups of young people. Conversely, it might be argued that the policy adjustment was made to ensure that at a time of limited resources, the most vulnerable young people continued to be supported. This would mimic the very early days of youth work when activities predominantly took place in very poor communities. The dichotomous nature of youth work emerges, whether it is a top-down, State agenda driven, verses grassroots, and youth led.

This trend was only heightened when the New Labour government came to power in 1997. The emphasis at this time appeared to be on dealing with social exclusion and focusing on services for youth rather than a youth service (Jeffs & Smith, 2001). This period of time saw a clear increase in public discussions around the need to create more cohesive services (Smith, 2013). The youth service began to observe much more managerialism. Youth work became noticeably more targeted and required 'measurable outcomes' (De St Croix, 2018). In order to illustrate this, key influencing documents at this time included Resourcing Excellent Youth Services (DfES, 2002) and Every Child Matters (DfES, 2003).

Interestingly, at the same time, Smith (2013) found that 21% of churches in England employed a full-time youth worker. This fact made churches the largest employer of youth workers in 1998. These both illustrate the connection with the historical significance that religious groups played in the development of youth work alongside the continuing importance placed on youth work within faith communities. This is despite the Office of National Statistics (ONS) reporting of an overall decline in religion in the UK (Sherwood, 2021). Supporting young people in community spaces has been maintained as a critical part of the support services from religious communities in England ever since the eighteenth century.

Around the time of the late twentieth century, the countries that make up the UK had begun to significantly diverge (Davies, 2008). When devolution occurred, whereby some legislative powers were passed over to Scotland, Wales, and Northern Ireland, policy and structural differences became more apparent. For example, Wales moved to recognize the importance of gaining a youth work qualification alongside being paid appropriately in recognition of that skillset (ETS Wales, 2020). However, this has not been implemented across the UK. As a result, the focus for the remainder of this work, particularly in relation to GYW, largely focuses on England.

Possible Ramifications Beyond England

There are some beliefs that these early beginnings of youth work may have influenced the models and approaches adopted elsewhere in the world. Certainly, the UK State's dominant perspectives on what constitutes good youth work may have manifested itself through international infrastructure organizations. De St Croix (2018) argues that 'the phrase of good youth workers is associated with evidence of impact, value for money and improved outcomes' (p. 427). Certain apparatus, such as UK International Voluntary Sector Organisations and International Aid Organisations may well have perpetuated UK-centric ideas regarding what should be constituted as good youth work. The domination of measurable outcomes is largely aligned with the spread of influence of the neoliberal system which dominates the world. Consequently, it is understandable that many organizations, State and voluntary sectors alike, may have endured and even promoted an impact-based approach to youth work. This would be especially the case when the ability to access funding is reliant upon the measurable impact agenda.

As government departments, funding agencies, and private philanthropists throughout the world become more outcome-focussed, it is having a significant influence on youth work practice (De St Croix, 2018, p. 415).

It would be beneficial for youth work in England to look to other countries for the practices and language required to adequately explain youth work. In Scotland, youth work is often incorporated into the term of community work. In Europe, the language of youth work tends to be more focussed on 'social pedagogy'. De St Croix (2018) suggests that the European term 'open youth work' is useful as it emphasizes an open admissions policy, open-ended engagement with young people in peer group settings, work that begins from the young people's starting points rather than from pre-defined outcomes and crucially that young people will be engaged with for as long as they choose to participate. This contrasts with "programmatic, time-limited, or evangelical youth projects" (de St Croix, 2018, p. 418). Davies (2008) argues that the entire history of the development of youth work in England has "formulated and refined an unfinished definition of a distinctive practice which we now call youth work" (Taylor, n.d.). This begins to elucidate the benefits of looking to models of youth work outside of England. More is discussed in the remainder of this chapter on the implications of the history of youth work on how youth work can be defined.

Contemporary Situation of Youth Work in England

The profound changes to the youth services in England in recent years may never be recovered from. The consequence of the measurable impact agenda is pervasive. Some stakeholders continue to value youth workers, such as Pupil Referral Units (PRUs), where young people that have been excluded from mainstream education are placed. However, the job title of youth worker and its associated pay scales usually related to JNC recognition are diminishing (Smith, 2013). The decline of youth work in State-sponsored services in England was accelerated by austerity measures following the banking crisis of 2008 (Smith, 2013). De St Croix (2018) adds that "in the wake of the 2008 financial crash, youth work suffered disproportionately from cuts, redundancies, and service closures" (p. 419). According to a recent report from the YMCA (2022), £1.1 billion has been cut from the youth services funding over the past ten years in England. The remaining support for young people is often carried out by voluntary sector organizations that are competing for limited available funds. Capacity for voluntary sector organizations is often diminished as they try to meet the needs of young people left wanting after so many closures of youth services. Following cuts to youth services around 2010, many youth work providers tried to adjust their activities to meet the dominant policy demands of the time, such as counter extremism. Overwhelmingly, this was done because of a desire to secure core funding for their organizations.

Unfortunately, the utilization of commissioning has weakened local community providers and favored larger organizations with bid-making infrastructure. According to Davies (2008), "well into the twentieth century youth work in the UK lacked a coherent national policy framework" (p. 15). With the impact of the global Covid-19 pandemic, young people have been hugely affected. Furthermore, "the attainment gap has widened for disadvantaged children" (Education Endowment Foundation, 2021). Additionally, it has been evidenced that young people's mental and physical wellbeing issues have considerably increased (The Lancet, 2021, cited in National Youth Sector Advisory Board, 2022). The dominant social, economic, and environmental issues that existed pre-pandemic have continued through the pandemic and throughout the recovery initiatives. In England, the cost-of-living and energy crisis appear set to marginalize many more people whilst continuing with an increasingly worsening disparity between the rich and the poor (The Guardian, 2022). A key concern questions whether the current predicament that youth work finds itself in in England is equipped to support young people in facing these challenges into the future.

Consequences of an Impact Obsessed Agenda

"Within less than a decade, youth work had moved from qualitative practice-centered forms of evaluation to a system of externally imposed targets" (De St Croix, 2018, p. 419). Performance targets were introduced by the New Labour government (1997–2010) which normalized systems of measurement and monitoring that had previously been unusual in youth work. This then enabled further quantitative based developments under the Coalition government from 2010 to 2015 and the Conservative government (2015 to present). During this time, getting paid for numbers has become increasingly normalized in youth work (De St Croix, 2018).

Policymakers, managers, and some youth workers have welcomed the move toward more quantitative and measurable outcomes because they view them as helpful in increasing the youth sector's accountability and driving up quality. Anecdotally, many youth workers working directly with individuals and communities, found the new measurement regime to be deeply alienating (Davies, 2008; De St Croix, 2018). The National Youth Agency (NYA) stated in their summary of a national census of the youth sector that "measures of economic value are not necessarily compatible with or reflective of social value" (NYA, 2021, p. 3). Despite this, in the Ten-Year Strategy for the youth sector, the National Youth Sector Advisory Board (2022) suggested that future youth services need to provide "demonstrable difference to young people's lives and life chances" (p. 2).

The youth impact agenda has been actively supported by successive UK governments throughout its development but not explicitly imposed through legislation or compulsory performance targets. This is the argument made by De St Croix (2018) who refers to this phenomenon as an example of policy 'steering at a distance' where they suggest that it is a key technique of neoliberal governments. In addition, the widely promoted 'theory of change' has also been criticized for reinforcing deficit and individualized views of young people, whilst obscuring structural inequalities (De St Croix, 2018). Arguably, all facets of life for populations in England have been economized. Historically, the core thrust of youth services in England was to help the very communities negatively affected by the structural inequalities that were generated through neoliberalism. Very often the key groups 'losing' are young people from disadvantaged communities. There is limited evidence to suggest that mimicking these top-down systems of power will result in different outcomes especially for marginalized and disadvantaged young people (Evans et al., 2005).

Davies (2008) is not alone in raising concerns that youth work has been diluted to the point whereby in England it is not viewed as a profession within its own right but as a set of skills that can be attached to teams from more highly regarded professions, such as social work. Within this narrative, youth work has failed to meet both the requirements of the State as well as the needs of young people. However, this might not be surprising when the turbulent history of youth work is considered where competing perspectives have seemingly always fought to take ownership of youth work. For example, Christian rooted initiatives, class activists, social and political campaigners, and military proponents.

The exploration of the history of the roots of youth work creation in England helps elucidate why qualitative tools are better suited to youth work rather than an impact agenda because the focus on process and soft skills is more evident (De St Croix, 2018). Qualitative measurements have not been absent in youth work. Previously, qualitative tools were employed, such as reflective team meetings, peer reviews, and meaningful youth participatory activities. These approaches did not view young people as outcomes but began where and how those young people dictated. Recent publications by Doherty and De St Croix (2021) offer practical tools to youth workers to evidence their impact without an over emphasis of quantitative tools.

Defining Youth Work

There continues to be debate regarding the understanding and defining of youth work. Certainly, in England, youth work should be viewed as distinct from other related professions, such as teaching and social care. Youth work has its own accredited qualifications up to undergraduate and postgraduate degree levels. Currently, many youth workers are unqualified and the majority are unpaid volunteers (De St Croix, 2018). Recently there has been an array of reports regarding youth work in England such as from those organizations mentioned in the introduction. This could be a positive sign for the youth sector in England. Although, whilst national organizations are liaising closely with the current government, many local youth workers fear that this posturing will not benefit young people most in need or help them in their work.

Within the recent Ten-Year Strategy, the National Youth Sector Advisory Board (2022) has offered an enticing definition of youth work when they state that:

> Youth work is a mosaic of local uniformed and faith organizations, youth clubs, out-reach work with young people on the streets, youth councils, social action projects, youth services, and safe places to meet. It is a rich blend of statutory, voluntary, and community provision, reflective of local need, community initiative, and political commitment (p. 6).

This definition highlights the diverse approaches to meeting the needs of young people and importantly, that localized responses are critical.

It is positive in this discussion and framing of youth work in England that Davies (2008) has argued that "debate and revision are permanent features" (p. 2). Linked to this Davies (2008) continues that youth work is a social construct whose creation has to be understood in the context of the wider political, economic, and social conditions in which it is developed. This might be suggestive that the definition would then inevitably change over time. The exploration of youth work history in the UK represents a convincing case that the structural inequalities that affected young people at the inception of youth work are still very much having an effect on the young people of today. However, in relation to this Davies (2008) stated that "the one [definition of youth work] which is deeply rooted historically and widely embraced is not one which the most influential policymakers want to hear least of all implement" (p. 2). Although some proponents of the measurable impact agenda might suggest that this is the best iteration of youth work in order to ensure that the sector is sustained in the current economic and political climate. Despite this, Davies (2008) continues by adding that:

> Organic forms of learner participation and commitments to their [young people's] empowerment which make the currently fashionable UK versions look insipid and manipulative (p. 6).

Recently, spearheaded by the NYA, a Youth Work Curriculum was developed for England (NYA, 2020). Within this curriculum, it is argued that youth work involves "seemingly disparate and varied activities but linked by the goal of being there for young people on their journey to adulthood" (NYA, 2020). The NYA (2020) suggests that with the curriculum they have generated 'for the first time in a generation the building blocks and themes that underpin good quality youth work have been pulled together in a single document'. Importantly, and maybe echoing the assertions made by Davies (2008) regarding youth work as a social construct, the NYA states that the curriculum is a framework and therefore should avoid a set stasis that could be found with more formal syllables. However, the curriculum has not been without its dissenters. Ord (2022) states that the curriculum "does not fit with youth works focus on process over content, and that more flexible alternatives were possible" (p. 1).

A Department for Education (2011) document for consultation entitled 'An education for the 21st Century: A narrative for youth work today' was developed with youth sector partners in England and the then Minister for Children and Families, Tim Loughton. Within this collaborative literature on youth work, it states that:

> Youth work practice engages young people in meaningful personal and social development processes which are challenging, rewarding, and enjoyable. Youth workers facilitate the abilities of young people to think, act, change, create, and grow, making a difference to their own lives, those of their peers and communities (p. 3).

As emphasized previously, the interplay between direct demands placed on services by young people and communities can often distort with the powerful requirements made by the State and policy. The conflicting agendas create a complex environment to sift out the definition of youth work. It is this chapter's assertion that if the definition of youth work is to be in line with one of youth work's most indisputable principles, namely, to be youth led. Consequently, at times, youth work may operate in juxtaposition to what state and organizational leaders might desire. Even if they believe that they know best and operate with the best of intentions for young people. Youth work definitions are at the center of a quandary that asks if it is most beneficial to adjust to fit within dominant social norms or challenge them whilst endeavoring to create new forms.

Introducing Global Youth Work (GYW)

Global Youth Work (GYW) grew out of the principles and values that are purported throughout youth work history as well as more recently in the youth work curriculum which emphasizes the importance of global citizenship (NYA, 2020). GYW can be defined as:

> Informal education with young people aims to encourage a critical understanding of the links between personal, local, and global issues. It seeks young people's active participation in bringing about change toward greater equity and justice (DEA, 2009, p. 5).

The then CEO of the Development Education Association (DEA), Hetan Shah, remarked that:

> In order to meet the multiple challenges that we face as a society around sustainable development, community cohesion, and international development, we need to ensure that all young people are given opportunities to think critically about these issues and to take action on them" (Connect Challenge Change, 2010, p. 3).

Consequently, GYW seemingly offers the synthesis of youth work developments across history in England as well as providing an opportunity for a way forward. The future of youth work in England through a GYW lens provides a support mechanism for young people growing up in an increasingly complex and challenging world as well as example tools to be utilized by youth workers. Furthermore, if this GYW approach became international language and seeded international sharing, it could become a truly reciprocal and useful global approach to supporting young people worldwide.

'Connect' is the first phase of the GYW framework of Connect, Challenge, Change (3Cs). Within 'Connect' the youth worker gets to know the young people better as well as the group getting to know one another better. This is the trust building stage of the process that creates the building blocks for even more meaningful activities later on. 'Connect' begins to introduce various topics to the group and starts to scope which areas they are most interested in exploring further. 'Connect' ends with a group decision on what topic the group wants to focus on and explore as part of their continuing engagement. The decision-making process at this stage can rely on creative approaches to decision making, explore the processes of consensus and democratic decision-making.

Following this initial stage of 'Connect', the framework then moves into 'Challenge'. The Challenge stage is about generating a deeper exploration of the information regarding the topic chosen by the young people. 'Challenge' can involve taking young people outside of their comfort zone. The multiple perspectives that exist when discussing a topic are explored in 'Challenge'. This stage requires regular times checking in with the young people for how they are feeling and how this potentially new information or differing perspectives are impacting on them. As the 'Challenge' stage draws to a close the group is encouraged to review their learning journey, what has been learnt, what has resonated, and an overall position that they now take in relation to their chosen topic. This stage is particularly useful in generating awareness of valuing different viewpoints, how to respond positively to challenges as well as developing critical thinking skills.

The final stage of the 3Cs approach is 'Change'. Having selected a topic and explored it in depth the youth group usually have some ideas about what action they believe should be taken. This is a great time to introduce the idea of Personal, Local, National and Global change. The young people can be shown examples of actions that young people from across the world have taken in relation to these different levels of social change. It can be emphasized that any level of approach to change is valuable. Different people at varying stages in their life journeys might have varied capacities for action. As a group, within this 'Change' stage, the young people then decide what 'Change' they would like to create. This stage can be a fantastic opportunity to introduce SMART (Specific, Measurable, Achievable, Realistic and Time-Bound) objectives and planning skills. The group are encouraged to consider critical factors in their planning such as health and safety as well as budget.

The culmination of the 3Cs framework is the young people's chosen action. It can be positive for young people to gain recognition for their actions, for example, with a story in the local press. This can also help in challenging the sometimes biased and negative representations of young people. The beauty of the framework is that it is flexible and allows freedom to be adapted to the needs of the young people and the locales of where they are situated. The "Connect, Challenge, Change approach helps ensure quality in global youth work" (Connect, Challenge, Change, 2010, p. 14).

Returning to the historical development of the definition of youth work in England, it is important to highlight that young people's voluntary participation should remain central (Davies, 2008). This is echoed in the more recently developed youth work curriculum (NYA, 2020). The 3Cs framework within GYW is ultimately a process-orientated and practice-centred approach that has its roots in the earliest iterations of youth engagement. Whilst the process is open to monitoring and evaluation with clearly illustrated objectives and outcomes it is inherently a qualitative and youth-led process. This situates the 3Cs in contrast to impact obsessed agendas that trump qualitative measures of youth work (De St Croix, 2018). The 3Cs framework creates space for the youth work approach to harness youth-led and participatory ethos which is so valued by youth workers. It is entirely possible that this works alongside an impact-based approach which would have the potential to soothe those that require measurement as a core part of their viewpoint on accountability.

The Relevance of Global Youth Work to International Partnerships

Most importantly, the 3Cs approach provides a framework for youth workers to utilize in supporting young people *today*. Young people across the world are struggling to make sense of their worlds. Young people across the world are facing a multitude of challenges from topics such as climate change to economic inequality. Young people across the world want to act to help make the world a better place not just for them but for future generations (Children's Commissioner, 2021). Whilst formal education and social care services are, rightfully so, preoccupied with meeting the immediate needs of young people, youth work can help young people to be considered more holistically through topics such as their positionality, identity, and citizenship. Critically, the 3Cs approach can assist young people to have a critical understanding of the relationship between personal and structural processes whilst assisting them to feel empowered to decide how they can act in response to the issues that they experience. The 3Cs is an approach that can harness the development of youth work in England and provide a map for moving forward. However, this progression of youth work in England, particularly GYW, would hugely benefit from greater connectivity with international partners and ensuring that sharing of good practices emerges as opposed to another UK-centric export to the world.

Evidence provided in this chapter emphasizes that there have been "concomitant policy shifts which may threaten the nature and long-term survival of grassroots open youth work practice" (De St Croix, 2018, p. 414). This has certainly taken place within England but is arguably a global trend as the financial crisis had world-wide ramifications, neoliberalism has dominated international infrastructure such as the World Trade Organisation (WTO) and more recently Covid-19 has affected the majority of young people. The 'deficit-based tropes' (De St Croix, 2018; Muirhead, 2020; Smith, 2013) alongside impact obsessed funding strategies are likely to have a universal effect on young people. Current approaches to accountability tend to be managerial rather than democratic. They rely on surveillance, comparison, and routine administrative practices, which are likely to restrict and undermine the potential contribution of youth work in young people's lives (De St Croix, 2018). Those that purport to want to support young people, such as youth workers, need to think locally in terms of the young people they walk alongside but also consider the global partnerships that exist, share examples of good practice, and foster solidarity with young people everywhere. The GYW approach and 3Cs framework can be the tools to assist with this.

Exploring the history of the development of youth work in the UK is important. As the great Maya Angelou commented, "if you don't know where you've come from, you don't know where you're going" (GFTU, 2021). Many of the challenges that gave rise to youth work in England have sadly remained the same, such as poverty. Both wealth and income inequality in the UK are at a post-war high (Dorling, 2011). In 2016, the Office of National Statistics (ONS) calculated that the richest 10% of households hold 44% of all wealth whilst the poorest 50%, by contrast, own just 9% (The Equality Trust, 2019). Unfortunately, the economic inequality that blights the UK is also mirrored globally. Oxfam (2022) have emphasized that Covid-19 has accentuated inequality around the world. "Since the pandemic began, the wealth of the world's ten richest men has doubled yet the incomes of 99% of humanity are worse off" (Oxfam, 2022). Whilst the world has evolved, young people have continued to face unique challenges, such as increased social media use, climate change, and greater concerns over mental health and well-being (Children's Commissioner, 2021). England has a contentious history, but now holds a different status on the world stage. Relationships with international partners must be built on mutual aid and reciprocity to ensure that there are purposeful moves away from neo-colonialism and the dangerous elements of patriotism that divide rather than unite. Tangible actions should be made to move beyond prior colonial and post-colonial attitudes that put the UK on a pedestal, such as when Baden Powell, creator of the Scouts Movement stated, "we must all be bricks in the wall of that great edifice – the British Empire" (Davies, 2008, p. 12). Now is the time, and this is particularly possible through youth work, to humbly illustrate that England needs to learn from partners overseas.

Conclusion

Prior to the global financial crisis and the austerity measures that have been implemented in the UK since 2010, GYW was a respected and critical part of the mosaic that made up youth work. GYW, and with that the wider citizenship agenda, were working hard alongside young people to continue to support youth work as an essential tool. As a result of the financial crisis and the subsequent scrabble to survive, youth provisions have become fixated on illustrating their need and following State policy in terms of targeted themes. Consequently, the importance and benefit of a specific branch of youth work, GYW, has begun to fade.

There are still many passionate supporters of youth work, and this is evidenced from the amount of work that takes place, despite insurmountable barriers as well as the flurry of consultations and reports influencing national level debate. It is essential to not lose sight of the crucial role that youth work plays for young people. Harnessing GYW approaches ensures that essential elements of a definition of youth work such as being young person led, process based, reflective, and critical thinking remain central. Furthermore, embracing a GYW approach equips young people today with the skills to navigate an increasingly complex world and challenge the array of issues that they witness. Additionally, the international partnerships developed around this topic bring the youthful populations across the world together on the topics that they are universally concerned about.

The approach of GYW is rooted in good youth work, adaptable, and effective in a diverse range of settings. This chapter has produced an argument that suggests that the UK must engage much more with youth work. Furthermore, this chapter suggests that the UK should proactively enter a process of learning about youth work from other countries. GYW would be an effective tool for the UK to utilize in reinstating the importance of youth work. Through increased reciprocity and global partnership working, youth work should grow to the benefit of all.

References

BBC News. (2022, July 29). Commonwealth: Seven things you might not know. *BBC News*. https://www.bbc.co.uk/news/uk-43715079

Children's Commissioner. (2021). *The big ask: The big answer*. The Children's Commissioner for England. https://www.childrenscommissioner.gov.uk/the-big-answer/

Commonwealth Secretariat. (2017). *Youth work in the commonwealth. A growth profession*. The Commonwealth. https://production-new-commonwealth-files.s3.eu-west-2.amazonaws.com/migrated/events/documents/YouthWorkintheCW_9781849291736.pdf

Davies, B. (2008). *Defined by History: Youth work in the UK*. https://pjp-eu.coe.int/documents/42128013/47261821/Davies.pdf/1d30eca5-3d68-427c-a87d-f8de81d43966

Davies, B. (2013). Youth work in a changing policy landscape: The view from England? *Youth and Policy, 110*, 6–32. https://www.youthandpolicy.org/wp-content/uploads/2017/06/yandp110.pdf

DEA. (2009). *Global youth work in the UK: Research report*. Development Education Association. https://think-global.org.uk/wp-content/uploads/dea/documents/GYW%20Research%20Report%20May09.pdf

DEA. (2010). *Connect challenge change: A practical guide to global youth work*. Retrieved July 23, 2022, from https://think-global.org.uk/resource/connect-challenge-change-a-practical-guide-to-global-youth-work/

Department for Education. (2011). *An education for the 21st century: A narrative for youth work today*. Development Education Association. https://assets.publishing.service.gov.uk/government/uploads/system/uploads/attachment_data/file/210380/a-narrative-for-youth-work-today.pdf

DfES. (2002). *Transforming youth work: Resourcing excellent youth services*. The Department for Education and Skills. DfES/Connexions.

DfES. (2003). *Every child matters*. Department for Education and Skills. https://assets.publishing.service.gov.uk/government/uploads/system/uploads/attachment_data/file/272064/5860.pdf

De St Croix, T. (2018). Youth work, performativity and the new youth impact agenda: Getting paid for numbers? *Journal of Education Policy, 33*(3), 414–438. https://doi.org/10.1080/02680939.2017.1372637

Doherty and de St Croix. (2021). *Valuing youth work—Research-informed practical resources for youth workers: Reflecting on the value and evaluation of youth work*. Kings College London. https://www.kcl.ac.uk/ecs/assets/rethinking-impact/valuing-youth-work-research-informed-practical-resources-for-youth-workers.pdf

Dorling, D. (2011). Underclass, overclass, ruling class, supernova class. In A. Walker, A. Sinfield, & C. Walker (Eds.), *Fighting poverty, inequality and injustice* (chap. 8). Policy Press.

Education Endowment Foundation. (2021). *Closing the attainment gap*. The Education Endowment Foundation. https://educationendowmentfoundation.org.uk/support-for-schools/bitesize-support/closing-the-attainment-gap

ETS Wales. (2020) *Professional youth worker endorsement guidelines*. Employment Training Standards Wales. https://www.etswales.org.uk/resource/ETS-Endorsement-Guidelines-Final-150520.pdf

Evans, B., Richmond, T., & Shields, J. (2005). Structuring neoliberal governance: The nonprofit sector, emerging new modes of control and the marketisation of service delivery. *Policy and Society, 24*(1), 73–97. https://doi.org/10.1016/S1449-4035(05)70050-3

GFTU. (2021). *Celebrating GFTU's 120 years supporting the labour movement*. General Federation of Trade Unions. https://gftu.org.uk/120-years-of-gftu/

Jeffs, T., & Smith, M. K. (2001). Social exclusion, joined-up thinking and individualization—new labour's connexions strategy. The encyclopaedia of pedagogy and informal education. In *Defence of youth work*. http://www.infed.org/personaladvisers/connexions_strategy.htm

Legane, R. (2018). Knife crime: The state and society is killing our young people. *Huffington Post*. https://www.huffingtonpost.co.uk/entry/knife-crime-the-state-and-society-is-killing-our-young_uk_5a6dd8a7e4b0290826014ae8

Muirhead, A. (2020). The Albemarle Report, 1960: A story of its full transcription 60 years later. *Youth and Policy*. https://www.youthandpolicy.org/articles/the-albemarle-report-1960/
National Occupational Standards. (2008). *National occupational standards for youth work*. Lifelong Learning UK. http://www.youthworkessentials.org/media/2859/national_occupational_standards_for_youth_work.pdf
National Youth Sector Advisory Board. (2022). *Ten year strategy*. National Youth Agency. https://www.nya.org.uk/wp-content/uploads/10-Year-Strategy-v5.i.pdf
Nicholls, C. (2011). Fifty years on: Lessons from the Albemarle Report. *Children and Young People Now*. https://www.cypnow.co.uk/opinion/article/fifty-years-on-lessons-from-the-albemarle-report
NYA. (2020). *NYA national youth work curriculum* [Video]. National Youth Agency. https://www.nya.org.uk/quality/curriculum/
NYA. (2021). *Initial summary of findings from the national youth sector census. First Report: November 2021*. National Youth Agency. file:///C:/Users/User/Desktop/Ruth/Writing/Youth%20Dev%20Chapter/Chapter%20Reading/Summary-Report-v5.pdf
NYA. (n.d.). *What does the joint negotiating committee do?* National Youth Agency. https://www.nya.org.uk/youth-work/jnc/
Ord, J. (2022). The national youth work curriculum: A process-based curriculum? *Youth and Policy*. https://www.youthandpolicy.org/articles/the-national-youth-work-curriculum/
Oxfam. (2022). *Inequality kills: The unparalleled action needed to combat unprecedented inequality in the wake of COVID-19*. Oxfam. https://policy-practice.oxfam.org/resources/inequality-kills-the-unparalleled-action-needed-to-combat-unprecedented-inequal-621341/
Richmond, P. (2008). A level playing field. In L. Firth (Ed.) *A classless society?* Independence (pp. 1–2).
Scouts. (2023). How scouting grew. https://www.scouts.org.uk/about-us/our-history/
Sherwood, H. (2021, March 20). Less than half of Britons expected to tick 'Christian' in UK census. *The Guardian*. https://www.theguardian.com/uk-news/2021/mar/20/less-that-half-of-britons-expected-to-tick-christian-in-uk-census
Smith, M. K. (2013). What is youth work? Exploring the history, theory and practice of work with young people. In *Defence of youth work*. https://infed.org/mobi/what-is-youth-work-exploring-the-history-theory-and-practice-of-work-with-young-people/
Smith, M. K. (2019). Ragged schools and the development of youth work and informal education. In *Defence of youth work*. https://infed.org/ragged-schools-and-the-development-of-youth-work-and-informal-education/
Taylor, T. (n.d.). Defined by History: Youth work in the UK. In *Defence of youth work*. https://indefenceofyouthwork.com/2010/10/12/defined-by-history-youth-work-in-the-uk/
The Equality Trust. (2019). *The scale of economic inequality in the UK*. The Equality Trust. https://equalitytrust.org.uk/scale-economic-inequality-uk#:~:text=GB%20Wealth%20Inequality&text=In%202016%2C%20the%20ONS%20calculated,and%202013%2C%20reaching%209%25
The Guardian. (2022, July 20). Young people in the UK: How is the cost-of-living crisis affecting you? *The Guardian*. https://www.theguardian.com/society/2022/jul/20/young-people-in-the-uk-how-is-the-cost-of-living-crisis-affecting-you
UK Youth. (2020). *UK youth movement*. UK Youth. https://impact.ukyouth.org/2020/uk-youth-movement/
UK Youth. (2021). *The impact of Covid-19 on England's youth organisations*. UK Youth. https://www.ukyouth.org/wp-content/uploads/2021/02/UK-Youth-Fund-Report_1.pdf
UNISON. (2016). *Millions axed from youth service spending, says UNISON* https://www.unison.org.uk/news/press-release/2016/08/millions-axed-from-youth-service-spending-says-unison/
Wonder Foundation. (n.d.). *How to prevent burnout in youth workers. Building a better future for women and girls*. https://wonderfoundation.org.uk/how-to-prevent-burnout-in-youth-workers/

World Association of Girl Guides and Girl Scouts. (n.d.). *Our History*. https://www.wagggs.org/en/about-us/our-history/#:~:text=In%201909%2C%20a%20group%20of,of%20girls%20and%20young%20women

YMCA. (2020). *History and heritage*. https://www.ymca.org.uk/about/history-heritage

YMCA. (2022). *Devalued: A decade of cuts to youth services*. https://www.ymca.org.uk/wp-content/uploads/2022/02/ymca-devalued-2022.pdf

Ruth Richardson is a Ph.D. student in the College of Business, Law and Social Sciences at the University of Derby in England. Their research topic takes a mixed methods approach to explore young people's relationship to the social category of class whilst considering the increasing economic inequality experienced in the United Kingdom (UK). Alongside these studies, Ruth also works as a lecturer in the College of Health and Social Care at the University of Derby. Their own academic background spans exploration, training and project work in Human Rights, Citizenship, Global Youth Work and Community Cohesion. Ruth has supported field trips to the Gambia, Senegal, Tanzania, and the United Nations in Geneva as well as working for over two years on projects addressing Child Rights in Mongolia. Previously Ruth worked as a Youth and Community worker for Local Authority based services alongside charitable organizations particularly in relation to Global Youth Work. Ruth was herself engaged in Voluntary Service Overseas (VSO) and later delivered training for British young people volunteering overseas through the International Citizenship Service (ICS). Currently, Ruth's work takes a particular interest in identity formation and the reliance on creating an 'other' to understand who we believe ourselves to be.

Chapter 6
Sport in Physical Education for Bullying, Harassment and Violence Prevention

Shane Pill and Phillip T. Slee

Abstract Well-designed sport programs provide the environment for leadership development, personal development, and community development. Research suggests these well-designed programs can positively affect self-esteem and self-worth (Hillyer in Women's softball in Iran: an autoethnographic journey. PhD thesis, University of Tennessee, 2010). Participation in youth sports programs with a development focus beyond technical and tactical game skill development, such as programs provided by a youth development focus, can address various social and emotional needs of adolescents: including having a sense of belonging, a sense of mastery, a sense of 'mattering', and reframing self and adult perceptions from the deficit 'being a problem' to agents that can make a difference in their social worlds (Agnew and Pill in Sport J, 2016; LeMenestrel and Perkins, in Special Issue: Sports-Based Youth Development 115:13–25, 2007). Historically and ideologically, there would appear to be strong support for the role of team games in promoting socio-moral development (Theodoulides and Armour in Eur Phys Educ Rev 7:5–23, 2001). Youth development through sport is a mechanism through which to promote peace and harmony (Mandigo et al. in Positive youth development through sport, Routledge, pp 110–121, 2008). While youth sport programs as avenues for positive youth development have been well considered (see Fraser-Thomas et al. 2005), the deliberate use of sport in Physical Education for bullying, harassment, and violence prevention is an area where little theorizing or program trialing has occurred. This lack of research exists despite physical activity opportunities generally, and sport in physical education as an area of physical activity provision, long being identified as an effective medium for the development of social harmony, inclusion, and resilience (Bailey in Educ Rev 57:71–90, 2005; Martinek and Hellison in Quest 49:34–49, 1997). In this chapter, the main objective is to highlight a strengths-based perspective on the role sport can play in promoting young people's wellbeing, particularly in terms of reducing bullying and promoting positive social relationships.

Keywords Sport · Physical education · Bullying · Harassment · Violence · Prevention

S. Pill · P. T. Slee (✉)
Flinders University, Adelaide, SA, Australia
e-mail: phillip.slee@flinders.edu.au

S. Deb and S. Deb (eds.), *Handbook of Youth Development*,
https://doi.org/10.1007/978-981-99-4969-4_6

Sport for Youth Development

Globally, sport continues to be one of the most popular activities among youth. When designed and enacted with specific intent, it is associated with a variety of physical, mental, and social benefits. Sport participation can be a context for the development of valued competencies, such as self-esteem, associated with a range of socially valued positive developmental outcomes (Jones et al., 2017). Positive youth development is a popular lens applied to sport for development research and practice (Jones et al., 2020). Holt et al. (2017) suggested that positive youth development is ideally a strength-based conception of development that positions youth as individuals with resources to be cultivated and developed, rather than positioning youth as 'problems to be solved'. An important objective of this chapter is to highlight a strengths-based perspective using sport as a medium for promoting harmony and wellbeing and addressing interpersonal violence including that of bullying and harassment.

Sport-specific approaches to positive youth development often focus on building 'life skills' and/or 'leadership'. Life skills are the physical, social, emotional, and cognitive skills that assist a person to succeed with the demands of 'everyday life' (Hodge & Danish, 1999). They can be "behavioral (communicating effectively with peers and adults) or cognitive (making effective decisions); interpersonal (being assertive) or intrapersonal (setting goals)" (Danish et al., 2004, p. 40). Examples of these programs include:

- *Youth Leadership in Sport and Phy sical Education* (Hellison & Martinek, 2009): A sport-based leadership program.
- *Hokowhitu Program* (Heke, 2001): A sport-based program to teach life skills such as decision-making, time management, task-related discipline, and goal setting, the program was developed by New Zealand Maori to use Maori language and culture in program development, implementation, and evaluation.
- *Sports United to Promote Education and Recreation* (SUPER; Danish, 2002): A community sport intervention with workshops taught like sport clinics with sport-specific skill development alongside or integrated with life skills development workshops.
- *The First Tee* (Petlichkoff, 2004): A program to introduce golf and the values of the game while at the same time exposing participants to life skills designed to enhance the ability to set goals and self-evaluate progress.
- *Play It Smart* (Petitpas et al., 2004, 2005): A framework for planning psycho-social development in youth sport programs.
- *Going for the Goal* (GOAL) (Danish, 1997; Goudas et al., 2006): A program to teach adolescents personal control and confidence about their future to enable them to make better decisions and become better citizens.
- *Captain's Leadership Development program* (Gould, 2008). A program to teach potential school sport captains' leadership and communication skills.

Danish et al. (2005) suggested that secondary school sport contexts may be appropriate for teaching youth life skills in addition to sport game and athletic skills. The appropriateness is predicated on an assumption that learning to play sport and learning life skills are similar (Danish et al., 2002) in that both skill sets are acquired through demonstration, modeling, and practice (Danish & Hale, 1981). Further, it is assumed that there is some overlap in the type of skills needed for success in sport and in other community settings, like the workplace (e.g., goal setting, problem-solving, persistence, resilience, and performance under pressure), creating the potential for transfer (Danish & Nellon, 1997). However, it cannot be assumed that participating in sport 'naturally' or 'automatically' leads to youth development of physical, social, emotional, and cognitive skills (Trudell & Bernard, 2013). The experience of sport may facilitate positive youth development when planned and enacted with this goal in mind (Papacharisis et al., 2005). An essential element of life skill and/or leadership skill development in or through sport is that the skills developed in the program can be transferred from the sport context to non-sport contexts (Knudsen et al., 2020). However, typically, there is little direct teaching of life skills in youth sport settings, including secondary school physical education (Danish et al., 2004; Holt et al., 2008).

Sport for Development in Physical Education

Sport is recognized globally as a focus area of Physical Education, providing content and key contexts for teaching and learning (Lopez et al., 2009). In connection with school Physical Education, sport has been described as pivotal (Green, 2000), integral (Bailey & Kirk, 2009), and legitimating the existence of Physical Education (Laker, 2003). Sport in Physical Education provides many youths a point of connection between what is learned in school and a social practice they value beyond the school gate (Drummond & Pill, 2011). As a focus area of school Physical Education, sport in Physical Education is distinguished from community and school sport provision by having an educative purpose—explicit student learning (Pill, 2012, Australian Curriculum, 2022a). Student learning in Physical Education includes outcomes across the domains of learning; psychomotor, cognitive, and affective domains (Hansen, 2008). In the Australian context in which the author's work, Arnold's (1979, 1988) knowledge base for developing the physically educated person encompasses the three domains of learning. The knowledge bases are:

- Education in movement to develop movement competency for participation objectives;
- Education about movement for theoretical and factual understanding; and
- Education through movement to achieve objectives other than movement, such as personal and social skill development.

Pill (2012) adapted Arnold's work to develop the concept of Sport Literacy as the functional use of sport knowledge. Sport literacy provided two themes for sport teaching in Physical Education: (1) Sport in Physical Education can enhance students' access to practices and ideas enabling them to positively contribute to society; and (2) Sport helps students understand self and the society in which they live (Pill, 2015).

Within the concept of Sport Literacy, education through sport included the intentional use of sport for personal, social, and community health outcomes. An example of a school program used this way was Pill et al. (2009) use of sport education as a model for boys' personal and social development. This program developed from a need to address bullying and a denial of play space and opportunities by older students to younger students at recess and lunch. This intervention comprised multi-year level interaction to develop friendship and respect across year levels. The program resulted in a reduction of referral of students during recess and lunch to the deputy principal by the teachers on duty.

Life Skills Development in Physical Education

Physical Education is an ideal context for youth development through sport. In a context like the Australian curriculum applicable to where the authors work, Physical Education is coupled with Health Education in the Learning Area, Health and Physical Education (HPE). This means there is both the opportunity and imperative where possible to integrate the objectives of the two subjects of the Learning Area for student learning of movement and physical activity ability together with the learning of personal, social, and community health knowledge, skills, and understandings (ACARA, 2022a).

Studies have demonstrated how Physical Education can be planned and enacted purposefully to develop students' life skills (e.g., Ennis, 1999; Goudas et al., 2006; Hastie & Buchanan, 2000; Holt et al., 2012). A recent overview of the existing literature on 6- to 18-year-olds personal and social development within the context of Physical Education and sports found that many consider the social character of Physical Education and sports an appropriate means of developing personal and social skills, such as personal and social responsibility, cooperation, and other prosocial skills. Most of the studies in this area report a positive relationship between participation in Physical Education or sports and a range of personal and social skills. The teacher and coach are integral in structuring the curriculum and pedagogical environment from which positive outcomes and the transfer of skills can be achieved (Opstoel et al., 2020).

In summary,

> Youth sports programs that promote psycho-social development are those that use sports as a vehicle to provide experiences that promote self-discovery and teach participants life skills in an intentional and systematic manner. In addition, these programs have clearly defined goals and strategies to enhance the generalizability and transfer of life skills to other important life domains (Petitpas et al., 2005, p. 66)

Sport for Development and Peace

The use of sport to address social issues related to human justice and equality through explicit peace and development objectives is referred to as Sport for Development and Peace. Non-sport-based activities attached to or integrated with sport activities deal with social issues such as gender equality, peace building and conflict resolution, social inclusion, crime and violence, racism, social inequality, and health education (Cárdenas, 2013).

There is limited scholarly or empirical literature discussing sport for development and peace in Physical Education. One such program was developed by Ennis and colleagues (1999). Ennis and colleagues developed and trialed a Sport for Peace program in an urban high school. The program was derived from the Sport Education model but enhanced and emphasized the responsibility concept attached to team roles and persisting team affiliation of the Sport Education model. Additional emphasis on conflict negotiation and care and concern for others was added. The Sport for Peace curriculum intentionally reflected the characteristics of peace education with goals and curricular structures specifically focused on promoting nonviolent behavior, a sense of community, and student ownership or empowerment. The results suggested that the Sport for Peace program fostered shared responsibility for learning, trust, respect, and a sense of family (Ennis et al., 1999).

Sport for Development and P.E.A.C.E (Preparation, Education, Action, Coping and Evaluation) in Physical Education: The deliberate use of sport in Physical Education for Bullying, Harassment, and Violence Prevention).

Bullying in schools is an international problem. It is widely regarded as a recognizable and destructive form of aggression, with harmful physical, social, and emotional outcomes for bullies, victims, and bystanders. The Preparation, Education, Action, Coping, and Evaluation (P.E.A.C.E.) the program was developed to address the problem of bullying in Australian Schools (Slee, 1996; Slee & Mohyla, 2007). The name of the program represents the order of the stages in the process for initiating, conducting, and evaluating a program for reducing school bullying (Slee & Mohyla, 2007).

Theoretically, the P.E.A.C.E. program draws on principles of systems thinking. School bullying is seen as nested within relationships and understood in terms of social constructivist thought. In broad terms, this means interventions may involve 'first-order' change whereby individuals caught in the bully–victim cycle may need to acquire some new skills, and 'second-order' change whereby the system itself begins to change. For example, school relationships, roles and interactions, and communication change meaning attitudes, perceptions, and beliefs, and the approach to the issue of bullying change (Slee & Mohyla, 2007). Interventions in primary and secondary schools in Australia, Japan, and Italy using the P.E.A.C.E. Pack showed the program to be effective in reducing the level of school bullying (Guarini et al., 2020; Slee, 1994, 1996, 2017; Slee & Mohyla, 2007; Slee & Taki, 1998). Since 2001, evaluations of the P.E.A.C.E. Pack have been made in primary and secondary schools in Australia (over 100 schools), and translated and implemented in Japan, Malta, Greece, and Italy. The evaluations have involved pre and post testing and longitudinal studies across 1–3 years. Over 15,000 students and their teachers have been involved in the evaluations. Typically, there are significant reductions in self-reported victimization (17–33%), reductions in bullying of other students (5–10%), increases in coping skills, feelings of safety at school, school belonging, and benefits to the reported wellbeing of students (see, Slee, 2017, for details).

In Australia, emphasizing the extent of the problem of school bullying, an Alanna and Madeline Foundation report by Price Waterhouse Corporation (PWC: 2018) indicated that 25% of school students, or an estimated 910,000 children, experience bullying at some stage during their time at school. The costs associated with bullying incurred while children are at school and the lingering effects for 20 years after school completion were estimated at $2.3 billion. The costs include medical and psychological treatment for associated effects such as depression and anxiety and costs associated with non-completion of schooling.

Most anti-bullying programs are conducted in the school context, with many of the programs relying on external professionals to the school to deliver the programs as an intervention. However, the central role of teachers in addressing bullying has been highlighted internationally, though in the extant literature, there are few teacher-led interventions reported (Guarini et al., 2020). The limited research to date suggests that Physical Education programs purposefully designed to focus on bullying and/or violence prevention have the potential to be effective for the promotion of attitudes and behaviors that decrease instances of violence and bullying (Benítez-Sillero et al., 2021). The International Year of Sport and Physical Education Final Report (United Nations, 2006) identified physical education as a way to establish the foundations of a more peaceful society. We propose that sport in Physical Education programs provides an ideal 'vehicle' to foster positive youth development, which can in turn lead to the ultimate goal of peace education. However, as we have explained so far, the deliberate use of sport in Physical Education for bullying, harassment, and violence prevention is an area where little theorizing or program trialing has occurred.

We therefore propose the P.E.A.C.E Pack as a sport for the development and peace curriculum for Health and Physical Education (HPE: Fig. 6.1).

The rationale for HPE is that:

> students develop personal and social skills through interacting with others in classroom and movement contexts. They use health and physical activity resources to enhance their own and others' wellbeing. Health and Physical Education addresses factors that influence the health, safety, relationships, wellbeing, and physical activity patterns of individuals, groups, and communities. Students develop the understanding to challenge discrimination, assumptions, and stereotypes. They gain skills to take positive action regarding diversity, inclusion, consent, and respect in different social contexts (Australian Curriculum, 2022a)

Included in the aims for students is that they "develop and use personal, social and cognitive skills and strategies to promote self-identity and wellbeing, and to build and manage respectful relationships" (Australian Curriculum, 2022a). Table 6.1 provides the Australian Curriculum links for the Sport for P.E.A.C.E in secondary school Physical Education programs.

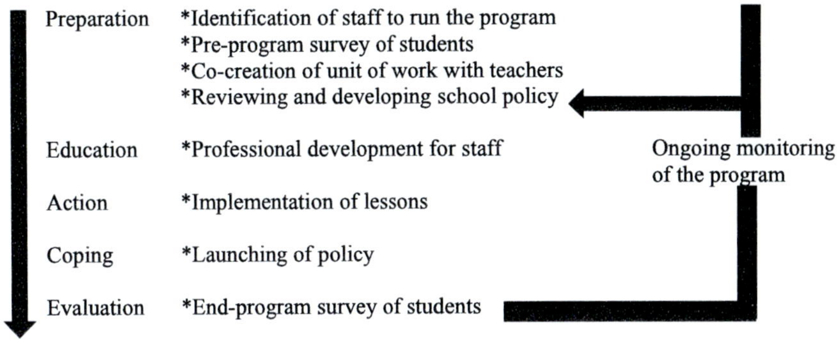

Fig. 6.1 Sport for P.E.A.C.E in Physical Education (adapted from Slee & Mohyla, 2007)

Table 6.1 The Australian Curriculum HPE Version 9 (Australian Curriculum, 2022b) curriculum links to the sport for P.E.A.C.E in physical education program

Movement and physical activity strand	Personal, social, and community health strand
Learning through movement sub-strand Year 7–8 Standard	**Interacting with other's sub-strand Year 7–8 Standard**
Practice and apply leadership, collaboration, and group decision-making processes when participating in a range of physical activities	Examine the roles of respect, empathy, power, and coercion in developing respectful relationships
	Analyse factors that influence emotional responses and devise strategies to self-manage emotions
Learning through movement sub-strand Year 9–10 Standard	**Interacting with others sub-strand Year 9–10 Standard**
Demonstrate fair play and reflect on how ethical behavior can influence physical activity outcomes for individuals and groups	Evaluate the influence of respect, empathy, power, and coercion on establishing and maintaining respectful relationships
Devise, implement, and refine strategies for decision-making when working in groups or teams that demonstrate leadership and collaboration skills	Evaluate emotional responses in different situations to refine strategies for managing emotions

Each HPE lesson comprises a significant element of social and emotional learning. Social and Emotional Learning (SEL) highlights the role of resilient and inclusive classrooms which provide new opportunities for group membership and creation of effective learning environments. In facilitating inclusion, it is important that all class members as well as their teachers develop the skills to understand one another, and to communicate and work together effectively. Social emotional learning (SEL) is aimed at developing these skills and is generally defined as a process by which individuals learn to understand and manage their own feelings, understand and empathize with the feelings of others, communicate, resolve conflicts effectively, respect others, and develop healthy relationships. These skills are important to all children, both children with special/complex needs and to those without, in terms of overall social development, perceptions of belonging, and promotion of overall mental wellness, as well as mitigation of the development of mental illness. Five competencies that are generally agreed to be core to Social & Emotional Learning (SEL) are included in the lessons. The lessons seek to develop in children the skills that promote:

- **Self-awareness**—accurately assessing one's feelings, interests, values, and strengths; maintaining a well-grounded sense of self confidence;
- **Self-management**—regulating one's emotions to handle stress, control impulses, and persevere in overcoming obstacles; goals; expressing emotions appropriately;
- **Social awareness**—being able to take the perspective of and empathize with others; recognizing and appreciating individual and group similarities and differences; recognizing and using family, school, and community resources; walking in someone else's shoes;
- **Relationship skills**—establishing and maintaining healthy and rewarding relationships based on cooperation; resisting inappropriate social pressure; preventing, managing, and resolving interpersonal conflict; seeking help when needed; developing and maintaining friendships; and
- **Responsible decision-making**—making decisions based on consideration of ethical standards, safety concerns, appropriate social norms, respect for others, and contributing to the well-being of one's school and community; making decisions based on what is right and wrong as well as in consideration of others.

The school HPE lessons focus on factors which research shows are significantly associated with positive relationships and well-being. The topics include friendship, resilience, self-concept, optimism, conflict management, and positive relationships. As described earlier Pill (2012) adapted Arnold's work to develop the concept of Sport Literacy as the functional use of sport knowledge. Education through sport includes the intentional use of sport for personal, social, and community health outcomes. The revised draft program (Table 6.1) is based on the pilot research of Pill et al. (2009) which utilized sport education as a model for student's personal and social development.

Conclusion

In this chapter, we have shown that there is a history of youth development in sport programs for the development of life skills. Mostly, these programs have run as interventions in community settings or school physical education. We argue that to make youth sport development programs sustainable and scale-able is possible by shifting program design from interventions to Physical Education curriculum providing for teachers what to teach, how to teach it, and how to assess if the students are at standard. A significant development of the revised draft program is the incorporation of key elements of Social and Emotional Learning as a significant part of the HPE lessons delivered by teachers in the school setting as part of the school curriculum.

References

Agnew, D. & Pill, S. (2016). "I think it's going to save lives." Sport administrator perspectives on youth development through sport. *The Sport Journal.* http://thesportjournal.org/article/i-think-its-going-to-save-lives-sport-administrator-perspectives-on-youth-development-through-sport/

Arnold, P. J. (1979). *Meaning in movement, sport, and physical education.* Heinemann.

Arnold, P. J. (1988). Education, movement, and the rationality of practical knowledge. *Quest, 40*(2), 115–125.

Australian Curriculum. (2022a). *Understand this learning area: Health and physical education.* ACARA. https://v9.australiancurriculum.edu.au/teacher-resources/understand-this-learning-area/health-and-physical-education

Australian Curriculum. (2022b). *Health and physical education.* ACARA. https://v9.australiancurriculum.edu.au/f-10-curriculum/learning-areas/health-and-physical-education/year-7_year-8_year-9_year-10?view=quick&detailed-content-descriptions=0&hide-ccp=0&hide-gc=0&side-by-side=1&strands-start-index=0&subjects-start-index=0

Bailey, R. (2005). Evaluating the relationship between physical education, sport and social inclusion. *Educational Review, 57*(1), 71–90.

Bailey, R., & Kirk, D. (2009). Introduction. In R. Bailey & D. Kirk (Eds.), *The Routledge physical education reader* (pp. 1–6). Routledge.

Benítez-Sillero, J. D., Corredor-Corredor, D., Córdoba-Alcaide, F., & Calmaestra, J. (2021). Intervention programme to prevent bullying in adolescents in physical education classes (PREBULLPE): A quasi-experimental study. *Physical Education and Sport Pedagogy, 26*(1), 36–50.

Cárdenas, A. (2013). Peace building through sport? An introduction to sport for development and peace. *Journal of Conflictology, 4*(1), 4.

Danish, S. J. (2002). *SUPER (Sports United to Promote Education and Recreation) program leader manual* (3rd ed.). Life Skills Center.

Danish, S. J. (1997). Going for the goal: A life skills program for adolescents. In G. Albee & T. Gullota (Eds.), *Primary prevention works* (pp. 291–312). Sage.

Danish, S. J., & Hale, B. D. (1981). Toward an understanding of the practice of sport psychology. *Journal of Sport Psychology, 3*, 90–99.

Danish, S. J., & Nellon, V. C. (1997). New roles for sport psychologists: Teaching life skills through sport to at-risk youth. *Quest, 49*(1), 100–113.

Danish, S. J., Fazio, R. J., Nellen, V. C., & Owens, S. S. (2002). Teaching life skills through sport: Community based programs to enhance adolescent development. In J. L. van Raalte & B. W. Brewer (Eds.), *Exploring sport and exercise psychology* (pp. 269–288). American Psychological Association.

Danish, S., Forneris, T., Hodge, K., & Heke, I. (2004). Enhancing youth development through sport. *World Leisure Journal, 46*(3), 38–49.

Danish, S. J., Forneris, T., & Wallace, I. (2005). Sport-based life skills programming in the schools. *Journal of Applied School Psychology, 21*(2), 41–62.

Drummond, M., & Pill, S. (2011). The role of physical education in promoting sport participation in school and beyond. In S. Georgakis & K. Russell (Eds.), *Youth sport in Australia* (pp. 171–184). Sydney University Press.

Ennis, C. D. (1999). Creating a culturally relevant curriculum for disengaged girls. *Sport, Education and Society, 4*(1), 31–49.

Ennis, C. D., Solmon, M. A., Satina, B., Loftus, S. J., Mensch, J., & McCauley, M. T. (1999). Creating a sense of family in urban schools using the "Sport for Peace" curriculum. *Research Quarterly for Exercise and Sport, 70*(3), 273–285.

García López, L. M., Contreras Jordán, O. R., Penney, D., & Chandler, T. (2009). The role of transfer in games teaching: Implications for the development of the sports curriculum. *European Physical Education Review, 15*(1), 47–63.

Goudas, M., Dermitzaki, I., Leondari, A., & Danish, S. (2006). The effectiveness of teaching a life skills program in a physical education context. *European Journal of Psychology of Education, 21*(4), 429–438.

Gould, D. (2008). *Becoming an effective team captain.* Michigan State University.

Green, K. (2000). Exploring the everyday 'philosophies' of physical education teachers from a sociological perspective. *Sport, Education and Society, 5*(2), 109–129.

Guarini, A., Menabò, L., Menin, D., Mameli, C., Skrzypiec, G., Slee, P., & Brighi, A. (2020). The P.E.A.C.E. Pack Program in Italian High Schools: An Intervention for Victims of Bullying. *International Journal of Environmental Research and Public Health, 17*(14), 5162.

Hansen, K. (2008). Teaching within all three domains to maximize student learning. *Strategies, 21*(6), 9–13.

Hastie, P. A., & Buchanan, A. M. (2000). Teaching responsibility through sport education: Prospects of a coalition. *Research Quarterly for Exercise and Sport, 71*(1), 25–35.

Heke, I. (2001). *The Hokowhitu Program: Designing a sporting intervention to address alcohol and substance abuse in adolescent Maori.* Unpublished doctoral thesis, University of Otago, Dunedin, New Zealand.

Hellison, D., & Martinek, T. (2009). *Youth leadership in sport and physical education.* Springer.

Hillyer, S. (2010). *Women's softball in Iran: An autoethnographic journey.* PhD thesis, University of Tennessee.

Hodge, K., & Danish, S. J. (1999). Promoting life skills for adolescent males through sport. In A. Horne & M. Kiselica (Eds.), *Handbook of counselling boys and adolescent males* (pp. 55–71). Sage.

Holt, N. L., Tink, L. N., Mandigo, J. L., & Fox, K. R. (2008). Do youth learn life skills through their involvement in high school sport? A case study. *Canadian Journal of Education/Revue canadienne de l'éducation, 31*(2), 281–304.

Holt, N. L., Sehn, Z. L., Spence, J. C., Newton, A. S., & Ball, G. D. (2012). Physical education and sport programs at an inner city school: Exploring possibilities for positive youth development. *Physical Education & Sport Pedagogy, 17*(1), 97–113.

Holt, N. L., Neely, K. C., Slater, L. G., Camiré, M., Côté, J., Fraser-Thomas, J., MacDonald, D., Strachan, L., & Tamminen, K. A. (2017). A grounded theory of positive youth development through sport based on results from a qualitative meta-study. *International Review of Sport and Exercise Psychology, 10*(1), 1–49.

Jones, G. J., Edwards, M. B., Bocarro, J. N., Bunds, K. S., & Smith, J. W. (2017). An integrative review of sport-based youth development literature. *Sport in Society, 20*(1), 161–179.

Jones, G. J., Edwards, M. B., Bocarro, J. N., Svensson, P. G., & Misener, K. (2020). A community capacity building approach to sport-based youth development. *Sport Management Review, 23*(4), 563–575.

Knudsen, J., Elkrog-Hansen, L., & Christiansen, L. (2020). Life skills through school sport: A participatory teacher development program. *Advances in Physical Education, 10*, 293–310.

Laker, A. (2003). The future of physical education: Is this the 'new pedagogy'? In A. Laker (Ed.), *The future of physical education: Building a new pedagogy* (pp. 153–170). Routledge.

LeMenestrel, S., & Perkins, D. F. (2007). An overview of how sports, out-of-school time, and youth well-being can and do intersect. *New Directions for Student Leadership, Special Issue: Sports-Based Youth Development, 115*, 13–25.

Mandigo, J., Corlett, J., & Anderson, A. (2008). Using quality physical education to promote positive youth development in a developing nation: Striving for peace education. In N. Holt (Ed.), *Positive youth development through sport* (pp. 110–121). Routledge.

Martinek, T. J., & Hellison, D. (1997). Fostering resiliency in underserved youth through physical activity. *Quest, 49*(1), 34–49.

Martinek, T., & Hellsion, D. (2009). *Youth leadership in sport and physical education.* Palgrave Macmillan.

Opstoel, K., Chapelle, L., Prins, F. J., De Meester, A., Haerens, L., van Tartwijk, J., & De Martelaer, K. (2020). Personal and social development in physical education and sports: A review study. *European Physical Education Review, 26*(4), 797–813.

Petitpas, A. J., Van Raalte, J. L., Cornelius, A., & Presbrey, J. (2004). A life skills development program for high school student-athletes. *The Journal of Primary Prevention, 24*, 325–334.

Petitpas, A. J., Cornelius, A. E., Van Raalte, J. L., & Jones, T. (2005). A framework for planning youth sport programs that foster psychosocial development. *The Sport Psychologist, 19*(1), 63–80.

Papacharisis, V., Goudas, M., Danish, S. J., & Theodorakis, J. (2005). The effectiveness of teaching a life skills program in a sport context. *Journal of Applied Sport Psychology, 17*, 247–254.

Petlichkoff, L. M. (2004). Self-regulation skills for children and adolescents. In M. R. Weiss (Ed.), *Developmental sport and exercise psychology* (pp. 273–292). Fitness Information Technology.

Pill, S. (2012). *Rethinking sport teaching in physical education.* PhD thesis. University of Tasmania.

Pill, S. (2014). Sport literacy: Providing PE teachers a "principled position" for sport teaching in PE and a process through which to frame that teaching according to situated contextual needs. *The Global Journal of Health and Physical Education Pedagogy, 3*(1), 47–68.

Pill, S. (2015). Valuing learning in, through, and about sport-physical education and the development of sport literacy. In H. Askell-Williams (Ed.), *Transforming the future of learning with educational research* (pp. 20–35). IGI Global.

Pill, S., Sluggett, S. & Priest, T. (2009). Sport education as a curriculum model for boys' personal and social development. In T. F. Cuddihy & E. Brymer (Eds.), *Edited proceedings of the 26th ACHPER international conference*, 7–10 July, Queensland University of Technology.

Slee, P. T. (1994) I'm a victim—stop bullying. In K. Oxenberry, K. Rigby, & P. T. Slee (Eds.), *Conference proceedings: Children's peer relations—cooperation and conflict*, 19–22 January. University of South Australia, Adelaide.

Slee, P. T. (1996). The PEACE Pack: A programme for reducing bullying in our schools. *Journal of Psychologists and Counsellors in Schools, 6*(S1), 63–70.

Slee, P. & Taki, M. (1998). The PEACE Pack: evaluations of interventions to reduce school bullying in Japan. In *Paper presented at the ISSBD conference*, 15–19 August. Berne, Switzerland.

Slee, P. T., & Mohyla, J. (2007). The PEACE Pack: An evaluation of interventions to reduce bullying in four Australian primary schools. *Educational Research, 49*(2), 103–114.

Slee, P. T. (2017). *School bullying*. Routledge.

Theodoulides, A., & Armour, K. M. (2001). Personal, social and moral development through team games: Some critical questions. *European Physical Education Review, 7*(1), 5–23.

Trudell, P., & Bernard, D. (2013). A case study of a high school sport program designed to teach athletes life skills and values. *The Sport Psychologist, 2013*, 188–200.

United Nations. (2006). *Sport for a better world: Report on the international year of sport and physical education, 2005.* United Nations. https://www.un.org/sport/sites/www.un.org.sport/files/ckfiles/files/Electronic_Version_IYSPE_book.pdf

Dr. Shane Pill is an Associate Professor: Physical Education and Sport, at Flinders University, Kaurna Yerta (commonly referred to as Adelaide, SA). He researches and teaches in curriculum pedagogy, educational leadership and sport. Shane is a Life Member and Fellow of the Australian Council for Health, Physical Education and Recreation for his services to physical education and sport. He remains an active sports coach. Prior to working at Flinders university, Shane was a Health, Physical Education and Science teacher in secondary schools for eighteen years. For more information about Shane and his work see https://www.flinders.edu.au/people/shane.pill.

Prof. Philip T. Slee is in human development in the College of Education, Psychology and Social Work at Flinders University of SA. He is a trained teacher and registered psychologist. He has published in the fields of child development, bullying, school violence, and well-being.

He has extensive research and statistical analysis skills including multi-level modeling and qualitative data analysis. He has a particular interest in the practical and policy implications of his research. He has presented his work nationally and internationally in workshops and lectures. His research teams have undertaken national consultancies and evaluated the Kids Matter Primary mental health initiative http://caef.flinders.edu.au/kidsmatter/ and the Kids Matter Early Childhood mental health initiative. He is also the Director of the Flinders Centre for "Student Well-being and Prevention of Violence" (SWAPv) (https://www.flinders.edu.au/student-wellbeing-prevention-violence). His international research projects have involved the countries of India, Japan, Korea, China, Canada, England, Malta, Chile, and the USA. His website is http://www.caper.com.au.

Chapter 7
Involvement in Sports and Exercise Behavior: Developing a New Culture for Youth

Anjali Gireesan and Sibnath Deb

Abstract Sports and exercise behavior are dynamic fields that have multiple positive consequences for different age groups. The Youth of a nation have a two-way relationship with sports and exercise behavior. They derive benefits from it as well as contribute to it to make sports one of the strong pillars of the nation. In this chapter, the characteristic of the present youth population has been elaborated. Then, the reasons because of which the youth may be inactive in this field have been discussed. Categorization of sports indulgence and the changes associated with it are deliberated on and how these may be effectively used to change the perception and participation of youth towards sports have been discussed. The chapter concludes with recommendations that are required to be brought into focus to understand the emphasis being laid upon sports and Exercise behavior.

Keywords Youth · Sports culture · Exercise · Health behavior · Intervention · Change

Introduction

The Youth today are a dynamic group of individuals who are a powerhouse of potential and can use their strengths to benefit themselves and the nation at large simultaneously. In order to bring out this potential, they need to be active and realize this potential. Sports and exercise behavior is one of the ways that can channelize their energy positively and make them more self-actualized.

A. Gireesan
Defence Research and Development Organisation (DRDO), Ministry of Defence, Government of India, New Delhi, India

S. Deb (✉)
Department of Applied Psychology, Pondicherry University (A Central University), Puducherry, India
e-mail: sibnath23@gmail.com

S. Deb and S. Deb (eds.), *Handbook of Youth Development*,
https://doi.org/10.1007/978-981-99-4969-4_7

Characteristic of Youth Today

The youth is an interesting developmental age category that has fascinated many research groups and it has been studied from various perspectives. The age group being considered in this chapter fundamentally forms part of two developmental stages in Psychology. These are Adolescence and Young adulthood. In Erickson's stages of psychosocial development, two major conflicts characterize this age group: (1) Identity versus role confusion and Intimacy versus isolation. Though this theory has undergone many studies and changes, its basic principles still hold true today as the theory is itself around the major change that takes place in each of the developmental stages. The stages correspond to two opposing psychological tendencies the resolution of which leads to a positive outcome (virtue). These are the strengths of our Ego. Contrarily, in case the resolution is incomplete, it results in a negative outcome (maldevelopment). In the age groups being considered for this chapter, the virtues are fidelity and love. Fidelity refers to one's firm confidence in the self-constructed moral and belief system even though the environment may present contradiction to the same. It emphasizes that one has achieved a stable identity, to which one present a strong sense of belongingness, in the society. Development of fidelity is a significant contributor in positive youth development and makes them well-adjusted and active members of their society (Brittian & Lerner, 2013). Fidelity makes one sure about self. On the other hand, Love, makes us seek out positive relationships in our social surroundings. Both of these Ego strengths strive to maintain better intrapersonal as well as interpersonal relationships of the youth. Both these developments take place in the mesh of socio-ecological factors surrounding the individual. Thus, the individual has multiple dynamic relationships to regulate (Table 7.1; Fig. 7.1).

There have been a lot of changes over the past many years in terms of physical, psychological, social, and ecological processes that surround an individual. These

Table 7.1 Erickson's stages of psychosocial development

Sl. No	Developmental period	Psychological tendencies	Virtue	Maldevelopment
1	Infancy	Trust versus mistrust	Hope	Withdrawal
2	Early childhood	Autonomy versus shame, doubt	Will	Compulsion
3	Play age	Initiative versus guilt	Purpose	Inhibition
4	School age	Industry versus inferiority	Competence	Inertia
5	Adolescence	Identity versus identity confusion	Fidelity	Repudiation
6	Young adulthood	Intimacy versus isolation	Love	Distanitation
7	Adulthood	Generativity versus stagnation/Self-absorption	Care	Rejectivity
8	Old age	Integrity versus despair	Wisdom	Disdain

Source Orenstein and Lewis (2021)

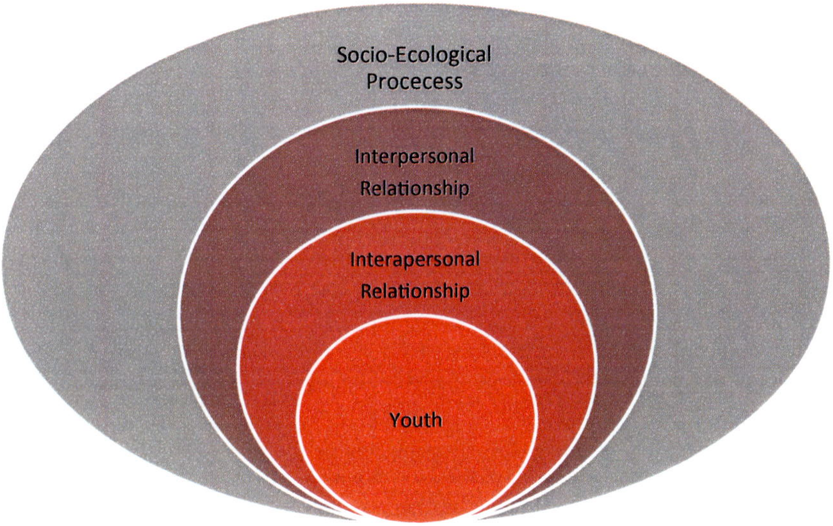

Fig. 7.1 Ego strength development during the youth

changes need to be ascertained from time to time so that the nature and needs of different populations may be effectively considered and worked upon. As a part of the report published by the Committee on Improving the Health, Safety, and Well-Being of Young Adults (Bonnie et al. 2015), some key findings have been deliberated on as the characteristics of youth today. These are as follows:

- **Major Developmental Milestone**: Youth has been viewed as a major developmental milestone as a lot of changes take place in this age group. There are physical alterations (visible as well as invisible), brain maturation, psychological adjustments with transition between multiple roles, and handling of some amount of independence that is very restricted in childhood. The degree of independence varies from culture to culture (Individualistic and Collectivistic) as well as family dynamics (dominant parenting styles). While physical changes pave the way for an adult-like appearance, different parts in the brain areas mature to handle the surroundings better. There are developments observed in the prefrontal areas (executive functions) as developments commensurate to a more controlled limbic system (emotional regulation and reward-seeking behavior). It is important to come in terms with all the changes that are happening simultaneously for the youth.
- **Unpredictability**: Youth today are less predictable than the previous generations. In earlier times, resources were limited and accessibility to different opportunities varied from place to place. More often than not, the path of the life cycle was more fixed and unidirectional. It flowed from completing education to a constructive job to a stable marriage to family management and then reaching old adulthood and relaxation. But this dynamic has shifted now. It's not necessary to follow these

steps in a routine manner. One can attain an education up to higher secondary, then do a job, and then when felt needed, can come back to education again. There are also many members of this population who choose other dyadic forms of co-existence rather than marriage. Having children and finding intimacy in the family has also gone down. In a way, the psychological milestones of youth like fidelity and love last for a longer period of time as compared to the milestones of the later age groups. Thus, it is difficult to ascertain the developmental trajectory that they are going to adopt.

- **Bridging Role**: The youth adopts characteristics of both the previous and the present generation. It comes as a part of the role transitions that are required to be fulfilled by them. For example, a youth who has recently taken up a job as a teacher has so many different sets of populations to interact with. He has to manage his parents and the principal (previous generation) as well as his peers (present generation) and children (Future generation). Compared to him, others have a more limited population subset to interact with. Hence, they need to be prepared to act as a bridge between the different generations.
- **Unhealthy Life Patterns**: There has been a trend of deteriorating health in the youth of today. This majorly branches off from the unhealthy life patterns being followed. As they transition from one role to another and their need to be accepted in all social groups, compromises more often than not happen in the health sector. The eating patterns are not fixed. Focus is on ease and availability rather than proper nutrition, which leads to problems of both malnutrition and obesity. Risk behaviors like drinking and smoking are adopted more easily because of new independence as well as the norms of the group that these individuals are a part of. Work schedules are erratic. As the hormones accompanying the changes are not channelized in an effective manner, they are more prone to many mental health issues as well as lifestyle disorders.

Looking at all of the above characteristics, the need of the hour is that the youth take responsibility for their well-being in all sectors of life and become active members of the society. A focused approach is needed to fulfill all the major tasks at hand. This makes it imperative that the youth today are in control of both their physical as well as mental resources so that they are equipped to take on the different kinds of challenges in front of them.

Inactive Youth

Inactivity in youth is a cause of great concern. It predisposes them toward various issues. Apart from having a direct effect on physical health, the mental health of these individuals is also in jeopardy. For example, lower levels of physical activity pave the way for higher risk of developing anxiety and depression (Denche-Zamorano et al., 2022). Inactivity also promotes adoption of unhealthy and risky practices like the use of tobacco (Monga et al., 2018). There are many reasons because of which we have observed that the youth is participating and contributing less towards sports. Some of the major reasons are as follows:

- **Use of Digital Resources**: The advent of the digital world has come with a lot of positive consequences. It has made many types of resources available as well as more easily accessible. The resources include social (Facebook, Twitter, Whatsapp, Linkedin, etc.), economical (digital payments and saving applications like Paytm, UPI, GROW, etc.), educational and physical amenities that are now available on all types of digital devices. Although these have made life better and were highly beneficial, especially during the COVID pandemic, their negative consequences cannot be ignored. Our brain has been programmed to choose the resources that make our survival easy as well as viable. A balance is required in the use of such resources. While online classes, fitness applications, and social media facilitated life during the pandemic, the same are the reasons that now youth are finding it difficult to leave their comfort zone and become productive again in the physical world.
- **Pediatric Inactivity Triad**: The pediatric inactivity triad is a relatively new concept and attempts to understand the reasons for inactivity stemming from three interrelated components (Faigenbaum et al., 2020). These components are: (1) Exercise Deficit Disorder; (2) Pediatric Dynapenia; and (3) Physical Illiteracy. Exercise deficit Disorder refers to a condition where more and more youth are engaging in lesser physical activities on a daily basis. Here the standard taken is that of Moderate to vigorous Physical Activity (MVPA) levels of less than 60 min. It has been observed across many studies that activity level below this standard has long term negative outcomes for children and youth. Pediatric Dynapenia is a condition characterized by lower muscular strength in an individual without any apparent organic basis for the same. This imposes limitations on the individuals to engage in physical activity and exercise on a long term basis as they get tired easily. Physical illiteracy majorly points at psychological factors of one's self belief, awareness, and motivation to engage and excel in a sport or exercise program. A stimulating environment and consequent opportunities are necessary for the children and youth to realize their competencies in this field. This promotes awareness and motivation devoid of which, there are less chances for the youth to participate in physical activity. All these components are surrounded by socio-ecological factors that facilitate or impede this process of engaging in physical activity. For example, the microsystem (inactive parents), mesosystem (inactive schools), and macrosystem (inactive communities) around the individual are important determinants of this triad.
- **Promotion of Sedentary Behaviors**: Technological advancements have also led to advancing of sedentary behaviors and lifestyles among the youth (Monteiro et al., 2019). Easy access to infrastructural resources is one of the many reasons that this behavior is promoted. For example, even for the shortest of the distances, today's youth will choose to use some mode of motor transport rather than choose walking or cycling. For managing household groceries and amenities, more often

than not, online mode of shopping is preferred where doorstep delivery is available. Even for the non-essentials, shopping offline for clothes, accessories, and house decorations during special occasions is discouraged. So, both fun and essential activities are managed and regulated with just a few clicks from home. The advent of pandemic has made the situation worse. Now, even the employed youth are adopting these behaviors because of the work-from-home paradigm of employment. It is important to become aware of engagement in such behaviors and reduce the incidences of inactivity.

- **Handling Performance Pressure**: Sports and exercise are generally highly competitive areas of interest for many individuals. Regardless of it being performed in isolation or in a group, it entails with it the pressure to perform. This is mainly because of the highly observable nature of these activities. Smallest of the discouragements and humiliations may hinder the performance and thus propel an individual to inactivity altogether. Moreover, interpersonal perfectionist pressures are high in sports. Fear of failure, once induced, increases the perception of pressure from multiple sources like parents and coaches and results in negative effects (Pineda-Espejal et al., 2019).
- **Increased Emphasis on Academics**: It is often observed that the youth today are compelled to excel in their academics in order to procure a good employment and make their place in the society. Parental expectations to perform in academics are high. At the same time, there is competition from the peers as well which is sometimes healthy and sometimes unhealthy. Apart from the regular academic work, they also have to perform well on entrance tests of different universities as well as common examinations like UGC-NET, CSIR, UPSC, and other related examinations. For these, they devote extra time to go for coaching in order to enhance their practice and knowledge. In such a scenario, sports and exercise are viewed as very low on priority because of paucity of time as well as the physical and mental exhaustion leading from engaging continuously in academics.
- **Perception of Sports and Exercise Behavior**: Sports and exercise behavior often receive an objective and passive appreciation from a distance. Unless it's an ingrained practice of an individual, there is a tendency to distance one from the same and appreciate that others are doing it. We often engage in rationalization and intellectualization when it comes to explaining to ourselves the reasons because of which one is not in exercise behavior. Also, if it's not being practiced in our environment, we do not feel the need to engage in it. That is because practicing a behavior that is not present in one's own social environment is perceived to make you lonely, which is not a desirable condition for many. For example, one is more likely to begin to go to the gym if there is expectation of some company rather than a total absence of it. Acceptance of such behaviors needs identification, awareness, and correction.

In view of the characteristics of the youth that we have discussed and the reasons because of which they are becoming relatively inactive in the society, it is necessary to introduce a change in the culture so that they become more active and leave their stand of passive participation in life alone. The following sections will explore the ways to identify and understand this process and an attempt will also be made to suggest interventions that might bring the positive behaviors into practice.

Health Behaviors and Sports Culture in the Youth

Sports or exercise behavior is not at the forefront for the youth today. It's mainly because of the commitments that they have in their daily lives. Even though there have been attempts to introduce the areas of sports and exercise behavior to them (For example, in the form of introduction of Physical education as a subject), it has not become a part of their schedule. Health behaviors also are planned behaviors that need to be consciously brought into practice. According to the Theory of Planned behavior, both healthy and unhealthy behaviors are governed by an individual's different psychological constructs. These include:

- **Belief**: This constitutes the cognitive schemas and repertoire that we have about a particular behavior and situation. In the theory of Planned Behavior, three types of beliefs have been considered- behavioral beliefs, normative beliefs, and control beliefs.
- **Intention**: This is the part that gives the motivational impetus to perform a behavior.
- **Behavior**: The actual constitutes the behavior paradigm of this model.

Let us consider two examples to understand this theory and maintenance of behaviors. For our discussion, we will take the case of three individuals- A, B, and C. Their process of running will be viewed across six different constructs of this theory (Table 7.2).

- *A runs regularly*
- *B runs occasionally and*
- *C does not run.*

In the above example, we observe certain processes that help three individuals maintain their behavior.

A. Continuously engaged in the behavior of running because his belief system, attitude, and perceptions are in the same direction. This translates into the intention to perform the behavior and thus we actually see the manifestation of the behavior in the form of running on a daily basis.
B. Occasionally engaged in running though has a favorable disposition towards running. In this individual, though the belief system is in place for running to take place, other factors are relatively weak. For example, not having a peer group that supports or participates in the activity may be a major concern to the individual because the person does not want to become lonely because of the practice of running. Along with that, the perception of having a difficult

Table 7.2 Comparison of individuals engaged in running as health behavior

	Attitude	Behavioral intention	Subjective norms	Social norms	Perceived power	Perceived behavioral control
A	(a) Views Running as a favorable behavior (b) Views it as having positive outcomes in daily life	Has strong motivation to perform the behavior on daily basis	Friends and family fully support and encourage practice of running	Is a part of running group, takes part in Marathons, and is a part of running groups on Social media as well	(a) Has made running a part of daily schedule (b) Has pre-decided route for running	Since running is a daily practice, it is perceived as a fun activity and can be performed happily
B	(a) Views Running as a favorable behavior (b) Views it as having positive outcomes from time to time	Has moderate motivation to perform the behavior on daily basis	Family supports the practice but does not have friends who support the practice	Runs individually and is not a part of any group that supports running as such	(a) Runs occasionally (b) Lives in a neighborhood where running is difficult	Running is an activity that is performed with moderate to great difficulty
C	(a) Views Running as an unfavorable behavior (b) Views it as having no outcomes of consequence for life	Has low motivation to perform the behavior on daily basis	Running is not relevant to family and friends also	Is not a part of group that supports or accepts running	Does not run	Running is viewed as an activity of severe difficulty which does not have much consequence in life

neighbourhood to run and running activity as such being moderate to great difficulty further weakens the intention to run. Hence, we observe that the B runs from time to time rather than regularly.

C. Does not engage in the behavior at all. For C also the belief system, attitude, and perceptions are in the same direction. But it is the opposite in nature as compared to A. Thus, C keeps maintaining the behavior of not indulging in running as a practice.

Thus, in order to understand the health behaviors of the individuals one has to look beyond the obvious and apparent reasons. There is a need to identify the area of reinforcement and accordingly, a program needs to be constituted if health behaviors are to be instilled in our youth. From this discussion, we arrive at the premise that categorization of sporting and exercise behavior is generally oversimplified. In the example described above, we observed the scenarios where attitude, belief system, and behavior are generally in the same direction. If this was always true, then we have three clearly distinct and understandable sporting attitude categories: (1) Very interested (2) Mildly Interested, and (3) Not interested (Fig. 7.2).

From the discussion that we had on the characteristics of the youth today, it is derived that youth today are dynamic and have changing needs. There is a lot of dynamism going on within each of them amongst the different psychological processes that finally manifest in behaviors of different forms. Hence assuming that

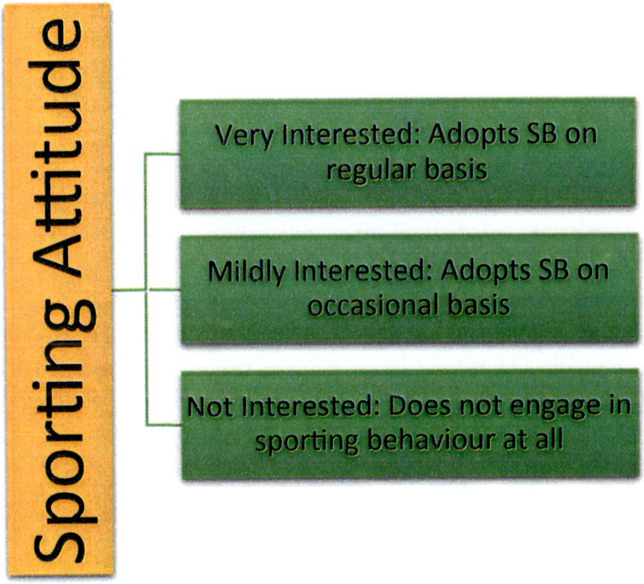

Fig. 7.2 Traditional categories of sporting attitude

the internal processes are consistent and homogenous may actually impede the effectiveness of the program being designed for them. Let us now look at another set of examples where attitude, belief system, and perceptions are not in a similar direction.

Though the behavior is same for A, B, and C in Table 7.3 as well, here we see some differences in their inherent attitude, behavior, and perceptions (beliefs).

A. Engages in running and has a strong motivation to pursue the same. Here we see that his control beliefs are not in tandem with his normative beliefs. But the control beliefs are strong enough to drive the favorable attitude and behavioral intent to run. Hence, the behavior is manifested strongly.
B. Engages in occasional running. Views running as a favorable but moderate to difficult activity and has low motivation to practice it. Since he does not have friends who support the behavior but on the other hand has power over resources that facilitate running, engages in the same. Also, is a part of social groups that support running. So maybe engaging in the same to reduce cognitive dissonance.
C. Does not practice running though has a favorable attitude towards the behavior. This is because of the perception of running being too difficult to be practiced by the individual, which affects the behavior though he feels like running (Intention) when he sees his favorite athletes perform during different championships.

All of the above individuals come in the interested and mildly interested categories of sporting attitude. They cannot be a part of the not interested in sports category just because of the incidence of the observable behavior. A more comprehensive way of looking at the sporting attitude would be by viewing the value and degree to which a particular sport or exercise behavior contributes to the life of an individual (Fig. 7.3).

Thus, in order to create a sports culture amongst youth and inculcate active behavior amongst them, one has to go beyond a generalized physical fitness initiative and programs aimed at masses based on overt data. A research base needs to be established and accordingly, an intervention plan needs to be implemented so that sports and youth can develop a two-way relationship so that both the sectors benefit from each other. Some of the key points while formulating such intervention strategies are as follows:

1. The characteristics of the young people need to be kept in mind while formulating the intervention strategies. For example, it has been discussed that the youth today have an unpredictable nature. Thus, any experience that is predictable, mundane, and cannot fit into their social environment will be received with reluctance and may not be considered important.
2. The Youth today are technologically oriented. Everything is available to them a click away. Hence, the programs have to be interactive and creative so that the youth do not get easily bored by the same. The experts delivering the intervention programs need to be trained in such a way that it becomes easy for the youth to identify with them.
3. The programs need to be designed in a way that does not add undue pressure on the youth to perform. They already are under their fair share of pressure because

Table 7.3 Comparison of individuals engaged in running as health behavior with attitude, behavior, and perceptions in different directions

	Attitude	Behavioral intention	Subjective norms	Social norms	Perceived power	Perceived behavioral control
A	(a) Views Running as a favorable behavior (b) Views it as having positive outcomes in daily life	Has strong motivation to perform the behavior on daily basis	Friends and family do not support and encourage practice of running	Runs individually and is not a part of any group that supports running as such	(a) Has made running a part of daily schedule (b) Lives in a neighbor-hood where running is difficult	Since running is a daily practice, it is perceived as a fun activity and can be performed happily
B	(a) Views Running as a favorable behavior (b) Views it as having positive outcomes from time to time	Has low motivation to perform the behavior on daily basis	Family supports the practice but does not have friends who support the practice	Is a part of running group, takes part in Marathons, and is a part of running groups on Social media as well	(a) Runs occasionally (b) Has pre-decided route for running	Running is an activity that is performed with moderate to great difficulty
C	(a) Views Running as a favorable behavior (b) Views it as having some positive outcomes	Has moderate motivation to perform the behavior on daily basis	Running is relevant to family and friends also but as passive participants	Is not a part of any specific group that supports or accepts running	(a) Does not run but watches and enjoys Athletics on television	Running is viewed as an activity of severe difficulty performed by only athletes and star performers

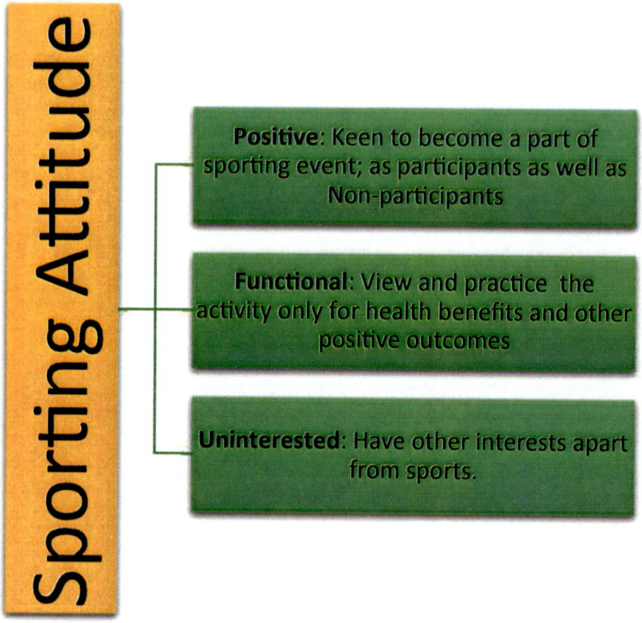

Fig. 7.3 Revised categories of sporting attitude. *Source* LSR27 Sport England—The challenge of growing youth participation in sport.pdf

of the other sectors of their life. The introduction of exercise behavior and sports should be seen as a channel to release this pressure rather than create space for more self-doubt.

4. Person and performance dimensions need to be considered while making intervention plans. These are represented in Table 7.4.
5. Changes in the behavior need to be checked on a periodic basis. Introduction of sports and exercise behavior is a lifestyle change that will require efforts from facilitators as well as the youth who are receiving it. This change will not happen over a short period of time if long term changes are needed to be observed. Hence, Impetus needs to be provided at every stage of change. We can attempt to understand the stages of change in the context of an intervention plan with an example. Though there are many models of change, here we are taking the Transtheoretical model of change (Prochaska & Vilicer, 1997) as the constructs are comprehensive and may aid in the formulation of a good intervention plan. This model consists of six stages of change, the processes with which change may be brought into force, and the decisional balance in which the individual assesses his own capabilities in view of the change. The six stages of change are: Precontemplation, Contemplation, Preparation, Action, Maintenance and Termination.

Table 7.4 Dimensions to be considered while formulating the intervention plan

S. No	Person dimensions	Performance dimensions
1	Physical capacity and endurance	Resources available for efficient training and practice
2	Status of mental health	Training schedule and ease of performing behavior on daily basis
3	Experience of psychological safety while engaging in the exercise behavior or sport	Management of performance pressure presence as well as absence of significant others
4	Physical precautions while engaging the exercise behavior or sport	Formulation of relevant goals and targets in discussion with experts as well as based on previous experience
5	Perseverance and Intrinsic motivation to pursue the activity	Conducive environment for practicing the sport or the exercise behavior

Let us take the example of bringing Yoga in Daily life of the Youth. In each stage, the process of change that may be applied is indicated in bold.

I. *Precontemplation*: Yoga is considered to be a slow exercise which does not give instant results to our fast moving youth. At this stage, they are still novices when it comes to practice of Yoga and are not considering making it a part of their own lives. The process of change that may be utilized here is **Conscious Raising**. Here a workshop may be organized to understand the barriers that may keep them from practicing Yoga in daily lives. Also, awareness about the myths and misconceptions associated with Yoga may be created. A sound database that provides information about which stage of change maximum of the youth may be obtained that will aid in propelling the intervention plan in the right direction. Also, this stage can be utilized to divide the participants of the program into Positive, Functional, and Uninterested categories. Each of them will spend different amounts of time in each stage of change and a different modality of the process of change may be required to facilitate transition through the different stages.

II. *Contemplation*: This is the stage where the intention to change is introduced. Left to own devices, the youth may take very long to come out of this stage. It may last up to six months. A combination of many techniques may be employed here to make the intent stronger and get them toward the next stage of change. For example, **Conscious raising**- make them aware about the apps that are available and promoting Yoga which is available at home itself (apps like Asana, Rebel, etc.), **Dramatic relief**- Providing them with explicit consequences of practicing yoga on daily basis like testimonies of popular celebrities and sadhgurus or make a reel of supporting Yoga in Instagram as well **self-revaluation** where they can be taught to visualize themselves as having practiced Yoga and envision the consequences of the same.

III. *Preparation*: In this stage, the youth are now prepared to take the action definitely. In this stage, they can be provided with multiple options of practicing different types of Yoga (**Self-liberation**). Difficulty level of each may be surmised and presented to them, so that they may choose the option that is most relevant to them.
IV. *Action*: This is the stage where the practice of Yoga should be physically monitored and regulated. Participants can be asked to keep a record of their practice through an application (For example, Strava, smart bands, etc.) or manually. They may be asked to put up lists or pictures of the goals that they want to achieve in their room (**Stimulus control**). In order to ensure that the behavior is intrinsically motivated, they can be asked to keep a diary of the changes that are taking place in their life because of the practice of yoga (**Contingency management**). They may be divided into groups where they will interact with group members periodically about their activity and then there can be inter-group discussion as well.
V. *Maintenance*: In this stage, the practice has become relatively more automatic, and less monitoring is required to ensure that the behavior is being implemented. The routine is streamlined and the practice of Yoga has been successfully introduced and implemented. This is a long lasting stage where the frequency of monitoring keeps reducing. A periodic check needs to be kept so that individuals do not get complacent. Along with a check on personal resources, a time-based **Environmental re-evaluation** is also necessary. Guidance may be provided when they are not able to practice the same because of new schedules and some changes in the environment.
VI. *Termination*: Termination of the program indicates that individuals have successfully implemented the change in their lifestyle and now are not in need of any external support or stimulation to practice the behavior. This stage indicates the efficacy of the program as well. Fig 7.4 indicates the summary of the steps explained.

Recommendations to Develop Culture of Sports and Exercise Behaviour

Implementation of a new program needs time and effort. Understanding the desirable behavior, its genesis, and being in the individual and its positive results is a systematic process. All of the above discussion puts emphasis on the point that in order to bring in a new culture of sports and exercise behavior, attention should be given to the process and not on the outcome (Fig. 7.5).

- Endeavor of the program and intervention should be to promote self-growth which gradually leads to healthy competition between equally equipped Youth. An integration of exercise behavior and positive sporting attitude into the self-concept of the individual is required to ensure the maintenance of behavior. This will make

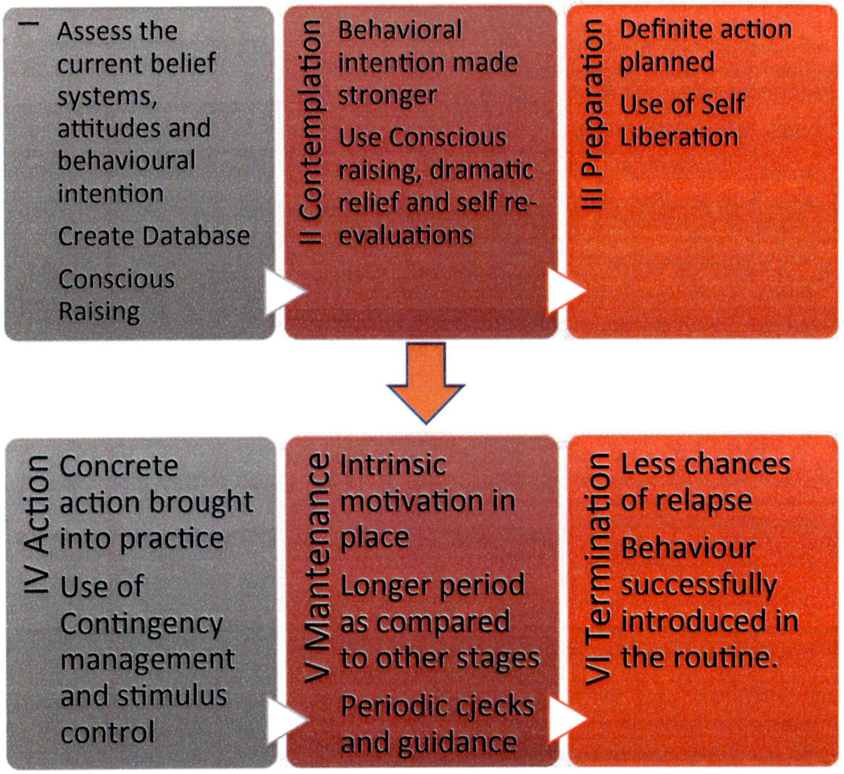

Fig. 7.4 Suggested modality of intervention plan for behavior change

Fig. 7.5 Bidirectional relationship of sports and exercise behavior and social networking

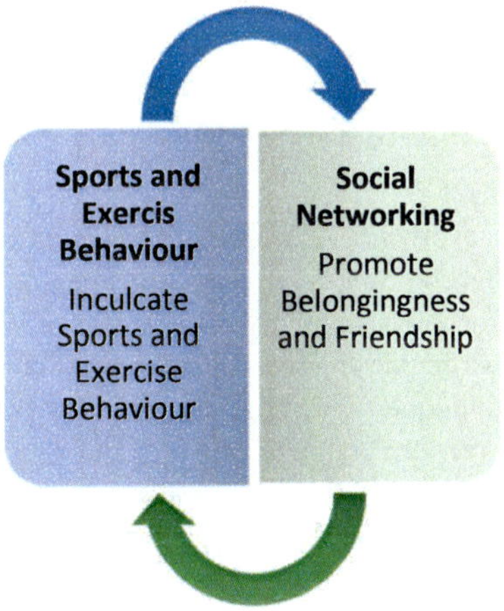

them more competent and willing to participate in sports at various levels with the capacity to handle performance pressure effectively.

- It is important to pave the way for natural growth in this area. There needs to be an opportunity for the youth to play and excel in the exercise behavior (For example, walking, running, cycling, gymnastics, etc.) and sports of their own choice. Mass popularity (both physically and digitally) may aid in this scenario. For example, a national campaign to promote the 'Fit India Movement' organized by the youth will give face validity to the endeavor and motivate more youth to pick up sports and exercise behavior.
- Reactivation of Indigenous sports and activities will help in easy adoption and maintenance of the sporting attitude and behavior. The physical disposition is a big part of ensuring participation in sports. Thus, indulging in activities that are a part of our collective unconscious will result in facilitating a positive sporting attitude and manifest in the form of behavior. Sports like Malkhamb, Kho-kho, and Kabaddi should be represented adequately and opportunities need to be created to play the same. Khelo India Youth Games (KIYG) is one such program that gives an opportunity to play such indigenous games at various levels and has given positive outcomes as well (Singh & Bali, 2020).
- Preparation of body and mind is necessary to inculcate a habit of exercise behavior and sporting attitude in daily life. Hence, it is important to ensure and promote self- awareness, mindful eating and nutrition, and appropriate physical literacy amongst the youth. The schedules should also be flexible in which variation may be permitted in frequency, duration, and intensity of the physical activity being adopted.
- Sports and exercise behavior will receive more value if they are embedded in the social context. Enhancing social networking through these will instill a sense of belongingness and friendship which in turn will reinforce the sports and exercise behavior.

Conclusion

Developing A culture of sports and exercise behavior amongst youth is a physical and psychological process. The change has to take place in multiple stages. Each stage is characterized by the developmental milestone the Youth is supposed to attain at a particular change, dynamic social environment, barriers to these developments, and a unique psychological process. Therefore, an intervention to change the existing practices requires changes not only at the physical level which includes policies, schemes, and opportunities but also at the interpersonal level. This should consider both person and performance dimensions in the appropriate context. A combined effort in all these areas can bring successful outcomes and make our youth more competent, healthy, and productive in various aspects of their lives.

References

Bonnie, R. J., Stroud, C., Breiner, H., Committee on Improving the Health, Safety, & National Research Council. (2015). Young adults in the 21st century. In *Investing in the health and well-being of young adults*. National Academies Press (US).

Brittian, A. S., & Lerner, R. M. (2013). Early influences and later outcomes associated with developmental trajectories of Eriksonian fidelity. *Developmental Psychology, 49*(4), 722.

Denche-Zamorano, Á., Franco-García, J. M., Carlos-Vivas, J., Mendoza-Muñoz, M., Pereira-Payo, D., Pastor-Cisneros, R., Merellano-Navarro, E., & Adsuar, J. C. (2022, January). Increased risks of mental disorders: Youth with inactive physical activity. *Healthcare, 10*(2), 237. MDPI. https://doi.org/10.1249/FIT.0000000000000584

Faigenbaum, A. D., MacDonald, J. P., Carvalho, C., Rebullido, T. (2020). RialACSM's. *Health & Fitness Journal, 24*(4), 10–17.

Monga, D., Goel, S., & Padhy, S. K. (2018). Level of physical activity and its relationship with tobacco use among youth: a cross-sectional survey in North India. *Indian Journal of Community Health, 30*(4).

Monteiro, D., Machado, S., Moutão, J., Bento, T., Vitorino, A., Alves, S., Rodrigues, F., Maciel de Lima, J. C., Teixeira, D., Murillo-Rodriguez, E., & Cid, L. (2019). Physical exercise and sedentary lifestyle: Health consequences. *Espiral. Cuadernos del profesorado, 12*(25), 75–88.

Orenstein, G. A., & Lewis, L. (2021). Eriksons stages of psychosocial development. In *StatPearls [Internet]*. StatPearls Publishing.

Pineda-Espejel, H. A., Morquecho-Sánchez, R., Fernández, R., & González-Hernández, J. (2019). Interpersonal perfectionism, fear of failure, and affects in sports. *Cuadernos de Psicología del Deporte, 19*(2), 113–123.

Prochask, J. O., & Velicer, W. F. (1997). Transtheoretical model of health behavior and changes. *American Journal of Health Promotion, 12*(1), 38–48.

Singh, G., & Bali, A. (2020). Play India youth games (Khelo India): Scheme for promotion of sports in India. *Website: www. ijpot. com, 14*(2), 261.

Dr. Anjali Gireesan from Pondicherry University (A Central University), has been working as Scientist 'C' in the capacity of a Psychologist in Selection Centre North, Jalandhar, Defence Research and Development Organization (DRDO), Ministry of Defence, Government of India. She has five years of full-time teaching and research experience. She has authored six original articles mainly in the area of student mental health and childhood disability. Also, she has authored book chapters in edited books published by SAGE, Routledge and Taylor and Francis. These include varied topics of importance ranging from Improving learning outcomes for students, Disability laws and their relevance, Counseling techniques useful for managing childhood trauma, importance of Sports in Youth Development and how the construct of belongingness has evolved over a period of time and its relevance in Psychology. She has also co-authored a Social Psychology textbook, titled "Social Psychology in Every Day Life" published by SAGE (2019). Her areas of research interest include child development, childhood disability, child abuse and neglect, and student's mental health.

Prof. Sibnath Deb is Professor of the Department of Applied Psychology, Pondicherry University (A Central University), Puducherry, India. Prior to that, Prof. Deb was serving the Rajiv Gandhi National Institute of Youth Development (An Institute of National Importance), Ministry of Youth Affairs and Sports, Government of India as Director for three and half years (January 8, 2020 to June 30, 2023). Professor Deb was also acting as Director (I/C), Directorate of Distance Education, and Dean (I/C), School of Law, Pondicherry University. He also taught at the University of Calcutta. In 1994, Professor Deb did an intensive course on 'HIV/AIDS and Qualitative Research' from the University of Western Australia. From April 2009 to August 2009, Professor

Deb visited the School of Public Health, Queensland University of Technology (QUT), Brisbane, Australia, as Visiting Faculty. Currently, he is also an Adjunct Professor at the School of Justice, QUT, Australia. During 2004–2008, he served the International Society for the Prevention of Child Abuse and Neglect (ISPCAN) as Council Member. In brief, he has 32 years of teaching, research and administrative experience and has produced 22 Ph.D.s in addition to publishing more than 100 research articles/book chapters in the leading national and international journals. Professor Deb has written nine books and edited 11 books. Some of his latest published books are (a) Child Safety, Welfare and Well-being: Issues and Challenges (2nd Edition, 2022, Springer Nature, Singapore); (b) School-based Family Counseling For Crisis and Disaster (Routledge, California, in press); (c) Health and Well-being: Challenges, Strategies and Future Trends (2022), Springer Nature, Singapore; (d) Youth Development in India: Future Generations in a Changing World (2021), New Delhi, Routledge. Professor Deb has received three national and three international awards in recognition of his contribution in the field of psychology including "Visitor's Award-2019" from the Hon'ble President of India Shri Ram Nath Kovind. His current areas of research interest include family dynamics, parenting styles, child safety, students' mental health, adolescent reproductive health and applied social psychology.

Chapter 8
Wrestling Out Youth Development Through Indigenous Sports and Games: An Account of Naga Wrestling

Avinu Veronica Richa, Neivikuolie Khatsu, and Amenu Richa

Abstract Naga wrestling or *Kene* is an indigenous sport of the Nagas and largely popular among the *Tenyimia* tribes like the Angami, Chakhesang and Zeliang of Nagaland, and the Mao, Maram and Poumai Naga tribes of Manipur. It is played only by the menfolk and the participants are considered as 'brothers' or 'friends' rather than opponents. So the very nature of participation in the game goes beyond the act of showing one's wrestling prowess or with the intent to defeat the other party, but most importantly it was considered as an act of extending friendship amongst individuals, villages and communities. Thus, the game is lauded for its non-conventional approach of what it means to compete and conveys a different perspective to the idea of games and sports, and competition altogether and known for promoting 'brotherhood' and friendship. This traditional game has seen its steady institutionalization with the formation of the formal bodies like the Naga Wrestling Association (NWA) which is laudable and timely. While such a move is imperative for the survival of traditional sports and games (TSG), the present article makes the case that in the haste to professionalize TSG, the true spirit of the game for which it was laid down should not be lost. India's respective National Youth Policies and other development programmes do lay emphasis on the promotion of indigenous games and sports to promote youth development. Intangible cultural forms as TSG are the key to attaining the sustainable development goals as rightly argued by UNESCO and with the amount of young talents in TSG it is an apt ground for harnessing positive youth development.

Keywords Naga wrestling · Traditional sports and games · National youth policy · Youth development · Sustainable development

A. V. Richa (✉)
Rajiv Gandhi National Institute of Youth Development (RGNIYD), Sriperumbudur, Tamil Nadu, India
e-mail: veronicarg100@gmail.com

N. Khatsu
Nagaland Olympic Association, Office Complex, Kohima, Nagaland, India

A. Richa
North East Initiative Development Agency (NEIDA), Kohima, Nagaland, India

S. Deb and S. Deb (eds.), *Handbook of Youth Development*,
https://doi.org/10.1007/978-981-99-4969-4_8

Introduction

> *"The practice of physical education, physical activity and sport is a fundamental right for all,"* International Charter of Physical Education, Physical Activity and Sport, Art.1.

Naga wrestling or '*Kene*' in *Tenyidie* language is an indigenous sport of the Nagas. *Tenyidie* is spoken by the Tenyimia Nagas which is a conglomeration of several Naga tribes, namely, Angami, Chakhesang, Zeliang, Poumai, Mao, Maram, Rengma, and Pochury. *Kene* is believed to be integral to the *Tenyimia* Nagas since time immemorial and largely popular among the *Tenyimia* tribes where Naga wrestling was confined to the respective villages of the Tenyimia group (Kense, 2020; Nagaland Wrestling Association [NWA], 2016; Yhokha, 2017).

Naga wrestling is different from other wrestling styles in its form and technique, and involves a lot of energy. The game is played by two wrestlers with no accessories except for a coloured cloth (*Pfhephrie*) tied around the waist for easy grip. The players try to topple each other and balance in such a way to avoid falling on the ground, because if any upper body part from above the knees such as the chest, shoulder, back, buttock, or thigh of the player touches the ground it was considered a 'fall' (Ambrocia, 2018; Yhokha, 2017).

However, the sport is also said to have a close semblance with the traditional national sport of Korea, *Ssireum* (Wikipedia, 2022) and *Alysh* which is the traditional Kyrgyz style of belt wrestling. For instance, in the recent International Sports Festival 'Pearl of Kyrgyzstan' (belt wrestling) held at Cholpan-Ata, Kyrgyzstan, during 15–20 June 2022, two of the Naga wrestlers, namely, Keduovilie Zumu and Nlumrai Hegwang representing the Nagaland Wrestling Association (NWA) bagged a bronze medal each in the competition (Nagaland Post, 2022). *Kene*, is not only one of the most popular but a much loved sport among the Nagas young and old. This is evident with the packed audience it draws during any of its sporting event and implies that people sincerely make time to enjoy the sport.

Naga wrestling is played only by the menfolk and the participants are considered as 'brothers' or 'friends' rather than opponents. The game is lauded for its non-conventional approach of what it means to compete and conveys a different approach to the idea of games and sports, and competition altogether. Along this line, it is significant to mention that the competing partners refer to each other as '*Khrietho-u*' which in *Tenyidie* means 'beloved friend', and signifies that the very spirit of the sport is friendship and comradeship and not the mere display of strength and power over others (Ambrocia, 2018; Tsukru et al., 2021; Yhokha, 2017). So the very nature of participation in the game goes beyond the act of showing one's wrestling prowess or with the intent to defeat the other party, but most importantly it was considered as an act of establishing bonds amongst individuals, villages and communities. Thus, Naga wrestling goes beyond the narrow confines of competition and muscle power, and known for promoting the spirit of 'brotherhood' and friendship which the Nagas consider as old as their history (Yhokha, 2017).

Traditionally, the sport was not restricted to any age or weight category, it was open to anyone young or old, light or heavy, all were considered same/equal, which reiterates the cultural significance of the game and the partakers were '*akhrietho-u*' friends to each other.

Nonetheless, generally it was young men in their prime teenage and youth participated in the sport though not limited to a specific age bracket. So the participants age may vary from early teenage to thirties but not exclusive.

Given such flexibility, the wrestlers maintain a heavy diet and can finish large quantities of meat in a single meal. They predominantly train the traditional way by carrying water and firewood to build their stamina though in contemporary times the usage of the gym and the like is slowly infiltrating, yet the majority of them still train the old way (Ambrocia, 2018). Besides, it could be lifting heavy stones, chopping and carrying firewood, etc., which are traditional ways of training in itself. The wrestlers are trained in their own local ways without much professional training continuing to be more or less self-trained.

In the traditional Naga society, wrestling matches were conducted in the open fields over hard soil and ground in the village squares and held during a specific time of the year. Men with strong body build-up and adept with the skills and techniques of wrestling participated. Every good wrestler was said to command respect and valour in the village (NWA, 2016). The people enjoyed the game as part of their leisure activity. A sacred character was attributed to the wrestling field which was accessible only to those considered as '*kemete*,' or pure, and when it comes to the question of gender, women could watch the sport only from a distance and were prohibited to come into contact or access the wrestling area (Yhokha, 2017). Besides, there was a ritual element associated with the game and it was a taboo for the villagers to go for any agriculture or related works once the sport commenced in the village. The wrestlers' diet is generally protein rich comprising primarily of various meat-based products like chicken, pork, dog meat, etc. to keep their body strong and fit. Wouters (2020) comments that clans showered much care on their wrestlers and collectively invested for their maintenance with a supply of rice, rice-beer, and meat to build their bodies, and abled bodied wrestlers were selected to represent the clan, and during the preparation phases even exempted from any agricultural works. This is significant because clans were also known by the number of strong wrestlers they had (Wouters, 2020).

As per tradition, the wrestler is required to strictly observe certain moral principles and behaviour during the entire duration of his participation in any wrestling match. The sanctity of the game was preserved in such a manner that it was a taboo for the family/ clan members of the wrestler to partake in any agricultural activities especially on the day of the event. Essentially, the wrestlers were required to observe strict celibacy for the entire duration prior and during the events. Such restriction was observed to avoid any untoward incident, ward off bad omen, and with the belief that any violation would bring bad luck and dismiss the chance of winning, etc. The wrestlers followed a certain cultural code of conduct to preserve the sanctity of the game (Tsukru et al., 2021).

Naga wrestling is unique in itself due to the 'humanity associated' with the sport remarked journalist Alice Yhoshii (cited in Yhokha, 2017). Reiterating the socio-cultural significance of Naga wrestling, Neivikuolie Khatsii, Former President,

Nagaland Wrestling Association (NWA) remarked, "Inside the arena, they may be rivals but outside, they become friends" (cited in Yhokha, 2017). Perhaps its cultural significance is best reflected in the history of this indigenous game.

History of Naga Wrestling

Traditionally, wrestling played a vital role in the Naga society in conflict resolution regarding land and water disputes, or settling antagonisms between individuals, families, clans, or villages which were assuaged and settled through wrestling matches played under close supervision of elders (NWA, 2016; Tsukru et al., 2021; Yhokha, 2017). It also aided in building intra and inter-tribal relations and whenever any dispute or disagreement arose between individuals or groups, it was resolved through a wrestling match with the onus on the loser to gracefully compromise and ended the matter on a good note (Yhokha, 2017). Elders invited individuals to wrestle out their rivalry or differences and settle the matter amicably to ensure that there was no room for hostility later. In such a context, male children in the village were expected to wrestle to safeguard the honour and dignity of the family, and sons were imparted wrestling skills right from childhood to be ready to stand up for the family honour as and when the situation demanded (NWA, 2016).

However, on a different note, Wouters (2020) states that employing wrestling as a means to settle social tensions was more of an intra-village affair and not for inter-village conflicts possibly owing to the constant inter-village feuds, raids and retaliations in the Naga hills which was a matter of power, prestige and domination, and with such a history, it could not be settled through the social ritual of wrestling.

However, over the course of Naga history, wrestling was also employed as a mechanism for conflict-resolution even for inter-village conflicts, and as such, among the Chakhesang Naga, three major mass wrestling events were held during the period 1940 and the early 1970s with an aim for peace-making between two large historically antagonistic villages (Wouters, 2020).

Institutionalization of Naga Wrestling

Naga wrestling as handed down over generations was practiced in the region for several centuries. However, organized wrestling is of recent origin and is believed to have commenced sometime during the late 1930s and 1940s when the Highway road constructions between Kohima and Imphal brought together many *Tenyimia* villages to earn some cash income in order to pay house tax (*Khazana*) to the British administration, and wrestling matches were held during lunch breaks from amongst well-built men encouraged and selected by the respective village leaders which brought the first ever inter-village wrestling matches among the *Tenyimia* people (NWA, 2016).

Furthermore, after the Second World War, while laying the foundations of Naga Hospital (present day Naga Hospital Authority Kohima [NHAK]) the villages in and around Kohima were invited to participate in the site levelling work, which saw the coming together of many villages for the work and during which able-bodied individuals wrestled during intervals. The get together of people from different villages of the *Tenyimia* areas afforded a good platform for wrestling at the inter-village and community level and the wrestling matches conducted during the site levelling of the said Hospital witnessed the first ever wrestling among villages held on a larger scale (NWA, 2016).

Likewise, realizing the need to safeguard the traditional sport and also to further better relations amongst the *Tenyimia* tribes, in 1965, the Federal Government of Nagaland (FGN) under *Japfu* state is said to have organized the first wrestling meet at Shepoumaramth to honour their republic day and to provide a platform to the wrestlers from various villages of the *Tenyimia* Nagas, and FGN went on to organize the first ever wrestling competition in 1966 at Phezu, Jotsoma and later at Thizami in 1967 (Kense, 2020; NWA, 2016; Yhokha, 2017). Within such a context, the institutionalization of Naga wrestling formally took shape when the Naga Wrestling Board (renamed as Naga Wrestling Association [NWA]) was established in 1969 which subsequently organized the first Naga Wrestling Championship in 1971 which was limited to multiple championships, and later in 1972, individual championship was introduced for the first time and continued till today (Kense, 2020; NWA, 2016; Yhokha, 2017). However, realizing the amount of resources and logistics required to organize such a mega event, from 1976 onwards, the NWA tournament was held biennially instead of annually except for the years 1972, 1973 and 1974. The Naga Wrestling Championship being organized by the NWA draws participants from its three affiliated units, namely, the Angami Wrestling Association, Chakhesang Wrestling Association and Zeliang Wrestling Association. Additionally, since 1994, besides the NWA tournament, the Association has been organizing 'Open Championship' biennially as well (NWA, 2016) for participants from non-affiliated members of the NWA under open category.

Such a scenario led to the steady professionalization of the game in the 1990s, and with it, it also opened doors for Naga women particularly in freestyle wrestling which is a major break away from its traditional approach. Mr. Khatsu, Former President, NWA is optimistic that given the opportunity for its international recognition, even though the conservative Naga society may take time, a more liberal outlook towards the game is hoped for in this regard (Yhokha, 2017).

Over the years, efforts have been made not only to revive this indigenous game but to make it more professional and institutionalized which is evident with the establishment of the Nagaland Wrestling Association (NWA) with three constituent units under its fold, namely, Angami Sports Association (ASA), Chakhesang Wrestling Association (CWA) and Zeliang Wrestling Association (ZWA). Besides, the NWA is an affiliate body of the Naga Olympic Association and the Wrestling Federation of India since 1999 which speaks volumes of its professionalization journey. Additionally, the Government of Nagaland has been taking efforts to promote the sport in a big way and since 2004 during the Hornbill Festival of Nagaland held in December every year, the NWA has been organizing the Hornbill Open Wrestling Championship which is sponsored by the Department of Tourism, Government of Nagaland, and which to a certain extent elevates the game at the National and International levels with international participants from Japan, Korea, USA, etc. (NWA, 2016).

Today, Naga wrestling has evolved in a more professional manner. With its institutionalization coupled with the State's efforts for its promotion, it is steadily establishing itself which is evident from the increasing number of wrestling events organized by the residents at various levels from the village to the State level. However, in spite of its steady prominence it is vital to ensure that all is not lost in the quest for the sports' formalization and expansion lest we forget the player and the spirit of the game. For the Nagas, wrestling also communicated fundamental cultural ideals of strength, valour, and pride embodying kinship and social networks besides playing an important role in the social and political sphere (Wouters, 2020).

Extending Training and Support Services

The Nagaland Wrestling Association (NWA) as the apex body organizes the official Naga wrestling tournaments and as per a report in the Morung Express, it garners huge revenue amounting to Rs. 70 lakhs or more per tournament which makes wrestling the highest revenue generating sports in Nagaland as compared to other popular sports like football which makes about Rs. 10–15 lakhs per tournament and also offers the highest prize money (Kense, 2020). For instance, during the 12th International Hornbill Naga Wrestling Championship held in December 2018, twenty two men participated under professional category and the winners took home cash awards which ranged from Rs. 20,000 up to Rs. One Lakh of prize money (Ambrocia, 2018).

Traditionally, with no professional training or financial support to maintain their physicality or keep healthy, wrestlers were all by themselves and bore the full expenses and hardships when it came to any injury suffered as a result of the game and the onus fell on their families. In recent times, with the steady formalization of the game while winners are awarded some prize money it may be inadequate to make a livelihood or sustain their families out of it, or help their dietary requirements, health care, etc.

According to Yhoshii, "Today the game has become more professional but the spirit remains the same and wrestlers share a strong sense of camaraderie with one another" (cited in Yhokha, 2017). As efforts by the NWA to take the indigenous sport beyond the regional and state level towards larger platforms at national and international levels (or its inclusion in the Olympics) gain momentum, such efforts while are much needed and welcome should sustain the real essence of the game which is of high significance especially in today's times where participants are high contenders and opponents. If institutionalization means the loss of its former cultural significance, it will only remain a competitive game devoid of its meaning and history. The spirit of any sport should be to foster peace, friendship and better human relations.

May the process of its professionalization be to forge stronger human relationships and bring humanity together. It also brings to attention that indigenous sports and games which house many youth participation be given due recognition in terms of training, financial support, health care, etc., in order to aid and nurture positive youth development.

Young traditional sports talents need to be identified and nurtured by providing them an enabling environment and a support system by both the government and the society at large. Along this priority, identification, preservation and promotion of indigenous games and sports could enable many young people to be meaningfully engaged contributing not only to their individual growth and development but which ultimately lends to the development of the family, community, and towards nation building. At the same time, a strong policy mechanism should be in place for the revival of these sports and games in order to sustain the rich intangible cultural systems of conflict resolution, peace building and youth empowerment.

Policy Perspectives: Traditional Sports and Games (TSG) for Youth Development

The respective National Youth Policies (NYP) of India underlines the importance and need for the promotion of youth development across various sectors with a thrust on nurturing young sports talents. However, the recognition of indigenous sports and games and skilling young people along this line needs greater acknowledgement and inclusion. For instance, the National Youth Policy (NYP) 2014 identifies 11 priority areas of action to promote youth development, and one of the key areas is sports. The policy underscores the development and access to various sports facilities, training; encourage sports among young people; extend support services to sports talents to enable a productive and healthy generation of young Indians besides many other measures. "Youth must also be encouraged to engage in sports and recreation in order to ensure their physical well-being," states NYP 2014 (p. 21). It also highlights the need to enable youth to pursue sports as a profession and calls for a greater focus on sports activities and its inclusion in the school and college curriculum.

While the draft NYP 2021 (Ministry of Youth Affairs and Sports, 2022) mentions five priority areas for youth development across sectors such as education, employment, leadership, health, sports and social justice, it underlines the viability of sports as a career option among the youth and the importance of sports in education. Most notable is the policy's reference for the popularization and promotion of indigenous sports in both educational institutions and in the community to enable youth development.

During the Khelo India Youth Games (KIYG) 2021 held in Haryana, four indigenous games from different parts of India found its inclusion as approved by the Ministry of Youth Affairs and Sports, namely, *Thang-Ta*, a form of martial art which originates from Manipur, *Kalaripayattu* from Kerala; *Mallakhamba* from the states of

Maharashtra and Madhya Pradesh; and, *Gatka*, a traditional sport and a self-defence art of Punjab; and where in Shri. Kiren Rijiju, then Union Minister of Sports and Youth Affairs had remarked, "India has a rich heritage of indigenous sports, and it is a priority for the sports ministry to preserve, promote and popularize these games… In the coming years we will be able to add more indigenous sports at the Khelo Games" (*The Hindu*, 2020). Such an inclusion and approach will go a long way in promoting healthy lifestyles among the youth given that sports is one such vocation where one must practice the highest discipline at all times. Besides, the very inception of National Sports Day on 29th August commemorating the birth anniversary of Major Dhyan Chand, the hockey legend of India, aims to raise awareness about the values of sports such as discipline, perseverance, teamwork, and to encourage the public at large to take up games and sports as an integral part of their lives while also emphasizing the importance of being fit and healthy.

Sports-Integrated Education for Holistic Development

In addition, the National Education Policy (NEP) 2020 locates students as the primary stakeholders in the education system and envisages an all-round development for every student in the academic as well as non-academic domains. Following which, Sports-integrated education including indigenous sports to enable the development of various skills of collaboration, self-initiative, self-direction, self-discipline, teamwork, responsibility, citizenship, etc. among students is highlighted.

The Right to Education (RTE) Act 2009 which mandates every school to have provisions for recreation and playgrounds can be a starting point where sports events and cultural programmes can incorporate indigenous games and sports which will not only document but also inculcate positive youth engagement and cultural appreciation from an early age. However, this will materialize only when state policies encourage and recognize the significance and potential of indigenous sports as a resource pool to shape youth development among young talents.

Investing in Traditional Sports and Games (TSG) for Sustainable Development

At the international front, UNESCO's commitment towards the promotion and preservation of the world's cultural heritage includes both tangible and intangible cultural forms. Most notably, its many activities and programmes for the promotion of cultural diversity, cultural exchange and preservation of intangible culture for sustainable development encapsulates the promotion and protection of TSG as sports practices and as forms of intangible cultural heritage. Reaffirming the importance of preserving TSG which can augment greater intercultural understanding and conciliation, strengthen youth empowerment, and instil the values of just sports practices, the *World Sports Encyclopaedia* as a "worldwide list of traditional games and sports" was published in 2003 which emerged out of a joint effort of UNESCO with Prof. Wojciech Liponski and documents more than 3000 sports and sporting games from around the globe consisting of various traditional and indigenous sports and games which are local or extreme in nature, historical and other sports which have died out, sports of the Olympics, international sports, martial arts, school and children's sports and games. Besides, the Collective Consultation on the promotion of TSG which took place in January 2009 in Tehran (Islamic Republic of Iran), invokes TSG's cultural heritage and its potential to promote healthy ambience amongst nations in its definitional framework of TSG, "Traditional sport and games are motor activities of leisure and recreation which can have a ritual character. They are part of the universal heritage diversity. They are practiced in an individual or collective manner, deriving from regional or local identity; they are based on rules accepted by a group that organizes competitive or non-competitive activities… The practice of traditional and games promotes global health" (UNESCO, 2017).

UNESCO's International Charter of Physical Education, Physical Activity and Sport lays emphasis that physical education, physical activity and sport can benefit individuals, communities, and society as a whole in a variety of ways. Stressing its intention, Article 1.3 of the Charter calls for, "Inclusive, adapted and safe opportunities to participate in physical education, physical activity and sport must be available to all human beings, notably children of preschool age, women and girls, the aged, persons with disabilities and indigenous people," and Article 1.5 states, "The diversity of physical education, physical activity, and sport is a basic feature of their value and appeal. Traditional and indigenous games, dances, and sports, also in their modern and emerging forms, express the world's rich cultural heritage and must be protected and promoted."

An incisive article by Bruner et al. (2016) talks about the potentialities of physical activity and sport and how it can be better conceptualized to shape the development of Aboriginal youth. While stating that despite much enthusiasm on how physical activity and sport can positively impact Aboriginal youth development in terms of their physical, mental, spiritual and emotional health, it underlined that there is a dearth of available resources to establish the same. The research highlighted that in order to facilitate positive youth development, a serious exercise collating literature resources which can assist programme planning, delivery, and intervention regarding physical activity and sport was much needed.

A study by Luchoro-Parrilla et al. (2021) in the context of Traditional Sports and Games (TSG) in Canary Islands, Spain established that TSG was a true reflection of traditional culture which had a huge advantage of sustaining both material and non-material cultural heritage. It highlighted the crucial role of physical education which can provide sustainability education via TSG especially in educational settings. Stressing that TSG are cultural treasures in themselves and key assets of physical education which can enrich local cultures, it reiterated that several studies support TSG can promote basic social values of peaceful co-existence, social inclusion, gender sensitivity, social and emotional health, and sustainable practices which are beneficial to the environment and people (Luchoro-Parrilla et al., 2021).

Perhaps, the potential of intangible cultural heritage which encompasses various forms of arts, manifestations of TSG, etc. can facilitate and realize sustainable development is best consolidated by the UNESCO's (2018) *2030 Agenda for Sustainable Development* which rationalizes the need to turn to culture for sustainable development. The inter-linkage and connectedness between culture and development is made for the first time in the 2030 Agenda which includes particular goals for preserving the world's cultural and ecological legacy, ensuring that our educational institutions promote respect for and understanding of our cultural diversity, and defending fundamental freedoms and participation in cultural activities. It further recognizes that intangible culture heritage are banks of resilience and knowledge which can help address the many problems that we face today such as poverty, climate change, illiteracy, etc., and intercultural dialogue and respect for cultural diversity are powerful tools for reconciliation and the creation of peaceful societies (UNESCO, 2018).

Traditional sports and games can be the central stage for appreciating cultural diversity, encourage global understanding and build cultural assets, and the varied presentations of traditional sports and games at the 5th World Sport for All Games 2012 which was held in Siauliai, Lithuania, indicates that such sports can be effectively employed to promote cultural dialogue and for the preservation of heritage in modern times (Brownikowska & Prabucki, 2014).

Conclusion and Way Forward

While Traditional Sports and Games (TSG) can be a powerful tool to shape youth development, it also demands a political will to initiate policy directives for its identification, preservation and promotion in order to support and align it with the youth's aspirations, talents, foster life values, and encourage healthy lifestyles for positive youth development. Besides, indigenous sports development and its revitalization is a potential sector for promoting youth development and to reach the rural, marginalized and most unreached communities which generally is home to a rich and vibrant cultural history. Scouting and nurturing young talents skilled in TSG who are readily available amongst local communities and its institutionalization can be an initial step.

However, in the effort to preserve and formalize TSG, its essence of fostering relationships, social coherence, conflict resolution, harmony, cultural plurality and a potential tool for peace building should continue to be sustained. Our youth development policies and sports programmes should definitely look this way for real transformation on the ground which can help materialize the true spirit of sustainable development and strengthen the attainment of the Sustainable Development Goals through the preservation and promotion of our rich cultural resources spreading friendship and community spirit as pillars of intangible cultural forms and so is Naga wrestling. While the traditional game continues to enjoy much popularity and gradual institutionalization, its socio-cultural distinctiveness as a catalyst for harmonious community living and transformative change should trigger positive youth development to pave way for many more young talents as ambassadors of peace, social harmony, and sustainability agents. As rightly stated by Roque et al. (2017, p. 97), "Indigenous peoples are still the keepers of this knowledge, which can ensure better quality of life worldwide. The World Indigenous Games are an important contribution to disseminate such knowledge and ways of life." May it open an era of positive youth engagement and sustainable development. Long live the era of Traditional Sports and Games.

Strategies for Way Forward

1. Identification, promotion and implementation of Traditional Sports and Games (TSG) across all educational institutions with the support of both the central and state government institutions/departments such as, Sports Authority of India, Sports Universities and Colleges, Sports Training Institutes, Department of Youth Resources and Sports, etc.
2. Initiate the documentation of TSGs in India in partnership with local communities, NGOs, government institutions, and any other relevant bodies.
3. Conduct training programmes, workshops, and conferences with various stakeholders to sensitize, disseminate and popularize the potential and prospect of TSG at the international, national, regional and local levels for promoting positive youth development and its scope for enabling sustainable development.
4. Mobilize and build a cadre of TSG community trainers as master trainers to mentor and coach young people.
5. Identification and extension of various support services to enable young talents to pursue TSG as a profession.

References

Ambrocia, M. (2018, December 5). How this indigenous Naga wrestling act won hearts at Hornbill Fest: More than just muscle power, the ancient sport is also about the spirit of brotherhood. *East Mojo*. https://www.eastmojo.com/news/2018/12/05/how-this-indigenous-naga-wrestling-act-won-hearts-at-hornbill-fest/

Bronikowska, M., & Prabucki, B. (2014). TAFISA and UNESCO joint effort for building cultural capital through traditional sports: An analysis of the 5th World Sport for All Games. *Studia Humanistyczne AGH, 13*(1), 29–40. https://doi.org/10.7494/human.2014.13.1.29

Bruner, M. W., Hillier, S., Baillie, C. P. T., Lavallee, L. F., Bruner, B. G., Hare, K., Lovelace, R., & Le'vesque, L. (2016). Positive youth development in Aboriginal physical activity and sport: A systematic review. *Adolescent Research Review, 1*(3), 257–269. https://doi.org/10.1007/s40894-015-0021-9

Ministry of Youth Affairs and Sports. (2022). *Draft National Youth Policy 2021*. Government of India. https://yas.nic.in/sites/default/files/Draft%20National%20Youth%20Policy%2029.09.2022.pdf
Government of India. (n.d). *National Education Policy 2020*. Ministry of Human Resource Development. https://www.education.gov.in/sites/upload_files/mhrd/files/NEP_Final_English_0.pdf
Government of India. (n.d). *National Youth Policy 2014*. Ministry of Youth Affairs and Sports. https://www.rgniyd.go
Kene (Naga wrestling). (2022, March 16). *Wikipedia*. https://en.wikipedia.org/wiki/Kene_(Naga_wrestling)
Kense, A. T. (2020, February 12). Naga wrestling: The highest grossing sport in Nagaland. *Morung Express*. https://morungexpress.com/naga-wrestling-highest-grossing-sport-nagaland
Luchoro-Parrilla, R., Lavega-Burgues, P., Damian-Silva, S., Prat, Q., Saez de Ocariz, U., Ormo-Ribes, E., & Pic, M. (2021). Traditional games as cultural heritage: The case of Canary Islands (Spain) from an ethnomotor perspective. *Frontiers in Psychology, 12*(153). https://doi.org/10.3389/fpsyg.2021.586238
Nagaland Wrestling Association. (2016). *Nagaland Wrestling Association (NWA): 25th tournament anniversary*. Nagaland Wrestling Association.
Roque, L., Terena, M., Calfin, J.A., & Terena, T. (2017). *World indigenous games: Celebrating is what matters*. UNDP.
Sports Ministry approves inclusion of four indigenous games in Khelo India Youth Games. (2020, December 20). *The Hindu*. https://www.thehindu.com/sport/sports-ministry-approves-inclusion-of-four-indigenous-games-in-khelo-india-youth-games/article33378223.ece
Tsukru, V., Khesoh, V., Dkhar, J. W., Limbu, D. K., & Mary, K. K. (2021). Body physique and nutritional status of Naga wrestlers: A case study of the Chakhesang tribe of Nagaland, India. *International Journal of Physical Education, Sports and Health, 8*(3), 374–379. https://doi.org/10.22271/kheljournal.2021.v8.i3f.2110
Two Naga wrestlers win bronze at International Sports Festival in Kyrgyzstan. (2022, June 19). *Nagaland Post*. https://www.nagalandpost.com/index.php/2-naga-wrestlers-win-bronze-atintl-sports-festival-in-kyrgyzstan/
UNESCO. (2017, July). *Concept note on traditional sports and games: Traditional sports and games, challenge for the future*. https://unesdoc.unesco.org/ark:/48223/pf0000252837
UNESCO. (2018). *Culture for the agenda 2030*. UNESCO. https://unesdoc.unesco.org/ark:/48223/pf0000264687
UNESCO. (n.d). International charter of physical education, physical activity and sport. https://unesdoc.unesco.org/ark:/48223/pf0000235409
UNESCO. (n.d). *Traditional sports and games*. https://en.unesco.org/themes/sport-and-anti-doping/traditional-sports-and-games
Wouters, J. J. P. (2020, September 22). Wrestling for peace: A physical duel has traditionally been an important tool for conflict resolution in Naga society. *The Statesman*. https://www.thestatesman.com/supplements/north/wrestling-for-peace-1502925231.html
Yhokha, V. (2017, March 10). Naga wrestling: The embrace of brothers. *The Hindu*. https://www.thehindu.com/thread/arts-culture-society/naga-wrestling-the-embrace-of-brothers/article17441800.ece

Avinu Veronica Richa is an Assistant Professor in the Department of Sociology, RGNIYD, Sriperumbudur. She has a Master's in Anthropology from North Eastern Hill University, Shillong. She imparts gender training to youth functionaries (NSS, NYKS), Police, Prison Officers, NDRF Personnel, youth and women worked as Field Investigator for the project, '*Cultural History, Ethnography & Physical Characteristics of Nagas of Nagaland*' under the Directorate of Art and

Culture, Govt. of Nagaland and Anthropological Society of Nagaland; and as Project Coordinator for the projects, '*Promoting Environmental Education through the Ethical Value of Conservation*,' and '*Women Promoting Sustainable Livelihoods through the use of Eco-friendly Technology*' at C-CERP, Dimapur. She has undergone the British Council's *Management Development Programme on Young Women Social Entrepreneurship Development Programme*, and has organized similar workshops for young women besides organizing capacity building programs on Women Managers in Higher Education, ToT on Gender Equity, Women Connect for Leadership and Change, Entrepreneurship with eSheBee Enterprises, Bangladesh, Youth-led development programs, etc.

Neivikuolie Khatsu is the Assistant Secretary General of the Nagaland Olympic Association. He is Advisor to the Nagaland Wrestling Association (NWA) and former President of NWA. Under his leadership, promoting Naga wrestling at the grassroots and at international level besides the regular forums was enhanced wherein team Nagaland participated in the 5th Asian Indoor and Martial Arts Games held in Ashgabath, Turkmenistan in 2017 which was the first ever international level participation, and subsequently in 2018, led the team's participation in the 3rd World Nomad Games held in Issykyl region, Kyrgyzstan. In 2020, together with his team, the first ever Naga wrestling under 16 category was introduced to encourage participation of school going children and to streamline the competition, and winners were awarded a one year scholarship. He has more than a decade of teaching experience having served as a lecturer in the Department of History at St. Joseph's College, Jakhama and Sazolie College, Jotsoma.

Amenu Richa works at NEIDA, Kohima as a Project Associate overseeing projects related to Springshed Management, Springshed-based Watershed Development, Internet of Things (IoT) Rural Smart Water Management, and Diversion-based Irrigation projects; provides capacity building training to Water and Sanitation Committees and communities under Jal Jeevan Mission; and liaises with various stakeholders, partners and government agencies for project implementation. She interned with the United Nations Development Program (UNDP) for the *UNDP-NBA Biodiversity Samrakshan Internship Programme 2020* during which she assisted communities in the project villages with tasks related to the constitution of Biodiversity Management Committees and preparation of People's Biodiversity Register, and assisted the GOI-NBA-UNDP India Biodiversity Awards 2020. She holds an M. Tech in Water Resources Engineering from NIT, Calicut.

Chapter 9
India's Demographic Dividend and Policy Implications

Sanjay Kumar, Shivendra Singh, and Jaydeep Biswas

Abstract Though India has achieved replacement levels of fertility (a Total Fertility Rate of 2 children per woman) in 2020, the absolute population size will continue to increase due to population momentum. The demographic transition, from high fertility and mortality conditions to low levels over a period, brings about changes in the age structure of the population with a shift towards a smaller share of the young population (0–14 years) and an increasingly share of the working-age population (15–59 years), which lowers the dependency ratio. After a lag of a few decades, eventually the share of older persons increases, which results in the increase in the dependency ratio. The period of potential demographic dividend occurs when the dependency ratio remains low. However, the demographic dividend phases do not automatically translate into economic growth. To harness the demographic dividend fully, policies and programmatic measures are required on an urgent basis. This chapter brings out the importance of higher investments in health and education, focusing more on vocational and skill-oriented education for young people, making reproductive health care services accessible on a rights-based approach with a focus on the marginalized population, women's empowerment, reducing gender inequality and increasing female workforce participation. Inter-regional diversity in demographic transition in India provides a unique situation, whereby the north-central region of the country

Authors are from UNFPA-India working as (1) Population Dynamics & Research Specialist; (2) Data Analyst and (3) Chief, Policy and Partnerships. The views expressed in the paper are that of the authors and does not necessarily reflect those of the organisations with which they are affiliated. The paper was presented in 'Youth Global Summit: An International Conference' during March 15–17, 2022 organized by Rajiv Gandhi National Institute of Youth Development, Chennai.

S. Kumar (✉)
Population Dynamics and Research Specialist, United Nations Population Fund (UNFPA), 55, Lodi Estate, New Delhi 110003, India
e-mail: skumar@unfpa.org

S. Singh
Data Analyst, United Nations Population Fund (UNFPA), 55, Lodi Estate, New Delhi 110003, India

J. Biswas
Chief, Policy and Partnership, United Nations Population Fund (UNFPA), 55, Lodi Estate, New Delhi 110003, India

S. Deb and S. Deb (eds.), *Handbook of Youth Development*,
https://doi.org/10.1007/978-981-99-4969-4_9

will serve as the reservoir of the working age population in future. Considering such diversities, a differential planning approach is needed to reap the benefits of demographic dividend.

Keywords Youth · India: demographic dividend · Policy · Implications

Introduction

The twentieth century has witnessed remarkable changes in India's demographic arena. The population has increased by four times; from 238.3 million at the beginning of the century, to one billion at the end of it (Office of the Registrar General and Census Commissioner, India, Census, 2011). In 2022, with 1.4 billion persons, India accounts for 18% of world population and is expected to be the most populous country surpassing China in the year 2023 (UNDESA, World Population Prospects, 2022 Revision).

Though India has achieved replacement levels of fertility (a Total Fertility Rate of 2 children per woman) in 2020, the absolute size will continue to increase due to the phenomenon of population momentum. The country will reach its peak of population figure of 1.69 billion in 2063. In other words, an additional 280 million people will be added to the country's population in the next forty years, before India achieves its population stabilization. Therefore, the increase in the future size of the population is inevitable.

Demographic Transition

The historic shifts in fertility and mortality rates over a period are known as demographic transition. The term demographic transition refers to the several phases of change those countries undergo, that is, from a period of high mortality and high fertility to one of low mortality and, with a lag, low fertility. Death rates tend to decline first, and therefore there is a high natural increase during this period. After a lag of time, fertility declines as societies adjust to improvements in survival rates among infants and children. Consequently, population growth slows down given that both mortality and fertility rates have fallen. The demographic transition is clearly distinguished by a country's birth and death rates and any country's progression is mostly shaped by changes both in fertility and mortality.

In the nineteenth century Frank W. Notestein, an American demographer described the demographic transition theory which has four stages of the demographic transition, while some others have also included the fifth stage of transition as well. The first stage is called pre-transition and characterized by high birth and death rates and as a result the natural increase in population remains low (Fig. 9.1). The population growth rate remains slow in this stage. Stage two which is also known

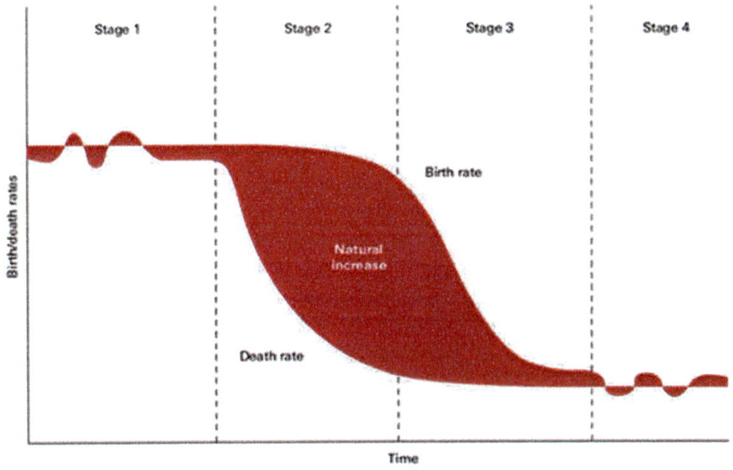

Fig. 9.1 Stages of demographic transition

as the early transition state, when death rate starts declining due to improvements of food supply, sanitation and improvements in public health and advancement in medical science. In this stage, although death rates begin to decline, the birth rate remains high for some period. This is the phase of rapid increase in population size as more numbers are added to population while due to lower death rates, people tend to live longer. In stage 3, the birth rate also starts declining due to various factors such as availability of contraception, urbanization, technological use in farming, increase in wages, an increase in women's education and their societal status, and improvement in the public health system etc. During stage four, both birth rate and death rate fall. Birth rates drop to reach below replacement levels of fertility. Even after reaching the replacement levels of fertility, the population size increases for a few decades due to population momentum phenomenon. Due to changes in age structure of population during the demographic transition period, the high fertility cohort moves in the reproductive ages and even with replacement levels of fertility, the size increases before it reaches to a peak and thereafter the population size starts shrinking.

India's Demographic Transition

In the case of India, both birth and death rates have registered declines. A steep fall in death rate was observed, especially during the middle of the twentieth century, without much decline in fertility for the first few decades (Fig. 9.2). Consequently, the rate of population growth was initially low, but accelerated after the 1950s, rising to two percent per annum. The birth rate gradually started declining, which resulted in slower growth of population.

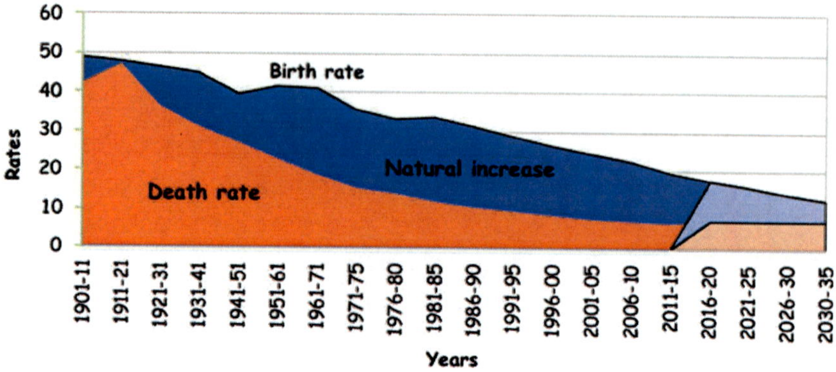

Fig. 9.2 Trends in birth rate, death rate and natural increase in India, 1901–2035

The total fertility rate (TFR), which is a more refined indicator and is defined as the average number of children that would be born to a woman, if she was to experience the current age-specific fertility rates through her reproductive span (usually referring to women aged 15–49 years). In India, after a long stall, fertility levels began to decline in the late 1970s-early 1980s. The TFR was more than 5 children per woman in 1971, which declined to 2.3 by 2016, and to 2.0 by 2019–2020, and reaching below replacement levels by 2020 (Fig. 9.3).

India is currently in the third stage of the demographic transition with almost steady death rates (Carl & Gribble, 2011). Over the course of demographic transition, the population of India has increased more than 2.5 times in the last 50 years from 548 million in 1971. Today, with 1.4 billion persons, India accounts for 18% of world

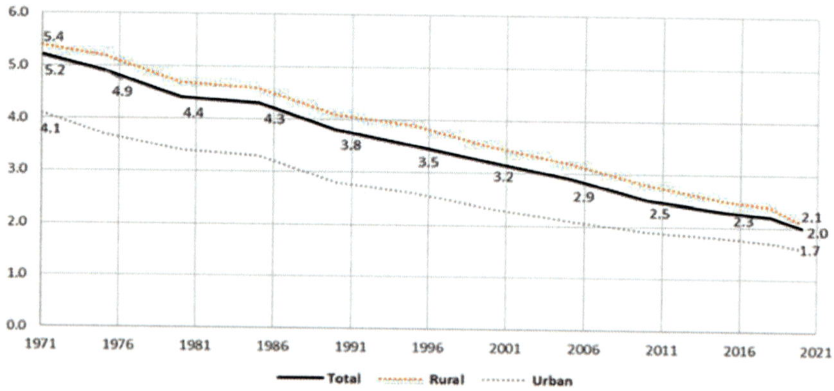

Fig. 9.3 Trends in Total Fertility Rate (TFR) in India by place of residence, 1971–2020. *Source* Sample Registration System, Registrar General of India, 2015 (from 1971 to 2018) and International Institute for Population Sciences, (IIPS), National Family Health Survey (NFHS-5), 2019–21 for 2020

population and is expected to be the most populous country surpassing China in the year 2023.

Though India has achieved replacement levels of fertility (a TFR of 2 children per woman), the absolute size of the population will continue to increase due to the phenomenon of population momentum. This happens in a relatively youthful age structure like that of India's, when births produced by its large number of women of reproductive age outnumber the number of deaths taking place in the total population, even if average TFR is at the replacement level.

Age Structure Transition

One of the consequences of the demographic transition is the transformation of age structure. Following the sustained decline in fertility, there has been a shift in the age-structure towards a smaller share of the young population aged 0–14 years, an increasingly larger share of the working-age population (15–59 years), and an increase in the share of older persons. The share of the age group 0–14 years to the total population, which was 42% in 1971, declined to 31% by 2011. The share of the working age population on the other hand had increased from 52 to 60% during the same period, while those 60 years and above increased their share from 6 per cent to 8.6%.

To understand the changes of age structure in future, population projections are required to be made based on most likely trends in population parameters. In India, the Government of India undertook population projections until 2031, while to study the demographic dividend, UNFPA prepared population projections till 2061. Both sets of the projections are used to understand the future trends of population as well as age structure transition and demographic dividend.

The age-structure transformation that accompanies the demographic transition is reflected in the population pyramids for 2011, 2036 and 2061 (Fig. 9.4). The base of the 2061 pyramid will be much narrower than in 2011, indicative of slower population growth due to sharp fertility reductions and moderate mortality changes. There will also be a shrinking share of the school going population and a widening bulge at the center indicating a bigger share of the working age population and those in the middle-ages. The top of the pyramid will also be wider on account of more people entering the ranks of the elderly population given longer life expectancy, as well as the longer-term effects of declining fertility trends.

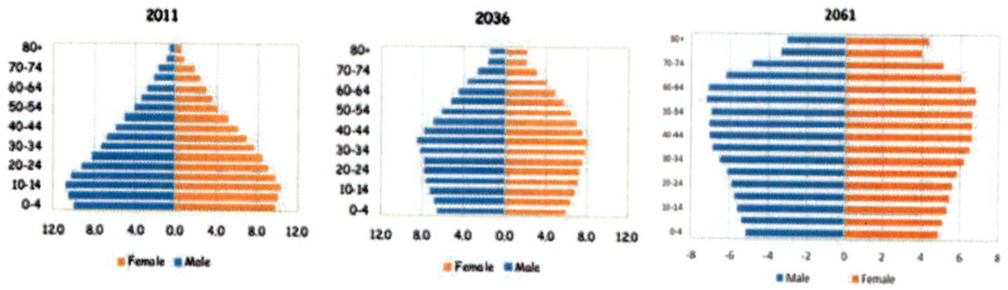

Fig. 9.4 Changing age-pyramid India: 2011, 2036 and 2061

Demographic Dividend

Demographic dividend depends on the age structure of the population. An important consequence of this rapid fertility decline is the accruing of demographic dividend due to rise in the share of the working age population, implying a fall in the dependency ratio,[1] these two are reciprocal in nature. After a decline in fertility, the share of the working age population increases but after some time, it declines as the share of the elderly rises. The period during which the dependency ratio is low, is the period of demographic dividend (window of opportunity). As evidenced elsewhere, the ensuing reduction in the dependency ratio because of the increasing share of the working population and a decrease in young dependents provide an opportunity for wealth creation and increased economic growth through higher levels of savings and investment. The resources that would otherwise have gone to the support of dependents were able to be channelled towards other productive investments which then boosted economic growth. The rise in the rate of economic growth due to the rising share of the working age population, relative to dependents, is what the demographic dividend is all about. But the dividend is only a given opportunity. To convert it into a benefit, actions will have to be taken on several fronts.

A country's development is interlinked to its population and its population significantly impacts its development (James & Srinivas, 2017). It has been a well-established fact that population size, structure, and composition have a critical impact on economic development (James & Srinivas, 2017). Changes in the age distribution of the population can have important economic effects (James & Jason, 2012). These effects reflect the influence of changes in the number of working-age individuals per capita, it depends on many policies, institutions, and conditions that determine an economy's capacity to equip its people with human and physical capital and to absorb them into productive employment (Agarwal, 2016; Bloom et al., 1999).

Fertility decline gives rise to two kinds of demographic dividend (Lee & Mason, 2006). The first is the consequence of falling child dependency ratios and the rise of the working age population. The dividend arises when the growing labour force has to support fewer dependents. The second demographic dividend builds up on

[1] Dependency ratio is defined as the ratio of young population (0–14 years of age) and old (60 + years of age) to the population in working ages (15–59 years), and is expressed in percentage.

savings for old age and retirement; the increased savings can contribute to capital accumulation and economic growth.

With declining fertility and an increasing population of working age groups, India is witnessing a change in its age distribution where the proportion of adults are increasing and the share of children shrinking at the same time (James, 2011). If the fertility decline is rapid, the increase in the population of working ages is substantial yielding the 'demographic dividend' (Bloom et al., 2003). The smaller share of children permits greater investment per child further increasing productivity. As a result, future entrants into the labour force can boost per capita income. With the passage of time, the share of the old age population rises and that of the working age population begins to fall and hence the dividend is available for a period of time, which is called 'the window of demographic opportunity'. Therefore, the dividend period is a window of opportunity rather than a guarantee of improved standards of living.

The age structure of the population will change substantially. The share of the young ages (below 15) will fall, from 30.9% in 2011 to 15.9% in 2061 and of the old ages (60 and above) rise, from 8.4 to 25.7% over the same period. During the process, the share of middle ages, or working ages, will rise for some time, reaching a peak of nearly 65.1% around 2031.

India will experience a higher labour inflow in the coming decades. The period during which dependency ratios are falling and remaining low would indicate the period of the demographic dividend. Taking the working age population as those in the 15–59 age-group, the dependency ratio of less than 67% (or less than two-thirds) is considered as the period when the demographic dividend accrues (Kulkarni, 2017). For India, the dependency ratio was quite high, 75%, in 2001 but fell to 65% by 2011. Thus, India has already begun to derive the dividend before 2011 and the dependency ratio is projected to fall further to 55% by 2021 and remain around that level for about 20 years (Fig. 9.5). However, after 2041, the dependency ratio would rise, and the dividend would not be as large. Moreover, by 2061, the ratio would rise above the critical 67% point and the dividend would no longer be available.

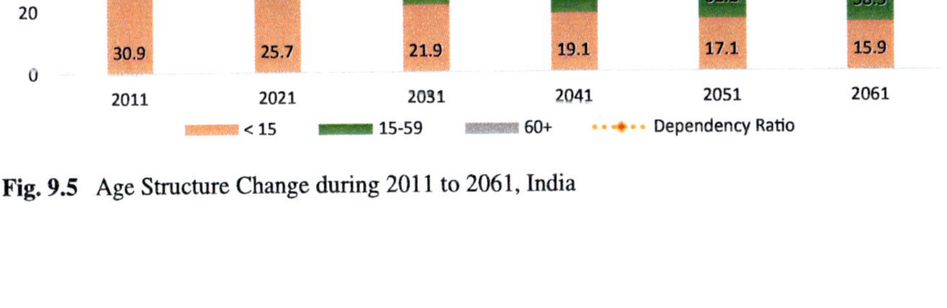

Fig. 9.5 Age Structure Change during 2011 to 2061, India

Different States Are at Different Stages

India is a diverse country even in terms of its demographic characteristic. Various states are at different stages of demographic transition. As a result of the variation in initial fertility and mortality levels and age distributions and projected trajectories, the growth will vary across the states. In the case of some states, Tamil Nadu and Kerala, the projected 2061 population will be only marginally higher (by less than 20%) than the 2001 populations. In Punjab, Himachal Pradesh, West Bengal, and Andhra Pradesh and Telangana, it will be higher by 20–30% and in Maharashtra and Karnataka, by just over 30%. On the other hand, it will more than double in Bihar, and nearly so (80% or higher) in Uttar Pradesh, Rajasthan, Madhya Pradesh and Jharkhand.

The state wise share of working and elderly population for the year 2021, 2041 and 2061 is provided in Fig. 6a, b, c respectively. It is clearly evident that many states will have more than 65% of the working population in 2021 (Fig. 9.6a) and after two decades, the share of the working age population in many states will shrink, with the exception of Uttar Pradesh—with around 65% of the working age population. While these states will have a larger share of elderly population (Fig. 9.6b), by 2061, only Madhya Pradesh, Uttar Pradesh and Bihar will have more than 60% of their population in the working age group, while majority of the states will have substantial higher share of elderly population (Fig. 9.6c).

Due to the different pace of demographic transition of states, the age structure composition is also different, which results in varying levels of dependency ratios. States ahead in demographic transition had begun to derive dividends before 2001 or did so soon after 2001, as they had lower dependency ratio by that time. Tamil Nadu, Kerala, Delhi, Karnataka, Andhra Pradesh, and Gujarat had ratios below 67% in 2001 and were soon joined by Himachal Pradesh, West Bengal, Punjab, and Maharashtra. By 2011, the ratios in these states had fallen below 60%. In these states, the dependency ratio will rise above two thirds (due to rise in the elderly population) before 2051. Thus, these states, ahead in the transition, have begun to gain dividends since early 2000, but will start losing it in the next 2–3 decades. Kerala and Tamil Nadu, the leaders among these, will lose the dividend sooner, before 2040 whereas the rest will do so around the mid-2040s. On the other hand, states lagging in the transition process had not begun to get dividends by 2001. But the dependency ratio was rapidly declining in these and by 2011 some of these, Odisha, Haryana, Assam, Chhattisgarh, and Uttarakhand had also begun to gain dividend (Kulkarni, 2017).

When the working age is taken as 15–59 years, the dependency ratio of less than two-thirds (67%) is considered advantageous, and the demographic dividend accrues[2]

[2] The cut-off dependency ratio, to be considered as advantageous has been derived from the stationary age distributions from the Model Life Tables (four tables produced by Coale-Demeny and five by the UN). The share of working age population remains around 60% in the middle and high life expectancy ranges and then it declines at very high life expectancy levels. Hence, when the dependency ratio is less than 40% or two-thirds (40/60), the dividend may be considered to accrue.

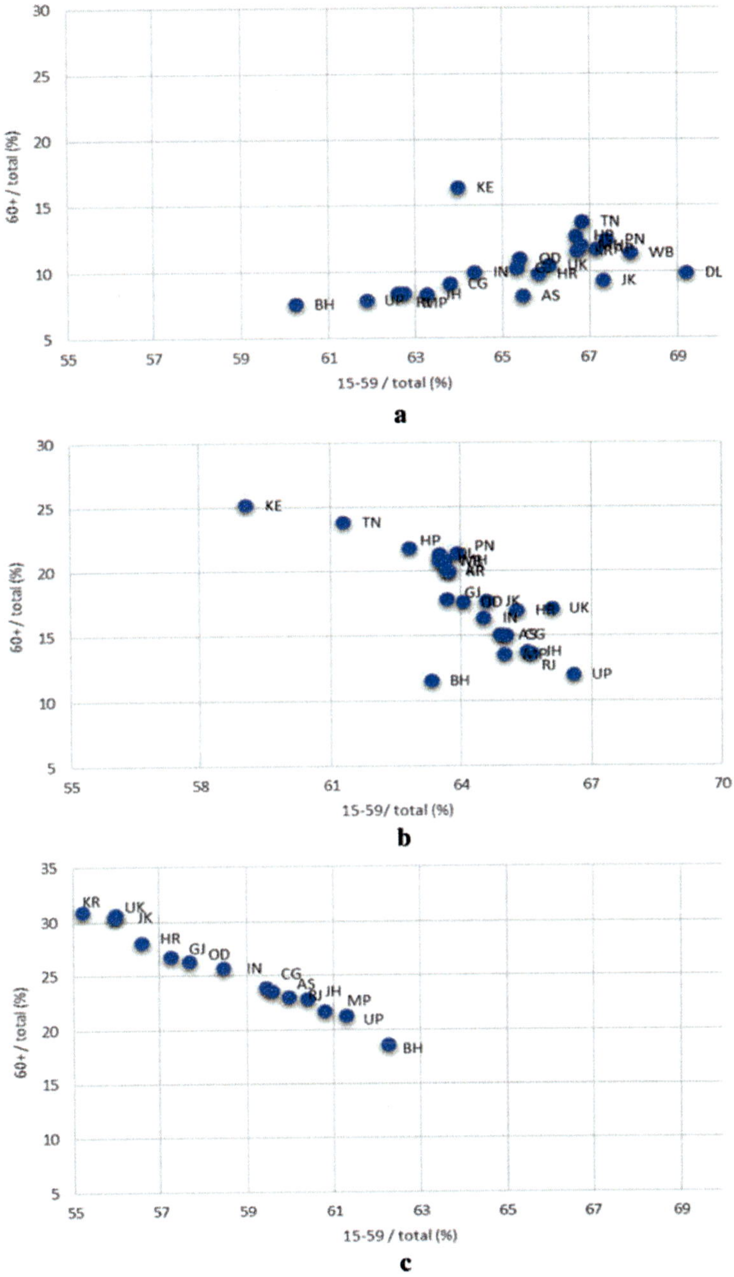

Fig. 9.6 **a** Share of Working Age and Elderly Population, India and States, 2021. **b** Share of Working Age and Elderly Population, India and States, 2041. **c** Share of Working Age and Elderly Population, India and States, 2061

at this stage. Saad (2009) has identified three stages of demographic dividend: Dividend 1: dependency ratio above two thirds and declining, Dividend 2: dependency ratio below two thirds and declining, and Dividend 3: dependency ratio below two thirds but increasing. During the first phase, the population is yet to begin to gain the dividend but is moving towards it (dependency ratio declining but above two thirds). During the second phase, the dividend is available and increasing (dependency ratio declining); which may be called the 'waxing' phase; the window of opportunity has opened and is widening. In the third phase, the dividend is still being derived but it is now closing (dependency ratio is rising); which may be called the 'waning' phase, and the window is gradually closing. Once the dependency ratio goes above the critical level, the third phase has ended, and the window will be closed.

Due to differential demographic transitions, the states are in different stages of demographic dividend phases and their trajectory has been estimated based on the projected trends in the share of population in the 15–59 age group and corresponding dependency ratios. The demographic dividend will be staggered spatially. This is inevitable given that the demographic transition is itself staggered. While the leading states will be gaining peak dividend, the lagging states will not have begun to get a dividend, and by the time the lagging states enter the phase of high dividend, many leading states will be in the waning phase of dividend. A consequence of the staggered dividend is that for India as a whole, the dependency ratio will not be very low; it will not fall below 54%. Thus, while India will certainly get a dividend, the intensity will not be very large. This is in contrast to China which experienced a very rapid fertility decline, the TFR halved within just one decade, the 1970s, and thereby gained a huge dividend (Kulkarni, 2010).

The states are arranged in order of entry into Phase II, when the dividend begins to be derived in Fig. 9.7. Most of the states which had entered Phase II before 2001 will have been out of Phase III before 2051 (with closed window of opportunity) and all the states which had begun to gain dividend before 2011 will have been out of Phase III before 2061. On the other hand, the late entrants into dividend, Jharkhand, Madhya Pradesh, Rajasthan, Uttar Pradesh, and Bihar, will continue to derive some dividend even beyond 2061. However, at that time, these will be in the Phase III with dividend declining and will run out within a short time after that.

One of the features of the state wise phases of demographic dividend in India is that those states which would have shortage of working age population, will attract it from those which have surplus and in terms of better economic opportunities and prospects, inter-state migration will intensify more in future.

Capturing the Dividend

The demographic dividend phases do not automatically translate into economic growth. To avail the dividend, a country's policy makers and administrators must invest in policies, strategies and programs in education and skill training, health, and other population development efforts aimed at strengthening the population's human

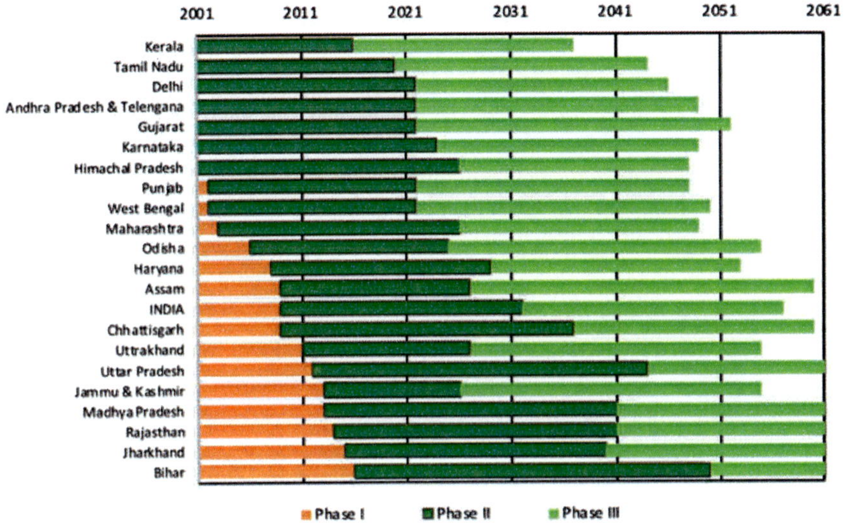

Fig. 9.7 Phases of demographic dividend in selected States of India. *Source* Kulkarni (2017)—Report of United Nations Population Fund, India. Phase I: Window opening—Dependency ratio above two-thirds (66.7%) and declining. Phase II: Window fully open—Dependency ratio below two-thirds (66.7%) and declining. Phase III: Window closing—Dependency ratio below two-thirds (66.7%) but increasing

capital. Investments in human capital are known to improve worker productivity and the economy's competitiveness. This is especially critical in view of the rapid growth of the working population as new youth cohorts enter the labour market. There is a need to provide decent and remunerative jobs that will allow the work force not only to support themselves and their dependents but in addition increase their savings that will enable the economy to invest and grow. Workers would also have spent longer time in education and training before entering work and be in good health. With the advent of new and emerging technologies, skills get obsolete quickly. India's workers will have to learn and unlearn to keep abreast of the rapidly changing job and skill requirements. Skills and knowledge acquisition must be continuous. The working ages are also the period in the life cycle when the propensity to save is highest. Financial literacy on the part of the households on one hand and the accessibility to strong financial institutions and intermediaries to convert these savings into productive investments are absolutely critical for the country to benefit from both the dividends (UNFPA, 2021).

Since different states in India will be passing through different stages of demographic dividend, it is important to have a differential approach towards achieving the dividend involving three clusters of states. The first cluster being states where the period of the demographic dividend will close in a decade, the second for those states where the dividend is already underway and will close soon, and the third for those states where the window is yet to open (UNPA, 2018).

In seven demographically advanced states,[3] the focus of the policies and programmes should be on ageing and creating a conducive work environment for migrant workers from outside. Another set of eight states[4] will have about a decade after which the dependency ratio will start increasing. The aim should be to empower young people. Even though some states[5] are lagging in demographic transition, these will have an edge of supplying a greater share of the working age population in future. A three-fold policy focus is required on ensuring universal access to quality sexual and reproductive health information and services; provisioning of education, life and vocational skills to young people; and addressing harmful practices against women and girls.

Conclusion and Way Forward

India has achieved replacement levels of fertility (a TFR of 2 children per woman) in 2021 and has passed through the demographic transition with historic declines in fertility and mortality rates. However, the absolute size of the population will continue to increase due to the phenomenon of population momentum. This will provide a situation with relatively youthful age structure, and with rise in the share of working age population, India is poised to face a phenomenon of 'demographic dividend', a potential opportunity with lower dependency ratios, which might boost economic growth if proper investments are done in the education, skills and health of the population.

One of the important consequences of the demographic transition is the changes in the age structure of the population. India is a diverse country and various states are at different stages of demographic transition. As a result of the variation in initial fertility and mortality levels and age distributions and projected trajectories, demographic parameters will vary by state. The Inter-regional population dynamics in India presents a unique situation, which can be turned into a powerful engine for the overall socio-economic development by adopting a differential planning approach. This calls for time-bound investments to empower, educate and equip young people before they enter the workforce. It is equally imperative to ensure an investment climate and labour policies to expand and sustain safe and secure employment.

The urgent first step would be to review existing policies and programmes of each group of states vis-à-vis the status of demographic window of opportunity. While group-specific actions would be required for states, a national body should be established to coordinate between the groups of states, as demographic shifts in one part of the country are usually impacted by changes in other areas.

---

[3] *Kerala, Tamil Nadu, Delhi, Andhra Pradesh, Gujarat, Punjab, West Bengal.*

[4] *Karnataka, Maharashtra, Himachal Pradesh, Odisha, Assam, Uttrakhand, Haryana, J&K,*

[5] *Uttar Pradesh, Bihar, Chhattisgarh, Jharkhand, Madhya Pradesh, Rajasthan,,*

To reap the benefits of the demographic dividend, forward looking policies need to be put in place now. Below are some of the important aspects which may be considered while evolving policies and programmes to take full advantage of demographic dividend.

1. **Undertake an updated National Transfer Accounts (NTA) assessment in 2022**. The NTA provides estimates of labour income, consumption, saving, and the flow of resources across age groups. One of the important contributions of the NTA analysis is to broaden our understanding on linkages between population dynamics and development. These accounts, influenced by demographic structures and trends, provide very rich and useful information for analysis and policy applications.

   Using NTA methodologies (Lee & Chen, 2016; Narayana, 2021), found that India's per capita consumption pattern deviates from the average of the Asian countries. For instance, a child in India consumes around 60% of the consumption by an adult aged 20–64, while a child in South Korea consumes about 90% of a prime-age adult's consumption on an average. The NTA data for India needs to be updated to understand consumption and production patterns to inform evidence-based policies and programmes.
2. **Address Inequalities**: India ranks poorly in terms of private human capital spending, and second to last in terms of public human capital spending in Asia (Lee & Chen, 2016). The country needs to invest more significantly in children and adolescents, particularly in early childhood coupled with nutrition components requiring careful assessments of investments vs outcomes. A greater focus needs to be on transitioning from secondary education to universal skilling and entrepreneurship, as done in Korea (Hanam, 2017).
3. **Higher Health Investments Will Be A Game Changer**: Health spending has not kept pace with India's economic growth. The public spending on health has remained flat at around 1% of GDP (average 0.9% between 2010 and 2018 compared to the global average of 5.8 and 4.5% for East Asian countries). This is now changing with the target of 2.5% of GDP by 2025. Evidence suggests that better health facilitates improved economic production, thus pointing to the importance of policies to promote health during the demographic dividend. We need both more finance for health and better health outcomes.
4. **Making reproductive health care services accessible on a rights-based Approach**: There is a need to bring quality and assured access in the free primary education and public healthcare currently provided. The high unmet need for family planning in India at 9.4% as per latest NFHS-5 (2019–2021) is high as compared to 3.3% in China, and 6.6% in South Korea or 8.0% in Thailand (World bank data), needs special attention which will eventually help women to contribute more towards economic development of the country. The burden of family planning on women needs to be reduced considerably.
5. **Education and Skill Development Are Enablers**: The gender inequality of education is a concern for India (Mason & Lee, 2013). In India, boys are more likely to be enrolled in secondary and tertiary school than girls. Though again

this is changing in the positive direction, concrete updated data from surveys is needed. In the Philippines, China and Thailand, it is the reverse. In Japan, South Korea, and Indonesia, the gender differences are rather minimal. India is one of the few countries in Asia where a large gender gap in enrolment is observed, though this gap has closed at primary levels. The focus should be on vocational and skill-oriented education which will equip the present generation to contribute more meaningfully towards economic growth of the country. The upgrading of human capital plays an important role in increasing employment, productivity, and income growth along with physical capital and technology. The estimates of the growth accounting between 1981 and 2010 suggest that human capital contributed directly as a productive input of about 22% of annual gross domestic product per worker growth in India. During the same period, it contributed around 21% in Bangladesh and 16% in Sri Lanka (ADB, 2017).

6. **Increase Female Workforce Participation**: In India, as in many countries, the Labour Force Participation Rates (LFPR) is high for males during the working ages and nearly universal in the range 25–49 but this is not the case for females. The female LFPR needs to be raised to utilise the opportunity provided by the favourable age structure. As of 2019, 20.3% of women in India are working or looking for work, down from 34.1% in 2003–04 (MOSPI, 2019). A recent study (Oxfam, 2022) which focuses on differential access to labour market (absorption and wages), factor market (access to credit) and endowment market (access to hospitalisation) indicate gender-based discrimination to be extremely high in all categories of employment in both rural and urban areas. The high degree of gender discrimination is explained by the existence of a large segment of well-qualified women not 'wanting' to join the labour market because of household responsibilities or "social status" within the community or in caste hierarchy. It is thus patriarchy that makes a large segment of women, who have the same or even higher qualifications as compared to men, stay outside employment, and this has shown no improvement over time.

   New skills and opportunities for women and girls befitting their participation in India's USD three trillion economy is urgently needed. For example, a girl who passes class X, needs more choices to undertake skills that will help her find appropriate work and meet her aspirations. South Korea's female workforce participation rate is 50% as a result of various policies including compulsory gender budgeting to analyse gender disaggregated data and its impact on policies, increasing childcare benefits, and boosting tax incentives for part time work. It is predicted that if all women engaged in domestic duties in India who are willing to work had a job, female labour force participation would increase by about 20%.

7. **Addressing Diversity between States**: While India as a whole is a young country, the status and pace of population ageing vary between the different States. Southern States, which are advanced in demographic transition like Kerala and Tamil Nadu, already have a higher percentage of older population. These differences in age structure reflect differences in economic development and health—and remind us of states' very different starting points at the outset of the 2030

Agenda. But this also offers boundless opportunities for States to work together, especially on demographic transition with the north-central region as the reservoir of India's workforce.

Acknowledgements The support, inputs and constant encouragement provided by Ms. Andrea M. Wojnar, UNFPA India Representative & Bhutan Country Director, is gratefully acknowledged.

References

Agarwal, A. K. (2016). A challenge for India to take advantage of demographic transition dividends. *Indian Journal of Health Sciences and Biomedical Research, 2016*(9), 27–30.

Asian Development Bank (ADB). (2017). Human Capital Development in South Asia. Achievements, Prospects, and Policy Challenges" Manila, Philippines. https://www.adb.org/sites/default/files/publication/385696/hcd-sa.pdf

Bloom, D., Canning, D., & Sevilla, J. (2003). *The demographic dividend: A new perspective on the economic consequences of population change* (p. 2003). RAND Corporation.

Bloom, D. E., Canning, D., & Malaney, P. N. (1999). Demographic change and economic growth in Asia (Working paper, no. 15, Center for International Development, 1999)

Carl, H., & James, G. (2011). The World at 7 Billion. *Population Bulletin, 66*, 2. For permission to reproduce portions from the Population Bulletin.

Hanam, S. P. (2017). Demographic dividend and labour force transformations in Asia: The case of the republic of Korea.

International Institute for Population Sciences and ICF. (2021). National Family Health Survey (NFHS-5), 2019–2021: India. IIPS.

James, K. S. (2011). India's demographic change: Opportunities and challenges, *Science, 333*, 576.

James, K., & Goli, S. (2017). Demographic changes in India: Is the country prepared for the challenge? *The Brown Journal of World Affairs, 23*.

James, N. G., & Jason, B. (2012). Achieving a demographic dividend. *Population Bulletin, 67*(2), 16.

Kulkarni, P. M. (2017). An assessment of demographic dividend in India and its large states, Report of United Nations Population Fund, India, UNFPA.

Lee, R., & Mason, A. (2006). What is the demographic dividend? *Finance and Development, International Monetary Fund, 43*(3).

Lee, S.-H., & Chen, Q. (2016). The economic impact of demographic change in China and India. In K. Eggleston (Ed.), *Policy challenges from demographic change in China and India* (pp. 11–31). Shorenstein Asia-Pacific Research Center.

Mason, A., & Lee, S.-H. (2013). Youth and their changing economic roles in Asia. *Asia-Pacific Population Journal, 27*(1), 61–82.

MoSPI, Government of India. (2019). Annual report: PLFS, 2017–2018, Ministry of Statistics and Programme Implementation.

Narayana, M. R. (2021). Economic inequality by age and its implications for inequity for living generations in India: Evidence based on national transfer accounts. *Asia-Pacific Journal of Regional Science, 5*, 373–396. https://doi.org/10.1007/s41685-020-00184-2

Office of the Registrar General and Census Commissioner, India. (2011). Ministry of Home Affairs, Government of India, Available at: http://www.censusindia.gov

Oxfam India. (2022). India Discrimination Report 2022, Unit. No. 412, NSIC New MDBP Building, 4th Floor, Okhla Industrial Estate.

Saad, P. M. (2009). Demographic Trends in Latin America and the Caribbean, Paper Prepared for the Workshop on Demographic Change and Social Policy organized by the World Bank at Washington.

The world Bank, https://data.worldbank.org/

United Nations Department of Economic and Social Affairs (UNDESA), Population Division. (2022). World Population Prospects 2022: Summary of Results. UN DESA/POP/2022/TR/NO. 3.

UNFPA. (2021). Population Situation Analysis–India, unpublished report.

UNFPA India. (2018). Policy brief: Harnessing India's Demographic Dividend. A differential Approach for sustainable Development.

Sanjay Kumar is working as Population Dynamics and Research Specialist at the United Nations Population Fund (UNFPA) in India. He has more than two and half decades of experience in research on population dynamics, reproductive health, nutrition and gender. He holds a Ph.D. in Demography from IIPS, Mumbai and has extensive experiences of undertaking demographic analyzes including demographic dividend, population projections, estimation of sex ratio at birth and using indirect estimation of demographic parameters. He has published many articles in reputed journals. He has been closely working with various ministries on SDG indicators and its monitoring and proving technical inputs to the large-scale data systems such as the National Family Health Survey.

Shivendra Singh is working as Data Analyst at United Nations Population Fund (UNFPA) in India. He is an experienced Monitoring and Evaluation professional with nine years of experience in research, large-scale survey design, and data analysis related to maternal and child health, sexual and reproductive health, nutrition and population dynamics. He has rich experience in program implementation and providing data-driven evidence for strategic planning and advocacy in Uttar Pradesh under UPTSU in partnership with Bill Melinda Gates Foundation. He has been involved in developing several interventions related to family planning, women and child health and strengthened the labor room facilities and family participatory care system in Odisha, and worked closely with government counterparts for implantation and capacity building programs related to family planning and maternal-child health. He is a master's graduate in Population Studies from the International Institute for Population Sciences, Mumbai, India.

Jaydeep Biswas is the Chief of Policy, Advocacy and Partnerships, UNFPA India, which includes leading policy work, population dynamics and research, communications and media, innovation and technology and strategic partnerships. Previously, he was Senior Governance Advisor and Acting Team Leader (DFID India Global Program) for the FCDO/DFID India. As Governance Adviser in UK DFID he led program and policy work in multiple sectors (health and nutrition, urban development, governance and institutions, public financial management and anti-corruption, civil service reforms and civil society) and countries (India, Nepal, Ethiopia, Bangladesh, Sierra Leone, Myanmar and the UK). Jay has a Master's in Governance and Development from IDS, University of Sussex, UK. He is a British Chevening Scholar. He speaks English, Hindi, Bengali and moderate Odiya and Nepali. Other interests include; music, cricket, traveling, poetry, physics and history

Chapter 10
Positive People and Confident Competitors: Resilient Youth Development Through Sport and Physical Activity

Sahen Gupta and K. Jayasankara Reddy

> *Sports teaches you character, it teaches you to play by the rules, it teaches you to know what it feels like to win and lose- it teaches you about life—Billie Jean King*

Abstract In the altering world scenario, there is a necessity to plan, prepare and progress with youth development. Research has associated positive youth development with the 5Cs model (competence, confidence, connection, character and caring) (Lerner et al., The Journal of Early Adolescence 25:17–71, 2005) to build resilience in youth. Over the past 35 years, sport psychology has established that sport helps in developing necessary psychological skills and attributes among youth. Youth sport is an extracurricular activity that provides young people with unique negative and positive experiences. Within these experiences, the individual goes beyond the self and has to work with a diverse group of others for self-development and achievement of shared goals. In this chapter, our primary objective is to review the foundations of literature concerning confidence, resilience and identity as cornerstones for positive youth development through sport. To achieve this objective, we adopt a global approach blending field experience from participatory sport, developmental sport and elite sport to provide an intervention framework grounded in applied sport psychology. Intervention framework provided is aligned to the COM-B behaviour change model (Michie et al. 2011) for sustainable change. The focus is on a balance between developing stable protective factors for mental health and positive youth development to ensure appropriate cognitive, social, emotional and

S. Gupta (✉)
Sport & High-Performance Psychologist/Lecturer in Applied Sport Psychology, University of Portsmouth, Portsmouth, UK
e-mail: sahen.gupta@port.ac.uk

School of Sport, Health & Exercise Sciences, University of Portsmouth, Portsmouth, UK

K. J. Reddy
Department of Psychology, CHRIST (Deemed to be University), Bengaluru, India

S. Deb and S. Deb (eds.), *Handbook of Youth Development*,
https://doi.org/10.1007/978-981-99-4969-4_10

behaviour skills to thrive in an evolving world. Implications for transferring this learning cross-culturally and in non-sport contexts such as schools and grass-root programs are discussed with recommendation for good practice.

Keywords Positive youth development · Adaptation · Life skills · Mental health · Intervention

Introduction

For decades sport has been touted as a domain where children not only acquire physical skills, but also attain important psychosocial milestones that generalize to life situations (Wiggins, 2013). This is perfectly illustrated in the quote above by Billie Jean King. However, scientific studies dating back to pre-1950s illustrate that sport participation does not *automatically* lead to favorable outcomes. Rather, there are just as many examples of negative maladaptive experiences due to misguided/inappropriate coach behaviors, parental and peer pressures as well as other adversities that are present in the environment of sport and physical activity (Fraser-Thomas & Côté, 2009). This has led to the focus on structured research on sporting context and its related social and environmental factors associated with the development of positive behavioral and psychosocial traits in youth (see Weiss & Gill, 2005; Weiss, 2016). Tracing historical developments in sport as a context for youth development, Weiss titles this body of scientific inquiry in sport as "old wine in a new bottle" (Weiss, 2016, p. 7).

Positive youth development (PYD) is a strengths-based approach in which the youth are facilitated to identify their own competencies, interests to ensure consistent psychosocial developmental growth. Some foundational work in this area originated from Larson's (2000) work on initiative development via structured voluntary activities of sport, art and others to encourage individuals to experience deep attention, psychosocial growth and intrinsic motivation. In the years since, greater perspectives have been integrated within PYD in the larger field of psychology (see Damon, 2004; Lerner et al., 2009; Shek et al., 2019). Within this chapter, we align ourselves to the framework provided by Petitpas et al. (2005a, 2005b) that integrated the PYD framework with youth sport literature. The key definitions of the same include: (a) *Context* as any intrinsically motivated sport/physical activity based activity in a psychologically safe environment; (b) *External Assets* as compassionate, caring, empathetic coaches, adults, peers; (c) *Internal* aspects of skills that are learned (both life skills and sport skills). Building upon Petitpas et al. (2005a, 2005b) we differentiate youth sport from performance sport. *Youth sport* refers to the participation, engagement and acquisition of skills via skill-building activities whereas *Performance Sport* refers to contexts where there is a deliberate focus on mastering sport and mental skills to compete against peers at high skill levels with constant evaluative conditions. This distinction is important, because the pressures associated with performance sport typically do not lead to favorable conditions for PYD on its own.

In this chapter, our primary objectives are (a) To outline PYD in sport and physical activity; (b) Outline the outcomes of PYD in sport; (c) To showcase the impact of PYD elements with case based examples. We do not limit ourselves to outcomes in the sport context. Rather, we look at youth development holistically, by focusing on mechanisms that create positive people and confident competitors in the face of failures, difficulty, and adversity. By adopting this lens, we look at resilient youth development- resilience in the context of adaptation post adversity but also resilience to maintain mental health and achieve developmental milestones. We start with outlining the role of resilience in PYD before exploring the relationships between PYD and sport/physical activity. Following this theoretical overview, we focus on showing case examples from applied sport psychology practice of first author (SG) and literature to contextualize the *how-to* achieve PYD to develop positive people, confident competitors and resilient youth.

Positive Youth Development Through Sport and Physical Activity

Positive Youth Development (PYD) is an area of study that has sparked increased interest recently (Qi et al., 2022). However, PYD is backed up with nearly a century of research in what was known as 'youth development via sport' (see Weiss, 2016). Briefly tracing the historical development of this area, C.H. McCloy was one of the earliest proponents of youth development in sport, discussing the role of physical education in the character building of youth (McCloy, 1930). McCloy (1930, 1933) focused on 'character education' i.e., "learning basis of conduct, or the determiners of conduct" (McCloy, 1930) highlighting that it is the duty of the physical educator to oversee the development of youth in the appropriate direction (McCloy, 1930). Following on in the 1950s, explorations were initiated into the relationship between sociometric status and athletic ability was found to be moderately high (McCraw & Tolbert, 1953). Sociometric status was defined as the extent to which individuals gain or fail to gain status in the group linking it to youth development (McCraw & Tolbert, 1953). Building upon the work of McCloy and others, Gould defined youth sport research as "studies focussing on sports programs for children and youth, typically between the ages of 7 and 18 years" (Gould, 1982, p. 204).

In the 1990s, the literature trends were focused on the deficit model of adolescent development which viewed youth as "problems to be managed" (Burkhard et al., 2019). The attention was mainly on dealing with problems such as conflicts, drug abuse, alcohol consumption and mood disruptions (Arnett, 1999). PYD, defined as the "process of growth and increasing competence" (Larson, 2000, p. 170) emerged as a prominent area of scientific research to counter this deficit model (Burkhard et al., 2019). The early 2000s saw a shift in focus to Athletic Participation (AP) in school which is purposeful and active participation in sports-related physical activities (Deelen et al., 2018). It was observed that AP had a positive impact on various variables like school grades, coursework selection, self-esteem, subsequent college enrolment, and highest educational level (Marsh & Klietman, 2003; Robst & Keil, 2000). Evidence also indicated links between athletic participation and competence to belongingness and social status (Smith, 2003).

In recent years, PYD is a multidimensional concept viewed as an umbrella term centered around how children and adolescents achieve optimal developmental experiences through involvement in organized activities (Neely & Holt, 2011). For example, sport as a medium for fostering PYD has started to evolve with programs incorporating life skills (Danish et al., 2005), sport and mental health among disadvantaged marginalized youth (Gupta & Sudhesh, 2019; Parker et al., 2019; Sudhesh et al., 2021). Sudhesh et al. (2021) designed and implemented a long-term intervention program for children and adolescents with HIV/AIDS using sport as an intervention element to help individuals form effective relationships, positive interaction experiences and develop self-concept. Other studies have shown sports to be an effective medium via which information on HIV/AIDS and safe sexual practices can be provided to the youth (Coalter, 2010; Coakley 2011). Therefore, PYD is seen to promote positive long-term psychosocial outcomes (Allan et al., 2017).

Consolidated, this body of research on PYD has demonstrated outcomes such as emotional regulation, resilience, and the achievement of development milestones (Vandell et al., 2015; Zarrett et al., 2009). This has impacted well-being research since PYD has been explicitly related to subjective well-being (SWB) (Park, 2004; Pilkauskaite-Valickiene & Gabrialaviciute, 2015). SWB includes how people view, appraise, and evaluate their own life (Diener et al., 2018). It also includes both reflection in terms of cognitive judgements, such as life satisfaction, and emotional responses to ongoing life (Diener et al., 2018) and is a key indicator of positive youth development (Park, 2004). Another associated outcome with successful PYD is emotional regulation (Wang et al., 2015) defined as the conscious and unconscious strategies used to maintain and control one or more components of an emotional response (Gross, 2001, 2020). It helps youth manage impulses, make informed decisions and be persistent towards goals (Buckley & Saarni, 2009). Additionally, emotional regulation facilitates self-efficacy, prosocial behavior and maintains supportive relationships with family and/or peers (Buckley & Saarni, 2009). PYD via sport participation has also been identified to promote resilience in young people with numerous adverse childhood experiences (Norris & Norris, 2021) or emergency situations such as the ongoing global pandemic (Gupta & McCarthy, 2021). Exposure to sport within a supportive framework increases environmentally relevant problem solving and behaviors that allow adaptation to stressors (Jacobson & Matthaeus, 2014), which has transferability as a life skill. Overall, recent literature indicates sport to be a context for youth's physical and psychosocial development (see Holt, 2016).

PYD, Sport and Physical Activity Through Developmental Periods

In India, nearly 36% of the population participated in sport or physical activity with the majority of them in the age bracket of 15–24 years (BBC, 2020). The representative statistics in the US ranges at about 45 million children and adolescents in regular sport with 75% of American families reporting that at least one school aged child participates in an organized sport (Merkel, 2013). In the UK, about 40% of youth of ages 16 years and older participate in at least one sport every week (Khan et al., 2012). Involvement in sport is shown to have positive effects on social interaction, building confidence, improving listening skills and overall health (Khan et al., 2012; Vierimaa et al., 2012).

PYD views youth as assets (Flanagan et al., 2007). It has its essence in the belief that healthy development can transform youth into competent resources that society can benefit from (Dillard et al., 2019). This allows a major focus on building competence which is one's positive views of one's actions in the different areas of life including social, academic, cognitive, health, and vocational contexts (Lerner et al., 2005). Through sport, PYD finds itself an avenue for change. Participation in sports has been linked to several positive outcomes (Bailey, 2006). Studies have found a relationship between sports participation and all indices of self-esteem i.e., our judgement and evaluations on how we perceive ourselves and our capacities (Bowker, 2006; Slutzky & Simpkins, 2009). Literature has also found that social responsibility has a positive outcome of sports participation. Participation in physical activity and active sports practice are associated with a higher development of personal and social responsibility (Cómez-Mármol et al., 2017). Increased sport participation is also positively related to improved mental health of children and adolescents (Hiremath, 2019; Steiner et al., 2000). The World Health Organisation defines mental health as "a state of well-being where an individual realises his or her own abilities and can cope with the normal stresses of life". In addition to the psychological, physical and social, and academic benefits described above, youth sport participation has also been associated with positive health behaviors such as right food choices and positive body image (Sabiston et al., 2019). There is evidence of pro-social behavior and reduced crime rates. For example, individuals who do not participate in sport and physical activities, exhibit higher levels of drunk driving, use of drugs, trespassing, shoplifting and juvenile criminal activities as compared to individuals who participate in sport (Taylor et al., 2015). Detailed outline of evidence is provided in Table 10.1 below.

The positive outcomes associated with PYD extend but are not limited to the factors mentioned in Table 10.1. Development within humans does not happen in isolation; there are developmental cascades interlinked with each other (Lewan-Bizan et al., 2010). The outcomes brought about because of PYD help with the overall development of youth. The next section outlines the emergent cognitive and psychosocial development outcomes for individuals achieved through sport and PYD.

Table 10.1 Positive outcomes as a result of participation in sport

Outcome	Summary of evidence	Further Reading
Social skills	Sport promotes outcomes like social skills and positive behaviors. It helps in facilitating personal growth and development among youth. Working towards sport development may also help with fostering personal development and increased social skills	Bruner et al. (2017), Taylor et al. (2015), Santos and Martinek (2018)
Emotional Skills	Literature has found links between sport and positive psychological development. A study revealed those involved in sports experienced higher levels of subjective well-being in their day-to-day life	Fraser-Thomas et al. (2007), Greenleaf et al. (2009)
Physical and psychomotor development	Participation in sport is seen to help develop motor coordination in childhood. This further helps in development of motor skills, which are required to perform everyday activities such as running, climbing, and other functional activities	Vandorpe et al. (2011), Brown and Fletcher (2017)
Decision making skills	Sports such as soccer, football, rugby and volleyball are seen to have significant contribution towards decision-making abilities among athletes	Kaya (2014), Khan and Khan (2019)
Problem solving skills	It has been found that physical exertion leads to short-term relaxation, enhanced creativity and memory, along with better mood, and improved problem-solving abilities	Douyon et al. (2010), Jacobson and Matthaeus (2014)
Attention and memory skills	Studies have suggested a positive relationship between participation in sports with attention and concentration	Voss et al. (2010), Howard et al. (2018), Nethravathi and Sreenivas (2020)

Psychosocial Development and Sport

"Psychosocial"—the term, was coined somewhere around the 1890s (Hayward, 2012). By definition, the psychosocial approach looks at combining the areas of influence due to social factors and a person's behavior (Vizzoto et al., 2013). Erikson's theory of psychosocial development gives a framework for studying human development through the lifespan (Cherry, 2020). Another pioneer in the field of development is Piaget, who gave an extended view on a person's cognitive or intellectual development. His theory was one of the first to focus on cognitive development, and it helped formulate a body of research in the area of children's thinking (Miller, 2011). We trace the outcomes through the psychosocial and cognitive development of individuals in relation to how it unfolds in the context of sport and physical activity.

The stages of development as they unfold as a consequence of PYD through sport are outlined below in Table 10.2.

Table 2 Psychosocial approach to development and links to sport participation

Age group	Eriksonian stages	Key markers	In sport	Piaget stages
18 months to 3 years	Autonomy versus Shame	Children begin to develop a sense of autonomy (e.g.; personal control). If encouraged by primary caregivers, they develop self-confidence. If not given the opportunity to express autonomy, they may become overly dependent on others	Actions like throwing a ball and running to stop an object on their own (autonomy) may begin	During Piaget's Sensorimotor stage, infants build reflexes in response to the environment. Learning to use their arms and legs together will have an advantage in sports where accuracy and speed are essential (Leppo et al., 2000)
4 to 6 years	Initiative versus Guilt	Children begin to take more initiative (eg; during play) and interact more with counterparts. If this is stopped by caregivers, children experience guilt	As children become more interactive and take initiative, they begin to indulge in team play. Starting team sports at this stage could help foster this further	Physical activity of some form at the Preoperational stage would allow children to develop verbal and non-verbal communication skills through interaction with peers
7 to 12 years	Industry versus Inferiority	As children begin to read and write, they develop a sense of competency (*industry*). If they are unable to develop a certain skill that their fellow peers may be developing, they may have a sense of inferiority	There is a desire to be good at what they do to develop competency. Sport participation and success will help foster that	At the concrete operational stage, starting individual training at this stage may be beneficial. Children are now capable of acquiring fundamental training, which will help develop their sport (Kushner et al., 2015)

(continued)

Table 2 (continued)

Age group	Eriksonian stages	Key markers	In sport	Piaget stages
13 to 18 years	Identity versus Role Confusion	There is a major transition, the one from childhood to adulthood. The (now) adolescent feels a certain need to fit in and develop a sense of identity. If this is not fostered, they may begin to get confused about who they really are	Interactions with peers in a team environment and sport participation helps develop a sense of identity. Although, balancing sport with academics may lead to some kind of role confusion	At the Formal Operational stage, there is now an improvement in reasoning abilities A more technical direction can now be applied to training to help develop the sport (Kushner et al., 2015)
19 to 39 years	Intimacy versus Isolation	There is a need to form intimate and loving relationships for the young adult. If there's a lack of intimacy, it may lead to loneliness		

A major focus of this theory was on the development of social identity during late childhood and through years of adolescence. Children begin to form relationships beyond the members of their family and derive their sense of self from these interactions with others. They go through a period of identity vs role confusion (Erikson, 1968). This framework and knowledge of the developmental trajectories of individuals is an important point of consideration, since PYD emphasizes on the importance of strengthening developmental assets in youth (Matos et al., 2018). The specific area of development that needs to be considered is resilience since evidence indicates links between resilience and psychosocial development in children (Luthar, 2013; Masten & Wright, 2010; Sunaina et al., 2019). Resilience and developmental outcomes have been found to be highly correlated concepts (Svetina, 2014). The section that follows provides a comprehensive outline of resilience and PYD, with areas of application.

Resilience and PYD: Existing Evidence and Applied Applications

In developmental psychology, a longitudinal study by Werner (1989) among a cohort of children in Kauai kicked off resilience research. This study followed children over a period of 10 years and found that one-third of the children did not exhibit delinquent/destructive behavior despite parental difficulty. They were labelled as 'resilient'. In the decades since, the scientific inquiry on resilience has sought to define resilience and find antecedent 'protective factors' that promote resilience in children, youth and adults. Masten (2007) traced this development across four waves with the current fourth wave focusing on assimilating existing knowledge and looking at integrative theoretical applications. PYD through resilience principles gleaned from sport psychology and developmental research is one such avenue.

What is Resilience?

There have been multiple definitions of resilience proposed in the diverse sub-disciplines of psychology. Resilience is viewed as a dynamic ability which can change over time as individuals learn and interact with the environment (Gupta, 2021; Gupta & McCarthy, 2021). Masten et al. (1990) highlighted resilience as a capacity to adapt in challenging/threatening circumstances with a significant part of resilience being the return to normal levels post failure/setback via 'bounce-back' (Wald et al., 2006). For example, an individual experiences a failure (personal loss of any magnitude, failure in academic/sport). Following the failure, the individual uses their resilience ability to process the event and adapt to return to normal functioning post failure.

Luthar et al. (2000) characterized resilience to be "a dynamic process encompassing positive adaptation within the context of significant adversity ... implicit within this notion are two critical conditions: (1) exposure to significant threat or severe adversity; and (2) the achievement of positive adaptation despite major assaults on the developmental process" (p. 545). This significant threat ranges from acute stressors such as major injury, personal loss, environmental disasters or violence (Masten & Narayan, 2012) or a string of low-intensity chronic stressors such as consistent academic stress, unsupportive parenting, racial/gender discrimination, lack of cultural acknowledge (Ungar et al., 2013). These may also take the form of significant challenges to the individual's developmental process such as loss of family members or constant movement of geographic location of a developing child (Walsh, 2020). In such cases, resilience protects against arrested development.

It is important to note that resilience is not static, but rather a result of interaction between dynamic processes that the individual uses to adapt in such adversity situations (Rutter, 2013; Masten, 2014). Luthar et al. (1993, 2000) conceptualized resilience as a continuum of adaptation resulting in success. This was further formalized in the evidence highlighting the 'trajectory' of resilience post adversity (see Bonanno & Diminich, 2015). Resilience is determined by a combination of socio-cultural, psychological and biological factors that interact with one another to determine the resilient response (Southwick et al., 2014). Research has revealed specific psychological (Bonanno & Diminich, 2013; Luthar et al., 2000; Tugade & Frederickson, 2004); environmental (Charney, 2004; Stassen et al., 2007); or genetic factors (Feder et al., 2008; Southwick & Charney, 2012; Tannenbaum & Anisman, 2003). Resilient individuals develop adaptive psychological resources for effective coping through this combination of factors (Giudice et al., 2011).

Resilience in Sport and Physical Activity

Resilience is the psychosocial variable that determines positive adaptation when faced with difficulties and adversities during the course of participation in sport and physical activity (Sarkar & Fletcher, 2014). Evidence in sport and exercise psychology indicates resilience to be a dynamic process where multiple factors and influences such as parents, coaches, rivals, athletes, environment among others play a role (Gupta & McCarthy, 2021, 2022; see also Montpetit et al., 2010; Stainton et al., 2019). Specifically, the definition of resilience in sport was initially proposed by Fletcher and Sarkar (2012) in a grounded theory study to be "the role of mental processes and behaviour in promoting personal assets and protecting an individual from the potential negative effect of stressors" (p. 675).

Developing on this conceptualization, Gupta and McCarthy (2022) proposed the meta conceptualization of 'Sporting Resilience' which is the interaction dominant, environmentally adaptable, dynamic process trajectory that incorporates "metacognitive-emotional-behavioural" capacities to allow the individual to operate at an equilibrium and positively adapt during adversity (Gupta & McCarthy, in-press A, p.7). Within this conceptualization, there are several protective factors of which determine the trajectory of resilience. These protective factors and how they aid PYD are outlined in detail in Table 10.3.

Resilience and PYD

The involvement of resilience in PYD can be classified into two connected but distinguishable levels. At the first level, resilience is a pre-requisite for successful PYD outcomes (Sanders et al., 2015). Individuals and service-delivery providers need to develop resilience to stay on course to adhere to the interventions and practices required for PYD (Camiré & Santos, 2019; Lerner et al., 2019; Spencer & Spencer, 2014). By its very nature, PYD is a long-term process ranging from late childhood to young adulthood (see Larson & Tran, 2014). This involves a planned but incremental approach to behavior change across months and years at a time. The transtheoretical model of change (Prochaska & DiClemente, 1984, 1997) is an important theoretical tool to help psychologists and professionals examine organizational and individual change for PYD across time. Furthermore, evidence indicates resilient systems and individual resilience abilities allow the individual to adhere to this change across the stages of change in emergencies (Mundorf et al., 2018), employment and occupation (Berstene, 2014); bereavement (Calederwood, 2011), physical activity and exercise behavior (Jiménez-Zazo et al., 2020; Nigg & Courneya, 1998; Ramenzanzade et al., 2016; Rostami et al., 2017; see for systematic review Spencer et al., 2006) and in psychological skills training in competitive sport (Keeler, 2006; Leffingwell et al., 2001). The process of change through the transtheoretical model and the role of resilience are illustrated in Fig. 10.1.

Table 10.3 Protective factors of resilience and PYD

Resilience protective resources	Definition	Role in PYD
Metacognitive-challenge appraisal	Process utilized to plan, monitor and assess adversity as challenging and having adequate ability and personal resources to grow and master from adversity experience (Fletcher & Sarkar, 2012; Gupta & McCarthy, 2021)	Assets and resources can be used to promote PYD in order to unearth the adaptations and strengths developed by youth under adversity (Barbarin et al., 2020)
Perceived/Tangible social support	The perception of and/or the actuality that an individual has the provision of assistance in the form of emotional/psychological support, informational and tangible support (Brown et al., 2015; Galli & Vealey, 2008; Fletcher & Sarkar, 2013)	PYD is seen to have a positive influence on the well-being of at-risk youth (O'Toole et al., 2019). This influence is facilitated by the support of family and community (O'Toole et al., 2019). Additionally, social support has been linked to having a healthy lifestyle (Lee & Sibley, 2019)
Self-regulation ability	The ability to control one's thoughts/emotions/behavior disruptive to the pursuit of their short- & long-term goals (Gupta & Sudhesh, 2019; Kegelaers et al., 2019)	The ability to intentionally self-regulate is seen to be a precursor of development across different contexts (Gestsdottir et al., 2017). An adolescent's ability to self-regulate may also facilitate the impact extra-curricular participation has on development of youth (Urban et al., 2010)
Sense of control	Broadly defined as mastery and sense of control over one's life circumstances within and outwith of sport (Fletcher & Sarkar, 2012; Gupta & McCarthy, 2021)	Participation in physical activities as a medium of promoting PYD may give the youth an opportunity to have real-world goals, along with giving them a sense of control (Ramey & Rose-Krasnor, 2011)
Facilitative environment	The physical and psychological sporting environment of the individual which adequately balances challenge and support to optimize positive growth, performance and resilience (Fletcher & Sarkar, 2016; Wagstaff et al., 2016)	A facilitative environment fosters the growth of PYD, including the promotion and transfer of life skills (Newman et al., 2021)

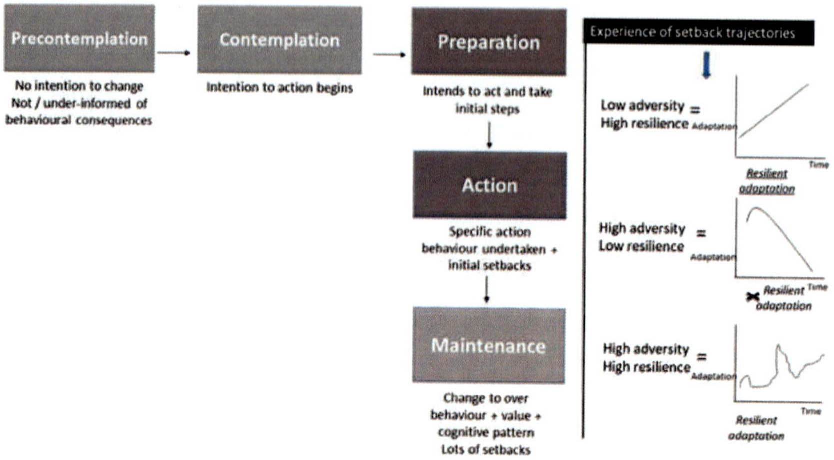

Fig. 10.1 PYD and resilience outcomes mapped in the transtheoretical model of change

At the second level, resilience is an *outcome* of PYD. By the process of effective PYD, children grow up to become resilient youths. Sport is one great arena where this can be established with effective and well-designed practices. Participation in sport and physical activity allows individuals to develop and practice several life skills (Danish et al., 2005; Gould & Carson, 2008) and existential skills (Ronkainen et al., 2021). For example, immigrant and refugee youth participation in sport allowed resilience development against the challenges to relocation to a new country and facilitated adaptation to related challenges (Kaya et al., 2014). Hughes et al. (2018) has indicated that youth sport participation allows individuals to build friendships/ social networks, access to role models all of which reduce lifetime mental illness. The mechanism of this 'resilient' PYD is the link of resilience with wellbeing and the healthy individual who can adaptively interact with specific environments (see Cowen, 1991). Regular physical exercise and sport acts as a 'controllable stressor' (Salmon, 2001). This allows the youth to dynamically interact with the environment to build the protective filter of resilience resources that facilitated positive adaptation (Gupta & McCarthy, 2022). Furthermore, sport participation also allows resilience resources to be accessed when sport is unavailable. For example, Gupta and McCarthy (2021) explored the narratives of resilience among athletes during COVID-19 and reported that sport support, identity and the challenge appraisal resources facilitated resilience even when sport was not regular. Sport also allows the building of emotional regulation mechanisms and behavioral regulation which is a protective factor promoting resilience (Bernstein & McNally, 2018). The defeat and failure experienced within controlled environments that promote facilitative learning led to the development of resilience in individuals (Fletcher & Sarkar, 2016).

Positive People and Confident Competitors: Resilience and Positive Development in Action

Building upon the literature on PYD reviewed above through the lens of PYD, human development models and resilience, we can illustrate that PYD through sport and physical activity is associated with positive outcomes. From SGs sport psychology practice, given below is the outline of a case. The case has two versions presented. The first provides the potential trajectory of where the development is headed, prior to SG's intervention. The second version shows SG's intervention and its succeeding outcome. We discuss with PYD, the impact of parental pressure, social relationships and peer support on youth via sport.

Case Vignette: *Diya Vanseka (pseudonym) is a 13-year-old female. She is currently studying in 8th standard in middle school and has no siblings. Diya's mother was an Indian cricketer, now coach and her father is a banker at the top of his profession. From an early age she had a passion for cricket and tennis as her sports and she was always encouraged at it. As a shy, reserved child she found sport to be a source of identity and self-belief as she was a 'natural'. t school, Diya has 2 friends, but finds it difficult to make new ones. She is often seen as the 'odd' one out and has proclaimed to her parents that 'she will never be confident'.*

Within the case vignette highlighted above, there are some key elements that are relevant to understanding how Diya could become a positive person and confident competitor through a focused intervention/support implementation of resilience based PYD. The client is at the age where psychosocial development is ongoing (see Pettipas et al., 2005), and within her social sphere she has two 'successful' examples of modelled behavior in her parents (Rouquette et al., 2020). As it stands, there is no pathology nor anything 'wrong' with Diya. Applying the principles of PYD, the focus should be on (a) facilitating an honest discovery of self-expression which links to her self-esteem (see Whitehead & Corbin, 1997); (b) social relationships and how she navigates them; (c) her relationship with others in the sporting environment and the sport environment as being facilitative (Fletcher & Sarkar, 2016); (d) focus on building the protective factors of resilience through direct or indirect interventions (see Table 10.3).

We explore the case through two alternate scenarios below. In one scenario, we trace the development of the individual with little or no application of PYD principles. Specifically, we highlight areas of deficiency which prevents Diya from becoming a resilient youth able to have the resources to adapt to adversity. In scenario B, we outline how Diya's development occurs when the principles of PYD and resilience youth development in sport are applied. In both scenarios, we frame the analysis of the applied case within the literature and following the cases provide recommendations for implementation in applied psychology practice.

Case Alternate A: No PYD Through Sport Principles

> Diya continued to take part in her sport. Her mother sees her natural talent in cricket and works to confirm an early specialisation in cricket and decides to coach Diya herself. By the time she is 14, Diya is committed to full-time cricket and plays nationals at age categories u16 and u18. She is touted as a 'future star'. Her father expects her to complete her education as well. Although her school is accommodating with her schedule due to performance sport, she slowly finds it difficult to manage a balance. The highly competitive nature of sport and her coach's insistence on 'total commitment to cricket' improves her skills greatly but internally she still does not feel confident enough. When she has a one-month gap in sport due to an ankle injury, she feels lost and has little to no sense of who she is. At age 16, Diya starts competing in the senior open category and does well which fast tracks her to the national squad for an international bilateral series. Diya's debut series is a challenge for her, and she feels unsupported. She feels a complete lack of positive influences in her life since everyone just wants her to be a cricketer. Being away from home and school has also meant that she barely has any time with her two close friends who Diya feels are 'moving on in their lives without her' and she cannot just be a teenage girl. Diya feels drained as now her sport demands more of her and she is experiencing more failures as well, but she struggled to adapt and bounce back. One day as she was waiting for an MRI scan, the technician asked her as they were setting up, 'so apart from cricket, what do you do?'. Diya had no answer, and genuinely felt that her life had no meaning as the one thing which she had given everything to, was the only thing which defined her.

Critical review evidence questions whether youth sport is a "friend or foe" (McKay et al., 2019, p. 141), since if inappropriately managed youth sport harms PYD. Despite its many known benefits, among females, sport participation declines through adolescence (Crane & Temple, 2015). Some factors associated with female sport dropout are competing academic and social commitments, development of alternative interests, issues around self-presentation as puberty occurs, gender roles and parental pressures which lead to nearly 70% female sport dropout (Crane & Temple, 2015; O'Sullivan, 2013). We see these competing difficulties in the case above which may increase performance pressure leading to pre-performance anxiety (Aravind et al., 2022). Diya has indirect parental pressure since her parents (especially mother) is a high-performance individual herself with a history in the sport. She also must balance sport and social competing causing strain on her relationship with friends.

Although there are no explicit gender role conformity issues, she does have to stop being 'just be a teenage girl' due to the pressures involved to succeed at sport. Her injuries also had significant physiological and psychological consequences with feelings of isolation, loss of motivation, fear of reinjury, stress and loss of identity (Podlog & Eklund, 2006; Wiese-Bjornstal et al., 1998). As she ages, the adolescent Diya transitions into late adolescence affording her a greater capacity to engage in abstract thinking, learning and sophistication reasoning (Blakemore, 2012a, 2012b). She is able to explore her emotions and identify the emotions of others as well. Diya is in a stage of identity vs. role confusion, according to Erikson's stages of psychosocial development. She is undergoing a major transformation from childhood to adulthood. She may feel a need to develop a sense of identity. Her interactions with peers in the team environment would play a major role in identity formation. According to

Piaget's theory, Diya is in the formal operational stage of development. At this stage, the reasoning abilities improve, and technicalities can be worked on in terms of sport.

A major area where the lack of PYD principles in her developmental support impacts her is her process of identity formation. Athletic and self-identity area key features in the ages of 15–18, within the developmental process of the individual (see Table 10.2). Athletic identity refers to the level to which being an athlete dominates the self-perception and social roles of the individual who partakes in sport and physical activity (Houle et al., 2010). A strong and exclusive athletic identity risks identity foreclosure where there is a loss of non-sport identity and could become an Achilles heel where the individual may pursue performance in sport at the detriment to their own mental health and well-being (see Brewer et al., 1993). When combined with the stressors in sport at the level Diya is competing (see Mellalieu et al., 2009), it severely compromises Diya's development of resilience resources and does not enable her holistic development according to PYD.

Diya has been exposed to the high stressors that are present in the elite competitive sport but has simultaneously lost her social support network, which is a major protective factor of resilience. The pressures and demands of top-level sport also mean that her time is also split between sport and academics, which does not afford her any time for self-regulation and self-reflection which is reported to be a key part of understanding one's identity and contributes to resilience (Crane et al., 2018; Gupta & McCarthy, 2021). Diya's parent is her coach, which may also impact the coach-athlete relationship adding to further stress and lack of space for parental support in sport (Burke et al., 2021). The environment Diya is focused on high performance and is not facilitative at all times. This increases threat appraisals of any setbacks and adversities allowing greater difficulty in resilient adaptation (Fletcher & Sarkar, 2016; Meijen et al., 2020).

This leads to a lack of PYD in Diya, a tough environment with minimal support, limited/no development of protective resources that promote resilience leading to a major compromise in her holistic development. Diya is already showing an externalized self-worth at age 17, where her self-esteem is linked to success in sport. Evidence indicates that this becomes a major issue when sport transition occurs or athletes as adults have to find a life outside sport (Findlay & Bowker, 2009; Newman et al., 2016). However, this need not be this way. Integrating the principles of PYD, we can use sport participation to benefit the development of a holistic self-esteem in the person (Fox & Lindwall, 2014; Richman & Shaffer, 2000; Slutzky & Simpkins, 2009; Smoll et al., 1993; Whitehead & Corbin, 1997).

When this lack of PYD and resilience resource development occurs, the individual gets stuck at the contemplation, preparation, or initial action stage in the transtheoretical model in their response to adversity and trajectory of development (see Fig. 10.2). Diya pre-contemplates change and begins to plan avenues for change. However, as she prepares and begins her initial action, she is faced with setbacks and adversities. Due to her lack of holistic positive perception of self, low mastery and high threat perception of these setbacks, the preparation and action is ineffective. This stunts her development and pushes her back at pre-contemplation for another avenue of action,

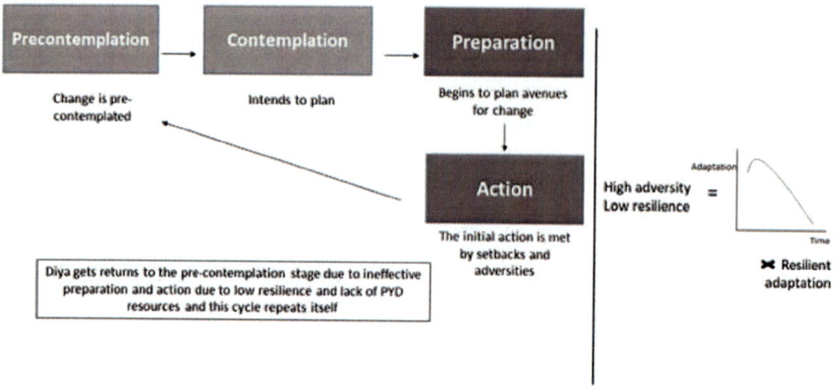

Fig. 10.2 Analysis of case alternate A with PYD and resilience outcomes

where the cycle repeats (see Fig. 10.2). As Diya develops, this will increase over-thinking and maladaptive perfectionism tendencies in Diya (Flett & Hewitt, 2016; Sellars et al., 2016). This will predispose her to anxiety symptoms and compromise her mental health (Flett et al., 2016) and leave her identity development unresolved (MacPherson et al., 2016).

Case Alternate B: Applying PYD Though Sport Principles in SG's Practice

> Diya continued to take part in her sport. Her mother sees her natural talent in cricket and works to confirm an early specialisation in cricket and decides to coach Diya herself. Both her parents emphasise that it is important for Diya to think about why she plays cricket and the values that she wants to have for the rest of her life. By the time she is 14, Diya has a long discussion with her parents who want her to take charge. She decides that she wants her mother to be her mother and not her coach. Her mother agrees and supports her as a parent. At this stage she decides to commit to 'trying her level best in cricket'. Diya (aged 14) plays nationals at age categories u16 and u18. She is touted as a 'future star'. At the age of 15, Diya realises that she needs to work on understanding herself more. Her coach recommends her to work with a sport psychologist. Working with the sport psychologist, Diya explores her values of hard work, being okay with failure, building mental models to adapt and how to understand her emotions. She considers sport to be a 'lab' since she 'gets to try out things and figure herself out'. Aged 16, Diya starts competing in the senior open category and does well which fast tracks her to the national squad for an international bilateral series. Diya makes it a point to actively communicate with her coach about her availability after understanding if her body and mind needs a break. During these moments she spends time with her friends and family. She has study groups with her two close friends to help her catch up with school, and also makes it a point to be available to them over call or text when she is away for sport. Often, she arranged for them to come visit during home matches as well. Diya slowly understands herself and is confident in her ability to compete and has accepted that she will sometimes fail. At her debut international bilateral series, Diya finds the step up

to be a challenge and fails to meet her own expectations. Although disappointed, she does not spiral but takes ownership of why that happened. Working with her sport psychologist and coach, she makes a plan on how to develop and learn further to keep competing at the highest level. Diya does not return to the international side till she is 19 but has kept an active communication loop with the governing body and coaches. She graduates school with her classmates and joins one of her friends at University studying history.

Literature shows that adult figures such as sports staff and parents play a crucial role in the development of life skills and facilitating learning (Hermens et al., 2017). In Diya's case, her parents showcase effective emotional and autonomy which promotes perceived self-control and social responsibility (McDonough et al., 2013). This is exemplified by her mother asking her what she wants to do with sport and allowing the space and support for Diya to autonomously make the decision about who she wants to be coached by and how she wants to proceed in sport. This case example from the field showcases what research evidence highlights in terms of parental/caregiver involvement and support in youth sports leading to PYD outcomes (Newman et al., 2016). Diya achieves two major PYD outcomes namely: (a) autonomy and decision-making in relation to sport and her life; (b) control and motivational processes regarding choices made in her support systems increasing social responsibility (Ryan & Deci, 2020). This is indicative of the resolution of the conflict between identity and role confusion.

Another key area of PYD outcomes seen in this case is the interpersonal relationship between the child and key adult figures in their life. In Diya's case her relationships are positive and well supported (e.g., mother, father, coach, sport psychologist). This facilitates her intrapersonal development and prosocial behaviour (Anderson-Butcher et al., 2004; McDonough et al., 2013). Specifically, she displays greater self-reflective ability, greater understanding and inclination to explore her values and self-esteem (cite). In this case, Diya works with a sport psychologist through her developmental period from a holistic paradigm which aids her positive youth developmental process (Petitpas et al., 2017). Acting as a facilitating agent, the sport psychologist helps Diya's social development, intrapersonal development and allows a space for emotional disclosure when needed to ensure her PYD is on track (Holt & Young, 2004). A clear indicator of this is her improved emotional regulation capacity which is linked to both sporting performance (Laborde et al., 2014) and PYD outcomes (Dvorsky et al., 2019). Diya participates in sport and at a competitive level too, which is an environment that leads to high-intensity emotions which are often difficult to manage and hampers normal development trajectories (Jones, 2012). Self-awareness and gradual engagement in honest self-reflection within a safe space facilitates emotional regulation and expression as needed (Silvia, 2002), which is shown to be a protective factor of resilience (Tugade & Fredickson, 2004) and facilitates positive emotional experiences (Tugade & Fredickson, 2004). Specifically, this demonstrates greater mastery ability to the individual imparting the belief that they can control elements of the difficulty they face (Robazza & Ruiz, 2018). This allows a better transition into the trajectory of resilience positive adaptation (Gupta & McCarthy, 2021).

On analyzing Diya's case, we can see that PYD does not happen in an instance. Rather, it is a culmination of psychological, developmental, and socio-environmental factors that converge to facilitate change. When this occurs, PYD and resilience resources are developed within the individual. Mapping this onto the transtheoretical model is their response to adversity. The individual engaged in pre-contemplation, contemplation, preparation and initial action. During this time and later, they experience adversity. However, since PYD outcomes have been met, the individual can (a) reflect on their controllable mastery elements in the situation; (b) have greater emotional awareness when adversity occurs, and effectively regulate as applicable; (c) have a greater sense of identity and values that can underpin their cognitive and behavioral response and (d) converge into stable self-esteem that helps the Diya define herself with elements in her self-concept that goes beyond success and failure metrics (Blattner et al., 2013). As such, Diya experiences failures of different kinds and intensities (e.g., failing in her debut bilateral series). However, this does not lead to a breakdown in resilient adaptation responses since through sport and environmental areas, her PYD outcomes and resilience has been developed over a period (see Fig. 10.3). Diya is now a confident competitor who does not define herself through win/loss outcomes, but rather through the process of 'applying herself' to her highest level. She is also a positive person, taking 'ownership of why that (failure) happened', and working on other controllable areas of her life that gives her meaning and joy (e.g., keeping in loop with the support staff and joining university).

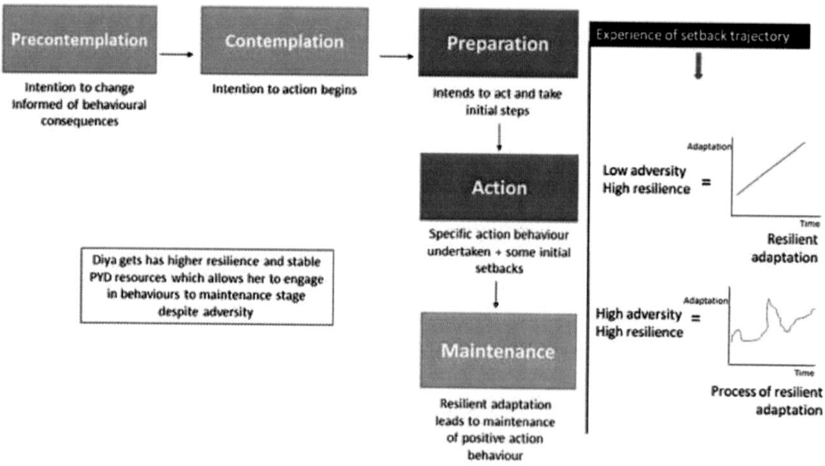

Fig. 10.3 Analysis of case alternate B with PYD and resilience outcomes

Recommendations for Applied Psychology Implementation

The outcomes of PYD and resilient youth development outlined above and discussed through the case have multiple applied psychology implementation potentials. Firstly, PYD is a longitudinal process. As such, effective planning and adjustment to the plan must be considered to ensure effective youth development. This process can range from an intensive 6-month period or intermittently through school-based or other organized activities over the span of a year or more (Gupta & McCarthy, 2022). Second, efforts should be made to coordinate and keep an effective communication flow between multiple stakeholders of PYD programs, especially since low levels of communication impacts athletes and development outcomes in sport (Henriksen et al., 2014). Third, we need to be conscious about integrating horizontal processes (i.e., different elements working together across states (Taylor et al., 2021) and vertical integration (i.e., mutually supportive working practices across a program (Abraham & Collins, 2011; Taylor et al., 2021). Finally, although integrated and multi-collaborative working is crucial, we need to be conscious of 'too many cooks' (cite the paper). A helpful way of doing so and engaging in best practice is to involve the youth itself within the development of the program in line with participatory research through the principles of co-production (Smith et al., 2022a, 2022b).

Conclusion

"Do what the person needs, not what you think they are in need of"—was a key reflection point from SG's applied work as a sport psychologist. It is one that is pertinent to PYD and resilient youth development. As demonstrated in this chapter, protective factors of resilience combined with specific PYD variables lead to effective outcomes. Put together, they allow for the development of positive people and confident competitors. However, this is not an automatic process, nor a quick one. Care needs to be taken to perceive the individual's PYD holistically, rather using the context of sport and physical activity as an overarching solution. Sport and physical activity are best considered as an ancillary field, where PYD principles can be developed, not one where it should be exclusively based.

Acknowledgements We would like to extend our thanks to Diya Valeja who supported SG in her capacity as a Research Assistant as part of Discovery Sport and Performance Lab.

References

Abraham, A., & Collins, D. (2011). Effective skill development: How should athletes' skills be developed. In *Performance psychology: A practitioner's guide* (207–229).

Allan, V., Turnnidge, J., & Côté, J. (2017). Evaluating approaches to physical literacy through the lens of positive youth development. *Quest, 69*(4), 515–530.

Anderson-Butcher, D., Cash, S. J., Saltzburg, S., Midle, T., & Pace, D. (2004). Institutions of youth development: The significance of supportive staff-youth relationships. *Journal of Human Behavior in the Social Environment, 9*(1–2), 83–99.

Aravind, R., Gupta, S., & RA, G. S. K. (2022). A pilot study on emotional intelligence and its impact on pre-competitive anxiety: How does it operate in the non-WEIRD Indian sport context?. *International Journal of Physiology, Nutrition and Physical Education, 7*(1): 08–16. https://doi.org/10.22271/journalofsport.2022.v7.i1a.2407

Arnett, J. J. (1999). Adolescent storm and stress, reconsidered. *American Psychologist, 54*(5), 317.

Bailey, R. (2006). Physical education and sport in schools: A review of benefits and outcomes. *Journal of School Health, 76*(8), 397–401.

Barbarin, O. A., Tolan, P. H., Gaylord-Harden, N., & Murry, V. (2020). Promoting social justice for African-American boys and young men through research and intervention: A challenge for developmental science. *Applied Developmental Science, 24*(3), 196–207.

Barlow, K. A., & Hickey, A. (2014). Academic achievement of NCAA Division III athletes. *Journal of Research in Education, 24*(2), 116–123.

Blakemore, S. J. (2012a). Imaging brain development: The adolescent brain. *NeuroImage, 61*(2), 397–406.

Blakemore, S. J. (2012b). The social brain during adolescence. *Biological Psychiatry, 71*(8), 128S–128S. Elsevier Science Inc.

Blattner, M. C., Liang, B., Lund, T., & Spencer, R. (2013). Searching for a sense of purpose: The role of parents and effects on self-esteem among female adolescents. *Journal of Adolescence, 36*(5), 839–848.

Bowker, A. (2006). The relationship between sports participation and self-esteem during early adolescence. *Canadian Journal of Behavioural Science/revue Canadienne Des Sciences Du Comportement, 38*(3), 214.

Brewer, B. W., Van Raalte, J. L., & Linder, D. E. (1993). Athletic identity: Hercules' muscles or Achilles heel?. *International Journal of Sport Psychology.*

Brown, D. J., & Fletcher, D. (2017). Effects of psychological and psychosocial interventions on sport performance: A meta-analysis. *Sports Medicine, 47*(1), 77–99.

Buckley, M., & Saarni, C. (2009). Emotion regulation: Implications for positive youth development. In Gillman, T. R., Huebner, E., & Furlong, M. (Eds.), *Handbook of positive psychology in schools.*

Burke, S., Sharp, L. A., Woods, D., & Paradis, K. F. (2021). Enhancing parental support through parent-education programs in youth sport: a systematic review. *International Review of Sport and Exercise Psychology*, 1–28.

Burkhard, B. M., Robinson, K. M., Murray, E. D., & Lerner, R. M. (2019). Positive youth development: Theory and perspective. *The Encyclopedia of Child and Adolescent Development*, 1–12.

Camiré, M., & Santos, F. (2019). Promoting positive youth development and life skills in youth sport: Challenges and opportunities amidst increased professionalization. *Journal of Sport Pedagogy and Research, 5*(1), 27–34

Cherry, K. (2020). Biography of Erik Erikson (1902–1994).

Coakley, J. (2016). Positive youth development through sport: Myths, beliefs, and realities. In *Positive youth development through sport* (pp. 21–33). Routledge.

Coalter, F. (2010). The politics of sport-for-development: Limited focus programmes and broad gauge problems? *International Review for the Sociology of Sport, 45*(3), 295–314.

Cómez-Mármol, A., Martínez, B. J. S. A., Sánchez, E. D. L. C., Valero, A., & González-Víllora, S. (2017). Personal and social responsibility development through sport participation in youth scholars. *Journal of Physical Education and Sport, 17*(2), 775.

Côté, J., & Fraser-Thomas, J. (2007). Play, practice, and athlete development. In *Developing sport expertise* (pp. 39–50). Routledge.

Crane, J., & Temple, V. (2015). A systematic review of dropout from organized sport among children and youth. *European Physical Education Review, 21*(1), 114–131.

Crane, M. F., Searle, B. J., Kangas, M., & Nwiran, Y. (2019). How resilience is strengthened by exposure to stressors: The systematic self-reflection model of resilience strengthening. *Anxiety, Stress, and Coping, 32*(1), 1–17.

Damon, W. (2004). What is positive youth development? *The Annals of the American Academy of Political and Social Science, 591*(1), 13–24.

Danish, S. J., Forneris, T., & Wallace, I. (2005). Sport-based life skills programming in the schools. *Journal of Applied School Psychology, 21*(2), 41–62.

de Oliveira, A. M., Buchain, P. C., Vizzotto, A. D. B., Elkis, H., & Cordeiro, Q. (2013). Psychosocial impact. In Gellman, M. D., Turner, J. R. (Eds.), *Encyclopedia of Behavioral Medicine.* Springer. https://doi.org/10.1007/978-1-4419-1005-9_919

Deelen, I., Ettema, D., & Kamphuis, C. B. (2018). Sports participation in sport clubs, gyms or public spaces: How users of different sports settings differ in their motivations, goals, and sports frequency. *PloS one, 13*(10), e0205198; Developmental experiences in sport. *The Sport Psychologist, 23*, 3–23

Diener, E., Oishi, S., & Tay, L. (2018). Advances in subjective well-being research. *Nature Human Behaviour, 2*(4), 253–260.

Dillard, R., Newman, T. J., & Kim, M. (2019). Promoting youth competence through balanced and restorative justice: A community-based PYD approach. *Journal of Youth Development, 14*(4), 14–35.

Dvorsky, M. R., Kofler, M. J., Burns, G. L., Luebbe, A. M., Garner, A. A., & Jarrett, M. A., et al. (2019). Factor structure and criterion validity of the five Cs model of positive youth development in a multi-university sample of college students. *Journal of Youth and Adolescence, 48*(3), 537–553.

Findlay, L. C., & Bowker, A. (2009). The link between competitive sport participation and self-concept in early adolescence: A consideration of gender and sport orientation. *Journal of Youth and Adolescence, 38*(1), 29–40.

Flanagan, C. A., Syvertsen, A. K., & Wray-Lake, L. (2007). *Approaches to positive youth development.*

Fletcher, D., & Sarkar, M. (2012). A grounded theory of psychological resilience in Olympic champions. *Psychology of Sport and Exercise, 13*(5), 669–678.

Fletcher, D., & Sarkar, M. (2013). Psychological resilience: A review and critique of definitions, concepts, and theory. *European Psychologist, 18*(1), 12.

Fletcher, D., & Sarkar, M. (2016). Mental fortitude training: An evidence-based approach to developing psychological resilience for sustained success. *Journal of Sport Psychology in Action, 7*(3), 135–157.

Flett, G. L., & Hewitt, P. L. (2016). Reflections on perfection and the pressure to be perfect in athletes, dancers, and exercisers: A focus on perfectionistic reactivity in key situations and life contexts. In *The psychology of perfectionism in sport, dance and exercise* (pp. 312–336). Routledge.

Flett, G. L., Nepon, T., & Hewitt, P. L. (2016). Perfectionism, worry, and rumination in health and mental health: A review and a conceptual framework for a cognitive theory of perfectionism. *Perfectionism, Health, and Well-Being*, 121–155.

Fox, K. R., & Lindwall, M. (2014). Self-esteem and self-perceptions in sport and exercise. In *Routledge companion to sport and exercise psychology* (pp. 58–72). Routledge.

Fraser-Thomas, J., & Côté, J. (2009). Understanding adolescents' positive and negative

Galli, N., & Vealey, R. S. (2008). "Bouncing back" from adversity: Athletes' experiences of resilience. *The Sport Psychologist, 22*(3), 316–335.
Gestsdottir, S., Geldhof, G. J., Lerner, J. V., & Lerner, R. M. (2017). What drives positive youth development? Assessing intentional self-regulation as a central adolescent asset. *International Journal of Developmental Science, 11*(3–4), 69–79.
Gould, D. (1982). Sport psychology in the 1980s: Status, direction, and challenge in youth sports research1. *Journal of Sport and Exercise Psychology, 4*(3), 203–218.
Greenleaf, C., Petrie, T., Reel, J., & Carter, J. (2010). Psychosocial risk factors of bulimic symptomatology among female athletes. *Journal of Clinical Sport Psychology, 4*(3), 177–190.
Gross, J. J. (2001). Emotion regulation in adulthood: Timing is everything. *Current Directions in Psychological Science, 10*(6), 214–219.
Gupta, S. (2021). Bouncing back! Clinical intersections of resilience, cognitive behavioural neuropsychology, and Psychoneuroimmunology (PNI); An Introduction. Resilience, Psychoneuroimmunology, Neuropsychology: Applications in Clinical Settings, 1.
Gupta, S., & McCarthy, P. J. (2021). Sporting resilience during COVID-19: What is the nature of this adversity and how are competitive elite athletes adapting? *Frontiers in Psychology, 12*, 611261.
Gupta, S., & McCarthy, P. J. (2022). The sporting resilience model: A systematic review of resilience in sport performers. *Frontiers in Psychology*, 6344.
Gupta, S., & Sudhesh, N. T. (2019). Grit, self-regulation and resilience among college football players: A pilot study. *International Journal of Physiology, Nutrition and Physical Education, 4*(1), 843–848.
Hermens, N., Super, S., Verkooijen, K. T., & Koelen, M. A. (2017). A systematic review of life skill development through sports programs serving socially vulnerable youth. *Research Quarterly for Exercise and Sport, 88*(4), 408–424.
Hiremath, C. (2019). Impact of sports on mental health. *International Journal of Physiology, Nutrition and Physical Education*, 14–18.
Holt, N. L. (Ed.). (2016). *Positive youth development through sport*.
Holt, N. L., Deal, C. J., & Pankow, K. (2020). Positive youth development through sport. *Handbook of Sport Psychology*, 429–446.
Houle, J. L., Brewer, B. W., & Kluck, A. S. (2010). Developmental Trends in Athletic Identity: A Two-Part Retrospective Study. *Journal of Sport Behavior, 33*(2).
Hu, T., Zhang, D., Wang, J., Mistry, R., Ran, G., & Wang, X. (2014). Relation between emotion regulation and mental health: A meta-analysis review. *Psychological Reports, 114*(2), 341–362.
Jacobson, J., & Matthaeus, L. (2014). Athletics and executive functioning: How athletic participation and sport type correlate with cognitive performance. *Psychology of Sport and Exercise, 15*(5), 521–527.
Jones, M. V. (2012). Emotion regulation and performance.
Kaya, A. (2014). Decision making by coaches and athletes in sport. *Procedia-Social and Behavioral Sciences, 152*, 333–338.
Kegelaers, J., Wylleman, P., Bunigh, A., & Oudejans, R. R. (2021). A mixed methods evaluation of a pressure training intervention to develop resilience in female basketball players. *Journal of Applied Sport Psychology, 33*(2), 151–172.
Khan, K. M., Thompson, A. M., Blair, S. N., Sallis, J. F., Powell, K. E., Bull, F. C., & Bauman, A. E. (2012). Sport and exercise as contributors to the health of nations. *The Lancet, 380*(9836), 59–64.
Kushner, A. M., Kiefer, A. W., Lesnick, S., Faigenbaum, A. D., Kashikar-Zuck, S., & Myer, G. D. (2015). Training the developing brain part II: Cognitive considerations for youth instruction and feedback. *Current Sports Medicine Reports, 14*(3), 235.
Laborde, S., Lautenbach, F., Allen, M. S., Herbert, C., & Achtzehn, S. (2014a). The role of trait emotional intelligence in emotion regulation and performance under pressure. *Personality and Individual Differences, 57*, 43–47.

Larson, R. W. (2000a). Toward a psychology of positive youth development. *American Psychologist, 55*(1), 170–183. https://doi.org/10.1037/0003-066X.55.1.170

Larson, R. W., & Tran, S. P. (2014). Invited commentary: Positive youth development and human complexity. *Journal of Youth and Adolescence, 43*(6), 1012–1017.

Lee, C. H., & Sibley, C. G. (2019). Sleep duration and psychological well-being among New Zealanders. *Sleep Health, 5*(6), 606–614.

Leppo, M. L., Davis, D., & Crim, B. (2000). The basics of exercising the mind and body. *Childhood Education, 76*(3), 142–147.

Lerner, J. V., Phelps, E., Forman, Y., & Bowers, E. P. (2009). *Positive youth development*. Wiley.

Lerner, R. M., Lerner, J. V., Almerigi, J. B., Theokas, C., Phelps, E., & Gestsdottir, S., et al. (2005). Positive youth development, participation in community youth development programs, and community contributions of fifth-grade adolescents: Findings from the first wave of the 4-H study of positive youth development. *The Journal of Early Adolescence, 25*(1), 17–71.

Lerner, R. M., Tirrell, J. M., Dowling, E. M., Geldhof, G. J., Gestsdóttir, S., & Lerner, J. V., et al. (2019). The end of the beginning: Evidence and absences studying positive youth development in a global context. *Adolescent Research Review*, 4(1), 1–14.

Luthar, S. S. (2013). Resilience at an early age and its impact on child psychosocial development. *Encyclopedia on Early Childhood Development*, 2nd edn.

MacPherson, E., Kerr, G., & Stirling, A. (2016). The influence of peer groups in organized sport on female adolescents' identity development. *Psychology of Sport and Exercise, 23*, 73–81.

Maree, J. G. (2021). The psychosocial development theory of Erik Erikson: Critical overview. *Early Child Development and Care, 191*(7–8), 1107–1121.

Marsh, H. W., & Kleitman, S. (2003). School athletic participation: mostly gain with little pain. *Journal of Sport and Exercise Psychology, 25*(2).

Masten, A. S., & Narayan, A. J. (2012). Child development in the context of disaster, war, and terrorism: Pathways of risk and resilience. *Annual Review of Psychology, 63*, 227.

Masten, A. S., & Wright, M. O. (2010a). Resilience over the lifespan: Developmental perspectives on resistance, recovery, and transformation. In J. W. Reich, A. J. Zautra, & J. S. Hall (Eds.), *Handbook of Adult Resilience* (pp. 213–237). The Guilford Press.

Matos, M. D., Santos, T., Reis, M., & Marques, A. (2018). Positive youth development: Interactions between healthy lifestyle behaviours and psychosocial variables. *Global Journal of Health Science, 10*(4), 68.

McCloy, C. H. (1930). Character building through physical education. *Research Quarterly. American Physical Education Association, 1*(3), 41–61.

McCloy, C. H. (1933). The case for physical education. *The Journal of Health and Physical Education, 4*(4), 3–63.

McCraw, L. W., & Tolbert, J. W. (1953). Sociometric status and athletic ability of junior high school boys. *Research Quarterly. American Association for Health, Physical Education and Recreation, 24*(1), 72–80.

McDonough, M. H., Ullrich-French, S., Anderson-Butcher, D., Amorose, A. J., & Riley, A. (2013). Social responsibility among low-income youth in physical activity-based positive youth development programs: Scale development and associations with social relationships. *Journal of Applied Sport Psychology, 25*(4), 431–447.

McKay, C. D., Cumming, S. P., & Blake, T. (2019). Youth sport: friend or foe?. Best practice and research. *Clinical Rheumatology, 33*(1), 141–157.

Meijen, C., Turner, M., Jones, M. V., Sheffield, D., & McCarthy, P. (2020). A theory of challenge and threat states in athletes: A revised conceptualization. *Frontiers in Psychology*, 126.

Mellalieu, S. D., Neil, R., Hanton, S., & Fletcher, D. (2009). Competition stress in sport performers: Stressors experienced in the competition environment. *Journal of Sports Sciences, 27*(7), 729–744.

Merkel, D. L. (2013). Youth sport: Positive and negative impact on young athletes. *Open Access Journal of Sports Medicine, 4*, 151.

Miller, P. H. (2011). Piaget's theory: Past, present, and future. In U. Goswami (Ed.), *The Wiley-Blackwell handbook of childhood cognitive development* (pp. 649–672). Wiley-Blackwell.
Neely, K., & Holt, N. (2011). Positive youth development through sport: A review. *Revista Iberoamericana De Psicologia De Ejercicio y El Deporte, 2*, 299–316.
Nethravathi, R., & Sreenivas, M. Relationship between self-concept and psychological skills among sports children.
New BBC research shows less than 30% of Indian women play any sports. (n.d.). Media Centre. https://www.bbc.com/mediacentre/latestnews/2020/indian-women-play-any-sports
Newman, H. J., Howells, K. L., & Fletcher, D. (2016). The dark side of top-level sport: An autobiographic study of depressive experiences in elite sport performers. *Frontiers in Psychology, 7*, 868.
Newman, T. J., Lower-Hoppe, L. M., Burch, M., & Paluta, L. M. (2021). Advancing positive youth development-focused coach education: Contextual factors of youth sport and youth sport leader perceptions. *Managing Sport and Leisure, 26*(4), 326–340.
O'Sullivan, J. (2013). *Changing the game: The parent's guide to raising happy.* Morgan James Publishing.
O'Toole, V., Martin, R., Fickel, L., & Britt, E. (2019). Emotional wellbeing as perceived and understood through the lenses of SEL and PYD: A qualitative commentary and suggestions for future research in Aotearoa New Zealand. *New Zealand Journal of Psychology, 48*(2).
Park, N. (2004). The role of subjective well-being in positive youth development. *The Annals of the American Academy of Political and Social Science, 591*(1), 25–39.
Parker, M. B., & Curtner-Smith, M. (2005). Health-related fitness in sport education and multi-activity teaching. *Physical Education and Sport Pedagogy, 10*(1), 1–18.
Petitpas, A. J., Cornelius, A. E., Van Raalte, J. L., & Jones, T. (2005a). A framework for planning youth sport programs that foster psychosocial development. *Sport Psychologist, 19*(1).
Petitpas, A. J., Cornelius, A. E., Van Raalte, J. L., & Jones, T. (2005b). A framework for
Petitpas, A., Van Raalte, J., & France, T. (2017). Facilitating positive youth development by fostering collaboration among community-based sport and physical activity programs. *The Sport Psychologist, 31*(3), 308–314.
Pilkauskaite-Valickiene, R., & Gabrialaviciute, I. (2015). The role of school context on subjective well-being and social well-being in adolescence. *Procedia-Social and Behavioral Sciences, 191*, 2588–2592.
Podlog, L., & Eklund, R. C. (2006). A longitudinal investigation of competitive athletes' return to sport following serious injury. *Journal of Applied Sport Psychology, 18*(1), 44–68.
Qi, S., Hua, F., Zhou, Z., & Shek, D. T. (2022). Correction to: Trends of positive youth development publications (1995–2020): A scientometric review. *Applied Research in Quality of Life, 17*(1), 447–448.
Ramey, H. L., & Rose-Krasnor, L. (2012). Contexts of structured youth activities and positive youth development. *Child Development Perspectives, 6*(1), 85–91.
Richman, E. L., & Shaffer, D. R. (2000). "IF YOU LET ME PLAY SPORTS" How might sport participation influence the self-esteem of adolescent females? *Psychology of Women Quarterly, 24*(2), 189–199.
Robazza, C., & Ruiz, M. C. (2018). Emotional self-regulation in sport and performance. *Oxford Research Encyclopedia of Psychology.*
Robst, J., & Keil, J. (2000). The relationship between athletic participation and academic performance: Evidence from NCAA Division III. *Applied Economics, 32*(5), 547–558.
Rouquette, O., Knight, C., Lovett, V., & Heuzé, J. P. (2020). Parent-athlete relationships: A central but underexamined consideration within sport psychology. *Sport and Exercise Psychology Review.*
Ryan, R. M., & Deci, E. L. (2020). Intrinsic and extrinsic motivation from a self-determination theory perspective: Definitions, theory, practices, and future directions. *Contemporary Educational Psychology, 61*, 101860.

Sabiston, C. M., Pila, E., Vani, M., & Thogersen-Ntoumani, C. (2019). Body image, physical activity, and sport: A scoping review. *Psychology of Sport and Exercise, 42*, 48–57.
Sanders, J., Munford, R., Thimasarn-Anwar, T., Liebenberg, L., & Ungar, M. (2015). The role of positive youth development practices in building resilience and enhancing wellbeing for at-risk youth. *Child Abuse and Neglect, 42*, 40–53.
Santos, F., & Martinek, T. J. (2018). Facilitating positive youth development through competitive youth sport: Opportunities and strategies. *Strategies, 31*(6), 47–49.
Sellars, P. A., Evans, L., & Thomas, O. (2016). The effects of perfectionism in elite sport: Experiences of unhealthy perfectionists. *The Sport Psychologist, 30*(3), 219–230.
Shek, D. T., Dou, D., Zhu, X., & Chai, W. (2019). Positive youth development: Current perspectives. *Adolescent Health, Medicine and Therapeutics, 10*, 131.
Silvia, P. J. (2002). Self-awareness and emotional intensity. *Cognition and Emotion, 16*(2), 195–216.
Slutzky, C. B., & Simpkins, S. D. (2009). The link between children's sport participation and self-esteem: Exploring the mediating role of sport self-concept. *Psychology of Sport and Exercise, 10*(3), 381–389.
Smith, A. L. (2003). Peer relationships in physical activity contexts: A road less traveled in youth sport and exercise psychology research. *Psychology of Sport and Exercise, 4*(1), 25–39.
Smith, B., Williams, O., Bone, L., & Collective, T. M. S. W. C. P. (2022a). Co-production: A resource to guide co-producing research in the sport, exercise, and health sciences. *Qualitative Research in Sport, Exercise and Health*, 1–29.
Smith, B., Williams, O., Bone, L., & Collective, T. M. S. W. C. P. (2022b). Co-production: A resource to guide co-producing research in the sport, exercise, and health sciences. *Qualitative Research in Sport, Exercise and Health*, 1–29.
Spencer, M. B., & Spencer, T. R. (2014). Invited commentary: Exploring the promises, intricacies, and challenges to positive youth development. *Journal of Youth and Adolescence, 43*(6), 1027–1035.
Steiner, H., McQuivey, R. W., Pavelski, R., Pitts, T., & Kraemer, H. (2000). Adolescents and sports: Risk or benefit? *Clinical Pediatrics, 39*(3), 161–166.
Storm, L. K., Henriksen, K., Larsen, C. H., & Christensen, M. K. (2014). Influential relationships as contexts of learning and becoming elite: Athletes' retrospective interpretations. *International Journal of Sports Science and Coaching, 9*(6), 1341–1356.
Sudhesh, N. T., Sreenath, K., Gupta, S., Nair, D., & Avnit. (2021). Snehagram model of an applied psychosocial intervention approach among adolescents living with HIV/AIDS: A blueprint. *Institutionalised Children Explorations and beyond, 8*(1), 98–119.
Sunaina, G. S., Gupta, S., & Sreenath, K. (2019). Resilience and well-being among adolescents living with HIV infection. *IAHRW International Journal of Social Sciences Review, 7*(5-III), 1646–1650.
Svetina, M. (2014). Resilience in the context of Erikson's theory of human development. *Current Psychology, 33*(3), 393–404.
Taylor, J., Collins, D., & Cruickshank, A. (2021). Too many cooks, not enough gourmets: Examining provision and use of feedback for the developing athlete. *The Sport Psychologist, 1*(aop), 1–12.
Taylor, S. J., Barker, L. A., Heavey, L., & McHale, S. (2015). The longitudinal development of social and executive functions in late adolescence and early adulthood. *Frontiers in Behavioral Neuroscience, 9*, 252; Bruner, M. W., Balish, S. M., Forrest, C., Brown, S., Webber, K., Gray, E., et al. (2017). Ties that bond: Youth sport as a vehicle for social identity and positive youth development. *Research Quarterly For Exercise and Sport, 88*(2), 209–214.
Tugade, M. M., & Fredrickson, B. L. (2004). Resilient individuals use positive emotions to bounce back from negative emotional experiences. *Journal of Personality and Social Psychology, 86*(2), 320.
Ungar, M., Ghazinour, M., & Richter, J. (2013). Annual research review: What is resilience within the social ecology of human development? *Journal of Child Psychology and Psychiatry, 54*(4), 348–366.

Urban, J. B., Lewin-Bizan, S., & Lerner, R. M. (2010). The role of intentional self regulation, lower neighborhood ecological assets, and activity involvement in youth developmental outcomes. *Journal of Youth and Adolescence, 39*(7), 783–800.

Vandell, D. L., Larson, R. W., Mahoney, J. L., & Watts, T. W. (2015). Children's organized activities. In M. H. Bornstein, T. Leventhal, & R. M. Lerner (Eds.), *Handbook of child psychology and developmental science: Ecological settings and processes* (pp. 305–344). Wiley.

Vandorpe, B., Vandendriessche, J., Vaeyens, R., Pion, J., Matthys, S., & Lefevre, J., et al. (2012). Relationship between sports participation and the level of motor coordination in childhood: A longitudinal approach. *Journal of Science and Medicine in Sport, 15*(3), 220–225.

Vierimaa, M., Erickson, K., Côté, J., & Gilbert, W. (2012). Positive youth development: A measurement framework for sport. *International Journal of Sports Science and Coaching, 7*(3), 601–614.

Voss, M. W., Kramer, A. F., Basak, C., Prakash, R. S., & Roberts, B. (2010). Are expert athletes 'expert'in the cognitive laboratory? A meta-analytic review of cognition and sport expertise. *Applied Cognitive Psychology, 24*(6), 812–826.

Walsh, F. (2020). Loss and resilience in the time of COVID-19: Meaning making, hope, and transcendence. *Family Process, 59*(3), 898–911.

Weiss, M. R. (2016). Old wine in a new bottle: Historical reflections on sport as a context for youth development. In *Positive Youth Development Through Sport* (pp. 7–20). Routledge.

Weiss, M. R., & Gill, D. L. (2005). What goes around comes around: Re-emerging themes in sport and exercise psychology. *Research Quarterly for Exercise and Sport, 76*(sup2), S71–S87.

Whitehead, J. R., & Corbin, C. B. (1997). Self-esteem in children and youth: The role of sport and physical education. In K. R. Fox (Ed.), *The physical self: From motivation to well-being* (pp. 175–203). Human Kinetics.

Wiese-Bjornstal, D. M., Smith, A. M., Shaffer, S. M., & Morrey, M. A. (1998). An integrated model of response to sport injury: Psychological and sociological dynamics. *Journal of Applied Sport Psychology, 10*(1), 46–69.

Wiggins, D. K. (2013). A worthwhile effort? History of organized youth sport in the United

Zarrett, N., Fay, K., Li, Y., Carrano, J., Phelps, E., & Lerner, R. M. (2009). More than child's play: Variable-and pattern-centered approaches for examining effects of sports participation on youth development. *Developmental Psychology, 45*(2), 368.

Dr Sahen Gupta is a Lecturer in Applied Sport and Exercise Psychology at the University of Portsmouth, UK and a Chartered Psychologist with the British Psychological Society with HCPC registration. His research centres on the resilience in sport for performance and mental health, psychotherapy, and cultural sport psychology. Specifically, Dr Gupta's work focuses on a) understanding and facilitating resilience in humans, b) athlete transitions and developmental experiences for mental health through psychotherapy (CBT, EFT), c) the development and assessment of interventions used in sport and performance psychology; and d) validation of sport psychology research cross-culturally. He is the Founder of Discovery Sport & Performance Lab based to aid in this mission.

K. Jayasankara Reddy has M.Sc and Ph.D. in Psychology in the area of NeuroPsychology, also has a Master degree in Clinical Neurophysiology and MBA in Higher Education Management. He has been an active teacher, researcher and practitioner in the field of Health, Cognitive Neuropsychology and Neuroscience since then. Presently, working as Professor of Psychology and Coordinator for Center for Research at Christ University, Bangalore, India. He has guided and graduated 12 Ph.Ds, 15 M.Phil by research and more than 90 postgraduate research project students in the area of Health, Neuropsychology and Cognitive Neuroscience. He has published more than 150 research articles in peer-reviewed journals, presented his research at more than 60 national and international conferences, and has also organized many conferences of national and international significance. Dr. Reddy is the recipient of Indian School Psychology Association (InSPA) – P K

Subaraja Trust Best Performance Award – 2017 for his valuable services and contributions to the promotion of school psychology in India. Also received National Stress Management Research Award 2017 in recognition of positive contribution to the subject of Stress Management from the International Stress Management Association (ISMA). All through his career, he is identified for successful contribution as a teacher in the field of Cognitive Neuropsychology and Neuroscience, and as academic administrator at various capacities while maintaining a very high level of research output in terms of quality as well as quantity. https://orcid.org/0000-0002-6071-0472

Part II
Youth, Education and Career

Chapter 11
A Review on the Impacts of Artificial Intelligence (AI) on Youth

Sabyasachi Mukhopadhyay and Amlan Chakrabarti

Abstract The influence of Artificial Intelligence (AI) is huge on the present young generation. Especially Gen Y and Gen Z are not only using AI-related applications in their daily lives, but also massively focusing the research and product developments related to it. The sectors like education, healthcare, automation, robotics, drone technologies, cloud, edge, and fog computing are immensely influenced by AI-related applications. Even in the quantum domain, AI is also progressing in a satisfactory manner and creating positive influences in parallel to the success of classical AI. By observing the ubiquitousness of AI, governments are also taking some serious steps to strengthen law enforcement related to AI. Undoubtedly, AI is going to be one of the trending technologies for the present and future generations due to its versatility in terms of applications. The goal of this chapter is to provide the readers with a brief overview of the impact of AI on current and future generations.

Keywords AI · Industry 4.0 · Automation · Process automation · Gen Y · Gen Z

Introduction

The term Artificial Intelligence deals with the concept of machine intelligence, considering the consequences of operational as well as social aspects (Horvitz, 2014). As per the predictions made by the experts, the AI market will reach $3 trillion by 2024, which results in massive funding from government and industry bodies (Russell & Norvig, 2009). In the present data-driven world, AI has already created impacts in a different range of sectors, which includes education (Chen et al., 2020), robotics (Mavridis, 2015), healthcare (Mukhopadhyay et al., 2017), process automation (Wooldridge & Jennings, 1995), drone technology (Atencia et al.,

S. Mukhopadhyay (✉)
Centre for Computational and Data Sciences, IIT Kharagpur, Kharagpur, India
e-mail: sabyasachi@kgpian.iitkgp.ac.in

A. Chakrabarti
A. K. Choudhury School of Information Technology, University of Calcutta, Salt Lake City, Kolkata, India

S. Deb and S. Deb (eds.), *Handbook of Youth Development*,
https://doi.org/10.1007/978-981-99-4969-4_11

2017), ChatGPT (Floridi & Chiriatti, 2020) and so on. According to the experts, the upcoming era of AI will be augmented intelligence, where Wearable devices, ubiquitous sensing systems and intelligent embedded systems can create a natural extension of human beings and our physical abilities (Horvitz, 2014).

The ChatGPT language model has a significant influence on today's youth (Floridi & Chiriatti, 2020). GPT stands for "generative pre-trained transformer," which has been developed by Open AI. It can write stories, poems, movie scripts, codes for software and app development, and so on (Floridi & Chiriatti, 2020; Kirmani, 2022).

Present-day youth are quite fancy about AI, forgetting the difference between science fiction and practical reality. In this article, we focus only on the rational aspects of AI in the present day's scientific progress scenarios, which have deeper impacts on youngsters. We strictly avoid unrealistic enthusiasm and unjustified fears related to AI.

To that end, we have provided readers with a brief overview of the impact of AI on current and future generations in this chapter.

Present Trends of AI

Presently, we are discussing the trending areas of AI that have a deeper impact on youth, as shown in Fig. 11.1.

Role of AI in Cloud Computing

There is a huge advantage to deploying AI in the cloud (Zheng & Wen, 2021). It easily removes the hardware dependencies and can take the help of the virtual GPUs present in a cloud. Therefore, there is a possibility of seamless virtualization. AI in the cloud is making business much easier for product development purposes. For instance, you can use AI algorithms for identifying the best-selling items depending on past purchase history, followed by recommendations to other customers. As a consequence, customer satisfaction levels are also increasing, which is creating positive impacts on customer relationship management (CRM) despite some challenges like data storage, data security, data privacy, integration, and so on.

The hybrid cloud is also playing a crucial role in taking advantage of the private and public clouds, where it can take the benefits of security, performance, and flexibility. Optimized use of hybrid clouds has already shown overall better growth in business. The adaptation of a hybrid cloud is facing several issues, which include data privacy concerns, non-adequate expertise on custom buildings, and high associated costs while using hardware resources like GPUs for complex deep learning problems (Zheng & Wen, 2021).

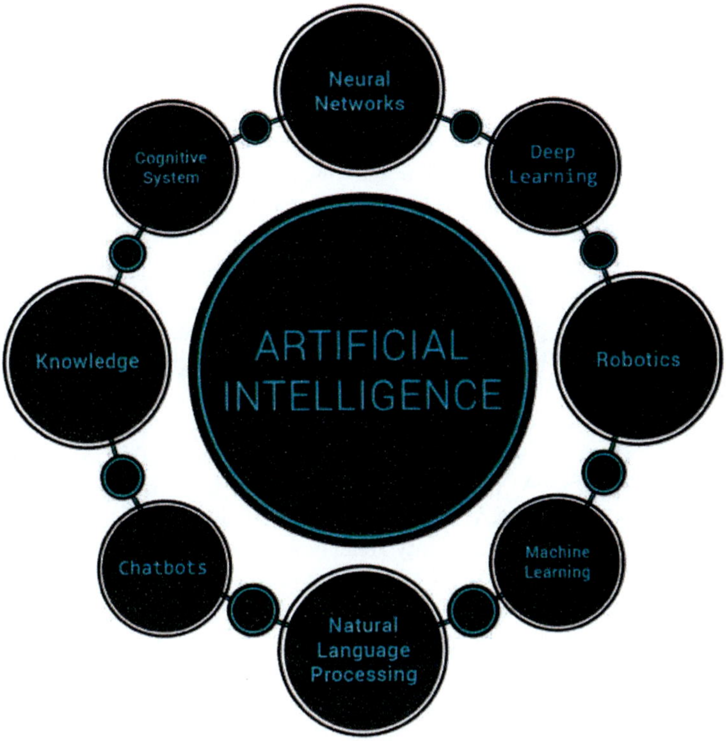

Fig. 11.1 A few important branches of Artificial Intelligence

Role of AI in Edge Computing

Zettabytes of data are being generated by billions of internet-connected things as the Internet of Everything (IoE) advances. As a result, sending all of that data to the cloud increases latency and bandwidth consumption. Edge Computing is becoming an optimal solution in terms of low latency and lesser bandwidth consumption due to the proximity of data sources. As a consequence, real-time data analytics, for instance, on text, video, images, the web, etc., is bringing promising solutions in order to improve healthcare, public safety and security, business intelligence, and so on. Even in the smart home, we observe the typical adaptation of IoE in the daily lives of human beings as a blessing of edge computing. Especially in healthcare, a small amount of latency can prevent patients from accessing vital services. Real-time analysis is critical in the healthcare domain, and it can only be accomplished through mobile edge computing. For instance, we can talk about the Edge AI software, which contains a large number of machine learning algorithms that can be executed on a physical hardware device (Chang et al., 2021).

AI in Healthcare

Disease diagnosis through artificial intelligence (AI) methods is an emerging area of research (Rovithakis et al., 2001). AI-based approaches, i.e., machine learning and deep learning techniques, can potentially discriminate between different stages of disease progression. We all know that the industry's gold-standard techniques, like biopsy, have an accuracy of 65–70% in the diagnosis of cancer and the approach is quite painful and takes 10–12 days to come up with the report. Therefore, painless and non-invasive techniques with higher accuracies are needed. However, the presence of fluorophores, scatterers, and absorption domains among tissues makes the task difficult for AI algorithms to diagnose diseases properly. Hence, deploying a robust and effective statistical biomarker as a feature extraction technique followed by an effective machine learning classifier was an integral part of the early diagnosis of diseases before the deep learning era. State-of-the-art techniques like principal component analysis (PCA) (Devi et al., 2014), multifractal detrended fluctuation analysis (MFDFA) (Das et al., 2016), and 2D multifractal detrended fluctuation analysis (2D MFDFA) (Sahoo et al., 2020) played a significant role in feature extraction and dimensionality reduction. Other data analytics tools, such as wavelets (Gharekhan et al., 2010), have demonstrated their effectiveness in identifying parameters that accurately represent disease progression. In terms of classification, machine learning algorithms such as Mahalanobis distance (Kumar et al., 2019), artificial neural networks (Rovithakis et al., 2001), support vector machines (SVM) (Mukhopadhyay et al., 2017), relevance vector machines (RVM) (Majumder et al., 2005), and the hidden Markov model (HMM) (Mukhopadhyay et al., 2017) have shown promise in the early detection of diseases such as cancer. Deep learning has already demonstrated its efficacy in classifying medical images for many types of medical data (Bhatt et al., 2021). Deep learning algorithms have also shown efficacy in the early detection of cancer (Gao et al., 2020). Quantum machine learning algorithms are gradually grabbing the attention of research communities in a pain-free early diagnosis of cancer.

Besides cancer, AI algorithms have been proven to be quite effective in the early diagnosis of chronic diseases like diabetic macular edema, diabetic retinopathy, COVID-19, heart-related diseases, and so on.

Impact of Quantum Machine Learning

Quantum data is a kind of data source that can take place in a natural or artificial quantum system. Hence, it can be classical data resulting from quantum mechanical experiments, or the data can be directly generated by a quantum device and then put into an algorithm as input. Already, there is evidence that hybrid quantum-classical machine learning applications on quantum data are capable of providing a quantum advantage over classical-only machine learning due to quantum mechanical properties where quantum data shows superposition and entanglement, which can lead to joint probability distributions requiring an exponential amount of classical computational resources for storage. The recent application of quantum machine learning is in quantum data, where actual states can be generated by quantum systems and processes. Many quantum machine learning algorithms are capable of finding patterns in classical data by mapping the data to quantum mechanical states, followed by manipulating them with the help of basic quantum linear algebra subroutines. Quantum machine learning (QML) algorithms are applied directly to the quantum states of light and matter to reveal their features and patterns. It is observed that quantum modes of analysis are better than the classical analysis of data taken from quantum systems (Mishra et al., 2021).

Robotics

Robotics is a kind of technology that consists of designing, constructing, and operating robots. These robots can implement a complicated set of tasks, followed by automating the movements. We have basic robots as well as completely autonomous vehicle-mounted robots. In general, a standard robot can execute a predefined program by operating on a single machine, whereas a collaborative robot can learn multiple tasks to assist human beings. We all know that industrial robots are machines with senses that can also collaborate with humans (Zhang et al., 2013).

These robots are capable of performing tasks in a factory like assembling parts, welding, material handling, picking and positioning, CNC milling, and so on (Alston, 2011; Mavridis, 2015).

These robots can also be seen in action by replacing humans in several hazardous situations like radioactive locations, high-temperature environments, environments with harmful gasses, and so on. Undoubtedly, these robots are quite adaptable and flexible, as well as budget-friendly, for different industries.

The vast amount of automation in the current market indicates hefty growth in the market share, and the valuation is expected to reach around 296.70 billion dollars in 2026, according to the report made by Fortune Business Insights. The appropriate choice of an automation system plays a vital role in accelerating the business under different labor conditions, competitive pressure, work requirements, the cost of labor, and so on (Gonzalez & Barr, 2000).

The Role of AI in Drone Technology

Our young generations are hugely influenced by drone technology (Floreano & Wood, 2015). Youngsters in engineering colleges and universities are coming up with a lot of interesting drone-related projects. In photography, videography, and delivery these drones are becoming an integral part of our lives. Even to make surveys in disaster zones, drones are used extensively. Unmanned aerial vehicles (UAVs), like drones controlled by a remote operator or by onboard computer systems, can be quite useful in military surveillance and other commercial aspects. The developers and researchers are working hard to automate these drones using AI. Eliminating human factors from drones can reduce the overall processing costs and other risk factors associated with this. This also enables the decision-making power of drones using AI (Atencia et al., 2017).

Developers are providing training to drones for thinking like themselves by using AI tools, for instance, machine learning, deep-learning, and so on. The main objective is to make drones smarter and completely autonomous, so that they can avoid obstacles and implement proper target tracking. The major challenge developers are facing while operating drones in an unknown environment where they do not have the proper information about the surroundings while flying.

Using machine learning and deep learning, researchers are trying to train drones in object recognition by interpreting the surroundings. Therefore, by following the predefined rules set by humans, these drones can easily make the necessary decisions. Computer vision tools and techniques can also play an important role in object identification for optimal navigation and obstacle avoidance. The sensor arrays present in drones can collect a large amount of data with the help of this data. These drones can be trained by using the supervised learning algorithm for flying automatically. Apart from avoiding the obstacles detected by the AI-powered sensors, these drones can fly effectively on the defined routes by avoiding wasting time (Atencia et al., 2017).

Automation (RPA)

Here, we are going to discuss two broader aspects of industrial automation, for instance; automation and software. Industrial automation can implement physical processes that can be completed by a human. Software automation can perform computer-based functions in such a way that humans can easily execute the operations with template-driven approaches.

Bespoke automation is applicable in such scenarios where you can observe defined and predictable production activities. In this situation, one requires specialist automation for incorporating the implementation to complete the entire process.

Bespoke automation plays important roles in processing several tasks like liquid filling, box filling, box erection as well as sealing, quality control, parts sorting, repetitive functions with few variables, production monitoring, carton, and product labeling, safety enhancements, and so on. Although the applications of bespoke automation are not limited, as we have discussed so far.

There are significant benefits of using bespoke automation, which can customize functionality according to the needs of customers. The use of this kind of automation can provide effective solutions for executing routine tasks at a much faster speed (Wooldridge & Jenning, 1995).

After gaining an idea about robotics and automation, a common query comes to mind: which one is to be given priority while providing customer services in the industry? In practical scenarios, the solution depends on the industrial requirements. It may happen that in some scenarios, one may have to deploy both tools i.e., robotics and automation to achieve a robust solution.

In a nutshell, robots are pieces of equipments that has the capability of implementing diversified operations with programming. Automation can be used to implement some sets of particular tasks. However, we should remember that robotics is also one of the forms of automation (Shidaganti et al., 2021).

RPA Versus Traditional Automation

Let us discuss the differences between RPA and traditional automation (Shidaganti et al., 2021).

- RPA can automate repetitive tasks and rule-based actions by mimicking human actions. On the other hand, traditional automation cannot mimic human actions but rather just execute predefined programmed instructions.
- In RPA, programming skills are not required due to its template-driven approach. On the other hand in traditional automation, programming skills are required.
- On being process-driven, RPA executes the task within a twinkle of an eye. Traditional automation takes several months to execute any task because of test design and feasibility studies.
- For integrating with other existing systems to execute tasks, RPA is quite suitable. Though traditional automation cannot do it due to a lack of API support.
- RPA can be a little costly in the initial phase but remains very cheap in the long run. Traditional automation is quite cheap in the initial phase though it becomes costly in the long run.
- RPA can execute any business process due to its simplicity, whereas, traditional automation faces difficulty to upgrade and update the scripts.

Intelligent Process Automation

The concept of intelligent process automation (IPA) was developed from AI, cognitive automation, and robotic process automation (RPA). The present technology adds optimized automation capabilities with self-decision-making power through an AI-based approach. For instance, UiPath is playing a pivotal role in the launch of IPA in the global market. The market size for IPA was 13.6 billion USD in 2022. It is expected that the market size will be 25.9 billion USD in 2027 (Shidaganti et al., 2021; Wooldridge & Jennings, 1995).

The Emergence of Super Chatbot

The emergence of the "super chatbot" is knocking at the door where chatbots will embrace RPA technology. As a consequence, this will result in an enhancement of the overall capabilities of chatbots and will make them "super chatbots." This kind of super chatbot will be able to understand the client's emotions, and in the backend, RPA technology will resolve customer issues by responding promptly. You may say that this category of chatbot will have cognitive abilities. Hence, it is quite evident that the emergence of a super chatbot will enhance the overall customer satisfaction level soon, which will be a huge boon for business (Nirala et al., 2022).

AI in Education

The efficacies of technologies in education are quite evident for the last few years which already have a very strong impact on the young generations. Hence, deploying AI in education has, therefore, no exceptions. The rise of AI in education is helping students a lot. For instance, the chatbots present on iPads, and laptops can help the students to understand a specific topic and they can even do the teaching progress analysis for each student if required. Considering the effectiveness of virtual reality (VR) technologies, they are helping a lot of the students understand different difficult concepts, including mathematical problems. Even staying remote, the students can stay connected with the help of a VR technology-generated three-dimensional environment by making the job of teachers quite easier. AI is also helping in the improvement of the learning management system (LMS), for instance, by assigning the coursework, tracking the progress among students, student performance report generations, and so on. Grading through AI can be done in a much faster way.

The main challenge is that teachers are required to learn these tools properly for effective teaching purposes. Therefore, a proper arrangement of training is required. On the other hand, there is no replacement for human-based teaching as AI robots can't sense emotions. Therefore, despite the presence of AI, human interventions will be required in the entire teaching-learning process (Chen et al., 2020).

AI in Agriculture

Agriculture is one of the major pillars of the economy in any country. AI has the potential to save the agriculture sector from various kinds of factors like climate change, the growth of population, safety related to food, and so on. Various kinds of AI-based algorithms can resolve agriculture-related problems like soil testing, crop predictions, food quality testing, detection of yield, and so on. Undoubtedly, the creation of AI-based predictive solutions for solving a real-world challenge in farming is the need of the hour. Here, we are discussing the key areas of AI-based applications in the agriculture domain (Talaviya et al., 2020).

- **AI in Precision Farming**. Precision farming reduces labor-intensive repetitive tasks in farming. For instance, we can talk about the reduction of plant stress levels, which can be implemented by analyzing the high-resolution images of various kinds of sensor data. For stress recognition, you can take input from that captured sensor data.
- **AI in Intelligent Spraying and Health Monitoring of Crops**. In smart spraying, AI sensors are playing pivotal roles by detecting weed-prone areas where herbicides can be sprayed to save cost and time. In this manner, AI sprayers can reduce the adverse effects of chemicals in the fields by improving overall crop quality and saving money. The researchers are working on building intelligent spraying robots. Nowadays, AI-based apps like Plantix can help monitor the health of crops.
- **Role of AI in the Forecasting of Weather and Price**. Farmers can still benefit from appropriate weather analysis. Proper price forecasting for crops can also be quite helpful to farmers in generating optimized revenue.
- **Disease Detection of Crops**. Disease detection in crops can be done by AI-based algorithms with the help of image analysis.

AI in Transportation

In the transportation sector, the development of fully autonomous vehicles is the area of main concern for AI. AI algorithms are applied to the cockpit to reduce the pilot's workload and achieve on-time performance. The challenges of deploying AI-based autonomous vehicles in crowded areas of countries like India and China. Researchers are working towards making the algorithms more robust (Iyer, 2021).

AI in Digital Marketing and E-Commerce

In the digital marketing and e-commerce sectors, AI is playing a pivotal role that ranges from the user experience to marketing and the distribution of products. There can be automated inventories as well as effective use of chatbots in aspects of AI-driven futuristic technologies. We can expect e-commerce with automated warehouses and inventory, shopper personalization, and the use of chatbots in the future (Kalia, 2021).

AI in Employment

AI can be used for employment purposes for job seekers by shortlisting the biodata according to the job descriptions (JD). Also, AI-based robots can take the interviews, followed by accepting or rejecting the job applicants. Therefore, AI is assisting HR activities quite well (Eubanks, 2018).

AI in Gaming Industry

The gaming industry is being revolutionized with the help of AI and is very popular in terms of controlling non-player characters (NPCs). Here, the characters interact with the player dynamically. AI also uses the virtual assistant for the playing of the game. These types of virtual assistants use NLP for understanding and responding to player requests. AI personalizes the gameplay for individual players based on their preferences. There are a few major challenges associated with the use of AI in the gaming industry. These factors are associated with cost, complexity, limited intelligence, a lack of creativity, and other ethical issues. In a nutshell, AI can improve the overall quality of gameplay (Millington, 2020).

ChatGPT

A concept like ChatGPT has been developed using unsupervised pre-training and supervised fine-tuning (Haque et al., 2022). This is an elegant chatbot that can understand and interpret user requests by responding in a natural human language. One can access ChatGPT via https://chat.openai.com/chat. ChatGPT can be a coding partner by writing software, capable of detecting security vulnerabilities. Besides, it can also be an app developer. The deployment of a virtual machine is also possible using a ChatGPT (Floridi & Chiriatti, 2020; Kirmani, 2022). While researchers are trying to explore the full technical side of this ChatGPT, one can even write a full manuscript using this tool (González-Padilla, 2022). As a result, determining ethical factors and implementing them in society for the use of ChatGPT is a major concern.

Conclusion

From the above discussions, we already know that AI is going to play a crucial role in the operations of the government and public institutions. It will also have an impact on the way interactions among citizens and their lifestyles. In spite of many hopes, there is a large amount of fear and growing concern related to human rights, the reliability of technologies, and other relevant ethical issues.

As we all know that the present generation is highly influenced by AI, therefore, it is quite expected that it will continue to create a strong impact on our social lives in the near future also. This is up to the young minds how they are planning to scale and fine-tune the capabilities of AI for global impacts. At the end of the day, we have to keep in mind that whatever autonomy we may bring through AI, it should shape our future in a positive direction.

References

Alston, P. (2011). Lethal robotic technologies: The implications for human rights and international humanitarian law. *Journal of Law Information and Science, 21*, 35.

Andreu-Perez, J., Poon, C. C., Merrifield, R. D., Wong, S. T., & Yang, G. Z. (2015). Big data for health. *IEEE Journal of Biomedical and Health Informatics, 19*, 1193–1208.

Atencia, C. R., Fernández, V. C., Pardo, A. G., & Camacho, D. (2017). New Artificial Intelligence approaches for future UAV Ground Control Stations. *CEC 2017*.

Bhatt, C., Kumar, I., Vijayakumar, V., Singh, K. U., & Kumar, A. (2021). The state of the art of deep learning models in medical science and their challenges. *Multimedia System, 27*, 599–613.

Chang, Z., Liu, S., Xiong, X., Cai, Z., & Tu, G. (2021). A survey of recent advances in edge-computing-powered artificial intelligence of things. *IEEE Internet of Things Journal, 8*(18), 13849–13875.

Chen, L., Chen, P., & Lin, Z. (2020). Artificial intelligence in education: A review. *IEEE Access, 8*, 75264–75278.

Das, N., Mukhopadhyay, S., Ghosh, N., Chhablani, J., Richhariya, A., Rao, K. D., & Sahooe, N. K. (2016). Investigation of alterations in multifractality in optical coherence tomographic images of in vivo human retina. *Journal of Biomedical Optics, 21*(9).

Devi, S., Panigrahi, P. K., & Pradhan, A. (2014). Detecting cervical cancer progression through extracted intrinsic fluorescence and principal component analysis. *Journal of Biomedial Optics, 19*, 127003.

Eubanks, B. (2018). *Artificial Intelligence for HR* (1st ed.). Kogan Page.

Floreano, D., & Wood, R. J. (2015). Science, technology and the future of small autonomous drones. *Nature, 521*, 460–466.

Floridi, L., & Chiriatti, M. (2020). GPT-3: Its nature, scope, limits, and consequences. *Minds and Machines, 30*(4), 681–694.

Gao, J., Guo, Y., Sun, Y., & Qu, G. (2020). Application of deep learning for early screening of colorectal precancerous lesions under white light endoscopy. *Computational and Mathematical Methods in Medicine.*

Gharekhan, A. H., Arora, S., Panigrahi, P. K., & Pradhan, A. (2010). Distinguishing cancer and normal breast tissue autofluorescence using continuous wavelet transform. *IEEE Journal of Selected Topics in Quantum Electronics, 16*(4), 893–899.

Gonzalez, A. J., & Barr, V. (2000). Validation and verification of intelligent systems-what are they and how are they different? *Journal of Experimental and Theoretical Artificial Intelligence, 12*, 407–420.

González-Padilla, D. A. (2022). Concerns about the potential risks of artificial intelligence in manuscript writing. *The Journal of Urology*. https://doi.org/10.1097/JU.0000000000003131

Haque, M. U., Dharmadasa, I., Sworna, Z. T., Rajapakse, R. N., & Ahmad, H. (2022). *I think this is the most disruptive technology: Exploring Sentiments of ChatGPT Early Adopters using Twitter Data*. https://doi.org/10.48550/arXiv.2212.05856 .

Horvitz, E. (2014). *One hundred year study on artificial intelligence: Reflections and framing.* Stanford University.

Iyer, L. S. (2021). AI enabled applications towards intelligent transportation. *Transportation Engineering, 5*, 100083.

Kalia, P. (2021). Artificial intelligence in E-commerce. In Bhargava, C., & Sharma, P. K. (eds.), *Artificial Intelligence* (1st ed.). CRC Press.

Kirmani, A. R. (2022). Artificial intelligence-enabled science poetry. *ACS Energy Letters, 8*, 574–576.

Kumar, P., Kanaujia, S. K., Singh, A., & Pradhan, A. (2019). In vivo detection of oral precancer using a fluorescence-based, in-house-fabricated device: A Mahalanobis distance-based classification. *Lasers in Medical Science, 34*(6), 1243–1251.

Majumder, S. K., Ghosh, N., & Gupta, P. K. (2005). Relevance vector machine for optical diagnosis of cancer. *Lasers in Surgery and Medicine: The Official Journal of the American Society for Laser Medicine and Surgery, 36*(4).

Mavridis, N. (2015). A review of verbal and non-verbal human–robot interactive communication. *Robotics and Autonomous Systems, 63*, 22–35.

Millington, I. (2020). *AI for games* (3rd ed.). CRC Press.

Mishra, N., Kapil, M., Rakesh, H., Anand, A., Mishra, N., & Warke, A., et al. (2021). Quantum machine learning: A review and current status. *Data Management, Analytics and Innovation: Proceedings of ICDMAI 2020, 2*, 101–145.

Mukhopadhyay, S., Das, N. K., Kurmi, I., Pradhan, A., Ghosh, N., & Panigrahi, P. K. (2017). Tissue multifractality and hidden Markov model based integrated framework for optimum precancer detection. *Journal of Biomedical Optics, 22*(10).

Nirala, K. K., Singh, N. K., & Purani, V. S. (2022). A survey on providing customer and public administration based services using AI: Chatbot. *Multimedia Tools and Applications, 81*, 22215–22246.

Rovithakis, G. A., Maniadakis, M., Zervakis, M., Filippidis, G., Zacharakis, G., Katsamouris, A. N., & Papazoglou, T. G. (2001). Artificial neural networks for discriminating pathologic from normal peripheral vascular tissue. *IEEE Transactions on Biomedical Engineering, 48*(10), 1088–1097.

Russell, S. J., & Norvig, P. (2009). *Artificial intelligence: a modern approach* (3rd ed). Prentice Hall.

Sahoo, G. R., Dey, R., Das, N., Ghosh, N., & Pradhan, A. (2020). Two dimensional multifractal detrened fluctuation analysis of low coherence images for diagnosis of cervical pre-cancer. *Biomedical Physics and Engineering Express, 6*(2).

Shidaganti, G., Salil, S., Anand, P., & Jadhav, V. (2021). Robotic process automation with AI and OCR to improve business process: review. *ICESC 2021.*

Talaviya, T., Shah, D., Patel, N., Yagnik, H., & Shah, M. (2020). Implementation of artificial intelligence in agriculture for optimisation of irrigation and application of pesticides and herbicides. *Artificial Intelligence in Agriculture, 4*, 58–73.

Wooldridge, M., & Jennings, N. R. (1995). Intelligent agents: Theory and practice. *The Knowledge Engineering Review, 10*, 115–152.

Zhang, L., Jiang, M., Farid, D., & Hossain, A. (2013). Intelligent facial emotion recognition and semantic-based topic detection for a humanoid robot. *Expert Systems with Applications, 40*, 5160–5168.

Zheng, Y., & Wen, X. (2021). The application of artificial intelligence technology in cloud computing environment resources. *Journal of Web Engineering, 20*(6).

Sabyasachi Mukhopadhyay is a Ph.D. Research Scholar at the Centre for Computational and Data Sciences (CCDS), IIT Kharagpur. He is also a Skills Development Manager (SDM) at the IIT Kharagpur AI4ICPS I Hub Foundation. He served as a University Faculty at MAKAUT (Govt. of WB), WB, India. He was also a Project Scientist at Nanoscope Technologies for a brief period of time. Mukhopadhyay received MS in Physical Sciences at IISER Kolkata and was the 'Topper' of 2015 batch.Mukhopadhyay delivered invited talks, served as panelist and judge of hackathons in leading IITs, IISERs, NITs, IIEST Shibpur and many leading state, central universities of India. He also delivered invited talks at foreign universities like 'University of Global Village, Bangladesh', 'Université Kofi Annan de Guinée, Guinea', and so on. Sabyasachi's research on biophotonics and AI-based cancer detection has been included in the current affairs syllabus of India's top Govt. official competitive exams like UPSC, IAS, IBPS, Banking, etc. Mukhopadhyay was also invited to deliver talks in 'ATAL AICTE Faculty Development Program' of IEM Kolkata, CEM Kolaghat, NIT Mizoram, NIT Durgapur, and 'Refresher Courses for Faculties in Calcutta University. He delivered invited talks in a number of student induction programs organized by IT Department of MAKAUT (Govt. of WB), Calcutta University, IEM Kolkata, and Netaji Subhash Engineering College.

Amlan Chakrabarti is a Full Professor in the A. K. Choudhury School of Information Technology at the University of Calcutta. He was a Postdoctoral fellow at the School of Engineering, Princeton University, USA during 2011-2012. He has 20+ years of experience in Engineering Education and Research. He is the recipient of the DST BOYSCAST fellowship award in Engineering Science (2011), the Indian National Science Academy (INSA) Visiting Faculty Fellowship (2014), the JSPS Invitation Research Award (2016), Erasmus Mundus Leaders Award (2017), the Hamied Visiting Professorship from University of Cambridge, UK (2018), Siksha Ratna Award by Dept. of Higher Education Govt. of West Bengal (2018) and has been awarded as the Fellow of West Bengal Academy of Science and Technology (2022). He has contributed immensely to the development of efficient computer algorithms and systems in multiple projects supervized by him at both International and National levels. He is the Series Editor of Springer Transactions of Computer Systems and Networks, the Series Editor of the Springer Book Series on "Water Informatics", an Associated Editor of the Elsevier Journal of Computers and Electrical Engineering and Guest Editor of the Springer Journal of Applied Sciences. He is a Sr. Member of IEEE and ACM, IEEE Computer Society Distinguished Visitor, Distinguished Speaker of ACM, Secretary of IEEE CEDA India Chapter, Member of the International Water Association, Vice President of the Data Science Society and Life Member of CSI India. His areas of research are Machine Learning, Computer Vision, Reconfigurable Computing, VLSI CAD and Quantum Computing.

Chapter 12
Youth as Teaching Professionals

Aleena Maria Sunny

> *The world needs almost 69 million new teachers to reach the 2030 education goals (UNESCO, 2016)*

Abstract 'Teacher as professional' has broader underpinning knowledge for practice. It is a profession that lies at the heart of social and economic development of a nation and is crucial in transmitting values and culture of that of equality and respect. However, latest reports from across the world show a steep decline in youth participating in teaching. This continues to become a matter of pressing concern as more practicing teachers are approaching their age of retirement. UNESCO estimated that the world needs almost 69 million new teachers to reach the 2030 education goals. Therefore, this chapter discusses the evolving roles a teacher has to play in the changing settings. An overview of topics such as reflective practice, theories and pedagogies in education, inclusive classrooms, teaching for social justice, and culturally-relevant pedagogy are provided. There is a session that discusses the need to promote subject-specific capital to the students as an effective means of enriching learning. The chapter ends with a few recommendations for policy makers and social scientists in making teaching an attractive profession.

Keywords Youth participation · Teaching professional · Education · Youth · Teachers

Introduction

The contribution of youth is crucial to two interrelated areas of nation building, namely, social development and policy formulation. At the moment, youth participation is mostly restricted to having formal dialogue and a few representative information gathering from them which is generalized to the whole population. Only a very limited portion of their potential is tapped and utilized and a huge lot is

A. M. Sunny (✉)
Department of Psychology, St. George's College, Weybridge, UK
e-mail: aleenasunny1993@gmail.com

S. Deb and S. Deb (eds.), *Handbook of Youth Development*,
https://doi.org/10.1007/978-981-99-4969-4_12

remaining untouched and unexplored. As per the guiding principles of the Universal Declaration of Human Rights, participation is a fundamental right for every individual. Encouraging active participation of youth is the first step to empowerment Lauritzen 2018. "Participation means to be involved, to have tasks and to share and take over responsibility. It means to have access and to be included" (Lauritzen, 2006). Participation is not only vital in the development of the youth participants, but also their whole community. Apart from the development of essential life skills, there would be an overall enhancement in the understanding of human rights and citizenship, which are essential to a country's development.

Upadhyay (2006) identified the key obstacles to youth participation in the 'Child and Youth Participation Guide' for UNICEF as inadequate education and training. Therefore, youth participation in education has to be motivated, particularly encouraging youth to enter the teaching profession.

> Teaching is a profession that lies at the heart of both the learning of children and young people and their social, cultural and economic development. It is crucial to transmitting and implanting social values, such as democracy, equality, tolerance, cultural understanding, and respect for each person's fundamental freedoms. (Education International, 2011)

Education is the one-way solution to address poverty and injustice as well as to attain peace, economic growth, and dignity in the world. To provide quality education to our children, we require a well-qualified, well-resourced and well-paid workforce. Is teaching an attractive profession? What proportion of youth get into teaching? As per the report of Organization for Economic Cooperation and Development teacher shortages is a pressing concern in many advanced economies. A large proportion of teachers are approaching the retirement ages and only unlimited proportion of youngsters are entering. It was further highlighted that even when the overall teacher supply and demand are in balance, there is a pressing shortage of specialist teachers serving in the disadvantaged communities (OECD, 2011). As per the Global Status of Teachers survey, only 4–25% of the teaching workforce is youth at all levels of education (Stromquist, 2018). More than three-fifths (68.70%) of participants reported that the teaching profession is not found as attractive to young people (OECD, 2011). Status in India is not different either. As per the Times of India report, enrolments of trainees to teacher training institutes all over India has also considerably dropped in the past 2 decades (Borwankar, 2017). Considering the facts mentioned as well as the changes in teaching profession happening across the world, more and more trained, well-qualified youth have to be motivated to enter into the teaching profession. These initiatives have to be made to make teaching into an attractive profession by governments across the world.

Evolving Roles of a Teacher

'Teacher as professional' has broader underpinning knowledge for practice. The various roles of a teacher are evolving with the time. Teachers can promote students' independent learning skills and active engagement in the subject through their classroom practice and teaching approach. Newer nuances of teaching and learning such as inclusivity, environmental sustainability and social justice are developing in education literature about which young teachers may need training.

Theories of Learning and Pedagogy

The seminal work title '*Active Learning: Creating Excitement in the Classroom*' by Bonwell and Eison defined active learning "as anything that involves students in doing things and thinking about the things they are doing" (1991, p. 19). Working on this broad definition, Mathie et al., added that "the active learning process helps students become critical, informed and autonomous builders and judges of different sophisticated worldviews" (1993, p. 190). A few examples of the simple-to-complex activities that promote active learning among students are debates, discussions, peer-teaching, observation, think-pair-share, and role-playing.

The active learning approach can be discussed from the perspectives of four theories. John Dewey, through his theory, criticized the traditional education approach as "passive and receptive" and advocated for student interaction with the environment as well as for learning through physical and mental action (1933, p. n.p). In other words, he defined learning as a continuous reconstruction of thoughts and modification of a learner's personal experience (Pardjono, 2002). Like Dewey, Piaget also rejected the traditional models of learning and appreciated the learners' interaction with the world. In the adaptation process proposed by Piaget, which is similar to Dewey's learning principles, learning is described as a continuous process of building and restructuring knowledge actively conducted by the learner. That is, the learner should actively construct knowledge using the stimulating environment provided by the teacher. However, learning, according to Vygotsky and Cole (1978) takes place through performing activities, but only with the help of others, thereby highlighting the need for social interaction. Therefore, for effective teaching, a teacher has to consider the students' interests and prior knowledge as well as provide a "vicarious form of consciousness" through scaffolding (Bruner, 1985, p. n.p.). Likewise, constructivists argue that people learn by making meaning by building on their previous learning using their higher-order skills (Cambridge International Education Teaching & Learning Team, 2015).

There are several ways in which active learning enhances the overall educational experience of the students. Firstly, the high student involvement demanded by such learning strategies is found to increase the students' interest in the topic (subject) and their intrinsic motivation for learning (McGee & Weimer, 1988). Several such studies on the effectiveness of active learning found an increase in students' involvement, attention, engagement, and motivation (Jensen & Owen, 2001; Wooldridge, 2006) and goal-directed behaviors (Bluestone, 2000; Perry et al., 1996). Additionally, in comparison to the traditional lecture style, active learning is found to be more effective in stimulating higher-order thinking (Wittrock & Farley, 2010) as well as in fostering thinking and writing skills among students (Bonwell & Eison, 1991). Given the solid theoretical ground and strong research evidence, teachers must be encouraged to apply active learning to practice.

Reflective Practice

Reflective teaching has been discussed as a paradigm shift in the field of education since the mid-1980s. As has been widely adopted as an effective method of improving quality of teaching by educators, curriculum designers and education and philosophers, there has been several attempts to apply and practice reflective teaching to deal with confusion and ambiguity faced by young teachers in their classrooms (Clift, 1991). There is no precise definition of reflective teaching, however, it can be understood as the ability of a teacher to engage thoughts based on their past experience and knowledge, to make informed decisions and actions in their classrooms (Shanmugavelu et al., 2020). There are three popular ways in which literature makes meaning out of reflective teaching, which are as follows: The first definition focuses on the ability of a teacher to analyse a practice to achieve the learning objectives of a lesson (Cruickshank, 1987). The second definition approaches reflective teaching as a competency of a teacher to handle an uncertain situation in the classroom in a problem-solving fashion. Schon (1983) defined it as "… we reveal it by our spontaneous, skill application of the performance: and are it verbally made to be characteristically explicit".

The third perspective is conceptualized by Zeichner and Liston (1987), where it is the application of professional knowledge and situational context based on which teacher reflects to choose their actions. This definition views a teacher as a professional and also highlights the moral and ethical standard teacher needs to attach to. The young teachers need to be trained in order to be 'transformative intellectuals' able to take into account the policies and context of the school while being guided by matters of justice and equality (Shanmugavelu et al., 2020). This also requires the teacher to be able to think about the overall goals of the curriculum, the social political context, and the long history of research findings in education.

Inclusive Classrooms

Understanding learner diversity is the first and foremost step in introducing and maintaining inclusive best practices in centers of learning. Diversity based on gender, regional, ethnic and linguistic minorities, students with exceptional learning needs as well as those suffering from illnesses such as HIV AIDS have to be taken into account (Possi & Milinga, 2017). According to Article 24 of the Convention on the Rights of Persons with Disabilities, inclusion is.

> a process of systemic reform embodying changes and modifications in content, teaching methods, approaches, structures and strategies in education to overcome barriers, with a vision to providing all students of the relevant age range with an equitable and participatory learning experience and the environment that best corresponds to their requirements and preferences (UN General Assembly, 2007).

Children with all these diverse needs and many more should be able to enroll and participate in regular education programs without facing any discrimination and ostracization. The aim has to be the complete elimination of exclusions based on religion, racism, language, sexual orientation, and ability. There are several strategies for inclusive education and classroom practices in western education system, which are well discussed. However not many of these strategies and recommendations can be put to practice in an under-resourced environment like that of India (Gale et al., 2022). The specific local context of the country coming from other disadvantageous factors such as poor socioeconomic and cultural factors and over population may make these policies realistic to be implemented (Forlin, 2013).

Bawane (2019) identified that a student with physical disability may have additional extensive education disadvantages to face which are stemming from their economic, cultural, caste, language, and gender. The 2009 Right to Education Act has mandated free and quality Elementary education for children between the age of 6 and 14 (Parliament of India, 2009). Special allocations have been made for girls and children from non-dominant language and religious backgrounds as well as for children from economically weaker sections as well as those with disabilities (Chaturvedi & Kuldeep, 2015). There is definitely a paucity of research in low and middle-income countries including that of India regarding inclusive education initiatives (Rose, 2017). A little LMIC research has recommended broad inclusion and positive teaching practices to develop a mature inclusive education system in the countries (Kundu & Rice, 2019). Of all categories of inclusivity, disability-based inclusivity seems to be more prominent than any other. This highlights the importance of taking up inclusive education as a topic for research, finding out context-specific needs to address this issue and also include teaching strategies and practices in teacher training programmes that equip the young teachers to be inclusive in their own platform.

Teaching for Social Justice

Teaching for social justice finds its space in the hidden curriculum that any teacher is trying to transfer to the students. It is definitely a difficult topic to communicate with the students because of the hypothetical nature of privilege and the advantage that may come to certain people or groups who are considered to be extra worthy in our society (Mcintosh, 2013). It becomes important for a teacher to understand the obstacles of learning and teaching about privilege. One should ensure that the myth of meritocracy or hopelessness in the face of injustice, which may be part of the teacher's belief system, should not get communicated to the students. A teacher should be equipped with strategies that they can adopt in their classroom practice which is more inclusive of diverse settings and contexts. Teaching for social justice may include strategies for more inclusive classrooms finding opportunities to discuss the various experiences of privilege and oppression in a meaningful manner, and also be able to quote research in the discussion taking place in a classroom setting (Mcintosh, 2013). A teacher can continue to teach for social justice even outside one's classroom by involving in ways and means to promote social inclusivity in the education institution, such as Anti-Bullying Committee, Gay-Straight Alliance etc. Case (2013). Once again, a teacher here goes beyond a classroom practitioner and becomes actively involved in the social justice activities of their educational institution. Therefore, the young teacher who enters into the profession needs to be sensitive, reflective and accommodative in order to address inequality and Injustice and teach for social justice.

Culturally Relevant Pedagogy

A popular educator Pewewardy (1993) opined that educators have traditionally inserted culture into education rather than education into culture, leading to experiencing difficulty in schools for Indian children. The concept of 'culturally-appropriate' (Au & Jordan, 1981) or 'culturally-responsive' (Cazden & Leggett, 1981) education can be found in the literature from the 1980s. These discourses have attempted to highlight the incongruence about their culture experienced by the students between their home and their educational institutions. Ladson-Billings (1995) has defined culturally relevant pedagogy as that allows the children to experience academic success while developing or maintaining cultural competency as well as critical consciousness. A young teacher aspiring to be culturally relevant should be able to utilize the culture to aid learning. A teacher can collaborate with the parents and other community members to plan and execute culturally relevant learning activities for the students. This can be seen from a social learning perspective, where children begin to learn how social relations are structured within and outside the classroom through the process of understanding the culture better (Ladson-Billings, 1995). Incorporating elements from the very many diverse social cultural backgrounds in

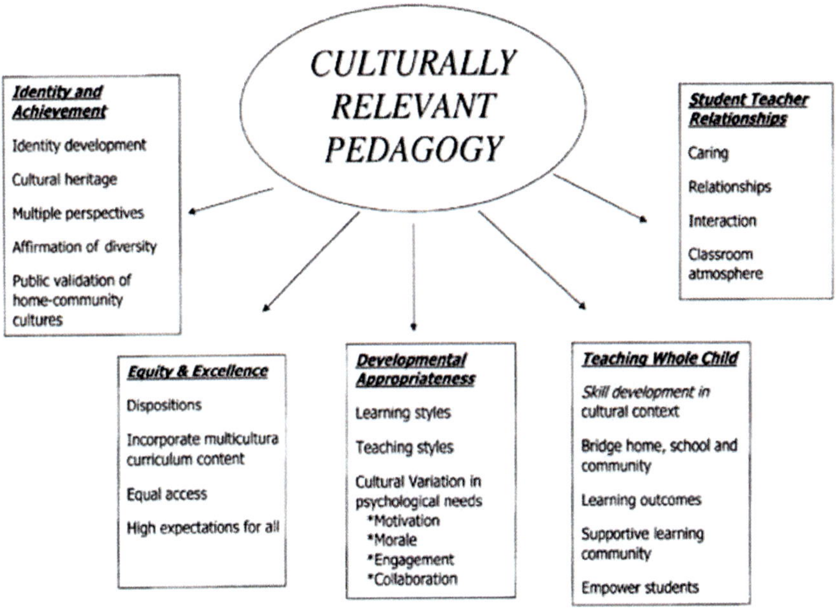

Fig. 12.1 The Principles of Culturally Relevant Pedagogy. Brown-Jeffy and Cooper (2011 *Source*). Toward a conceptual framework of culturally relevant pedagogy: An overview of the conceptual and theoretical literature. Teacher education quarterly, 38(1), 65–84

our country, a teacher can make learning more engaging for the students from that culture, as well as being able to provide an opportunity for other students to expose themselves to the diversity of India (Fig. 12.1).

By analyzing the various theories, Brown-Jeffy and Cooper (2011) developed a conceptual model for culturally relevant pedagogy which has five core themes, as shown below.

Being a multicultural society, diversity can be expected in the student population in Indian schools and colleges. The age-old tension that exists among multiple social layers based on language, caste, tribe and religion comes in the way of establishing inclusion in the pedagogy (Bagai & Nundy, 2009). The concept of culturally appropriate education came into the periphery of the Indian education system when Mahatma Gandhi highlighted the need for local knowledge in place of the British education system (Mukherjee, 2019). Thereafter there have been several culturally based revisions and policies that got endorsed and incorporated into our education system such as the National Policy of Education (1986), National Curriculum Framework for School Education (2005), and National Curriculum Framework for Teacher Education (2009). The scope for great deal of improvement continues even today as the burden on backwardness remains unaddressed (Chakrabarty, 2002). We can benefit from the cultural knowledge each student brings to the classroom for learning, recognize more local languages as a foundation for our curriculum, and involve more community-based learning as well as appreciating intercultural interaction. As suggested by Pare (2004), this will reflect on the participation of students and teachers from indigenous communities and languages, as well as the enrichment of our culture.

Professionalism and Ethics in Teaching

Any profession has its own social and moral context upon which the professional should work, and that is professionalism. The job of a teacher will be reduced to that of a skilled technician if transferring knowledge is its only purpose. If the focus is on making young teachers into a professional, then they should be capable of promoting the value dimension including the personal, social, and moral development of their students (Arthur et al., 2021). The young teacher must be trained to have the flexibility to adapt to the larger social setting in which they are out of hospital, be able to take for suspected based on the theory that education and human development they have learnt, keeping in mind the social policies towards working together as educators (Watkinson, 2013). As Elliott (1989) proposed:

> When teachers are viewed as practitioners of an ethic then they may be described appropriately as members of a profession. But when their activity is viewed as a kind of technology then their status may simply be reduced to that of the technician (Elliott, 1989, p. 9)

It goes without saying that teachers are a major influence on the value formation of their students. Halstead and Taylor (2000) study emphasized on warm, positive, and secure relationships that are shared between the student and the teacher to aid learning. So, a teacher who encourages the practice of ethics in one's classroom very clearly introduces and conveys values to their students. As students spend a significant amount of time with the teachers, they look for fairness and consistency in the character of a teacher. It is not an easy task for young teachers to adopt a model perspective into their teaching. This is where the importance of teacher training and teacher standards get highlighted. They should be trained to demonstrate competence in their classrooms and acquire professional values that will be committed to in the teaching profession.

How Can the Teaching Profession Be Made Attractive for the Youth?

Discussed based on statistics earlier, there is an evident and drastic decline in the number of young people getting into teaching professions. However, as we understand it is the need of the hour to make teaching an attractive profession and ensure sustainability.

Like every profession, there should be an opportunity for continuous and consistent professional development in teaching. Providing opportunities to progress in the various roles and responsibilities, based on interest can attract youngsters. Young teachers should be given the opportunity to progress into academic or managerial or pastoral roles in their employing institutions. Interested teachers should be provided with opportunities to do research, community services or other similar activities and may be encouraged to be involved in making policy level changes in their institution. Associated with this is the provision of sustainable salary policies. For teaching to be seen as an attractive profession, steps should be taken to increase the salary of teachers and provide financial benefits to compensate for the additional work they do in additional activities of their institution. production. These policies have to be made applicable for teachers working in both private and public sectors. To equip the young teachers to meet the growing demand, specialized and research-based teacher training programmes should be provided. Bursaries and scholarships can be given to deserving teacher trainees. Qualified and experienced teachers should be provided further opportunities for training and continued professional development in the form of conferences, workshops and exchange programs.

Promotion of Subject-Specific Literacy in Building Economy

Literacy is the overall ability and skill of a student to apply their learnings from the subject to benefit their wider life contexts. Therefore, the term 'literacy' in this context is not only the ability to read, write and understand a particular language, but the ability to apply the knowledge and skills attained from studying a subject to practice use. There is a growing body of evidence which defines and discusses literacy skills all subjects are capable of. For instance, psychological literacy is.

> being insightful and reflective about one's own and others' behaviours and mental processes and having the ability to apply psychological principles to personal, social and organization issues in work, relationships and the broader community (McGovern et al., 2010, p. 11)

The possibilities of various subjects in everyday lives are limitless, and the subject contributes to the economy through various job sectors such as criminal justice, health, education, human resources, sports, and entertainment. It is the concept of literacy that allows students to go beyond the traditional graduate workplace and contribute to other wider job sectors (Hulme, 2014). For instance, the Subject Benchmark Statement produced by Quality Assurance Agency (2019) contains a comprehensive list of generic and subject-specific skills a psychology student get trained, and are invaluable assets to on-going employability in the fast-changing job market. Likewise, in everyday life too, literate individuals are more likely to make informed decisions and choices (Barnett, 2010), and also more likely to engage in voluntary activities (HESA, 2016) and community projects (Harnish & Bridge). The engagement of such literate citizens, who are "critical scientific thinkers and ethical and socially responsible participants in their communities" (McGovern et al., 2010, p. 10) would be found to make positive contributions to society and the economy.

A teacher plays a key role in delivering the demands of the subject. It is the responsibility of the teacher to be aware of the aims of the curriculum as well as pass on the subject knowledge that suits the needs of the students. Teachers need to adapt their teaching approach and focus on the more active transfer of subject-specific knowledge and skills that have applicability beyond their classroom (Hulme, 2014). As Dunn et al. rightly stated "promoting literacy entails re-orienting what and how we teach students in a way that emphasizes psychology's relevance" (Dunn et al., 2011, p. 16). Therefore, a teacher cannot assume the students to apply their learnings to the real-world, unless they have been trained to do so in the classroom. Towards this, the literature suggests three possible ways that teachers can adapt. Firstly, teaching real-world applications of subject-specific skills in the classroom seems to be more beneficial in improving literacy, rather than always teaching theoretical contexts (Mair et al., 2013). Secondly, the curriculum has to explicitly align to the goal of promoting literacy among students (Biggs, 1994), and this has to be seen in learning outcomes, teaching practices as well as assessment objectives (Trapp et al., 2011). Finally, teachers may enhance literacy among students by practicing the disciplinary knowledge and transferable skills in their professional lives and using them to inform teaching practices, problem-solving, and ensuring inclusivity (Cranney et al., 2012; McGovern et al., 2010; Zinkiewicz et al., 2003). Therefore, teachers should take proactive measures in providing ample opportunities for students to exercise these transferable skills in their conducive classroom environments.

Recommendations

The scope of each subject is different and therefore, the teaching strategies to be adopted for each subject may vary. Therefore, subject-specific teacher training programs have to be provided. The curriculum of such training programmes should be based on the latest research findings in the education. Opportunities for hands-on training with the backing of mentors can help the teacher trainee to gain confidence. Similar support should be provided for the early career teachers during the initial years of teaching practice.

Teacher policies have to be made that ensure consistent professional development. Teacher standards have to be made which are relevant and expected of a practicing teacher. All teachers have to be observed on the basis of these set teacher standards and have to be evaluated based on their performance every year. The promotion and other professional development have to be based on their performances and not merely based on their experience alone.

Initiatives have to be taken by the government to make teaching an attractive profession and also to ensure that youth enter the professions. This could be through the institution of standardized pay packages applicable to both public and private sector, provision of bursaries and scholarship for teacher trainees, offering exchange programmes for teachers and inviting qualified teachers from other countries to practice in ours.

Conclusion

Reports from various studies across the world highlight the lack of young people in the teaching profession. The various roles a teacher needs to undertake is changing and evolving as per the demands of the changing world. The identity of a teacher as a professional broader is underpinning knowledge for practice. Practice should be made based on theories and latest research studies in education and pedagogy. Reflective practice should be made as a routine exercise and practice should also be able to share the hidden curriculum apart from the subject matter. Inclusivity, teaching for social justice, environmental sustainability, culturally relevant pedagogy are all relevant and evolving topics that a teacher needs training and understanding. Considering the pressing demand and reducing youth in teaching, ways have to be identified to make teaching into an attractive profession.

References

Arthur, J., Davison, J., & Lewis, M. (2021). Professional values and practices in teaching and learning. *Professional Values and Practice*, 11–28. https://doi.org/10.4324/9780203580530-5

Au, K. H., & Jordan, C. (1981). Teaching reading to Hawaiian children: Finding a culturally appropriate solution. *Culture and the bilingual classroom: Studies in classroom ethnography* (pp. 139–152)

Bagai, S., & Nundy, N. (2009). Tribal education: A fine balance. *Dasra: Catalyst For Social Change.*

Barnett, R. (2010). Life-wide education: A new and transformative concept for higher education? In N. Jackson & R. Law (Eds.), *Enabling a more complete education* (pp. 4–6).

Bawane, J. (2019). Teaching and teacher education. *Teaching and Teacher Education*, 1–15. https://doi.org/10.1007/978-3-030-26879-4

Biggs, J. (1994). Enhancing teaching through constructive alignment. *Higher Education, 32*(3), 347–364. https://doi.org/10.2331/fishsci.60.753

Bluestone, C. (2000). Feature films as a teaching tool. *College Teaching, 48*(4), 141–146. https://doi.org/10.1080/87567550009595832

Bonwell, C., & Eison, J. (1991). *Active Learning: Creating Excitement in the Classroom. 1991 ASHE-ERIC Higher Education Reports.*

Borwankar, V. (2017). 'Time to inspire youth to take up teaching.' *The Times of India, 1–7.*

Brown-Jeffy, S., & Cooper, J. E. (2011). Toward a conceptual framework of culturally relevant pedagogy: An overview of conceptual and theoretical literature. *Teacher Education Quarterly, 38*(1), 65–84.

Bruner, J. (1985). Vygotsky: A historical and conceptual perspective. In *Culture, Communication and Cognition Perspective* (pp. 21–35). Cambridge University Press.

Cambridge International Education Teaching and Learning Team. (2015). *Getting started with active learning techniques.* Cambridge International Education Teaching and Learning Team. https://www.cambridge-community.org.uk/professional-development/gswal/index.html

Case, K. A. (2013). Deconstructing privilege: Teaching and learning as allies in the classroom. *Deconstructing Privilege: Teaching and Learning as Allies in the Classroom*, 1–244. https://doi.org/10.4324/9780203081877

Cazden, C. B., & Leggett, E. L. (1981). Culturally responsive education: Recommendations for achieving Lau rem-Cazden. In H. Trueba, G. Guthrie, & K. Au (Eds.), *Culture and the bilingual classroom: Studies in classroom ethnography* (pp. 69–86). Rowley. https://www.researchgate.net/publication/269107473_What_is_governance/link/548173090cf22525dcb61443/download%0A; http://www.econ.upf.edu/~reynal/Civil wars_12December2010.pdf%0A; https://think-asia.org/handle/11540/8282%0A; https://www.jstor.org/stable/41857625

Chakrabarty, D. (2002). Habitations of modernity. *Essays in the Wake of Subaltern Studies, 173*. http://books.google.com/books?id=No-rdspJXhYC&pg=PR20&dq=intitle:Habitations+of+Modernity&hl=&cd=1&source=gbs_api%5Cnpapers3://publication/uuid/A070DD39-9CFA-4A60-AB2D-E717609E363A

Chaturvedi, A., & Kuldeep, N. (2015). Status of implementation of the RTE Act 2009 and challenges in the schools of Rajasthan. *International Journal of Economic and Business Review, 3*(3), 163–169.

Clift, R. T. (1991). Encouraging reflective practice in education: An analysis of issues and programs. *Teachers' College Press*. https://doi.org/10.12973/iji.2017.1011a

Cranney, J., Botwood, L., & Morris, S. (2012). *National standards for psychological literacy and global citizenship : Outcomes of undergraduate psychology.*

Cruickshank, D. R. (1987). Reflective teaching: The preparation of students of teaching. *Association of Teacher Education.*

Dunn, D. S., Cautin, R. L., & Gurung, R. A. (2011). Curriculum matters: Structure, content and psychological literacy. In Cranne & D. Dunn (Eds.), *The Psychologically literate citizen* (Issue 8.5.2017, pp. 2003–2005). Oxford University Press.

Education International. (2011). *6th World Congress Report Building the Future through Quality Education.*

Elliott, J. (1989). Teacher evaluation and teaching as a moral science. In M. L. Holly & C. MvLouglin (eds.), *Perspectives on teacher professional development*. Palmer Press. https://doi.org/10.1080/00220270701294210

Forlin, C. (2013). Changing paradigms and future directions for implementing inclusive education in developing countries. *Forlin Asian Journal of Inclusive Education, 19*. http://www.ajie-bd.net

Gale, L., Bhushan, P., Eidnani, S., Graham, L., Harrison, M., McKay-Brown, L., Pande, R., Shreeraman, S., & Sivashunmugam, C. (2022). Overcoming barriers to inclusion in education in India: A scoping review. *Social Sciences and Humanities Open, 5*(1), 100237. https://doi.org/10.1016/j.ssaho.2021.100237

Halstead, J. M., & Taylor, M. J. (2000). Learning and teaching about values: A review of recent research. *Cambridge Journal of Education, 30*(2), 169–202. https://doi.org/10.1080/713657146

HESA. (2016). Destinations of leavers from higher education in the United Kingdom for the academic year 2014/15. *Hesa*, 1–17. https://www.hesa.ac.uk/news/30-06-2016/sfr237-destinations-of-leavers

Hulme, J. (2014). Psychological literacy—from classroom to real world. *Psychologist, 27*(12), 932–935.

Jensen, E. J., & Owen, A. L. (2001). Pedagogy, gender, and interest in economics. *Journal of Economic Education, 32*(4), 323–343. https://doi.org/10.1080/00220480109596112

Kundu, A., & Rice, M. (2019). Indian educators' perceptions of their inclusion implementation practice in secondary schools. *International Journal of Information and Education Technology, 9*(2), 143–148. https://doi.org/10.4324/9781315008011-13

Ladson-Billings, G. (1995). But that's just good teaching! the case for culturally relevant pedagogy. *Theory into Practice, 34*(3), 159–165. https://doi.org/10.1080/00405849509543675

Lauritzen, P. (2006). Participation. *Training course on the development and implementation of participation projects at local and regional level.*

Mair, C., Taylor, J., & Hulme, J. (2013). An introductory guide to psychological literacy and psychologically literate citizenship. *The Higher Education Academy*, 1–22. http://www-new1.heacademy.ac.uk/assets/Documents/disciplines/psychology/MairTaylorHulme-intro-psyc-lit.pdf

McGee, R., & Weimer, M. G. (1988). Teaching large classes well. *Teaching Sociology, 16*(4), 477. https://doi.org/10.2307/1318184

McGovern, T. V, Corey, L., Cranney, J., Dixon, W., Holmes, J. D., & Kuebli. (2010). Psychologically literate citizens. In *Undergraduate education in psychology: A blueprint for the future of the discipline* (pp. 9–27). American Psychological Association. https://doi.org/10.1037/10515-000

Mcintosh, A. (2013). *Deconstructing privilege: Teaching and learning as allies in the classroom.* Routledge.

Mukherjee, M. (2019). Culturally responsive teaching learning in indian multicultural context : Review of contemporary policy and practice. In *International multi-disciplinary conference on arts, social science, management and technology* (pp. 158–185)

OECD. (2011). *Teacher Employment.* Organization of Economic Cooperation and Development. https://gpseducation.oecd.org/CountryProfile?plotter=h5&primaryCountry=TUR&treshold=5&topic=TA

Pardjono. (2002). Active learning: The dewey, piaget, vygotsky and constructivist theory perspectives. *Jurnal Ilmu Pendidikan, 9*(3), 163–178.

Pare, L. (2004). *Culturally appropriate quality education: Learner centered approaches. A statement by the Government of Canada at Indigenous Education In The 21st Century.*

Parliament of India. (2009). *The right of children to free and compulsory education act.*

Perry, N. W., Huss, M. T., McAuliff, B. D., & Galas, J. M. (1996). An active-learning approach to teaching the undergraduate psychology and law course. *Teaching of Psychology, 23*(2), 76–81. https://doi.org/10.1207/s15328023top2302_1

Pewewardy, C. (1993). Culturally responsible pedagogy in action: An American Indian magnet school. In J. K. Hollins & W. Hayman (Eds.), *Teaching in action: An American Indian magnet school.*

Possi, M. K., & Milinga, J. R. (2017). Learner diversity in inclusive classrooms: the interplay of language of instruction, gender and disability. *Malaysian Online Journal of Educational Sciences, 5*(3), 28–45. www.moj-es.net

Quality Assurance Agency. (2019). *Subject benchmark statement-Psychology* (Issue September). Quality Assurance Agency.

Rose, R. (2017). Seeking practice informed policy for inclusive education in India. *Asian Journal of Inclusive Education, 5*(1), 5–22. https://www.researchgate.net/publication/319205395

Schon, D. A. (1983). The reflexive practitioner. *In the Basic Book.* https://doi.org/10.17831/enq:arcc.v6i1.5

Shanmugavelu, G., Parasuraman, B., Arokiasamy, R., Kannan, B., & Vadivelu, M. (2020). The role of teachers in reflective teaching in the classroom. *Shanlax International Journal of Education, 8*(3), 30–33. https://doi.org/10.34293/education.v8i3.2439

Stromquist, N. P. (2018). The global status of teachers and the teaching profession. In *Education International Research* (Issue September). https://www.researchgate.net/profile/Vasileios_Symeonidis3/publication/305947470_The_Status_of_Teachers_and_the_Teaching_Profession_A_study_of_education_unions'_perspectives/links/57a7071308aefe6167b8c32e/The-Status-of-Teachers-and-the-Teaching-Profession

Trapp, A., Banister, P., Ellis, J., Latto, R., Miell, D., & Upton, D. (2011). *The future of undergraduate psychology in the United Kingdom* (Issue January).

UN General Assembly. (2007). Convention on the rights of persons with disabilities: Resolution adopted by the general assembly. In the United Nations. https://doi.org/10.1017/S0020818300029453

Vygotsky, L. S., & Cole, M. (1978). Mind in Society. In *The development of higher psychological processes.* Harvard University Press. https://doi.org/10.2307/1421493

Watkinson, A. (2013). Professional values and practice. In *Professional values and practice.* https://doi.org/10.4324/9780203822517

Wittrock, M. C., & Farley, F. (2010). Learning as a generative process. *Educational Psychologist, 45*(1), 40–45. https://doi.org/10.1080/00461520903433554

Wooldridge, B. R. (2006). The power of perception: An active/experiential learning exercise for principles of marketing. *Marketing Education Review, 16*(2), 5–7. https://doi.org/10.1080/10528008.2006.11488952

Zeichner, K., & Liston, D. (1987). Teaching student teachers to reflect. *Harvard Educational Review, 57*(1), 23–49. https://doi.org/10.17763/haer.57.1.j18v7162275t1w3w

Zinkiewicz, L., Hammond, N., & Trapp, A. (2003). Applying psychology disciplinary knowledge to psychology teaching and learning. *York, Learning and Teaching Support Network, 2.* http://scholar.google.com/scholar?hl=en&btnG=Search&q=intitle:Applying+Psychology+Disciplinary+Knowledge+to+Psychology+Teaching+and+Learning#0

Aleena Maria Sunny is a teacher of Psychology at St. George's College, Weybridge, UK. She did her Ph.D. under the supervision of Prof. Sibnath Deb. She is a qualified teacher and has completed her Postgraduate Certificate in Education from University College London (UCL). She has completed her Master's in Applied Clinical Psychology from Tata Institute of Social Sciences, Mumbai and Bachelor's in Psychology (Honours) from Christ University Bangalore. Her notable publications include Youth Development in India (Routledge Publishing) Community Psychology: Theories and Application (SAGE Publications India), Disadvantaged Children in India: Empirical Evidence, Policies and Actions (Springer Singapore) and Childhood to Adolescence: Issues and Concerns (Pearson Education).

Chapter 13
Current Trends in Career Decision in Youth: Opportunities and Challenges

Upasana Bagchi and K. Jayasankara Reddy

Abstract In today's times, career is a crucial life decision. Due to its paramount importance in our lives, the youth experience diverse kinds of stresses and pressures while choosing their career in life. Contrary to earlier handful career options, current trends offer an unlimited mix of traditional as well as unconventional career roles which further create confusion and anxiety while making the final decision. Newer factors, challenges and opportunities have forced a change of frameworks and perspectives to career decision-making. In career counselling, current trends are shifting away from the traditional practice of matching skill-sets to the job. Today's career decision-making takes an inclusive approach by discussing the various internal influences, emotional management, cognitive thinking styles, coping strategies, adaptability, etc. as well as external influences of uncertainty, evolving lifestyle demands, changing economic tapestry, etc. In addition, the influences of gender, family and culture affect the nature of the goals and their acceptability. The current chapter throws light on the evolving scenario in the field of career decision-making among the youth and attempts to offer solutions to the challenges being faced by the youth.

Keywords Career · Decision-making · Youth · Career decision-making

Introduction

Career is a pivotal decision in a person's life. Career selection starts from early youth and, more or less, settles down by the young adulthood stage in a person's life. Although, we may see clarity in career choices towards late adolescence and early adulthood, career decisions play a role through the lifespan. Our interests, preferences and attitudes towards different careers are guided by our early experiences and social influences. Hence career decision making involves choosing the most optimal field and role that ensures an individual's all round development as well as helps the

U. Bagchi (✉) · K. J. Reddy
Department of Psychology, CHRIST (Deemed to be University), Bengaluru, India
e-mail: upasana.bagchi@res.christuniversity.in

S. Deb and S. Deb (eds.), *Handbook of Youth Development*,
https://doi.org/10.1007/978-981-99-4969-4_13

individual to contribute towards the betterment of the society (Muniarti & Siahaan, 2019).

Earlier, there were limited choices available that required a certain set of skills to perform the job, but today there are a staggering number of limitless options. This has resulted in more career confusion as well as diversity in career choices for people who want to go beyond the traditional set roles or jobs. There are multilevel forces that interact amongst each other in career decision making that warrant in-depth analysis and investigation to understand the market scenario. Today's selection of career has its own set of challenges and stresses because of the paramount importance that the youth place on their careers. Thus, this chapter attempts to assimilate the various viewpoints and trends in career decision making among the youth.

Understanding Career

A comprehensive definition of career is that it is a "composition of activities" required to perform as part of our role as a human resource (Manodara et al., 2022). It is a complex process to decide the optimal career for any individual as there is an array of influences on the career decision making process ranging from psychological characteristics to the larger socio-cultural processes. Career decision making involves a complex decision making mechanism taking into account multiple controllable and uncontrollable forces and their multivariate interactions (Manodara et al., 2022). Thus career decision making processes are more complex than a linear decision making process due to which an organized body of research is required to study this evolving phenomenon.

A person choosing their career will have to first find their options, compile, compare, identify and finalize their chosen alternative. If the chosen career suits the person, it leads to career satisfaction and personal growth. However, if a person goes wrong in their attempt to finalize their career, they experience many work-life challenges which will result in poor professional satisfaction. This leads to internalized regrets and/or moving from job to job in the hope of finding the best fitting alternative as their career (Gati & Kulcsár, 2021). Career decisions are linked with a person's identity formation, personal growth, relationships, life satisfaction, quality of life and wellbeing which justify the turmoil and perplexity associated with career decision making (Manodara et al., 2022).

Paradigm Shift

Traditional career decision making was simplistic attempting to match the skill sets with the job role in the society. This oversimplified process of career decision making was not able to account for the psychological and socio-cultural aspects involved in this complicated process. The archaic standard of matching a person's skill set with the task at hand is a simplistic solution to a complex problem. This realization led to the evolution of our understanding of the different aspects of career decision making. Holland's view takes into account the personality characteristics that match for various trades, but categorizing everybody from the same trade as similar makes it insufficient to explain the career decision making process. Taking into account individual differences, the Decision Theory focuses more on the wants, needs and aspirations of the individual where choosing a career becomes a way of achieving personal goals like money, respect, fame, intellectual stimulation, motivation, success, etc. (Gati et al., 1996). However, there were more external influences found to affect career decision making apart from this utility-oriented explanation.

Bandura's Social Cognitive Career Theory introduces us to the concept of self-efficacy and how social factors interact and form cognitive beliefs about our capabilities with regards to our career and determine our attitudes (Bhatia & Babu, 2021). Super's developmental approach looks at the formation of one's self concept through the career decision making process. Among the individuals of about 15–17 years of age, a tentative direction and preferences form. By the age 18–21 years, these preferences crystallize and become clearer and by the early 20 s, the specificity of the vocation choice is finalized in congruence with one's self concept. This developmental approach looks at career maturity and development as a part of one's lifespan development with its own set of development tasks and challenges.

Today's vocational tapestry is more convoluted and intricately rich than just getting a job or finding a source of income like the yester years. The economies and societies have evolved and so have the job markets. The needs and demands have changed drastically. Given the dynamic nature of the economy, the "perfect fit" of skill to job role is more complex than a simple linear solution (Celik & Storme, 2017). In today's dynamic job market, the human factor is also taken into consideration apart from a person's skill set (Gati & Kulcsár, 2021). Thus there is a paradigm shift from conceptualizing "workforce" into "human resource" that has completely altered the way careers are being understood. The human resources viewpoint acknowledges that the workforce is ultimately "human" and focuses on physical, psychological, intellectual, emotional, social and personal growth and development at its core. Different approaches now explore how the human resource identifies their role in the entire system. This has incited interesting avenues of research over the recent years.

Current Trends in Career Decision Making

Career Decision Makers

According to Muniarti and Siahaan (2019) career decision makers largely involve high school students, undergraduates, graduates, interns and job seekers. Career thought starts seriously at the level of high school in choosing the subjects and streams. At the college and university level, the chosen subject becomes more specialised as interests find the right focus. Interns and job seekers have more clarity on the job role demands and expectations in the context of their reality. However career decision making may continue beyond these to the working professionals as well.

Career Conflict

Career decision making involves an awareness that an individual has to decide a career, the willingness to make that decision and the capability to make the final career decision (Gati et al., 1996). A problem with any of these aspects is experienced as a career decision making difficulty. Owing to the complex and complicated nature of the career decision making process, career indecision may be in the form of prevention of decision making altogether or making less optimal career decisions. The more complex the process is the more is the career decision making difficulty and career confusion. Celik and Storme (2017) proposed that career decision making difficulty is majorly due to general indecisiveness, lack of motivation and dysfunctional career beliefs which affect the decision making process.

Career conflict has been explained using different concepts by different approaches. The Psychodynamic approach explains career indecision as a result of internal conflict in the id, ego and superego which is not resolved. Id follows the pleasure principle of instant gratification while the superego follows the principle of morality and delayed gratification following the rules. Ego balances the id and superego by resolving the conflict. A failure to do so results in mental disturbances and can lead to this inability to decide until a choice is made by the ego. The developmental approach explores career indecision as a failure to attain vocational maturity by completing the developmental tasks that are expected by the individual. The Vocational Interests approach further proposes that insufficient crystallization of interests results in career indecision (Gati et al., 1996).

Career Choice Anxiety and Indecision

Another trend observed is career choice anxiety. Career choice anxiety can be understood as an "affective distress associated with career decision making" (Kaur & Kaur, 2017). This anxiety is specific to making any career decisions and can inhibit the person from making any progress in the decision making process. Career choice anxiety can broadly be classified as anxiety about the process of making career decisions, anxiety about uncertainty and ambiguity, anxiety about making a choice, and anxiety about the outcome (Gati et al., 2011).

According to researchers, lack of information and skills to choose can be the cause of career choice anxiety (Kaur & Kaur, 2017). Career indecisiveness may also be caused by factors like lack of mature decision making skills, lack of readiness, lack of information about self, insufficient information about other alternative available, ignorance about the ways to access this information, inconsistent information, ambiguous data, unreliable information, dysfunctional myths, dysfunctional career thoughts, dysfunctional career beliefs, unclear goals, value conflicts and perceived barriers (Amir & Gati, 2006; Fidan & Nas, 2021; Gati et al., 1996) On delving deeper, internal conflicts could be the psychological process which plays a role in this difficulty in making a career decision. In addition to this, taking too much stress about making the choice can lead to obsessions and panic in the person until the decision is taken. People with neurotic tendencies tend to experience higher anxieties including career choice anxiety (Gati et al., 2011).

Career Exploration

As per the current trend, career exploration is often cited as the problem as well as the solution. Career exploration can be explained as behaviors that provide an individual access to new information about their vocational characteristics, job or organizational characteristics (Celik & Storme, 2017). Career exploration facilitates more accurate information and increases the reliability of the source of that information. Knowing more about the range of career options can help one to make a crystallized decision regarding one's career. Career exploration can help to eliminate the issues that one would face in their career decision making process due to the inconsistency and insufficiency of information available to an individual. Thus career exploration reduces the difficulty in career decision making by reducing the uncertainty and ambiguity in the information available to an individual.

The job market is a complex and dynamic system where change is the only thing inevitable. The rate at which socio-economic and socio-cultural factors are changing is more rapid today. Hence to keep up with the changing times and conditions, one has to constantly evolve and update. So career exploration can give an individual the opportunity to update, change and evolve their career goals and expectations. Moreover, with the rapidly changing markets and socio-economic values, the impact of career exploration and career decision making has also altered drastically. This change in perspective is very important in the career decision making process to update oneself with the latest and more accurate information. This, in turn, increases one's confidence in their career decisions and career self-efficacy (Celik & Storme, 2017).

However, career exploration is an antecedent to career decision making as well as to career decision making difficulty (Muniarti & Siahaan, 2019). Career exploration is also found to increase career confusion (Celik & Storme, 2017). It is proposed that limited time and information can cause career confusion. Information overload can negatively impact the higher executive cognitive functions, which lead to errors in the information processing and decision making processes. These cognitive errors in inferential processing can lead to inaccurate beliefs and dysfunctional attitudes about one's career. This also reduces the motivation to make career decisions. For example, dysfunctional beliefs like there is only one right choice and only one perfect try can increase the negative affect and anxiety. Dysfunctional beliefs and general indecision can also be developed as psychological defenses during career exploration (Celik & Storme, 2017). Thus it is important to determine the "what", "where", "how" and "how much" career exploration is required by a person to facilitate smoother career decision making (Aftab & Malik, 2017).

Cognitive Trends in Decision Making

Decision making can be viewed as a problem-solving process involving the cognitive and affective processes needed to develop a plan" (Kaur & Kaur, 2017). This involves delving deeper into an individual's personal strengths, interests, ambitions, skills, values, scholastic aptitude as well as their higher cognitive functions of goals setting, planning, problem solving and decision making (Amir & Gati, 2006; Manodara et al., 2022). Muniarti and Siahaan (2019) observed that millennials have more open minded thinking capacity but have a neurotic nature of thinking. However, their ability to concentrate and focus on a task is hampered. This impacts their critical thinking ability negatively and causes issues in career decision making.

A good career plan reduces difficulties faced in arriving at the decision of a well-suited career. The challenges faced in career decision making may include both internal and external obstacles but a good career plan takes into account the possible barriers and obstacles that may be encountered by an individual in arriving at the final career choice. The readiness to decide is crucial in starting the process of career decision making. People with higher needs for cognitive closure tend to be more ready in making vital career decisions (Gati et al., 2011). By taking quick decisions, they try to avoid ambiguity and uncertainty and the anxiety associated with it.

Emotion and Personality in Career Decision Making

Gati et al. (2011) proposed that although deliberation is normal but it is a temporary phase. Pervasive and chronic career decision making difficulty may be related to emotional or personality related characteristics of the individual. People with negative cognitive biases and perceptions about the process of career decision making, about the world of work or about their own control were more likely to face career decision making difficulty and career indecision. This also negatively impacts the career decision making self-efficacy of an individual. Perfectionist people may experience higher career decision making anxiety. These processes are important for career identity formation in the individual.

On further exploring the BIG five personality traits, neuroticism was positively related to emotional and personality related career decision making difficulty as people with higher neurotic tendencies experience more emotional instability and psychological disturbances. Extroverts, on the other hand, were found to experience lesser career decision making difficulty than introverts because socializing with others improves self-efficacy in making career decisions by increasing access to information. People who rated high on agreeableness also faced less career decision making difficulty.

Conscientious people are believed to be more ordered in their approach and hence are less likely to be facing career decision making difficult. In fact, their investment and involvement in the career decision making process is found to be greater than others. Interestingly, people with higher scores in the openness to experience factor showed mixed responses. This indicates that flexibility and curiosity can be either positive or negative depending on the situation. For example, career exploration can result in reduced career decision making difficulty or increased career choice confusion depending on the context (Gati et al., 2011).

Muniarti and Siahaan (2019) observed that millennials faced more problems in concentration, engagement and socialization. According to their research, career decision makers today are more focused on their personal contribution rather than working together as a team. Since the locus of control is trending more towards intrinsics, they are more motivated by gainsharing and personal achievements rather than achievement of collective goals. As a result leadership styles are also changing because of the apparent inadequacy of elements of social competence. With changes in motivation, role models and focus also have changed drastically. Their expectations and reality of work-life balance have also changed a lot with the changing times and environments.

Decision Making Style

According to Mabel and Nagarenitha (2016), career decision making styles can be broadly classified as rational career decision makers, intuitive career decision makers, and dependent career decision makers. As the name suggests, rational career decision makers are very logical, organized and systematic in their way of arriving at a decision regarding their career. On the other hand, intuitive career decision makers tend to rely largely on their internal affective states. This may also result in impulsive and emotionally charged decisions regarding one's career. The third type of decision makers is the dependent career decision makers whose decisions about their career are contingent on other's reactions. They are often influenced easily by external factors like family influences, peer pressure, reactions of the society, etc.

Vocational decision styles and profiles have been developed to understand the underlying psychosocial interactions with various factors that affect our choice in career. As per the Career Decision Making Profile (Gati et al., 2012) information gathering, information processing, locus of control, effort invested, procrastination, speed of making the final decision, consulting with others, dependence on others, desire to please others, aspiration for an ideal occupation, and willingness to compromise were important characteristics in career decision making (Gati et al., 2012).

Muniarti and Siahaan (2019) have studied the cross-cultural differences in these factors. They found that Asian Americans have lesser difficulties in career decision making. Asian and Chinese students had a significantly high score on consulting with others compared to their counterparts, which contributed to easing their confusions and getting right guidance regarding their career decisions. They also had the tendency to please others, compromise, depend on others and procrastinate more than other Americans. White Americans on the other hand faced fewer obstacles in career decision making than their counterparts which helped them transition into their professional life easily and smoothly. However since more obstacles are faced by non-White Americans, their aspirations and achievements are lower in comparison. The locus of control is also found to be culturally very different in Eastern and Western cultures which impact the career decision making process.

Career Decision Making Self Efficacy

Bandura proposed that self-appraisal or self-efficacy becomes an important determinant in effective career decision making (Amir & Gati, 2006). Self efficacy is a way of cognitive regulation of motivation based on the expectations and determines the effort we spend towards the achievement of those expectations. While low levels of career decision making self-efficacy result in stress about career decisions, poor planning of career goals and career indecision, higher levels of career self-efficacy lead to stagnated growth and a lazy workforce (Fouad et al., 2009). Our previous personal experiences, past experiences in our career, past achievements, previous experiences of decision making, etc. play a key role in the formation of our cognitive beliefs (Manodara et al., 2022; Sud et al., 2020). The cognitive beliefs influence our attitudes towards a career by impacting our interests, preferences, passions, ambitions, gender beliefs, etc.

Career and Technology

With the advent and rapid evolution of technology, societies and markets have evolved with time to keep pace with the rapidly changing times. As the technology of the job markets change, the skills sets of the past soon become redundant and constant updation with the times becomes a necessity. The current trend of technological adaptation and advancement is a huge shift from the paradigm of the manual era. Social media which once was for entertainment has now become a priority requirement as a job skill set in most industries. Social media is also being used for profiling, tracking, hiring and recruiting human resources online and serves as a source of background check (Muniarti & Siahaan, 2019).

Current career decision makers have better access to information with the optimal utilization of technology. Due to the advancement and free access to technology in today's times, more career information is freely available. In fact, technology has transformed into a resource rather than just being a medium of information. Career decision makers need to be trained in utilizing and exploring the technological resources to their optimum levels. Prospective career decision makers can now make more informed decisions regarding the career options available. However, just like with any medium, information available online may not always be accurate and true always. Hence caution is required to process the information available online (Muniarti & Siahaan, 2019).

Changes in Education

With the advanced times, the pedagogical practices also have to adapt with the changing scenario. Currently, the approach to education is more practical and application-oriented than the previous trend of theoretical by-the-book education systems. Critical thinking and analytical abilities are further developed by the modern system of more open education that focuses on the learning rather than the lesson. Technological advancements have also contributed to developing more awareness and self-efficacy in making career decisions (Muniarti & Siahaan, 2019). Internships and other ways of career exploration activities further help individuals gain support and clarity in the demands, expectations and roles associated with a career option. This has led to increased acceptability of support seeking and help seeking behaviors in career decision making. The education system has also adapted to help the students in cognitive reframing and cognitive restructuring to avoid the pitfalls of faulty or less than optimal decision making (Mabel & Nagarenitha, 2016).

Ambiguity Tolerance

Ambiguity is present in different aspects of career decision making. With limited options and opportunities in the past, people were exposed to lesser ambiguity. However the modern World has increased ambiguities in various forms by opening more options and opportunities in the world of work. Hence to adapt to the changing world, tolerance for uncertainty and ambiguity is required as a skill to function smoothly in the world of successful and satisfying careers.

In the current fast-paced ever changing world, a very important factor is ambiguity tolerance where there is an overload of information of all kinds (Storme et al., 2017).

Socio-cultural Factors

Socio-cultural factors greatly influence the process of career decision making in youth. One of the most important socio-cultural influences is the influence of family on the career decision making process. Depending on the culture, families have different structures and hence different levels of involvement in the career decision making process. Fouad et al. (2016) found that people of color are more likely to be influenced by family expectations. Family background plays a key role in developing work values and perceptions of a career. Non-white career decision makers are more likely to have extrinsic family values due to higher family involvement in their career decisions. People with stronger sense of obligation to assist, support and respect the family's collective values and behaviors have strong influences on the family.

Another important aspect is the support that one receives from the family. In collectivistic cultures, family and society are greatly involved in career decision making of the individual. Since the individual receives financial, informational and emotional support from the family and society, the family expectations become the guiding force in the career decision making process which can also become a career barrier at times (Fouad et al., 2016). Parent's attitudes and wishes, involvement in the decision making process, awareness of options, socioeconomic status, experience in career, support, educational background, resources available, etc. (Bhatia & Babu, 2021; Manodara et al., 2022).

Family plays a crucial part in learning emotional regulation and expression that is approved by society (Sidek & Bakar, 2019). Work volition is the individual's perceived capacity to make career choices. Individuals from privileged backgrounds have greater access to career decision making opportunities and options. Individuals who come from strained and backward social backgrounds have limited options, limited opportunities and limited resources while making career decisions. Family and society becomes the final agency in deciding the career choice for the individual for the marginalized (Fouad et al., 2016).

External conflicts can arise from the involvement of social agencies like family and culture of the individual career decision maker. Loss of control and agency in making career decisions and choices can result in external conflicts with the family or society. Criticism, lack of support, loss of approval, fear of face loss, need to please others, etc. can influence external conflicts and the career decision making process (Gati et al., 2011). Lifestyle and life situation can be an important deciding factor in a career like family situation, locations, commitments, marital status, childbirth, family attitudes, etc. Professional life factors like stress, working hours, employment opportunities, work-life balance, income, mentorship, internship, prestige, peer influences, influence of teachers, etc. are taken into account while selecting a career (Sud et al., 2020). Vicarious observation and encouragement or discouragement can be a very powerful influence in career decision making.

Career Counselling

To help individuals struggling with the career decision making difficulties and career indecision, specialized and trained professional help is available in the form of career counselling. Just like other branches of psychological counselling, career counsellors are available to assist a person in making this important life decision. With the evolving markets and changing demands, career counsellors adopt a more inclusive and focused approach to help in selecting one's career. The tools available can help an individual who is struggling with this process by identifying their needs, evaluating their life roles, finding out their interests, identifying personal characteristics, exploring the influences of socio-cultural factors, overall decision making ability, obtaining career information, integrating the information regarding self with the career information, making a career choice, developing a career plan and implementing it to achieve their professional goals and satisfaction (Mabel & Nagarenitha, 2016).

In fact, after realizing the benefits of career counselling, various educational institutions as well as psychosocial organizations offer millennials an early and easy access to career counselling through their schools, colleges, Universities, internships and even in the workplace. This reduces the confusion and anxiety associated with the career decision making process and the individuals are able to make satisfactory career decisions and grow further in their chosen field. With the development in technology, there is widespread application of online career guidance and assessments available at the touch of a button (Muniarti & Siahaan, 2019).

Conclusion

Career is indeed a crucial decision that can make or mar a person's life. With the evolving World, career choices have also evolved and so have the challenges faced in career decision making with every option seeming enticing than the other. However, career decisions are a dynamic life long process where our interests will keep changing from time to time at every age and stage of life. The key to a happy career is to balance our internal wants and demands congruently with the external job markets. With the new problems, there are new solutions to the challenges and barriers in career selection and decision making. There is ample and free information available on various online platforms that help to increase awareness and decide. However careful interpretation of this information is warranted to protect against ambiguous and misleading information (Amir et al., 2008). Career courses and career guidance from counselors are an effective way to get clarity in making career decisions (Fouad et al., 2009). Prescriptive ways of career decision making is more congruent and builds resistance to tackle the challenges and low self-efficacy in making important career decisions.

References

Amir, T., & Gati, I. (2006). Facets of career decision-making difficulties. *British Journal of Guidance & Counselling, 34*(4), 483–503.

Amir, T., Gati, I., & Kleiman, T. (2008). Understanding and interpreting career decision-making difficulties. *Journal of Career Assessment, 16*, 281.

Aftab, S. R., & Malik, J. A. (2017). Mediating role of career thoughts for the effect of career exploration on career decision making. *Foundation University Journal of Psychology, 2*(1), 1–18.

Bhatia, S., & Babu, N. (2021). Parental involvement in the career decision making of adolescent girls. *Journal of Applied Research in Humanities, Language and Social Sciences, 1*(1), 111–120.

Celik, P., & Storme, M. (2017). Career exploration and career decision-making difficulties: The moderating role of creative self-efficacy. *Journal of Career Assessment, 20*(10), 1–12.

Fidan, V., & Nas, S. (2021). Career decision-making difficulties for high school students. *The Journal of International Education Science, 8*(29), 1–18.

Fouad, N., Cotter, E. W., & Kantamneni, N. (2009). The effectiveness of a career decision-making course. *Journal of Career Assessment, 17*(3), 338–347. https://doi.org/10.1177/1069072708330678

Fouad, N. A., Kim, S. Y., Ghosh, A., Chang, W. H., & Figueiredo, C. (2016). Family influence on career decision making: Validation in India and the United States. *Journal of Career Assessment, 24*(1), 197–212.

Gati, I., & Kulcsár, V. (2021). Making better career decisions: From challenges to opportunities. *Journal of Vocational Behavior, 126*, 103545.

Gati, I., Krausz, M., & Osipow, S. H. (1996). A taxonomy of difficulties in career decision making. *Journal of Counseling Psychology, 43*(4), 510–526.

Gati, I., et al. (2011). Emotional and personality-related aspects of career decision-making difficulties: Facets of career indecisiveness. *Journal of Career Assessment, 19*(1), 3–20.

Gati, I., Gadassi, R., & Mashiah-Cohen, R. (2012). Career decision-making profiles versus styles: Convergent and incremental validity. *Journal of Vocational Behavior, 81*, 2–16.

Kaur, S., & Kaur, K. (2017). Career decision making and career choice anxiety in students with learning disabilities. *International Research Journal of Commerce Arts and Science, 8*(4), 133–142.

Manodara, D. K., Tennakoon, W. D. N. S. M., & Lasanthika, W. J. A. J. M. (2022). Explanatory study on career decision making difficulties. *Asian Journal of Education and Social Studies, 9*(1), 1–11.

Mabel, S. B., & Nagarenitha, M. (2016). Career maturity and career decision-making—A review. *International Education and Research Journal, 2*(12), 56–57.

Murniarti, E., & Siahaan, L. I. (2019). Millennials' career decision-making difficulties (cdmd) in Indonesian university students. *Advances in Social Sciences Research Journal, 6*(9), 268–276.

Storme, M., Celik, P., & Myskowski, N. (2017). Career decision ambiguity tolerance and career decision making difficulties in a french sample: The mediating role of career decision self-efficacy. *Journal of Career Assessment, 12*, 1–16.

Sud, S., Wong, J. P., Premji, L., & Punnett, A. (2020). Career decision making in undergraduate medical education. *Canadian Medical Education Journal, 11*(3), 56–66.

Sidek, M. S., & Bakar, A. Y. A. (2019). Emotional intelligence and self-efficacy career decision making among high school students. *Education and Social Sciences Review, 1*(1), 1–7.

Upasana Bagchi is a Doctoral Research Scholar in the Department of Psychology, Christ University, Bangalore. She has a Master's degree in Counseling Psychology from Christ University and has been practicing as a counselor since the past eleven years. She is the author of the book

"Rediscover Life" and has also published multiple scholarly articles and book chapters in Scopus-indexed journals and international projects. She has been invited to deliver speeches and seminars on various interesting topics. She conducts practical workshops on topics of Psychology that synthesize her knowledge of Psychology with the experience of Counseling. Her area of special interest is stuttering. She enjoys working on unique phenomena that interest the Psychologist in her.

Prof. K. Jayasankara Reddy has M.Sc and Ph.D. in Psychology in the area of NeuroPsychology, also has a Master degree in Clinical Neurophysiology and MBA in Higher Education Management. He has been an active teacher, researcher and practitioner in the field of Health, Cognitive Neuropsychology and Neuroscience since then. Presently, working as Professor of Psychology and Coordinator for Center for Research at Christ University, Bangalore, India. He has guided and graduated 12 Ph.Ds, 15 M.Phil by research and more than 90 postgraduate research project students in the area of Health, Neuropsychology and Cognitive Neuroscience. He has published more than 150 research articles in peer-reviewed journals, presented his research at more than 60 national and international conferences, and has also organized many conferences of national and international significance. Dr. Reddy is the recipient of Indian School Psychology Association (InSPA)—P K Subaraja Trust Best Performance Award—2017 for his valuable services and contributions to the promotion of school psychology in India. Also received National Stress Management Research Award 2017 in recognition of positive contribution to the subject of Stress Management from the International Stress Management Association (ISMA). All through his career, he is identified for successful contribution as a teacher in the field of Cognitive Neuropsychology and Neuroscience, and as academic administrator at various capacities while maintaining a very high level of research output in terms of quality as well as quantity.

Chapter 14
Efficacy of Online Training on Internet of Things (IoT) and Automation Through Industry and Institute Partnership During COVID-19 Lockdown

Sibnath Deb, David Paul, Shikha Soni, Emily J. Hernandez, and Shayana Deb

Abstract COVID-19 forced all educational institutions to close down for the safety of students, educators, and community, and transformed the traditional face-to-face classroom teaching to a virtual mode of teaching and remote learning for the continuity of education. While this shift affected the overall process of traditional teaching, learning practices, and norms, many students made adjustments and managed to be engaged in the learning process and made progress towards gaining knowledge in this new modality. During the lockdown phase, a one week intensive training program was organized for students and young professionals with information technology (IT) backgrounds free of cost to provide them a hands-on orientation on Internet of Things (IoT) and Automation through an Industry and Institute Partnership. The resource persons i.e., teachers for the training were from premier technical institutions like the National Institute of Technology and Industry. A total of 262 participants completed the program. After the training program, 139 participants provided online feedback and shared their views about the experiences and effectiveness of the training. The objective of this article was to examine the participant perceptions of the effectiveness of the IoT and automation online training. About half of the participants were male (65.5%), below 25 years of age (74.1%), and studying at different levels including 10 Ph.D. scholars, and about four-fifths of them were current students of IT. Gaining knowledge was the main reason for 69.1% of participants while 18.7% attended the training with a notion that a training certificate will be beneficial for their career

S. Deb (✉)
Department of Applied Psychology, Pondicherry University (A Central University), R.V. Nagar, Puducherry 605 014, India
e-mail: sibnath23@gmail.com

D. Paul · S. Soni · E. J. Hernandez
Rajiv Gandhi National Institute of Youth Development (RGNIYD), Ministry of Youth Affairs and Sports (MoYAS), Government of India (GoI), Pennalur, Sriperumbudur 602 105, Tamil Nadu, India

S. Deb
University of Groningen, Groningen, The Netherlands

S. Deb and S. Deb (eds.), *Handbook of Youth Development*,
https://doi.org/10.1007/978-981-99-4969-4_14

growth. More than half of them found the training to be very effective (53.2%) while 45.3% found it to be effective ($\chi^2 = 6.94$, $p < 0.05$). About two-thirds (66.2%) of participants stated that all the resource persons were knowledgeable and experienced while 26.6% remarked that the majority of the resource persons were knowledgeable and experienced ($\chi^2 = 11.07, p < 0.01$). Hands-on training and sessions on practical applications were the most interesting part of the training as revealed by thematic analysis of qualitative data. The results of this study indicate that the online mode of training was a good option for knowledge dissemination and even hands-on training during the COVID-19 lockdown as pointed out by 94.2% of participants reporting that they would like to attend a similar training in the future.

Keywords Online training · Internet of things · Automation · Industry and institute partnership · India · COVID-19 · Impact

Introduction

The effectiveness of teaching and learning greatly depends upon the knowledge and experience of the teachers, their level of engagement with the class, along with their styles of teaching, personality, communication skills and passion for teaching (Yen, 2020). Besides the teacher's personal qualities, pedagogy also makes a big difference in teaching and learning outcomes. It helps to create a good teaching and learning environment if a teacher uses a visual for the class such as a power-point presentation (ppt), facilitates dialogue that provides stimulating context for learning and makes it interesting for the student. In turn, pedagogy helps in engaging students in the subject. Explaining the basic concepts of the topic in a simple form giving practical examples and allowing the students to ask questions and clarifying the queries of the students while teaching make students more comfortable to attend a class and gain knowledge resulting in better understanding of the subject. The more engaged students are with the content, class, and instructor, the more actively involved they are in the learning process.

Transitioning from face to face learning to virtual teaching and remote learning due to the COVID-19 pandemic lockdown was necessary in order to provide for continuity of the learning process and access to education for students across the world. A number of past studies have reported on the positive and negative aspects of online teaching and learning. Evidence related to the positive aspects of online teaching highlight that it was most successful when suitable pedagogy was adopted, there were no internet connectivity problems, and students could afford or have access to a smartphone and/or computer for attending online teaching (Bahasoan et al. 2020; Lapitan et al., 2021; Paudel, 2021) . For instance, Bahasoan et al. (2020) reported that "the online learning system carried out during the COVID-19 pandemic was effective and also inefficient. Effectively implemented because of the conditions that require online study and inefficient because the costs incurred more when compared with offline lectures." Based on a quantitative study, Yen (2020) reported that flipped classrooms (i.e., a type of blended learning where students are introduced to content at home and practice working through it at institute) for online teaching are effective and feasible to implement. In addition, engaging students before class, in-class and after-class activities were also found to be effective. Finding ways to enrich the content, making the class fun and engaging, including the sense of humor of instructors and a positive climate in the classroom were found to have additional positive benefits in the flipped classroom model for online teaching. Therefore, universities should develop policies to encourage teachers to encourage their adaptation of flipped classrooms. Further, Susilawati and Supriyatno (2020) observed that there are increasing trends in online learning in this current generation and post-pandemic Covid-19 by using platforms for additional engagement such as "WhatsApp", or other digital communication applications, to increase learning motivation by students with the premise that these are additional ways that increase student engagement with the learning content.

Additional aspects of online teaching and learning have also been found to be effective. Likewise, for teaching and learning purposes through the broadcast of pre-recorded lecture videos on internet platforms, such as "YouTube", to allow students to study and progress with learning at their own pace by using a five-component blended learning strategy referred to as "Discover, Learn, Practice, Collaborate and Assess" (DLPCA) was found to be effective (Lapitan et al., 2021). Overall, this study found that students were satisfied with the DLCPA strategy. Evidence concerning the negative aspects of online teaching demonstrates a number of factors which acted as barriers for an effective teaching and learning process and they included poor communication between teachers and students, lack of understanding of the material, poor internet connectivity, lack of motivation among students, and fatigue in attending the online classes continuously (Adnan & Anwar, 2020; Alawamleh, Al-Twait, & Al-Saht, 2020). In this regard, Tang et al. (2020) found that students were dissatisfied with online learning in general, and they were especially dissatisfied with the lack of communication with instructors and questions and answers modes on platforms. However, the combined model of online teaching with flipped learning improved students' learning, attention, and evaluation of courses. In another study Alawamleh et al. (2020) observed that students' lack of motivation in attending online mode of teaching was related to failing to get answers to their questions within a timely manner. Feelings of isolation caused by online classes were found to be another reason for poor motivation among students in online classes. Students from developing countries are in a disadvantageous position since their access to devices and regular internet connectivity is a big problem for their country. For example, in a study in Pakistan, authors examined the attitudes of Pakistani higher education students towards compulsory digital and distance learning university courses amid Coronavirus (COVID-19). The findings of the study highlighted that online learning cannot produce desired results in underdeveloped countries like Pakistan, where a vast majority of students are unable to access the internet due to technical as well as monetary issues (Adnan & Anwar, 2020). This is further applied to more developed countries in more rural areas and geographic regions with higher rates of poverty.

The Internet of things (IoT) is a very important subject in the present era of digital communication and networking. It refers to network interfacing and communication of physical objects, devices and peripherals. In summary, IoT is a networking technology which keeps the devices interconnected and helps in efficient utilization for economic benefits of the industries and end-users. IoT and automation have several valuable applications. For example, IoT helps in efficient traffic management and using GPS so one can find the traffic position in a particular route and ascertain the shortest possible routes and alternatives while industries use IoT for process management and tracking of products and for optimization of quality customer services to name a few. Likewise automation has many applications in our day to day life minimizing human efforts. Some of the applications of automation include the use of various control systems for operating equipment such as machinery, processes in factories, boilers, heat-treating ovens and so on.

Application of knowledge in different areas of IT in solving various daily life problems is very important. The students with information technology background need to be updated from time to time since advancement in various dimensions of IT is very rapid and they must acquaint themselves with the latest development so that they can probe their updated knowledge at the time of interview and apply the advanced knowledge in their workplace. Given this background and need, a one week intensive training program on "Internet of Things and Automation" was organized for the students with IT background to enhance their knowledge and skills about various applications of the subject in real life by providing hands-on training in addition to giving an overview of basic concepts in simple form. After the intensive training program, feedback from the participants was collected through an online mode.

The objective was to study the effectiveness of a one-week online intensive training on "Internet of Things and Automation" as perceived by the participants of the online training.

Methods

Sample: Students and young professionals with information technology (IT) and mathematics background attended the training on Internet of Things and Automation and provided online feedback about the same. Information about the training program was circulated through the website of the institute and personal network with other higher learning institutes and participation in the online training was voluntary.

Intervention: A one week intensive training was developed and organized by a National Institute of Youth Development in association with premier Institutes in the field of Information Technology in India and one industry during March 15–19, 2021. The training was designed combining the basic/theoretical concept and practical applications (hands-on exposure) after giving serious thoughts on the subject to make it more interesting and beneficial for the potential participants. Altogether, 20 sessions were arranged and each session was one and half hours in duration. Highly experienced specialized faculty/teachers from the premier technical institute in India and from the IT industry were engaged in the training program. All the resource persons delivered lectures with special interest using a visual medium such as a ppt and at the end there was a question and answer session for clarification of queries.

There was no course fee for participation for students. However, at the end of the training a certificate was issued only to those youth participants who attended 80% of the lecture. This information was communicated to potential participants in the information brochure indicating the level of professionalism, seriousness, and expectations of course participation.

Study Tool for Data Collection: At the end of the course, using a Google Form (Semi-structured Questionnaire) feedback was obtained from 139 youth participants of the courses through online mode based on voluntary participation. In addition to background information like age, gender, educational background and present occupation, their feedback about the courses and resource persons were collected. Some of the questions included the following:

What is the source of information i.e., how the participants came to know about the online training?

Why did you decide to attend the short-term training?

Did you attend all the sessions? If not, why?

Did you face internet connectivity problems while attending the on-line classes?

Did you find the course effective? Why did you say so?

Did you find the resource persons knowledgeable and experienced?

Did you find on-line mode of classes as a good option for teaching during this phase?

Would you like to attend a similar training programme in future?

Which aspect/lecture of the training was very stimulating for you?

What are the key messages you got attending the course?

The Semi-structured Questionnaire has both open and close ended questions and option for mode of response varies from question to question. For example, in case of one question like *"Did you face internet connectivity problems while attending the on-line classes?", mode of responses include Always….0.1; Sometimes………2; and Never………3 while in case of another question i.e., "Did you find the course effective?", response is captured in terms of Very Effective…….0.1; Effective……0.2; Not So Effective……….0.3.*

Data Analysis: Quantitative data was subject to calculation of frequency and percentages while qualitative data with respect two issues viz., (i) Which aspect /lecture of the training was very stimulating for you? and (ii) What are the key messages you got attending the course? were subject to thematic analysis. A Chi-square test was done to find the difference between variables while thematic analysis was used to examine the common responses and/or themes that are topics, ideas and patterns of meaning that came up repeatedly from the participants with respect to two different issues. The first step involved familiarization with the qualitative data to enable further analysis. Next, codes were identified in the data. After having identified codes, different themes based on qualitative data were noted, examined, defined, named and presented in the results section.

Results

Table 14.1 shows the information regarding the background of the participants who provided the feedback after participating in the training. The participation of males was significantly higher (65.5%) as compared to (34.5%) females in the training program ($\chi^2 = 5.27, p < 0.05$). The majority of the participants (74.1%) were aged below 25 years, 10.8% were aged 26–30 years, 6.5% were 31–35 years old and the remaining 8.6% were aged 36 and above years ($\chi^2 = 12.02, p < 0.01$). The percentage of the participants whose education was below graduation was significantly higher (47.5%) followed by post graduates (30.2%), graduates (15.1%), and Ph.Ds (7.2%) respectively ($\chi^2 = 7.57, p < 0.01$). Regarding the occupation, the participation of youth (79.9%) was significantly higher when compared with teachers (12.9%) and those employed in other jobs (7.2%), ($\chi^2 = 8.39, p < 0.05$). Less than half of the participants came from North East India (43.9) and more than half of the participants (56.1%) who took part in the training program were from other parts of India ($\chi^2 = 8.39, p < 0.05$).

Regarding the source of information about the training, more than one-third of the participants (38.1%) received the information from the website of RGNIYD, followed by faculty (22.3%), friends (19.4%), others (15.1%) and Department Notice Board (5.0%) ($\chi^2 = 8.39, p < 0.05$). Concerning the reason for attending the training, the majority of the participants (69.1%) attended it to gain knowledge followed by receiving course certificate (18.7%), re-skill to get re-entry in the job market (5.8%), to refresh knowledge (4.3%), clarify specific queries related to the subject (1.4%) and others ($\chi^2 = 7.98, p < 0.05$). An overwhelming percentage of the participants (93.5%) attended all the training sessions while the rest 6.5% did not attend all the sessions ($\chi^2 = 12.25, p < 0.01$). The majority of the participants faced internet connectivity problems sometimes, 12.2% always, and the remaining 18% did not face any internet connectivity problems while attending the online training ($\chi^2 = 8.12, p < 0.05$) (Table 14.2).

Table 14.3 depicts the perception of participants about the training and resource persons. More than half of the participants (53.2%) found the training to be very effective followed by effective (45.3%), and not so effective (1.4%) respectively ($\chi^2 = 6.94, p < 0.05$). The training was found to be effective because 41.5% found resource persons very effective, 40.7% learned a lot of new things, 14.8% reported coverage of good content and the rest 3.0% disclosed that they could clarify their queries while attending the training ($\chi^2 = 7.10, p < 0.05$). Two-thirds of the participants that is 66.2% reported that all the resource persons were knowledgeable, over a quarter (26.6%) found the majority of them knowledgeable, less than one-tenth (6.5%) found few of them knowledgeable and 0.7% found none of them knowledgeable ($\chi^2 = 11.07, p < 0.01$). More than ninety percent of the participants (94.2%) were of the opinion that online mode of training was a good option for teaching and learning during COVID-19 lockdown phase while 5.8% shared opposite views ($\chi^2 = 13.22, p < 0.01$). Almost all the participants (97.8%) showed interest to attend the similar training in future except 2.2% ($\chi^2 = 15.13, p < 0.01$).

Table 14.1 Background of the participants who provided feedback after the training ($n = 139$)

Variables	Mode of response		Chi-square
	f	%	
Gender			
• Male	91	65.5	5.27*
• Female	48	34.5	
Age			
• <25 years	103	74.1	12.02**
• 26–30 years	15	10.8	
• 31–35 years	9	6.5	
• 36 + years	12	8.6	
Education			
• <Graduation	66	47.5	7.57*
• Graduate	21	15.1	
• Post graduate	42	30.2	
• Ph.D.	10	7.2	
Occupation			
• Student	111	79.9	8.39*
• Teaching	18	12.9	
• Employed in other job	10	7.2	
Place of origin			
• North East India	61	43.9	3.47*
• Other part of India	78	56.1	

* *Significant at* $p < 0.05$ *level*; ** *Significant at* $p < 0.01$

Figures 14.1 and 14.2 reflect that over 98% of participants perceived the program to be effective with approximately 93% finding the resource persons to be knowledgeable and experienced.

Table 14.4 presents the participants perception about the training program wherein more than half of the participants (55.4%) felt that training program was highly effective in achieving its stated objectives while 38.1 and 6.5% felt it effective and moderately effective. Interestingly, none of the participants felt it ineffective in achieving its stated objectives ($\chi^2 = 7.88, p < 0.05$).

Qualitative Analysis of Data

Thematic analysis was carried out to examine the responses of the participants with respect to two issues, viz., (a) Which aspect/lecture of the course was very stimulating for you? and (b) What are the key messages you got attending the course? As

Table 14.2 Source of information about the training and reasons for attending ($n = 139$)

Variables	Mode of response		Chi-square
	f	%	
Source of information about the training			
• From the website of RGNIYD	53	38.1	6.27*
• From friends	27	19.4	
• From faculty	31	22.3	
• Department notice board	7	5.0	
• Others	21	15.1	
Reasons for attending the training			
• To gain knowledge in the subject	96	69.1	7.98*
• To refresh knowledge	6	4.3	
• To clarify specific queries related to the subject	2	1.4	
• To re-skill to get re-entry in the job market	8	5.8	
• Course certificate will be beneficial for career growth	26	18.7	
• Others	1	0.7	
Attended all the sessions			
• Yes	130	93.5	12.25**
• No	9	6.5	
Faced internet connectivity problems while attending the on-line training			
• Always	17	12.2	8.12*
• Sometimes	97	69.8	
• Never	25	18.0	

* *Significant at* $p < 0.05$ *level;* ** *Significant at* $p < 0.01$

discussed before the sub-themes in the following section with respect to each theme are presented:

Thematic analysis with respect to the first issue (i.e., which aspect/lecture of the course was very stimulating for you?) helped to identify the areas/sub-themes which were highly stimulating for the participants and explained in the following section. For example.

Sub-themes with respect to first issue after thematic analysis are as follows:

- *Practical implementation of the course*
- *Importance of Internet of Things (IoT)*
- *Emerging innovative technology of IoT*
- *Technology update*
- *Miscellaneous.*

Q: Which aspect/lecture of the course was very stimulating for you?

Table 14.3 Perception about the training and resource persons ($n = 139$)

Variables	Mode of response		Chi-square
	f	%	
Did you find the training effective?			
• Very effective	74	53.2	6.94*
• Effective	63	45.3	
• Not so effective	2	1.4	
Why did you say so?			
• Not at all effective	0	0	7.10*
• Resource persons were very effective	56	41.5	
• Learnt a lot of new things	55	40.7	
• Could clarify queries	4	3.0	
• Good contents covered	20	14.8	
• Others, specify	0	0	
Did you find the resource persons knowledgeable and experienced?			
• All of them	92	66.2	11.07**
• Majority of them	37	26.6	
• Few of them	9	6.5	
• None of them	1	0.7	
Did you find on-line mode of training as a good option for teaching during COVID-19 lockdown phase?			
• Yes	131	94.2	13.22**
• No	8	5.8	
Would you like to attend a similar training in future?			
• Yes	136	97.8	15.13**
• No	3	2.2	

* *Significant at* $p < 0.05$ *level;* ** *Significant at* $p < 0.01$

Practical Implementation of the Course

One of the most commonly observed themes is regarding practical implementation of IoT and Automation during the course. The majority of participants found the training very helpful. Below are few statements of the participants:

> Demonstration of practical implementation made this course even more interesting - a male IT student (25 years)

> All the sessions specially today's session…directly demonstrate with practical experience and skills - a female IT professional (27 years)

> The last day practical was amazing - a male IT student (22 years)

> Giving insight into the field and hands on knowledge with a session on opportunities - a female IT professional (32 years)

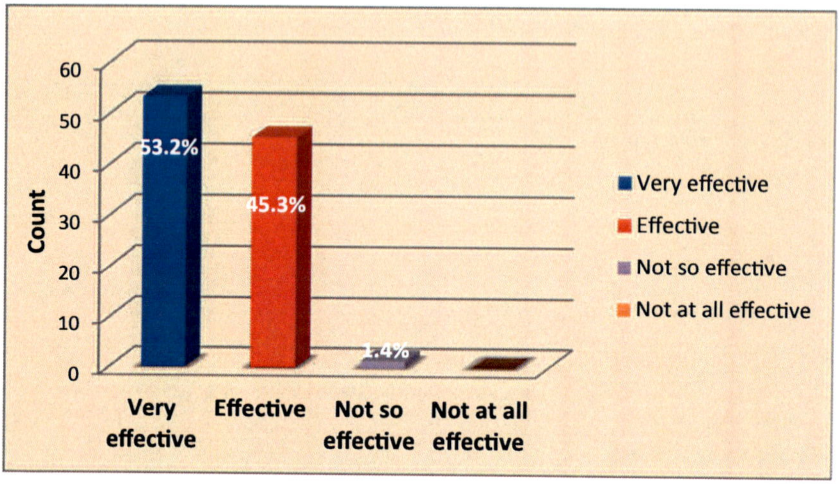

Fig. 14.1 Was internet of things (IOT) and automation training effective?

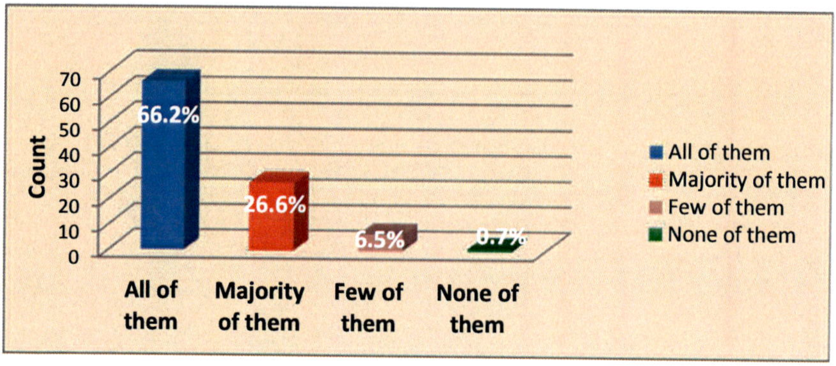

Fig. 14.2 Did you find the resource persons knowledgeable and experienced?

Table 14.4 Perception about the training program ($n = 139$)

Do you think that the training program was able to achieve its stated objectives?	Mode of response		Chi-square
	f	%	
• Highly effective in achieving its stated objectives	77	55.4	7.88*
• Effective in achieving its stated objectives	53	38.1	
• Moderately effective in achieving its stated objectives	9	6.5	
• Not so effective in achieving its stated objectives	0	0	

* *Significant at* $p < 0.05$ *level;* ** *Significant at* $p < 0.01$

Importance of Internet of Things

Another common theme was related to the Internet of things (IoT). Many participants reported that the information shared was valuable and technologically significant. Below are few statements of participants:

> As I am a bioinformatician so the lecture on IoT in smart health monitoring was most effective lecture for me… -a female IT faculty (34 years)

> Practical assignments related to IoT - a male IT student (21 years)

> Project on IoT and automation - a male IT professional (27 years)

> Smart home using IoT - a female IT student (20 years)

> IoT enabled WSNs for agricultural applications - a male IT faculty (36 years)

Miscellaneous

Additionally, there were other miscellaneous aspects of the lecture reported by the participants, such as lectures on automation, robotics techniques, Rasberry Pi Picco, drone technology, specific resource persons, etc. Following are few statements of the participants:

> Sensor topic and the robotic techniques used in hospitals and industries is very much stimulating for me - a male IT professional (33 years) working in a hospital

> The drone technology was very interesting and was worth investing my time - a female IT final year student (22 years)

> …and practical on Rasberry Pi Pico and micropython - a male IT faculty (29 years)

Apart from the themes mentioned above, many other participants said that all the lectures were helpful.

Participants were further asked to share their views about the key messages they got attending the training program. Thematic analysis of responses of the participants with respect to second issue (i.e., what are the key messages you got attending the course?) are broadly categorized into three groups and provided below with explanations:

- *Emerging innovative technology of IoT*
- *Technology update*
- *Miscellaneous.*

Q: What are the key messages you got attending the course?

- ***Emerging innovative technology of IoT***

The most common key message reported is regarding the development of new technology with changing times. IoT is one such technology that participants found to be growing in India. For instance, participants mentioned the following things that they learnt about the IoT:

> IoT has huge amount of financial benefits in India - a male IT students (21 years)

> Reskill oneself, and learning about IOT and other related technology - a male IT professional (29 years)

> IoT is going to be the future and learning this will make us more adaptive to analyze things in future - a female IT professional (26 years)

> 1) Sensors to collect the data for the IoT system to process it, (2) Connection and identification from the device to the IoT system through an IP address - a female IT professional (27 years)

> I had zero knowledge of IoT but with online courses held...now I know the use of IoT in health care, agriculture, smart everything, cloud computing, app development, the industrial IoT...India's acceleration in IoT... - a male IT professional (29 years)

> They key messages I got attending this course were the progression towards automation, improving precision through IoT and its role in growth in various sectors like healthcare, logistics etc., and opportunities in this field - a female IT professional (26 years)

Technology Update

Other than IoT, participants also mentioned it is important to be updated with the advanced and upcoming technology in the fast pacing world. This is reflected in following verbatims of participants:

> The tech world is growing at very fast pace, we need to learn and keep up with the world - a female IT professional (28 years)

> Technology keep advancing and we need to move forward with changing tech - a male IT student (22 years)

> We need to learn new skills to keep up with the level of innovation and experimentation going on in today's world - a female IT student (21years)

> Brand new waves of technologies are lying ahead of us to be tapped and used - a female IT PhD scholar (26 years)

Miscellaneous

The participants conveyed a few other miscellaneous key messages where participants conveyed about learning new things and applying it to their skill set and their overall development. Following are the few verbatim responses:

> Expand your knowledge in IoT and seeing forward to gain much more knowledge regarding it - a male IT PhD scholar (25 years)

> I have got good resources, knowledge about the internet of things like connecting sensors with medical instruments, with automobiles and drones also. One of the amazing facts was that Tesla cars work on the internet of things. It self-drawing mode is very fantastic and its safety measures is also amazing - a female IT professional (29 years)

> To explore bookish knowledge into real word - a male IT student (22 years)

...we don't need to be good at everything in this field. If we are good at at least one thing, we need to keep working on it and that itself will help us a lot. - a male IT PhD scholar (26 years)

Learning is the key to success - a female IT student (23 years)

Initially I have no deep knowledge of the subject, but, now I have vast directions to move in this subject further - a female IT PhD scholar (27 years)

In this modernization world it's good to know and gain some knowledge of how the technologies work and functions and use it for a betterment - a male IT professional (28 years)

Discussion

A one week intensive training program jointly conducted by the industry and institute partnership through virtual mode on Internet of Things and Automation was successful in enhancing the knowledge and skills of Indian youth as clearly indicated in the feedback form. Qualitative data also endorsed the quantitative data with respect to efficacy of the training. The resource persons for this training from the premier technical academic institutes with vast research experience took the sessions with special interest and presented the subject in a simple form providing many practical examples.

The findings of the present study corroborate with findings of some of the previous studies although the methodology for virtual/online mode of teaching and learning varied to some extent and they carried out the study among different branches of students at different levels (Tartavulea et al., 2020; Bahasoan et al., 2020; Yen, 2020; Susilawati & Supriyatno, 2020). For example, Bahasoan et al. (2020) observed that the online learning system carried out during the COVID-19 pandemic is effective. At the same time, Yen (2020) reported that flipped classrooms for online teaching are effective and it can be implemented in higher learning institutes. Further, the author suggested that some activities before and after the virtual classes and even during the virtual classes will make teaching and learning more interesting and engaging for the students. Similarly, Susilawati and Supriyatno (2020) found that there is an increase in online learning in this generation and post-pandemic Covid-19 by using different applications and platforms, such as "WhatsApp" to increase learning motivation and engagement. However, Nadeak (2020) reported that distance learning using social media is found to be effective for theoretical subjects only, not so effective for practical subjects. In another study students expressed their interest for the multimedia means of studies with availability of enough sources of soft study materials during COVID-19. However, the study also pointed out the poor internet connection problems causing interruption during the virtual education (Pandey et al., 2021). The study by Muthuprasad et al. (2021) indicates that the majority of the students (70%) were ready to opt for virtual mode of teaching for completion of the syllabus during COVID-19 pandemic. However, students wanted some flexibility in attending the virtual classes. In order to improve their performance, students wanted the recorded classes with a quiz at the end of each class. For practical oriented subjects, students wanted a hybrid mode.

Like other training and online programs particularly in the field of IT, the number of male participants was double the number of female participants. Interestingly the number of young participants i.e., below 25 years of age was more and most of them were current students of IT. A good number of the participants working in different IT industries also attended the training looking at the profile of the resource persons. The participation of ten Ph.D. scholars in the training is another indication of proper planning of the training on the subject and identification of suitable teachers. It is relevant to mention that in India there are a number of engineering colleges teaching IT related courses in addition to other engineering branches. However, Indian Institute of Technology (IIT) and National Institute of Technology (NIT) are the most sought after premier Engineering Institutes in India for studying any technical subjects including IT related courses. There is tough competition for admission in those institutes. Therefore information regarding the training on Internet of Things and Automation in association with two branches of National Institute of Technology—an institute of national importance under the Ministry of Education, Government of India—through partnership with an industry attracted a large number of youth mostly with IT background to register for the training since most of the resource persons are from NITs. In addition, training on such an important and job oriented subject without fee was another reason for more participation. Obviously experienced resource persons with research-based knowledge could meet the expectation of the participants and therefore most of the participants expressed their satisfaction after attending the training program as reflected in the online feedback. On and above, hands-on training provided by the resource persons from the industry complemented the sessions conducted by the academics. In between the sessions and end of each session, question and answer sessions made the teaching and learning process more interesting, understandable and engaging for youth.

Thematic analysis reflected that the practical implementation of the subject was the most interesting aspect of the training as reported by most of the participants, followed by valuable and technologically significant information shared by the resource persons during the training and some lectures on automation, robotics techniques, Rasberry Pi Picco, drone technology, specific resource persons and so on. As far as key messages from the training as perceived by the participants are concerned, IoT and automation is perceived to be an emerging innovative technology which has many applications in day to day life. For example, using IoT technology self-drawing mode cars are coming into the market and it is unique and safe.

It is relevant to mention that the New Education Policy (NEP) 2020 of the Government of India emphasized on multidisciplinary education, academic as well as industry and institute partnership for more innovative and start-up programs. Therefore the one week intensive training was in line with NEP, 2020. In the past, very few industry and institute partnership training programs were conducted in India. Hence academic partnership and partnership between the industry and academic institute added additional value in making the training more interesting, informative and educational.

Conclusion and Recommendations

A one week online training program on Internet of Things and Automation through Industry and Institute Partnership yielded positive results. Out of 264 participants, 139 provided online feedback which helped to assess the effectiveness of the training. Findings clearly indicated success of the training as more than half of the participants found the training to be very effective (53.2%) while 45.3% found it to be effective. Further two-thirds (66.2%) of participants stated that all the resource persons were knowledgeable and experienced while 26.6% were of the view that the resource persons were knowledgeable and experienced. Reportedly, the partnership between the academic institute and industry, hands-on training, sessions on practical applications of the subject and question and answer sessions for clarification of the queries were some of the most interesting parts of the training for participants. During the COVID-19 lockdown, the online mode of training on such an important subject to enhance the knowledge of participants and refresh their knowledge was a good option as pointed out by 94.2% youth and most stated they would like to attend similar training in future. Further, it is recommended to provide the visual content in power-point presentation (ppt) of all the training sessions prior to the training program to the participants along with a soft copy of relevant study materials. Given the positive experience and effectiveness results reported by participants, it would be recommended to continue to conduct similar short-term intensive training programs periodically and ensure similar results by inviting the best resource persons on the subject.

References

Adnan, M., & Anwar, K. (2020). Online learning amid the COVID-19 pandemic: Students' perspectives. *Online Submission, 2*(1), 45–51.

Alawamleh, M., Al-Twait, L. M., & Al-Saht, G. R. (2020). The effect of online learning on communication between instructors and students during Covid-19 pandemic. *Asian Education and Development Studies.*

Bahasoan, A. N., Ayuandiani, W., Mukhram, M., & Rahmat, A. (2020). Effectiveness of online learning in pandemic COVID-19. *International Journal of Science, Technology & Management, 1*(2), 100–106.

Lapitan, L. D., Jr., Tiangco, C. E., Sumalinog, D. A. G., Sabarillo, N. S., & Diaz, J. M. (2021). An effective blended online teaching and learning strategy during the COVID-19 pandemic. *Education for Chemical Engineers, 35*, 116–131.

Muthuprasad, T., Aiswarya, S., Aditya, K. S., & Jha, G. K. (2021). Students' perception and preference for online education in India during COVID-19 pandemic. *Social Sciences & Humanities Open, 3*(1), 100101.

Nadeak, B. (2020). The effectiveness of distance learning using social media during the pandemic period of covid-19: A case in Universities Kristen Indonesia. *International Journal of Advanced Science and Technology, 29*(7), 1764–1772.

Pandey, D., Ogunmola, G. A., Enbeyle, W., Abdullahi, M., Pandey, B. K., & Pramanik, S. (2021). COVID-19: A framework for effective delivering of online classes during lockdown. *Human Arenas,* 1–15.

Paudel, P. (2021). Online education: Benefits, challenges and strategies during and after COVID-19 in higher education. *International Journal on Studies in Education, 3*(2), 70–85.

Susilawati, S., & Supriyatno, T. (2020). Online learning through WhatsApp group in improving learning motivation in the era and post pandemic COVID-19. *Jurnal Pendidikan: Teori, Penelitian, Dan Pengembangan, 5*(6), 852–859.

Tang, T., Abuhmaid, A. M., Olaimat, M., Oudat, D. M., Aldhaeebi, M., & Bamanger, E. (2020). Efficiency of flipped classrooms with online-based teaching under COVID-19. *Interactive Learning Environments,* 1–12.

Tartavulea, C. V., Albu, C. N., Albu, N., Dieaconescu, R. I., & Petre, S. (2020). Online teaching practices and the effectiveness of the educational process in the wake of the COVID-19 pandemic. *Amfiteatru Economic, 22*(55), 920–936.

Yen, T.-F. (TF). (2020). The performance of online teaching for flipped classrooms based on COVID-19 aspect. *Asian Journal of Education and Social Studies, 8*(3), 57–64.

Prof. Sibnath Deb Ph.D. & DSc, is Professor of the Department of Applied Psychology, Pondicherry University (A Central University). Prior to that, Prof. Deb served the Rajiv Gandhi National Institute of Youth Development, Ministry of Youth Affairs and Sports, Government of India as Director for three and half years (January 8, 2020 to June 30, 2023). Professor Deb was also acting as Director (I/C), Directorate of Distance Education, and Dean (I/C), School of Law, Pondicherry University. He also taught at the University of Calcutta. In 1994, Professor Deb did an intensive course on 'HIV/AIDS and Qualitative Research' from the University of Western Australia. From April 2009 to August 2009, Professor Deb visited the School of Public Health, Queensland University of Technology (QUT), Brisbane, Australia, as Visiting Faculty. Currently, he is also an Adjunct Professor at the School of Justice, QUT, Australia. During 2004–2008, he served the International Society for the Prevention of Child Abuse and Neglect (ISPCAN) as Council Member. In brief, he has 32 years of teaching, research and administrative experience and has produced 22 Ph.D.s in addition to publishing more than 100 research articles/book chapters in the leading national and international journals. Professor Deb has written nine books and edited 11 books. Some of his latest published books are (a) Child Safety, Welfare and Well-being: Issues and Challenges (2nd Edition, 2022, Springer Nature, Singapore); (b) School-based Family Counseling For Crisis and Disaster (Routledge, California, in press); (c) Health and Well-being: Challenges, Strategies and Future Trends (2022), Springer Nature, Singapore; (d) Youth Development in India: Future Generations in a Changing World (2021), New Delhi, Routledge. Professor Deb has received three national and three international awards in recognition of his contribution in the field of psychology including "Visitor's Award-2019" from the Hon'ble President of India Shri Ram Nath Kovind. His current areas of research interest include family dynamics, parenting styles, child safety, students' mental health, adolescent reproductive health and applied social psychology.

David Paul has 21 years of experience as Research Associate at National Institute of the Visually Handicapped—Regional Centre (Govt. of India) and served as Training and Placement Officer where he undertook research studies pertaining to jobs identification for the visually impaired and their performance evaluation. He previously taught Career Counseling and Counseling Psychology at RGNIYD, an apex organization of the Union Ministry of Youth Affairs and Sports. He is currently a Training Officer at RGNIYD. His passion areas include training, teaching, research, documentation, and dissemination on youth issues and specialize in applied psychology, career counseling and disability rehabilitation.

Dr. Shikha Soni is a Rehabilitation Council of India licensed Clinical Psychologist, and currently, she is a Doctoral Research Scholar in Psychology in the Department of Liberal Arts at Indian Institute of Technology, Hyderabad. She has completed her MPhil in Clinical Psychology from Central Institute of Psychiatry, Ranchi, graduation and postgraduation in Psychology from Delhi University. She has been trained in various psychological testing like psychodiagnostic, intelligence tests, neuropsychology, and other tests (disability/psychopathology) and therapies like cognitive behavior therapy, supportive therapy, marital/family therapy, and various other therapies. Her research interests bridge the areas of positive, social, personality, and clinical psychology. She is currently researching in the area of positive adaptation to loss through the unique lens of life stories.

Dr. Emily J. Hernandez is an associate professor and program coordinator of the School-Based Family Counseling program at Cal State University, Los Angeles. She brings over 25 years of experience working in public education and mental health in the United States. Her professional background includes working directly with schools, families, and communities including school counseling and child welfare and attendance, K-12 school administration, clinical mental health, private practice, employee assistance services, and counselor preparation and education. She is a Licensed Marriage and Family Therapist with areas of expertize in working with children, couples and families, educators, victims of violence, trauma, and crisis counseling. As a leader in the field, she has presented locally, regionally, nationally, and internationally and has authored a variety of scholarly work. She has served on multiple organizational leadership boards advocating for the need for mental health services in education. She brings a unique lens to working with educators and school systems understanding the importance of bridging the gap towards more access to mental health in prevention and intervention in education. She holds a bachelor's degree in psychology and a master's degree in counseling in Marriage and Family Therapy and School Counseling from Cal State University, Los Angeles, and a doctoral degree in Educational Leadership with a concentration in educational psychology from the University of Southern California (USC).

Shayana Deb obtained M.Sc in Behavioral Science from the CHRIST (Deemed to be University), Bengaluru, India. She did her undergraduate with a triple major i.e., Biotechnology, Chemistry and Botany. Currently, she is pursuing second Master Degree on Youth Policy in the University of Groningen, The Netherlands. She attended a number of online courses on different subjects based on her areas of academic interest. She has a special interest in child protection and youth development. On a voluntary basis, she worked in two research projects which created interest in her on child welfare and well-being issues and positive development of adolescence and youth. She has published three articles, eight book chapters and one conference proceedings as co-author. Recently she has co-authored two book and they include (i) Social Psychology: Theories and Applications and (ii) Community Psychology: Emerging Issues and Challenges (in press, Routledge).

Chapter 15
Youth and Media Literacy in the Age of Social Media

Sukriti Pant, Bhuvana Manohari Nataraj, and K. Jayasankara Reddy

Abstract Living in the age of information means information is all pervasive, uncensored, unreliable, and with the potential to influence. The unfettered access to information and communication through social media is a double-edged sword in the hands of youth. The impact of this was explored from sociocultural and mental health perspectives. Specifically, the role of media literacy in combating the challenges posed by usage of social media was explored in this chapter. Various theories, frameworks, models, and components of media literacy were analysed. Impact of the various media literacy interventions on the youth, case studies of specific information literacy programs across regions, and other relevant critiques were reviewed and consolidated. Further to this, recommendations have been presented on creating robust in-school, and outside-school media literacy programs for the youth.

Keywords Media literacy · News literacy · Youth development · Youth education

Introduction

Information has never been as available as it is in the current times. With unfettered access to media and media devices, the youth of today deal with the constant availability of information at their fingertips. Kemp (2022) reported that 67% of the world's population has access to mobile phones, 63% were internet users, and 58% used social media. These statistics include 75% of social media users who are aged 13 years and above. While there are advantages, this unfettered access can also lead to numerous issues. The youth and young adults are the cusp of adulthood, where they are still developing physiologically and psychologically. The type, the quality, and the sheer quantity of information that they engage with each day can impact them

S. Pant
Via News Didi, Jalandhar, India

B. M. Nataraj · K. J. Reddy (✉)
Department of Psychology, CHRIST (Deemed to be University), Bengaluru, India
e-mail: jayasankara.reddy@christuniversity.in

S. Deb and S. Deb (eds.), *Handbook of Youth Development*,
https://doi.org/10.1007/978-981-99-4969-4_15

physically, mentally, and socially. While it is impossible to roll back the availability of information, media literacy may be the tool that the youth need to be equipped with so that the engagement with media will be more beneficial and less harmful. In this light, the impact of media on youth, the need for media literacy among youth, and ways to inculcate media literacy are explored in this chapter.

Impact of Social Media on Youth

As Carr and Hayes (2015) attempt to lay the ground to define social media, they remark that definitions of social media differ not just in the characteristics they emphasize, but also the disciplines they are defined in context of. With respect to definitions of social media originating from the communication discipline, Kaplan and Haenlein (2010) and Terry's (2009) definitions of social media, talk of digital technology platforms that center around user-generated content or interaction. Social media has also been defined through the exchange of messages (Kent, 2010) or through modes of interaction, in people's use of social networking tools like Facebook or Twitter (Howard & Parks, 2012). However, as Carr and Hayes (2015) explain, definitions that try to delineate the nature of social media in too simplistic a manner (such as a description of its tools) run the risk of equating it to other forms of communication like email, which lacks the nuance that these varied social media platforms do.

> Within the related discipline of public relations, Kent (2010) states that any interactive communication channel that allows for two-way interaction and feedback could be called a social medium… Modern social networks are characterized by the potential for real-time interaction, reduced anonymity, propinquity, short response times, and the ability to "time shift," or engage the social network whenever it suits each particular member. (p. 645)

This definition is notable in its differentiation between traditional media (commonly understood as print and online media) and modern social media, which has now become synonymous with the platforms that are used to engage in it.

What is visibly different between traditional and modern social media is the agency granted to the user. Gone are the days when all consumers could do was absorb the information given to them. With the advent of social media, users can now not only absorb the information they see or hear, but consciously (and sometimes unconsciously) add to the body of information that is at their disposal. This also means that regulation of this information is virtually impossible, since all one needs to have in order to become a creator of content is a smartphone and an internet connection, amenities that are no longer in short supply in households across the globe. Thus, social media comprises both devices such as mobile phones, tablets, computers, and of media platforms such as networking sites, messenger tools, and content creation applications. Also, social media users can both be content creators and users at the same time.

According to Erik Erikson (Batra, 2013), the stage of adolescence, which can last from the age of to 10–24 or 26 years, is a time when an individual is undergoing both physiological and behavioral changes, and are consolidating their identity, establishing relationships, and are developing their moral and ethical framework to understand the workings of the world. Media usage at this stage can have significant impact on the direction of development at this stage of the youth. Media devices and social media are currently designed to be addictive. With the use of intermittent reinforcement, affirmation, validation, attention-grabbing techniques such as notifications, social connection, competition, and the fear of missing out or being left out, individuals can be habituated to using media constantly, and thus, can create an addiction (Griffiths, 2018). Furthermore, the information available is oftentimes emotionally loaded with the intention to provoke, biased, with questionable veracity (Fox, 2018).

Social media usage impacts the youth physically, psychologically, and socially. A study conducted in Taiwan (Chang et al., 2016) reported that there was a relationship between exposure to alcohol and tobacco in media and consumption of alcohol and tobacco among them. A study done among American adolescents revealed that technology-based social comparison, and seeking reassurance was associated with depressive symptoms, and it was more so among females, and those who were less popular in school (Nesi & Prinstein, 2015). In a survey conducted in Ghana, the participants reported experiencing sleep deprivation, difficulties in concentrating at school, and cyberbullying among other things (Ocansey et al., 2016). Dunlop et al., (2016) analyzed the prevalence of marketing of harmful products on social media platforms, and found that, despite policies and regulations, marketers used subtle means to promote harmful products such as alcohol, tobacco, and unhealthy food. In another survey conducted among pre-university and university students in India, Singh et al., (2017) found that over 75% of them used social media for over three hours per day. While they reported that they found social media useful for communication, location-based services, outlet for creativity, and learning, they also stated that use of social media caused physical problems such as headache, eye pain, high blood pressure, and pain in hand, gastro-intestinal issues, and poor eating habits; psychological problems like anxiety, stress, mental exhaustion, and panic; social and academic problems like decreased interaction with others, disinterest in studies, and unproductive time spent on social media. An analysis presented by Abi-Jaoude et al. (2020) concluded that social media consumption affects mental health of the youth: mental health impact includes sleep deprivation, poor self-view, negative social interaction including cyberbullying, negative effects on cognitive functioning and attention, academic performance, socio-emotional functioning, self-injury, and so on. They also reported that there is a link between the amount of social media consumption and the extent of impact, and that some individuals are more susceptible than others. In a Mexican study among university students, social media addiction was found to be associated with depression, and suicidal ideation (Jasso-Medrano & López-Rosales, 2018). Khodabakhsh and Leng (2020) found that there was moderate association between social media consumption and negative body image among university students. Another negative impact of social media is that the anonymity has given rise to hate speech along political, religious, race, and other divisive lines.

While there are negative bio-psycho-social impacts of use of social media on youth, there are also positive impacts. Maamari and Zein (2014) found that the Lebanese youth, despite not engaging in the voting process, used social media to engage in political discussions. Social inclusion of youth on the fringe is another benefit available through social media. Ybarra et al. (2015) found that LGBT (lesbian, gay, bisexual, and transgender) youth found the online space as safe for finding friends and obtaining social support compared to their non-LGBT peers. Clark et al. (2018) suggest that social media can promote social well-being of adolescents. They make a distinction between connection promoting use of social media versus non-connection promoting usage, and propose that using social media can enhance quality of the relationship, and meet acceptance and belonging needs. However, when use of social media does not fulfill acceptance and belonging needs, it can lead to lower sense of well-being. Nesi et al. (2019) found that among youth that were psychiatrically hospitalized used social media to distract themselves from their difficulties, and some even sought social support from peers, though there were negative impacts like comparison with others, with feelings of exclusion as well. Harriman et al. (2020) found that with increased exposure to social media, there was an increased likelihood to hate speech. They also found that online space led to decrease in inhibition, thus, making it more likely to engage in hate speech encounters.

Thus, social media and internet platforms provide benefits and challenges to the youth of today. Prevalence of social media is here to stay, and equipping the youth with media literacy to navigate the world of social media will empower them to use it judiciously.

Media Literacy and Youth

What is Media Literacy

It is evident that social media is a place that has a lot to offer to the people that engage with it. As Brown (1998) argues, media presence in the youth's daily lives has become all-pervading, having an impact on not just on leisure time, but also on one's perception and judgment about society, as well as the political, economic and social environment that they are a part of. More than twenty years on, his argument still holds water, and brings to light the importance of media literacy for the youth. However, if social media can have such diverse definitions, then an intervention designed to equip the youth to combat its effects will surely have many interpretations.

Potter (2013), through his review of literature of media literacy studies, lays out several definitions of media literacy, postulated by both scholars as well as citizen action groups. Adams and Hamm (2001) state that

> Media literacy may be thought of as the ability to create personal meaning from the visual and verbal symbols we take in every day from television, advertising, film, and digital media. It is more than inviting students to simply decode information. They must be critical thinkers who can understand and produce in the media culture swirling around them. (p. 33)

Silverblatt and Eliceiri (1997) define media literacy as

> a critical-thinking skill that enables audiences to decipher the information that they receive through the channels of mass communications and empowers them to develop independent judgments about media content. (p. 48)

The Center for Media Literacy (n.d.) describes media literacy as

> a framework for accessing, analyzing, evaluating and creating media, as well as the ability to communicate competently in all media forms, print and electronic, as well as to access, understand, and analyze and evaluate the powerful images, words and sounds that make up our contemporary mass media culture.

Considine (1995) defines that media literacy

> as the ability to choose, to understand—within the context of content, form/style, impact, industry and production—to question, to evaluate, to create and/or produce and to respond thoughtfully to the media we consume.

Through an analysis of both categories of definitions of media literacy, it becomes clear that while the output of media literacy may vary, where all definitions of media literacy converge is in the inclusion of certain skills that they postulate their target audience will learn/imbibe. These skills range from critical thinking and interpretation to analysis and evaluation of the content that people consume. In a push towards a skill-based understanding of media literacy, Potter (2013) lists a set of seven specific skills that media literacy programs develop—"analysis, evaluation, grouping, induction, deduction, synthesis, and abstraction." Most definitions also align on the individual's increased ability to develop their own judgements about the content they are consuming post the intervention. In an attempt to also bring to fore the 'creatorship' of a user of social media, media literacy programs also seek to empower their target audience with the skills to responsibly and reflectively create content for their and others' viewership.

The way that media literacy has been approached has seen many changes in the past years. From a moralistic approach to media literacy in its early years, where the focus lay in the removal of objectionable content, to a more objective and dispassionate stand taken by researchers and educators, who sought to make media literacy less value-laden and more pluralistic, to media literacy espousing valuative judgements against mass media corporations, each of these standpoints have collectively shaped the face of media literacy today. Since a critical evaluation of media is not an isolated practice, elements of cultural studies, semiotics and Marxist theory also find their place in media literacy interventions (Brown, 1998). Lewis and Jhally (1998) also talk of textual and contextual approaches to media literacy, which revolve around the familiarity that a user displays towards the content that he/she consumes. A textual approach is found to be more beneficial in situations where the target audience is new to the idea of comprehension and textual analysis, whereas a contextual approach to media literacy has a greater impact on a target audience that is familiar with comprehension and analysis, and can begin to see the interlinkages between the context of the production and reception of the media they consume and engage with.

Arguments also exist on what the purpose of media literacy should be. While most scholars say that the purpose of media literacy is to improve the lives of individuals in some way, through the provision of greater control over how their consumption of media will affect them (Buckingham, 1993; Hobbs, 1998; Lewis & Jhally, 1998), others view media literacy as playing a role in an educational curriculum (Brown, 1998; Buckingham, 1993; Masterman, 1997), while still others view media literacy as having a role to play in social activism (Buckingham, 1993; Lewis & Jhally, 1998). To an extent, each of these three purposes are visible in existing media literacy interventions for the youth and general population.

Importance of Media Literacy for the Youth

Considering the pervasive availability of media, and the impact it has on the youth, it is imperative that the youth are equipped to use this powerful tool in a way that is beneficial to them, and does not harm them. In essence, media literacy empowers individuals to use media discerningly. Following are some research that elucidate the positive impact of media literacy on various aspects of youth development.

Media Literacy and Risky Health Behaviour: Two similar studies done among the youth in Taiwan (Chang et al., 2016), and in Argentina (Salgado et al., 2012) indicate that social media literacy acted as a protective factor in preventing the youth from consuming alcohol or tobacco. The Taiwan study showed that, while increased exposure to alcohol and tobacco use corresponded with increased likelihood of substance use, presence of media literacy helped reduce substance use intention. Through meta-analysis of various researches it was found that media literacy had a small to moderate impact on youth having a positive attitude towards risky health behavior (Vahedi et al., 2018). Equipping youth with critical skills to analyze media and product messages enabled them to make healthier choices. Austin et al. (2020) found that media literacy-based nutrition programs that included both parent and youth showed an increase in child-initiated discussion about food-related media messages, and food nutrition. There was also an increase in consumption of fruit among the youth. Pinkleton et al., (2012) found that media literacy intervention enhanced the youth's ability to think critically about the unrealistic nature of sexual portrayals in the media, which helped them to make healthier decisions regarding engaging in sexual behavior.

Media Literacy, Civic Engagement, and Political Participation: In a study conducted among high school and college students in California, (Kahne et al., 2012) found that over half of them engaged in online media literacy activities, and a major portion of this participation was in the form of consumption of civic and political information. However, those that engaged in content creation were fewer than a quarter of them. They also found that those who engaged in media literacy activities showed greater politically driven online participation. Participants of a news literacy educational intervention done to enhance civic competence in Amsterdam demonstrated increased news media literacy, political efficacy, and political knowledge (Geers et al., 2020). Kahne and Bowyer (2019) found that increased participation in "Digital Engagement Learning Opportunities" corresponded with increased online participatory politics, which means online activities where the youth expressed their views on issues of public concern, and with increase in targeted political pressure, which includes participation in online campaigns, online petitions, etc.

Media Literacy and Body Image Issues: McLean et al. (2016) found that educating participants in critical media literacy on thin-ideal body images offset the impact of media message on the youth internalizing the messages, and they had better body satisfaction outcomes. Kurz et al. (2021) analyzed that eating disorder and body image interventions that included media literacy were more effective than those that did not include media literacy.

It is evident that media literacy programs encourage critical thinking and equip youth with tools that enable them to make informed decisions. In essence, media literacy puts the power back in the hands of the media consumer.

Examples of Media Literacy Programs

Many different forms and types of media literacy interventions exist around the world. Media literacy programs follow two predominant modes—in-school programs, and out-of-school programs. Media literacy can be incorporated into regular school curriculum, or be offered as periodic training programs, like camps, after-school workshops, and the like. Online programs are also increasingly becoming popular. They can either be in the form of online or hybrid workshops, or can be self-paced learning programs. Following are descriptions of some of the programs, and they typically use a blend of different methods.

Interventions Offered by a Network of Organizations

The News Literacy Network is chaired by the National Literacy Trust (n.d.) and comprises media, education and charitable organizations like BBC Young Reporter, Discovery Education, The Guardian Foundation and The Economist Educational Foundation, among others. Their goal is to aid teachers and educational institutions to provide the best media literacy programs they can to their students. To this end, they have compiled resources from multiple providers that educators and institutions can choose from. For example, BBC Young Reporter and The Guardian Foundation run their own media literacy programs for students to critically engage with the news.

The Australian Media Literacy Alliance (n.d.) (https://medialiteracy.org.au/index.php/about-us/) is a group of organizations with closely aligned objectives in the area of media literacy. The seven partner organizations provide insight into content creation, information provision, education and media and information usage. Their Media Literacy Framework encourages people to ask critical questions about the media using a set of six concepts—institutions, audiences, representations, technologies, languages and relationships. Their focus on this process of asking and answering questions around these six concepts leads to critical understandings, and forms the basis for more successful media experiences.

The Dutch Digitalisation Strategy 2021. The Government of Netherlands (2021) proposed the Dutch Digitalisation Strategy 2021. It is a policy level program in the Netherlands that contains all national policies concerning digitalization. It specifically targets youth by increasing school curricula. As of 2021, the Netherlands was still in the process of incorporating digital literacy and practical skills in the new school curricula for primary and secondary education. It also aims to support institutes for secondary vocational education and higher education to improve students' digital skills. Among other things, lecturers are trained and supported to digitalize education. For example, Tilburg University (n.d.) examines the influence of digital resources on the balance between work and private life, school performance, social relations and welfare, with the aim to further develop courses and other services to enhance digital skills.

Interventions Offered by the Government

Department for Science, Innovation & Technology (n.d) curates a website detailing events, programs, free resources and contact details of organizations working in various domains like preventing online harassment, managing privacy, recognizing misinformation and disinformation, avoiding harmful content online etc. The UK government has also instituted a school subject called PSHE (personal, social, health and economic) education, whose curriculum includes media literacy and digital resilience.

Media literacy resources by the California State Department of Education, in conjunction with the California School Library Association (CSLA) and KQED has also curated resources not just for students to access and learn from, but also for educators to better understand media literacy and find ways to integrate it into the school's curriculum (Howerter, 2022). The website also contains a section where resources to support media literacy in a distance-education mode are curated.

Media Arts by the Australian Government. The Australian government has constituted a framework for media literacy education within the Australian curriculum called Media Arts. It mandates media literacy education for all students in preschool to year 6, and to provide a scope and sequence beyond these mandatory years, up to year 10, providing teachers with support to ask critical questions about news accuracy, believability, bias, misrepresentation and ethical practice, as well as opportunities for students to make their own news stories (Nettlefold & Williams, 2018).

Interventions by Targeted Organizations

The Centre for Media Literacy (n.d.) is a nonpartisan, non-denominational educational organization that is dedicated to promoting and supporting media literacy education as a framework for accessing, analyzing, evaluating, creating and participating with media content. Their program, the CML MediaLit Kit is designed for implementation in classrooms, teacher in-service training or community education. The program follows a four-step "inquiry" process of awareness, analysis, reflection and action. Youth that are a part of the program learn to access information from a variety of sources, analyze and explore how messages are "constructed" through different media, evaluate media's explicit and implicit messages against their own principles, create their own messages using a variety of media tools and hence participate in a global media culture.

UNESCO's (n.d.) Media and Information Literacy Curriculum provides a framework for educators worldwide to implement media literacy curriculum in school contexts where it is possible, often within other curriculum frameworks such as Arts, English and Social Studies.

MediaSmarts (n.d.) is a Canadian not-for-profit charitable organization for digital and media literacy. They develop digital and media literacy programs and resources for homes, schools and communities. Their work involves supporting adults with information and tools so they can help children and teens develop the critical thinking skills they need for interacting with the media they love. Their website houses games, tip sheets, activities, lesson plans, tutorials and workshops for educators, parents and children.

The Way Forward

Media literacy is still an emerging field, and that is continually evolving alongside technological development. Drawn from existing research and work done in media literacy, the following are some suggestions and observations that will be useful for developing media literacy programs.

1. Focused Programs: Media literacy programs that have a specific focus reach the youth better than those that are generic. Kurz et al. (2021) found in their analysis that those programs that targeted specific issues had better impact on the participants. According to Piaget's theory of cognitive development, youth is the

stage at which individuals are growing from concrete operational stage to formal operational stage, which means that they are still at the stage of generalizing from specifics, and their ability to think abstractly is still developing.

2. Critical Thinking: The common element in effective media literacy interventions was encouraging critical thinking in the participants. When individuals are equipped to analzse media content critically, they gain the ability to recognize manipulation and propaganda, which enables them to regain their agency in decision making.
3. Engagement in the Curricula: Allowing for active participation in the creation of media literacy programs make it more accessible, relevant, and allows for better reach among the youth.
4. Training to Create Content: Media literacy programs that go beyond equipping youth in analyzing content consumed to creating online content tend to increase critical thinking, and encourage more meaningful participation.
5. Inter-agency Collaboration: Media literacy programs that are developed through inter-agency collaborations tend to be more robust as multiple perspectives can be brought in.

Conclusion

Information always comes with the ability to influence attitude, beliefs, and behavior. With the advent of mass media, those in control of the media hold considerable power in shaping individuals specifically, and societies at large. The omnipresence of information in the hands of people, including the youth, means that their attention is at the disposal of the media and media devices. When access to information is unrestrained as we see in the current times, the potential for distortion of information and manipulation is manifold. While it is nearly impossible to restrict access to information, it is possible to empower individuals with the capacity to regain agency and autonomy in how they interact with social media, and gain autonomy in what information they consume. Media literacy, at its core, has the potential to fill this gap in this age of unfettered information access. Thus, alongside the development of social media and media devices, continual development of media literacy is essential to ensure healthy development of the youth in our societies.

References

Abi-Jaoude, E., Naylor, K. T., & Pignatiello, A. (2020). Smartphones, social media use and youth mental health. *Canadian Medical Association Journal, 192*(6), E136–E141. https://doi.org/10.1503/CMAJ.190434

Adams, D., & Hamm, M. (2001). *Literacy in a multimedia age.* Christopher-Gordon Publishers. https://books.google.com/books/about/Literacy_in_a_Multimedia_Age.html?id=BN3gT8ARw08C

Austin, E. W., Austin, B., Kaiser, C. K., Edwards, Z., Parker, L., & Power, T. G. (2020). A media literacy-based nutrition program fosters parent-child food marketing discussions, improves home food environment, and youth consumption of fruits and vegetables. *Childhood Obesity, 16*(S1), 1–12. https://doi.org/10.1089/CHI.2019.0240

Australian Media Literacy Alliance. (n.d.). *Media literacy framework.* https://medialiteracy.org.au/index.php/framework/

Batra, S. (2013). The psychosocial development of children: Implications for education and society—Erik Erikson in context. *Contemporary Education Dialogue, 10*(2), 249–278. https://doi.org/10.1177/0973184913485014

Brown, J. A. (1998). Media literacy perspectives. *Journal of Communication, 48*(1), 44–57. https://doi.org/10.1111/J.1460-2466.1998.TB02736.X

Buckingham, D. (1993). Going critical: The limits of media literacy. *Australian Journal of Education, 37*(2), 142–152. https://doi.org/10.1177/000494419303700203

Carr, C. T., & Hayes, R. A. (2015). Social media: Defining, developing, and divining. *Atlantic Journal of Communication, 23*(1), 46–65. https://doi.org/10.1080/15456870.2015.972282

Center for Media Literacy. (n.d.). *What is media literacy? A definition... and more.* http://www.centerformedialiteracy.com/reading-room/what-media-literacy-definitionand-more

Center for Media Literacy. (n.d.). *CML Framework.* https://www.medialit.org/cml-framework

Chang, F. C., Miao, N. F., Lee, C. M., Chen, P. H., Chiu, C. H., & Lee, S. C. (2016). The association of media exposure and media literacy with adolescent alcohol and tobacco use. *Journal of Health Psychology, 21*(4), 513–525. https://doi.org/10.1177/1359105314530451

Clark, J. L., Algoe, S. B., & Green, M. C. (2018). Social network sites and well-being: The role of social connection. *Current Directions in Psychological Science, 27*(1), 32–37. https://doi.org/10.1177/0963721417730833

Considine, D. M. (1995). Are we there yet? An update on the media literacy movement. *Educational Technology, 35*(4), 32–43. https://www.jstor.org/stable/44428286?casa_token=83C47Tdn7uEAAAAA%3Aa1rZw3eINCzlrd0pOUtBQmFmr9iyQhPfxroE2oBH3ZKVTDy6_ce4yMr_QOyyYhkn9ycRPZER-R4lXX5qCzhv5EahR7c3gLkIc-7KJoQ2Pxsy8wCDGs8B#metadata_info_tab_contents

Department for Science, Innovation & Technology. (n.d.). Government of UK Department for Science, Innovation & Technology. https://www.gov.uk/government/organisations/department-forscience-innovation-and-technology

Dunlop, S., Freeman, B., & Jones, S. C. (2016). Marketing to youth in the digital age: The promotion of unhealthy products and health promoting behaviours on social media, *4*(3), 35–49. https://doi.org/10.17645/mac.v4i3.522

Fox, J. (2018). An unlikeable truth: Social media like buttons are designed to be addictive. They're impacting our ability to think rationally. *Index on Censorship, 47*(3), 11–13. https://doi.org/10.1177/0306422018800245

Geers, S., Boukes, M., & Moeller, J. (2020). Bridging the gap? The impact of a media literacy educational intervention on news media literacy, political knowledge, political efficacy among lower-educated youth. *Journal of Media Literacy Education, 12*(2), 41–53. https://doi.org/10.23860/JMLE-2020-12-2-4

Government of Netherlands. (2021). *The Dutch digitalisation strategy 2021 (English).* https://www.nederlanddigitaal.nl/documenten/publicaties/2021/06/22/the-dutch-digitalisation-strategy-2021-eng

Government of the United Kingdom. Department for Digital, Culture, Media and Sport. (2021). *Online media literacy resource.* https://www.gov.uk/guidance/online-media-literacy-resources

Griffiths, M. D. (2018). Adolescent social networking: How do social media operators faciliate habitual use? *Education and Health, 36*(3), 66–69.

Harriman, N., Shortland, N., Su, M., Cote, T., Testa, M. A., & Savoia, E. (2020). Youth exposure to hate in the online space: An exploratory analysis. *International Journal of Environmental Research and Public Health 2020, 17*(22), 1–14. https://doi.org/10.3390/IJERPH17228531

Hobbs, R. (1998). Building citizenship skills through media literacy education. In M. Salvador & P. M. Sias (Eds.), *The Public Voice in a Democracy at Risk* (pp. 57–76). Praeger. https://books.google.co.in/books?hl=en&lr=&id=qLoFui46dO8C&oi=fnd&pg=PA57&dq=hobbs+1996+media+education&ots=hL2EDep1Ch&sig=17ub0QeecniVAfRKNBf2cS7gzPQ&redir_esc=y#v=onepage&q=hobbs1996mediaeducation&f=false

Howard, P. N., & Parks, M. R. (2012). Social media and political change: Capacity, constraint, and consequence. *Journal of Communication, 62*(2), 359–362. https://doi.org/10.1111/J.1460-2466.2012.01626.X

Howerter, J. (2022). *Media literacy resources: A collection of resources to support media literacy in classrooms*. https://www.cde.ca.gov/ci/cr/ml/

Jasso-Medrano, J. L., & López-Rosales, F. (2018). Measuring the relationship between social media use and addictive behavior and depression and suicide ideation among university students. *Computers in Human Behavior, 87*, 183–191. https://doi.org/10.1016/J.CHB.2018.05.003

Kahne, J., & Bowyer, B. (2019). Learning, media and technology can media literacy education increase digital engagement in politics? *Learning, Media and Technology, 4*(22), 211–224. https://doi.org/10.1080/17439884.2019.1601108

Kahne, J., Lee, N., & Feezell, J. T. (2012). Digital media literacy education and online civic and political participation. *International Journal of Communication, 6*(1), 1–24. https://www.researchgate.net/publication/279626069_Digital_Media_Literacy_Education_and_Online_Civic_and_Political_Participation

Kaplan, A. M., & Haenlein, M. (2010). Users of the world, unite! The challenges and opportunities of social media. *Business Horizons, 53*(1), 59–68. https://doi.org/10.1016/J.BUSHOR.2009.09.003

Kemp, S. (2022). *Digital 2022: Global overview report*. DataReportal—Global Digital Insights. https://datareportal.com/reports/digital-2022-global-overview-report

Kent, M. L. (2010). Directions in social media for professionals and scholars. In R. L. Heath (Ed.), *The SAGE Handbook of Public Relations* (First). SAGE Publishing.

Khodabakhsh, S., & Leng, C. S. (2020). Relationship between social media usage and body image evaluation in Malaysian youth. *Malaysian Journal of Medical Research, 4*(4), 62–67. https://doi.org/10.31674/mjmr.2020.v04i04.013

Kurz, M., Rosendahl, J., Rodeck, J., Muehleck, J., & Berger, U. (2021). School-based interventions improve body image and media literacy in youth: A systematic review and meta-analysis. *Journal of Prevention, 43*(1), 5–23. https://doi.org/10.1007/S10935-021-00660-1/FIGURES/3

Lewis, J., & Jhally, S. (1998). The struggle over media literacy. *Journal of Communication, 48*(1), 109–120. https://doi.org/10.1111/J.1460-2466.1998.TB02741.X

Maamari, B. E., & Zein, H. E. (2014). The impact of social media on the political interests of the youth in Lebanon at the wake of the Arab Spring. *Social Science Computer Review, 32*(4), 496–505. https://doi.org/10.1177/0894439313512777

Masterman, L. (1997). A rationale for media education. In R. Kubey (Ed.), *Media Literacy in the Information Age* (1st ed., pp. 15–68). Routledge. https://doi.org/10.4324/9781351292924-2

McLean, S. A., Paxton, S. J., & Wertheim, E. H. (2016). Does media literacy mitigate risk for reduced body satisfaction following exposure to thin-ideal media? *Journal of Youth and Adolescence, 45*(8), 1678–1695. https://doi.org/10.1007/s10964-016-0440-3

MediaSmarts. (n.d.). *Use, understand & engage: A digital media literacy framework for Canadian schools*. https://mediasmarts.ca/teacher-resources/use-understand-engage-digital-media-literacy-framework-canadian-schools

National Literacy Trust. (n.d.). *News literacy network: Find the right fake news and critical literacy teaching resources*. https://literacytrust.org.uk/policy-and-campaigns/all-party-parliamentary-group-literacy/fakenews/newsliteracy/

Nesi, J., & Prinstein, M. J. (2015). Using social media for social comparison and feedback-seeking: Gender and popularity moderate associations with depressive symptoms HHS public access. *Journal of Abnormal Child Psychology, 43*(8), 1427–1438. https://doi.org/10.1007/s10802-015-0020-0

Nesi, J., Wolff, J. C., & Hunt, J. (2019). Patterns of social media use among adolescents who are psychiatrically hospitalized. *Journal of the American Academy of Child and Adolescent Psychiatry, 58*(6), 635-639.e1. https://doi.org/10.1016/J.JAAC.2019.03.009

Nettlefold, J., & Williams, K. (2018). *Insight five: A snapshot of media literacy in Australian schools.*

Ocansey, S. K., Ametepe, W., & Fynn Oduro, C. (2016). The impact of social media on the youth: The Ghanaian perspective. *International Journal of Engineering Technology and Sciences, 6*(1), 90–100. https://doi.org/10.15282/ijets.6.2016.1.12.1062

Pinkleton, B. E., Austin, E. W., Chen, Y. C. Y., & Cohen, M. (2012). The role of media literacy in shaping adolescents' understanding of and responses to sexual portrayals in mass media. *Journal of Health Communication, 17*(4), 460–476. https://doi.org/10.1080/10810730.2011.635770

Potter, W. J. (2013). Review of literature on media literacy. *Sociology Compass, 7*(6), 417–435. https://doi.org/10.1111/SOC4.12041

Salgado, M. V., Pérez-stable, E. J., Primack, B. A., Kaplan, C. P., Mejia, R. M., Gregorich, S. E., & Alderete, E. (2012). Association of media literacy with cigarette smoking among youth in Jujuy, Argentina. *Nicotine and Tobacco Research, 14*(5), 516–521. https://doi.org/10.1093/NTR/NTR240

Silverblatt, A., & Eliceiri, E. M. E. (1997). *Dictionary of Media Literacy.* Greenwood Press. https://books.google.co.in/books?hl=en&lr=&id=SxuLleZCuVUC&oi=fnd&pg=PR7&dq=Siverblatt+and+Eliceiri+(1997)&ots=MVaxXUydxg&sig=vRAVivf1DKtanS82bSV4rDXn-WM&redir_esc=y#v=onepage&q=SiverblattandEliceiri(1997)&f=false

Singh, M. M., Amiri, M., & Sabbarwal, S. (2017). Social media usage: Positive and negative effects on the lifestyle of Indian youth. *UCT Journal of Social Sciences and Humanities Research, 5*(4), 39–44.

Terry, M. (2009). Twittering healthcare: Social media and medicine. *Telemedicine and E-Health, 15*(6), 507–510. https://doi.org/10.1089/TMJ.2009.9955

Tilburg University. (n.d.). *Digital Society.* https://www.tilburguniversity.edu/research/topics/digital-society

UNESCO. (n.d.). *Media and information literacy curriculum.* https://www.unesco.org/en/communication-information/media-information-literacy

Vahedi, Z., Sibalis, A., & Sutherland, J. (2018). Are media literacy interventions effective at changing attitudes and intentions towards risky health behaviors in adolescents? A meta-analytic review. *Journal of Adolescence, 67*, 104–152. https://doi.org/10.1016/j.adolescence.2018.06.007

Ybarra, M. L., Mitchell, K. J., Palmer, N. A., & Reisner, S. L. (2015). Online social support as a buffer against online and offline peer and sexual victimization among U.S. LGBT and non-LGBT youth. *Child Abuse and Neglect, 39*, 123–136. https://doi.org/10.1016/J.CHIABU.2014.08.006

Sukriti Pant is a Postgraduate student at Azim Premji University, Bengaluru, while also holding the position of Director of Programs at Via News Didi, a social enterprise imbibing media literacy and journalism skills in school students. Prior to this, she has worked with Teach for India as a Teaching Fellow at a Government Higher Primary School in Bengaluru, Karnataka. Her areas of interest include social studies curriculum and pedagogy, teacher professional development, child development and learning, media and news literacy for children and inclusive education.

Bhuvana Manohari Nataraj is a Ph.D. scholar pursuing her doctorate in psychology at CHRIST (Deemed to be University), Bengaluru, India. After completing her M. Sc. in Applied Psychology, and M. Phil in Psychology, she worked with corporate clients, and non-governmental agencies in the areas of psychological assessment, counseling and psychotherapy, and training and development. Her areas of interest include counseling and psychotherapy, positive psychology, mindfulness-based programs, school psychology, and psychosocial well-being. In the long run, she seeks to work towards enhancing well-being in schools and educational institutions.

Prof. K. Jayasankara Reddy has M.Sc. and Ph.D. in Psychology in the area of NeuroPsychology, also has a Master degree in Clinical Neurophysiology and MBA in Higher Education Management. He has been an active teacher, researcher and practitioner in the field of Health, Cognitive Neuropsychology and Neuroscience since then. Presently, working as Professor of Psychology and Coordinator for Center for Research at Christ University, Bangalore, India. He has guided and graduated 12 Ph.Ds, 15 M.Phil by research and more than 90 postgraduate research project students in the area of Health, Neuropsychology and Cognitive Neuroscience. He has published more than 150 research articles in peer-reviewed journals, presented his research at more than 60 national and international conferences, and has also organized many conferences of national and international significance. Dr. Reddy is the recipient of Indian School Psychology Association (InSPA)—P. K. Subaraja Trust Best Performance Award—2017 for his valuable services and contributions to the promotion of school psychology in India. Also received National Stress Management Research Award 2017 in recognition of positive contribution to the subject of Stress Management from the International Stress Management Association (ISMA). All through his career, he is identified for successful contribution as a teacher in the field of Cognitive Neuropsychology and Neuroscience, and as academic administrator at various capacities while maintaining a very high level of research output in terms of quality as well as quantity.

Chapter 16
Online Professional and Job Oriented Courses for Youth in India with IT Background During COVID-19 Lockdown: Examining Its Effectiveness

Sibnath Deb, Tusharika Mukherjee, and David Paul

Abstract COVID-19 shattered the life of human civilization across the world psychologically, physically, socially and economically. Quality education from primary level to tertiary level has been badly affected as all the educational institutions were closed down for prevention of further spread of COVID-19 and depend on online mode of teaching and learning as education should never cease. Given this situation, RGNIYD in association with NIT Jalandhar, India organised four professional and job-oriented short term certificate courses (one-week) on different dimensions of IT for youth with IT and related background in 2020. The broad objective of this article was to examine the efficacy of online professional and job oriented courses. Data was collected by using a Google Form through online mode. Findings disclosed that about half of the youth participants (50.4%) found all the courses very effective with some variations while 46.8% found them effective as they could learn a lot from the courses because of diverse contents covered and they could clarify their confusions. We assessed the role of participant's grit and emotional intelligence in determining the training outcome and observed that grit mediated the relationship between perceived stress and training efficacy among male participants with a Northeast domicile and female participants from the rest of India. Regarding the resource persons, 67.3% youth participants stated that all the resource persons were knowledgeable and experienced when 27.1% stated that the majority of them were knowledgeable and experienced. About 90% found online mode of teaching and learning as a good option during COVID-19 lockdown. Interestingly about 84.5% stated that they would like to attend a similar course in future. In fine, it might be stated that the courses were highly successful in disseminating knowledge and information

S. Deb (✉) · D. Paul
Department of Applied Psychology, Pondicherry University (A Central University), Puducherry, India
e-mail: sibnath23@gmail.com

T. Mukherjee
Work and Organizational Psychologist, Münster, Germany

Associated with Justus-Liebig University, Giessen, Germany

S. Deb and S. Deb (eds.), *Handbook of Youth Development*,
https://doi.org/10.1007/978-981-99-4969-4_16

about four different areas of IT and their practical applications. It is recommended to organise similar courses in future which will be beneficial for youth for gaining knowledge and for getting a job.

Keywords Information technology (IT) · Online IT related course · Training effectiveness · Youth · India · COVID-19

Introduction

E-learning was one of the effective methods of learning which was much popular and useful much before the CoronaVirus pandemic. Online courses and e-learning platforms have proved to be beneficial for individuals to pursue additional courses with an option of self-pacing, particularly by working people. Computer assisted technologies are constantly advancing and shaping our day-to-day lives. Particularly, online education has become inevitable and the only viable method of teaching–learning process during the COVID-19 pandemic phase. World over, the universities, higher educational institutions and even schools have switched over to online methods of imparting education as an attempt to contain the spread of coronavirus. There are several advantages for online learning which includes flexibility, less cost, option for self-pacing the learning programmes, transcending the geographical boundaries through technology, focussed opportunities for career advancement and improving technical skills and utilizing the time effectively (Bahasoan et al., 2020; Susilawati & Supriyatno, 2020; Lapitan et al., 2021). The other advantages include improved educational outcomes that provide an enjoyable experience, which is less strenuous. While the effectiveness of face-to-face learning programmes over online programmes cannot be ruled out, online learning is always regarded better than no learning.

Online Learning an Alternative Method During COVID-19 Pandemic

The coronavirus pandemic has locked doors of markets, factories, offices, schools and universities in India and people, particularly the young people, are forced to confine themselves inside their homes. However in this extended lockdown India is witnessing a positive trend as e-learning platforms have opened up hundreds of windows for learning. There is a massive upsurge in the traffic of online learning platforms as more and more Indians (of all age groups) want to engage in meaningful learning. College/University Students are more inclined towards widening their range of academic learning whereas young working professionals want to utilize their time to enhance knowledge, acquire new skills or re-skill and up-skill themselves so that they can stay relevant in the future. The flexibility and convenience offered by the digital platforms is the greatest advantage to the learners at large.

On the other hand, the rapid advancement in the information technology sector is largely influencing various disciplines, industrial and allied sectors through automation and digitization of various products and processes thereby enabling to increase the efficiency levels of performances, enhance productivity and reduce costs and inputs. These new-era technologies will drive the future economy of the entire world and provide a range of opportunities for different categories of people. Therefore, there is a dire need for skill development to meet the current and futuristic manpower requirements in the IT industries.

Further, going forward, re-skilling and up-skilling will be constantly required by working professionals and online courses will help them remain relevant in the fast-evolving employment scenarios. For working professionals to remain relevant and climb up their career ladders requires continuous up-gradation of skills, while the new entrants and students who are poised to enter into the world of work require certification from reputed education brands besides possessing hands on transferable skills. However, the transfer of knowledge and skills can be potentially augmented by individual differences, which in turn are instrumental in bringing forth differential training outcomes. Contemporary literature has discernibly affirmed the impact of grit and emotional intelligence on both performance and coping with stress. Grit (Duckworth, 2016) is a predictor of educational, professional, and personal prosperity (Fernández-Martín et al., 2020) and has been described as the resilience and passion towards goal (Kent et al., 2015) predicting achievement and well-being (Duckworth & Quinn, 2009; Salles et al., 2014). Similarly, literature is replete with evidence of emotional intelligence predicting achievement in different areas of functioning (e.g., Mavroveli & Sánchez-Ruiz, 2011; Parker et al., 2004). Emotional intelligence allows perception, management, and utilization of emotions, hence serving as a social skill assisting individuals in self-reflection in the area of emotional functioning targeted towards both career goals and management of crisis (Schutte & Malouff, 2002; Schutte, Malouff, & Bhullar, 2009). Emotional intelligence becomes particularly relevant during a crisis like the COVID-19 pandemic which has resulted in unprecedented amounts of stress across the demographic sections. Considering these parameters, RGNIYD has taken advantage of the time and situation to empower the young people in terms of education, skill building and fostering employability by offering chances to the disadvantaged youth to get trained in the modern trending IT skills.

Conduct of Online Courses by RGNIYD

During the period of COVID-19 pandemic, a large number of youth have lost their jobs and are looking for skilling/level up training or re-skilling programs to enhance their employability skills and to secure gainful employment. In order to empower the youth with the latest knowledge and information RGNIYD conducted five day short-term courses on IT related issues like cyber security, artificial intelligence and machine learning, recent advances in data sciences and cloud computing.

While there are opportunities provided by MOOCs, Coursera, Code Academy, Swayam platforms, EdX, Udemy, Hack Design, Udacity and the like, learners have a wide range of options to choose their online programmes. RGNIYD has become a choice for many underprivileged students across India, particularly among the youth of north-eastern region due to the fact that the free online cutting-edge short-term courses offered by RGNIYD were designed appropriately with inbuilt theory and application nexus which will not only enhance the knowledge of the youth but also level-up the skills for enhancing the employability.

With a view to strengthen and add more value to the course, RGNIYD partnered with the National Institute of Technology (NIT), Jalandhar, Punjab (an Institution of National Importance functioning under the Ministry of Human Resource Development, Government of India). The salient features of these short-term courses were that the sessions were handled by renowned faculty and experts of high acclaim from various NITs, Indian Institute of Technology (IITs), premier universities and apex higher educational institutions across the country.

While RGNIYD has been imparting these short-term certificate courses free of charge through online mode, it was felt imperative for RGNIYD to evaluate from the learners the effectiveness of online method of education and to assess whether RGNIYD should continue to offer such online programmes to the youth of the country. Further, this type of evaluation will also provide scope for RGNIYD to study the effectiveness of the online programmes and to appropriately revamp and restructure the online courses based on the perceptions of the learners.

Therefore, the participants who attended the five-day short-term certificate courses on cyber security, artificial intelligence and machine learning, recent advances in data sciences and cloud computing were asked to provide their feedback online through a semi-structured questionnaire floated as Google form after the training to record their learning experiences, formed the data for this present study. The broad objective of this article was to examine the effectiveness of four online short-term certificate courses.

Methods

Sample: Youth with mostly information technology (IT), mathematics, commerce and pure science background attended the short-term certificate course on different dimensions of IT and provided online feedback about the courses.

Intervention: One week short-term certificate course was organised by Rajiv Gandhi National Institute of Youth Development—an institute of national importance under the Ministry of Youth Affairs and Sports, Government of India in association with National Institute of Technology (NIT), Jalandhar—another institute of national importance under the Ministry of Education, Government of India in 2020 during the COVID-19 lockdown phase through online mode on four different dimensions of IT and they include Cyber Security (September 14–18, 2020), Artificial Intelligence & Machine Learning (September 28–October 2, 2020), Data Science (October 19–23, 2020) and Cloud Computing (November16–20, 2020). The courses were designed after giving serious thoughts on the subject so that they become interesting and beneficial for the potential participants. The online teaching methods adopted include presentation of basic concepts of each subject through power-point presentation, the practical orientation, use of flipped methods, online demonstration, troubleshooting, use of case-studies for problem solving online, working on online programming exercises and so on.

In each course, 18–22 lectures were arranged and each session was for one and half hours. Highly experienced specialized faculty from the premier technical institutes in India like Indian Institute of Technology (IITs), National Institute of Technology (NITs) and from some other institutes were involved in the courses and even some from Australia for enlightening the youth on the subject keeping practical applications of the subject into account. All the resource persons delivered lectures with special interest using a power-point and at the end there was a question and answer session for clarification of queries.

There was no course fee for participation. However, at the end of the course certificate was issued only to those youth participants who attended 80% of the lectures and this information was notified in the information brochure indicating the seriousness of the course.

Study Tool for Data Collection: At the end of the course, using a Semi-structured Questionnaire (Google Form) feedback was obtained from the youth participants of the courses through online mode based on voluntary participation. In addition to background information like age, gender, educational background and present occupation, their views about the courses and resource persons were collected. Some of the questions include

What is the source of information about the course?

Why did you decide to attend the short-terms course?

Did you attend all the sessions? If not, why?

Did you face internet connectivity problems while attending the on-line classes?

Did you find the course effective? Why did you say so?

Did you find the resource persons knowledgeable and experienced?

Did you find on-line mode of classes as a good option for teaching during this phase?

Would you like to attend a similar programme in future?

In addition, three questions were kept in the Google Form, to have an idea about mental health status and support facilities of the youth during the COVID-19 prolonged lockdown phase in 2020. For example,

Do you feel like consulting a mental health professional to reduce your stress and/or to discuss any mental health challenges?

Do you have anybody to discuss your personal issues and problems?

If so, with whom do you prefer to discuss your personal issues and problems?

The Semi-structured Questionnaire has both open and close ended questions and option for mode of response varies from question to question. For example, in case of one question like *"Did you face internet connectivity problems while attending the on-line classes?", mode of responses include Always....0.1; Sometimes.........2; and Never.........3 while in case of another question i.e., "Did you find the course effective?", response is captured in terms of Very Effective.......0.1; Effective......0.2; Not So Effective..........0.3.*

Along with the background information schedule and questions pertaining to the training, participants also undertook measurement of individual factors like grit and emotional intelligence.

Grit (S) Scale (Duckworth & Quinn, 2009) consists of 8 of the original 12-item scale Grit (O) Scale, and assess perseverance of efforts and consistency of interests. Four items measured the participants' consistency of interests (CI: e.g., "I often set a goal but later choose to pursue a different one"), and four items assessed the students' perseverance of effort (PE: e.g., "I am diligent"). The items were rated on 5 point scales (5 = very much like me, 4 = mostly like me, 3 = somewhat like me, 2 = not much like me, 1 = not like me at all). A number of previous studies ascertained the psychometric properties of Grit Scale and found it to be suitable (Duckworth & Quinn, 2009; Strayhorn, 2014). This scale was used by scholars and academics globally and they established its psychometric properties (Clark & Malecki, 2019; Rojas et al., 2012; Duckworth & Quinn, 2009). The Cronbach's alpha of Grit Scale with the present sample was 0.80 for the consistency of interest domain, and 0.64 for the perseverance of efforts domain.

The Assessing Emotions Scale (Schutte et al., 2009) comprises 33 items assessing how well respondents typically identify, understand, regulate, and harness emotions in themselves and others. Each item is rated on a 5-point scale from 1 (Strongly disagree) to 5 (Strongly agree), three of which (5, 28 and 33) are reverse-scored. The scale is divided into four subscales namely, Perception of Emotion (items 5, 9, 15, 18, 19, 22, 25, 29, 32, 33), Utilization of Emotion (items 6, 7, 8, 17, 20, 27), Managing Own Emotions (items 2, 3, 10, 12, 14, 21, 23, 28, 31), and Managing Others' Emotions (items 1, 4, 11, 13, 16, 24, 26, 30), are marked in the present study as EI1, EI2, EI3, and EI4, respectively. The scale has good internal consistency and evidence of construct validity through association with theoretically related constructs (Schutte et al., 2009). Higher scores indicate greater emotional intelligence. Internal consistency in the present sample, as assessed by Cronbach's alpha, was 0.933.

Data Analysis: In addition to calculation of frequency and percentages, inter-correlations between perceived stress, grit, emotional intelligence, training effectiveness, gender and North East Domicile was carried out.

Results

Data depicted in Table 16.1 highlights the number of youth registered for attending the online short-term Certificate Courses on four different IT related issues and finally the number of youth attending the courses. Data indicates that about half of the youth (47.2%) attended the four different courses with some course-wise variation.

It is clear from Table 16.2 that youth in India were more interested in artificial intelligence and machine learning courses ($n = 110$), followed by cloud computing ($n = 83$), data science and cyber security ($n = 44$). About two-third of them were male (67.6%) while one-third were female (32.4%). However, gender-wise variation has been observed from course to course. The majority of the youth belonged to the 19–22 years age group (38.7%), followed by 31.0 and 27.5% belonging to 27 year and above and 23–26 years age groups. The remaining 2.8% were below 18 years of age group. The majority of the youth were graduate or postgraduate. As far as occupation is concerned, more than half of them were IT students (53.5%) at different levels while about one-third (29.2%) was working in IT sectors. More than half of the youths were from the North East Region of India (53.2%) while 46.8% were from the rest of India.

Most of the youth came to know about the courses from the website of RGNIYD and the rest from faculty members of different institutes, friends, notice boards of different educational institutions and other sources like facebook (Table 16.3). The

Table 16.1 Number of participants registered, attended and provided feedback

Variables	Cyber security (Sept. 14–18, 2020)		Artificial intelligence & ML (Sept. 28–Oct.2, 2020)		Data science (Oct.19–23, 2020)		Cloud computing (Nov.16–20, 2020)		Total
	f	%	*f*	%	*f*	%	*f*	%	*f* (%)
No. of participants registered online	121	100	262	100	151	100	313	100	847 (100)
No. of participants attended the courses out of total registered	64	52.9	164	62.6	69	45.7	103	32.9	400/847 (47.2)
No. of participants provided the online feedback out of total attended the courses	44	68.8	110	67.1	47	68.1	83	80.6	284/400 (71%)

Table 16.2 Background of the participants who provided feedback after the course

Variables	Cyber security (n = 44)		Artificial Intelligence & ML (n = 110)		Data science (n = 47)		Cloud computing (n = 83)		Total (n = 284)
	f	%	f	%	f	%	f	%	f (%)
Gender									
• Male	32	72.7	60	54.5	32	68.1	68	81.9	67.6
• Female	12	27.3	50	45.5	15	31.9	15	18.1	32.4
Age									
• <18 years	1	2.3	7	6.4	0	0	0	0	2.8
• 19–22	13	29.5	51	46.4	16	34	30	36.1	38.7
• 23–26	15	34.1	26	23.6	14	29.8	23	27.7	27.5
• 27 + years	15	34.1	26	23.6	17	36.2	30	36.1	31.0
Education									
• <Graduation	11	25	41	37.3	9	19.2	15	18.1	26.8
• Graduate	19	43.2	33	30	20	42.6	28	33.7	35.2
• Post graduate	13	29.5	31	28.1	17	36.1	38	45.7	34.9
• Ph.D.	1	2.2	5	4.5	1	2.1	2	2.4	3.1
Occupation									
• Student	18	40.9	74	67.9	16	34	44	54.3	53.5
• Teaching	3	6.8	3	2.8	6	12.8	3	3.7	5.3
• Employed in other job	16	36.4	22	20.2	18	38.3	27	33.3	29.2
Place of origin									
• North East India	25	56.8	39	35.5	15	31.9	72	86.7	53.2
• Other part of India	19	43.2	71	64.5	32	68.1	11	13.3	46.8

main reason for attending the courses as cited by the youth was gaining knowledge about the subject (65.1%) while 21.1% thought that the attendance certificate of the course will help them for career growth. Other reasons include re-skilling for getting re-entry in the job market, refreshing knowledge and so on. An overwhelming percentage of the youth attended all the lectures (87%). Internet connectivity was found to be a regular problem for 14.4% of the participants while 68% faced the same problem sometimes. For 17.6% the internet worked well.

As individual difference variables contribute significantly to goal setting, training intentions, motivation, and performance and success, we assessed two factors—grit and emotional intelligence—in order to take into account perseverance and adaptive emotional functioning as being instrumental in training outcomes. Grit was found to bear a significant association with perceived stress as well as training effectiveness (Table 16.3). The emotional intelligence domain of perceiving emotions was observed to be significantly related to training effectiveness (Table 16.3).

Table 16.3 Inter-correlations and descriptive statistics

	Perceived stress	Grit	EI1	EI2	EI3	EI4	Training effectiveness	Gender	NE domicile
Perceived stress	–								
Grit	−0.416**	–							
EI1	036	0.127*	–						
EI2	016	243**	0.733**	–					
EI3	−0.051	0.252**	0.802**	0.771**	–				
EI4	−0.084	0.241**	0.793**	0.764**	0.827**	–			
Training effectiveness	0.068	−0.256**	−0.085	−0.064	−0.076	−0.120*	–		
Gender	−0.071	0.110	0.038	0.114	0.169**	0.166**	0.029	–	
NE Domicile	−0.112	0.045	0.074	0.041	0.044	0.047	0.067	−0.066	–
Mean	17.93	26.76	35.71	22.55	33.19	29.77	1.53		
SD	5.16	4.32	5.24	3.77	5.22	4.65	0.56		

* Correlation is significant at the 0.05 level (2-tailed)
** Correlation is significant at the 0.01 level (2-tailed)
Note Emotional Intelligence is measured through its fours subscales and marked as EI1: perception of emotions, EI2: utilization of emotions, EI3: managing own emotions, and EI4: managing others' emotions

Table 16.4 Source of information about the short-term courses and reasons for attending

Variables	Cyber security (n = 44)		Artificial intelligence & ML (n = 110)		Data science (n = 47)		Cloud computing (n = 83)		Total (n = 284)
	f	%	*f*	%	*f*	%	*f*	%	(%)
Source of information about the course									
• From the website of RGNIYD	11	25	28	25.5	23	48.9	42	50.6	50.6
• From friends	17	38.6	21	19.1	10	21.3	12	14.5	14.5
• From faculty	7	15.9	57	51.8	13	27.7	21	25.3	25.3
• Department notice board	3	6.8	4	3.6	0	0	4	4.8	4.8
• Others	6	13.6	0	0	1	2.1	4	4.8	4.8
Reasons for attending the short-terms course									
• To gain knowledge in the subject	21	47.7	72	65.5	31	66	61	73.5	65.1
• To refresh knowledge	2	4.5	4	3.6	2	4.3	5	6	4.6
• To clarify specific queries related to the subject	4	9.4	4	3.6	0	0	1	1.2	3.2
• To re-skill to get re-entry in the job market	2	4.5	7	6.4	4	8.5	2	2.4	5.3
• Course certificate will be beneficial for career growth	14	31.8	22	20	10	21.3	14	16.9	21.1
• Others	1	2.3	1	0.9	0	0	2	2.4	1.4
Attended all the sessions									
• Yes	37	84.1	93	84.5	43	91.5	74	89.2	87.0
• No	7	15.9	17	15.5	4	8.5	9	10.8	13.0
Faced internet connectivity problem while attending the on-line classes									
• Always	4	9.1	14	12.7	8	17	15	18.1	14.4
• Sometimes	25	56.8	77	70	35	74.5	56	67.5	68.0
• Never	15	34.1	19	17.3	4	8.5	12	14.5	17.6

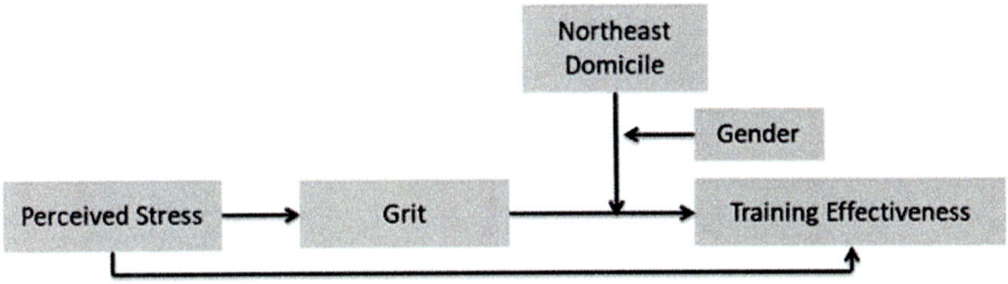

Fig. 16.1 The model representing the indirect effect of perceived stress on training effectiveness

Based on the preliminary analyses we purported to understand the relationship between the study variables in connection with two demographic factors namely, Northeast domicile and gender. We hypothesized that perceived stress relates to training effectiveness through grit and this mediation is conditional upon domicile and gender. As emotional intelligence via all its domains did not emerge as a significant predictor of training effectiveness, it was not included in the moderated-moderated mediation analysis as schematically represented in Fig. 16.1.

To test whether the indirect effect of perceived stress on training effectiveness through grit is moderated by the respondents' domicile and further moderated by gender, we tested a second stage moderated-moderated mediation model. To examine the conditional indirect effect, we used Model 18 in SPSS PROCESS macro (Hayes, 2018), with the interaction term comprising the product of mean-centered, using unstandardized variables and calculated 95% confidence intervals from 10,000 bootstrapped samples. Perceived stress was entered as a predictor, grit as a mediator, Northeast domicile as the second stage moderator, gender as the moderator for primary moderator, and training effectiveness as an outcome.

The moderated–moderated mediation index revealed a significant interaction (Index: −0.035, SE = 0.013, CI: −0.065; −0.012). The interaction of the two moderators is revealed by the significant indirect effects in two categories wherein the pathway from perceived stress to training effectiveness via grit has a positive significant index of moderated-moderated mediation for male participants with northeast domicile (Index: 0.033, SE = 0.010, CI = 0.016, 0.054) and female participants from domicile other than the northeast (0.014, SE = 0.005, CI = 0.005, 0.024). The index of conditional moderated mediation by domicile for female respondents ($b = 0.03$, SE = 0.01, $t = 2.16$, $p < 0.04$) indicates that the indirect effect of perceived stress on training effectiveness through grit was significant among female participants hailing from the Northeast states, however the same effects were not observed for the male respondents from the same region.

The results of the moderated mediation regression are presented in Fig. 16.2.

Regarding the perception of the courses, about half of the youth participants stated all the courses were very effective while 46.8% remarked effectiveness. The sole reasons for the very effective and effective course include Resource persons who were very effective (32.7%) and they could learn a lot from the course (45.1%). In addition, some of the participants were of the view that the course covered good contents and

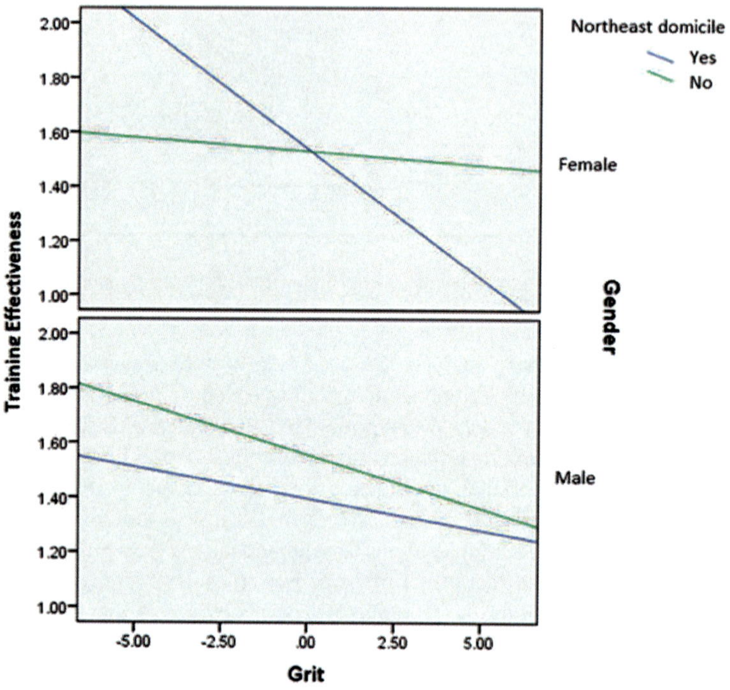

Fig. 16.2 Training effectiveness

they could clarify their queries. As far as resource persons are concerned, 67.3% openly stated that all the resource persons were knowledgeable and experienced when 27.1% stated that the majority of them were knowledgeable and experienced. About 90% youth participants found online mode of classes as a good option for teaching during the COVID-19 lockdown phase. Interestingly about 84.5% stated that they would like to attend a similar course in future (Table 16.5).

More than four-fifths of the participants (83.8%) stated that they would like to consult a mental health professional to reduce their stress and/or to discuss any mental health challenges. As far as support facilities are concerned, 85.9% reported that they have somebody to discuss personal issues and concerns and for this purpose a friend was the first option for 41.2% youth while for 34.9% it was parents. The rest were dependent on siblings and others (Table 16.6).

Table 16.5 Perception about the course and resource persons

Variables	Cyber security (n = 44)		Artificial intelligence & ML (n = 110)		Data science (n = 47)		Cloud computing (n = 83)		Total (n = 284)
	f	%	*f*	%	*f*	%	*F*	%	(%)
Did you find the course effective?									
• Every effective	29	65.9	45	40.9	27	57.4	42	50.6	50.4
• Effective	15	34.1	58	52.7	20	42.6	40	48.2	46.8
• Not so effective	0	0	6	5.5	0	0	1	1.2	2.5
• Not at all effective	0	0	1	0.9	0	0	0	0	0.4
Why did you say so?									
• Resource persons were very effective	13	29.5	27	25.5	17	38.6	36	43.9	32.7
• Learnt a lot of new things	23	52.3	52	49.1	18	40.9	35	42.8	45.1
• Could clarify queries	1	2.3	1	0.9	2	4.5	4	4.9	2.8
• Good contents covered	7	15.9	25	23.6	7	15.9	6	7.3	15.8
• Others, specify	0	0	5	4.5	3	6.3	1	1.2	3.2
Did you find the resource persons knowledgeable and experienced?									
• All of them	32	72.7	65	59.1	35	74.5	59	71.1	67.3
• Majority of them	10	22.7	35	31.8	12	25.5	20	24.1	27.1
• Few of them	2	4.5	9	8.2	0	0	4	4.8	5.3
• None of them	0	0	1	0.9	0	0	0	0	0.4
Did you find on-line mode of classes as a good option for teaching during this phase?									
• Yes	42	95.5	93	84.5	42	89.4	77	92.8	89.4
• No	2	4.5	17	15.5	5	10.6	6	7.2	10.6
Would you like to attend a similar programme in future?									
• Yes	40	90.9	89	80.9	43	91.5	68	81.9	84.5
• No	4	9.1	21	19.1	4	8.5	15	18.1	15.5

Discussion

The present study attempted to assess the effectiveness of four online certificate courses which aim at fostering professional and job oriented skills for youth during the COVID-19 pandemic. The feedback provided by the participants of all the four

Table 16.6 Perceived stress and support facilities

Variables	Cyber security ($n = 44$)		Artificial intelligence & ML ($n = 110$)		Data science ($n = 47$)		Cloud computing ($n = 83$)		Total ($n = 284$)
	f	%	*f*	%	*f*	%	*F*	%	(%)
Do you feel like consulting a mental health professional to reduce your stress and/or to discuss any mental health challenges?									
• Yes	36	81.8	96	87.3	38	80.9	68	81.9	83.8
• No	8	18.2	14	12.7	9	19.1	15	18.1	16.2
Do you have anybody to discuss your personal issues and problems?									
• Yes	40	90.9	97	88.2	42	89.4	65	78.3	85.9
• No	4	9.1	13	11.8	5	10.6	18	21.7	14.1
If so, with whom do you prefer to discuss your personal issues and problems?									
• Parents	16	36.4	37	33.6	18	38.3	28	33.7	34.9
• Sibling	5	11.4	16	14.5	4	8.5	8	9.6	11.6
• Friends	18	40.9	41	37.3	19	40.4	39	47	41.2
• Others	5	11.4	16	14.5	6	12.8	8	9.6	12.3

information-technology related courses were highly encouraging as almost all the participants expressed that they participated to gain new knowledge and refresh their knowledge during the lockdown period or re-skill themselves as a result of downsizing by their employers due to the consequence of coronavirus pandemic. Most of the participants felt that the online courses offered by RGNIYD were effective due to the structure, content and its delivery, resource persons besides other factors. The participants also felt that an online method of learning was the only best viable option for learning during such circumstances.

Numerous studies have been conducted on the effectiveness of online programs. However the courses conducted by RGNIYD are of paramount significance and were unique in many ways such as these courses were on trending subjects, highly job oriented, futuristicin nature, offered by premier institutions free of charge, centered on skill building and the certification will enrich their profile. Therefore, it was vital for RGNIYD to evaluate the effectiveness of its online courses.

While online learning is an alternative method of traditional teaching, it is to be reiterated that online learning was the only mode available for the students and learners who were keen on utilizing their time effectively for acquiring knowledge and skills. Our findings corroborate with some of the previous studies (Bahasoan et al., 2020; Lapitan et al., 2021; Mishra et al., 2020; Tartavulea et al., 2020). For example, Susilawati and Supriyatno (2020) through their study confirmed the increase in student learning outcomes as a result of online learning through use of WhatsApp. They further reiterate that online learning has the potential of increasing learning motivation among the students during difficult times like the COVID-19 pandemic.

While suggesting the effective use of online learning as an alternative method, the means and methods for effective online learning are to be considered as important factors. In this regard, Alawamleh et al. (2020) probed on the effectiveness of online learning during the COVID-19 pandemic with particular reference to the role of communication between the instructors and students. Their study revealed that students preferred real-time classroom learning over online programs due to the fact that the students lacked motivation to attend online classes, had difficulties in comprehending the online resource material and the decreased levels of communication between the student and teacher besides the making the students feel lonely due to the social restrictions posed by online classes. However, it is important to design each class or session by the educational administrators and teachers to suit the specific learning needs of the students with appropriate content, methodology with much flexibility.

Regarding the perceptions and preferences for online education in India, Muthuprasad et al. (2021), underpinned that the majority of students preferred the usage of smart phones for online learning and recording the sessions for future reference. They also favored the use of quizzes to evaluate their assimilation of online learning. Flexibility and convenience were found to be attractive factors while the challenges were mainly centered on internet connectivity issues, particularly for rural students. They also indicated that learners' levels of preparedness, design of the online program and its effectiveness were imperative factors which contribute to the efficacy of the online programs. It is pertinent to mention here that in RGNIYD's online program almost all the students use their smartphones to attend their classes which did not add problems for the students. The curriculum of the IT courses conducted by RGNIYD were customized to the specific requirement of the learners based on the details of expectations indicated by the participants at the time of registration. Further the timings of the sessions were scheduled in a very flexible manner to enable the participants to conveniently attend the sessions. The method of teaching by using multimedia presentations, PowerPoint presentations, videos, display of pictures, prototypes, models, use of online polls made a big impact on the effectiveness.

Beyond explaining the basic concept about each subject through power point presentation, the practical orientation, use of flipped methods, online demonstration, troubleshooting, use of case-studies for problem solving online, working on online programming exercises were the hallmarks of RGNIYD's courses. These methods fall in line with the study conducted by Yen (2020) who verified the procedures and effects of flipped classroom for online teaching during the COVID-19 period and found that flipped classroom for online teaching is workable. It was also studied that activities prior to the sessions and activities post session were found to enhance the learning capacities. Whereas, Nadeak (2020) opined that distance learning through online modes were suitable for theoretical courses and mentioned that for practical courses the online methods were found less effective. However, in the present course, the learners did not express any difficulty relating to the practical aspects due to the fact that all the practical problems were provided to the learners online and were demonstrated online. The computer programs were shared with them online and were demonstrated to fix the problems.

The effectiveness of teachers who deliver the content is equally important for any program to be effective. Sessions for all the four courses were facilitated by prolific experts from the National Institutes of Technology, Indian Institutes of Technology, premier universities and apex higher technical educational institutions across the country. The faculty who handled the sessions used appropriate methodologies, presentation, effective communication strategies, clarity in concepts, practical inputs which were the highlights of the online courses as indicated by the participants. George (2020) in his study demonstrated that effective teaching methods have enhanced the learning outcomes in the online programmes during the COVID-19 pandemic. His study also reiterated the fact that employing effective methods will prevent the degradation of students' performance in learning. Corroborating with this study, the courses conducted by RGNIYD utilized effective teaching methodologies which contributed to the effectiveness of the online courses as rated by the learners.

Studies quoted earlier have suggested the flexibility in online programs will be an advantageous factor. The RGNIYD's online courses were uniformly fixed for a duration of five days each with three focussed sessions per day. In the event where the participants felt that a session needed to be extended it was done based on mutual consent between the teacher and the learners to gain more insights into those particular topics or to work on practical exercises. The sessions were also paced with gap in between so as to enable the participants to attend their work or complete their regular academic requirements. The online link for the entire day remained the same so that the learner can easily join the session with much flexibility.

Tang et al. (2020) in their study of flipped classrooms with online based teaching during COVID-19 recorded the students' dissatisfaction regarding online learning. The major reasons for student dissatisfaction were the communication issues and the sessions were more of Q&A mode. However, in the RGNIYD's courses, the faculty encouraged more questions and doubts to be raised to be clarified. The students who were unable to articulate the questions were provoked to use the chat option to post their doubts without any hesitation. The Q&A sessions were the most satisfying component of the online program as most of the participants revealed their satisfaction that their doubts were cleared.

Another element for effective online learning is the adaptability of learners. The participants of RGNIYD's courses were highly adaptive to the online method of learning. The online platform used for imparting online education was Cisco Webex which was much user-friendly for interactions both through use of audio and chat means. This factor falls in line with the study conducted by Tartavulea et al. (2020). Their research revealed that the universities and students were quick to adapt to online methods of education in the wake of COVID-19 pandemic. The respondents of their study perceived online teaching to have a positive effect on the educational process. Further they also probed that institutional support, trust in the online education system were positively associated with the effectiveness of online education. As a contributory factor to the learners' adaptability, it is prudent to highlight the role of grit in enhancing the effectiveness of any training programme. Described as a malleable trait (Duckworth, 2016), grit is a significant mediator between perceived stress and training outcomes. Grit enables persistence in a crisis, aids in coping with stress, and facilitates achievement. However, as there can be several psychological antecedents to grit like interest, deliberate practice, and hope (Duckworth, 2016; Tang et al., 2019) there is not much consistency in the evidence supporting grit as a predictor of academic or training outcomes. In line with this, in the present study the association between stress and training effectiveness has been partially mediated by grit for just two segments of the sample as demonstrated in the moderated-moderated mediation analysis. The evidence holds true for the groups based on domicile and gender viz. the male participants with Northeast domicile and female participants from the rest of India. The group differentials can be viewed in the socio-cultural subtext of contemporary India, where women are exhibiting greater perseverance and striving for long term goals particularly due to the longstanding patriarchal control of technology-based disciplines. Similarly, the progress of male participants from the Northeast in enlarging their reach and strengthening their career prospects has been facilitated by the modernistic and inclusive cultivation of science and technology provided by the institutes like RGNIYD to foster skill development and career advancement of the youth despite the challenges levied by the pandemic.

Similar to regular classroom learning, a conducive learning environment is essential for learning to take place effectively (Vu et al., 2020). The students during the course had a stress-free learning environment as the teachers were highly resourceful, considerate on the needs of the students, provided additional resources to enhance the knowledge, closely interacted with the students, aroused the interest to learn new skills and their application teaching besides making the students to comprehend each concept with much clarity. Further, their study also underscored that the teacher's perspectives regarding the objectives of teaching activities during the pandemic, the extent of organizational support received by the teachers and the professional development of teachers were found to be contributing to the effectiveness of online learning.

Finally, the attitude of teachers and learners are very essential to the effectiveness of online programmes. Pandey et al. (2021) in their framework for effective delivery of online classes during lockdown explored various online teaching platforms, resource material, teaching and learning techniques and technologies. They suggested that the effectiveness of online programmes also lies in learners' satisfaction with the online study and the teachers' attitude towards delivery of online classes.

With the background presented above, online learning can be an effective method at all times, be it during the unprecedented pandemic situation or a disaster or even during a normal period. Online learning has several academic benefits to the learners such as learning and acquiring new knowledge, up-skilling or re-skilling and multi-skilling options, enhancement of IT skills to work with various online environment and platforms, promotion of research skills, connecting the young minds with practitioners and researchers to work on new projects, avenues for higher education, linkages for educational and vocational guidance by the faculty (Paudel, 2021).

While there are several advantages, few barriers and challenges haunt the online method of education. The chief factor hampering the effectiveness of online education is the cost involved and internet connectivity problem for some learners. Many institutions of higher learning, finishing schools and academies price their online programs skill development programs at a very high price. Bahasoan et al. (2020) on investigating the effectiveness of online learning during COVID-19 concluded their study that the online learning system carried out during the COVID-19 pandemic is effective and inefficient. Effectively implemented because of the conditions that require online study and inefficient because the costs incurred more when compared with offline lectures. Further, Adnan and Anwar (2020) in their study stressed that online learning cannot produce desired results in underdeveloped countries where a vast majority of students are unable to access the internet due to technical as well as monetary issues. Mahmood (2021) in his work on Instructional strategies for online teaching in COVID-19 pandemic reinforced that the appropriate government needs to take commensurate efforts to establish linkages with telecom departments/industries to provide internet access to the needy underprivileged students on preferential basis so as to enable them overcome such barriers to online education.

However, the online courses offered by RGNIYD were mainly for the underprivileged students and youth. The courses were imparted free of cost and the certificate provided by various institutions of national importance which will add more value to the participants. While such IT courses on the demand-driven skills are very costly, these programs were offered to the students and youth without any cost. Most of the participants attended the courses through their smartphones which made the participants attend the courses enthusiastically. However, internet connectivity issues were the only barriers as expressed by the participants that prevented them attending all the sessions.

COVID-19 resulting in continuous lockdown for more than a year in India caused a lot of stress for the younger population for which they felt the need to consult mental health professionals. In this regard, the findings of the present study corroborate with findings of some of the previous studies (Giannopoulou et al., 2021; Guessoum et al., 2020; Mohler-Kuo et al., 2021; Rehman et al., 2021; Rossi et al., 2020). Nevertheless, support facilities for sharing stress with friends over phone, parents and siblings helped them to deal with the situation and to remain emotionally strong.

Conclusion and Recommendations

The present study found that the online professional and job oriented courses for youth during the pandemic period were highly effective based on the feedback provided by the participants. The participants had a comfortable online learning environment with rare opportunity to utilize their time more effectively during the lockdown period. As the courses were free of cost, many students and youth across different states of India participated, particularly, the north-eastern youth who have such sporadic opportunities. The participants thoroughly enjoyed the courses more than regular classroom teaching due to the innovative teaching methodologies employed by the resource persons including the practical demonstrations. In addition to reskilling the participants on technical areas, the training provided scope for nurturing their social and emotional competencies like grit and emotional intelligence, especially catering to the needs of women across the country and male participants from the north-eastern states of India. As grit and emotional intelligence are malleable, training opportunities like the current program offer a conducive environ for enhancing such skills, thereby aiding effective coping with concurrent issues and progress in the future. Connecting experts from different locations including international experts was one of the advantages of the program. The participants had a chance to interact with the experts and establish professional connections for higher education, pursuing research, undertaking projects, and sought job related guidance. The online sessions were recorded for future reference of the participants and for the benefit of the underprivileged youth who did not get the opportunity to attend the courses which will be made available in the public domain on RGNIYD's website. Ultimately, the certificate jointly issued by RGNIYD and NIT Jalandhar will enhance the value of the skill set acquired by the participants to get entry into various jobs. Almost all the participants in the feedback expressed that they would like to attend many more online programmes in future to be conducted by RGNIYD and will also disseminate the details of the programmes among their contacts. However, the only limitation to the participants, particularly, those residing in rural and far flung villages including the north-eastern India was the internet connectivity issues. Though they were willing to attend, internet interruptions were the main reason that prevented a few participants attending all the sessions.

Quality oriented online courses cannot be sidelined and considered as a less rated method of learning. Therefore, the need of the hour is that the youth need to explore the world of online opportunities, experience the benefits of online learning and expand their horizons of knowledge and skills. The cost of an online programme for a small or large group will remain the same with the same expected learning outcomes for which a suitable interactive online platform needs to be chosen to include more number of participants. The contemporary period demands the educational and training institutions to concentrate and invest more on online methods of teaching with user-friendly tools and contents which will enable to realize the priorities as enshrined in the new National Education Policy, 2020 as well as the National Youth Policy of India in the real sense by expanding the access to quality education with lower costs thereby providing the student community a flexible educational trajectory apart from enabling higher educational institutions to stay prepared for imparting uninterrupted learning during unprecedented situations like COVID-19 pandemic.

References

Adnan, M., & Anwar, K. (2020). Online learning amid the COVID-19 pandemic: Students' perspectives. *Online Submission, 2*(1), 45–51.

Alawamleh, M., Al-Twait, L. M., & Al-Saht, G. R. (2020).The effect of online learning on communication between instructors and students during Covid-19 pandemic. *Asian Education and Development Studies.*

Bahasoan, A. N., Ayuandiani, W., Mukhram, M., & Rahmat, A. (2020). Effectiveness of online learning in pandemic COVID-19. *International Journal of Science, Technology & Management, 1*(2), 100–106.

Clark, K. N., & Malecki, C. K. (2019). Academic Grit Scale: Psychometric properties and associations with achievement and life satisfaction. *Journal of School Psychology, 72,* 49–66.

Duckworth, A. (2016). *Grit: The power of passion and perseverance* (Vol. 234). Scribner.

Duckworth, A. L., & Quinn, P. D. (2009). Development and validation of the short grit scale (GRIT-S). *Journal of Personality Assessment, 91*(2), 166–174.

Fernández-Martín, F. D., Arco-Tirado, J. L., & Hervás-Torres, M. (2020). Grit as a predictor and outcome of educational, professional, and personal success: a systematic review. Psicología Educativa. *Revista de los Psicólogos de la Educación, 26*(2), 163–173.

George, M. L. (2020). Effective teaching and examination strategies for undergraduate learning during COVID-19 school restrictions. *Journal of Educational Technology Systems, 49*(1), 23–48.

Giannopoulou, I., Efstathiou, V., Triantafyllou, G., Korkoliakou, P., & Douzenis, A. (2021). Adding stress to the stressed: Senior high school students' mental health amidst the COVID-19 nationwide lockdown in Greece. *Psychiatry Research, 295*, 113560.

Guessoum, S. B., Lachal, J., Radjack, R., Carretier, E., Minassian, S., Benoit, L., & Moro, M. R. (2020). Adolescent psychiatric disorders during the COVID-19 pandemic and lockdown. *Psychiatry Research,* 113264.

Hayes, A. F. (2018). Partial, conditional, and moderated moderated mediation: Quantification, inference, and interpretation. *Communication Monographs, 85*(1), 4–40.

https://daninstitute.com/blog/the-effectiveness-of-online-learning-13-reasons-why-online-courses-are-more-effective/

https://www.eurekalert.org/pub_releases/2020-04/nruh-aes040720.php

Kent, M., Rivers, C. T., & Wrenn, G. (2015). Goal-directed resilience in training (GRIT): A biopsychosocial model of self-regulation, executive functions, and personal growth (eudaimonia) in evocative contexts of PTSD, obesity, and chronic pain. *Behavioral Sciences, 5*(2), 264–304.

Lapitan, L. D., Jr., Tiangco, C. E., Sumalinog, D. A. G., Sabarillo, N. S., & Diaz, J. M. (2021). An effective blended online teaching and learning strategy during the COVID-19 pandemic. *Education for Chemical Engineers, 35*, 116–131.

Mahmood, S. (2021). Instructional strategies for online teaching in COVID-19 pandemic. *Human Behavior and Emerging Technologies, 3*(1), 199–203.

Mavroveli, S., & Sánchez-Ruiz, M. J. (2011). Trait emotional intelligence influences on academic achievement and school behaviour. *British Journal of Educational Psychology, 81*(1), 112–134.

Mishra, L., Gupta, T., & Shree, A. (2020). Online teaching-learning in higher education during lockdown period of COVID-19 pandemic. *International Journal of Educational Research Open, 1*, 100012.

Mohler-Kuo, M., Dzemaili, S., Foster, S., Werlen, L., & Walitza, S. (2021). Stress and Mental Health among Children/Adolescents, their parents, and Young Adults during the first COVID-19 lockdown in Switzerland. *International Journal of Environmental Research and Public Health, 18*(9), 4668.

Muthuprasad, T., Aiswarya, S., Aditya, K. S., & Jha, G. K. (2021). Students' perception and preference for online education in India during COVID-19 pandemic. *Social Sciences & Humanities Open, 3*(1), 100101.

Nadeak, B. (2020). The effectiveness of distance learning using social media during the pandemic period of covid-19: A case in Universitas Kristen Indonesia. *International Journal of Advanced Science and Technology, 29*(7), 1764–1772.

Pandey, D., Ogunmola, G. A., Enbeyle, W., Abdullahi, M., Pandey, B. K., & Pramanik, S. (2021). COVID-19: A framework for effective delivering of online classes during lockdown. *Human Arenas,* 1–15.

Parker, J. D., Creque Sr, R. E., Barnhart, D. L., Harris, J. I., Majeski, S. A., Wood, L. M., et al. (2004). Academic achievement in high school: does emotional intelligence matter?. *Personality and Individual Differences, 37*(7), 1321–1330.

Paudel, P. (2021). Online education: Benefits, challenges and strategies during and after COVID-19 in higher education. *International Journal on Studies in Education, 3*(2), 70–85.

Rehman, U., Shahnawaz, M. G., Khan, N. H., Kharshiing, K. D., Khursheed, M., Gupta, K., et al. (2021). Depression, anxiety and stress among Indians in times of Covid-19 lockdown. *Community Mental Health Journal, 57*(1), 42–48.

Rojas, J. P., Usher, E. L., & Toland, M. D. (2012). Creativity and grit as predictors of mathematics achievement in early adolescence. *Race/Ethnicity, 8*(05), 02.

Rossi, R., Socci, V., Talevi, D., Mensi, S., Niolu, C., Pacitti, F., et al. (2020). COVID-19 pandemic and lockdown measures impact on mental health among the general population in Italy. *Frontiers in Psychiatry, 11,* 790.

Salles, A., Cohen, G. L., & Mueller, C. M. (2014). The relationship between grit and resident well-being. *The American Journal of Surgery, 207*(2), 251–254.

Schutte, N. S., & Malouff, J. M. (2002). Incorporating emotional skills in a college transition course enhances student retention. *Journal of the First-Year Experience and Students in Transition, 14,* 7–21.

Schutte, N. S., Malouff, J. M., & Bhullar, N. (2009). The assessing emotions scale. In *Assessing emotional intelligence* (pp. 119–134). Springer.

Strayhorn, T. L. (2014). What role does grit play in the academic success of black male collegians at predominantly white institutions? *Journal of African American Studies, 18,* 1–10.

Susilawati, S., &Supriyatno, T. (2020). Online learning through WhatsApp group in improving learning motivation in the era and post pandemic COVID-19. *JurnalPendidikan: Teori, Penelitian, Dan Pengembangan, 5*(6), 852–859.

Tang, T., Abuhmaid, A. M., Olaimat, M., Oudat, D. M., Aldhaeebi, M., & Bamanger, E. (2020). Efficiency of flipped classroom with online-based teaching under COVID-19. *Interactive Learning Environments,* 1–12.

Tang, X., Wang, M. T., Guo, J., & Salmela-Aro, K. (2019). Building grit: The longitudinal pathways between mindset, commitment, grit, and academic outcomes. *Journal of Youth and Adolescence, 48*(5), 850–863.

Tartavulea, C. V., Albu, C. N., Albu, N., Dieaconescu, R. I., & Petre, S. (2020). Online teaching practices and the effectiveness of the educational process in the wake of the COVID-19 pandemic. *Amfiteatru Economic, 22*(55), 920–936.

Vu, C. T., Hoang, A. D., Than, V. Q., Nguyen, M. T., Dinh, V. H., Le, Q. A. T., et al. (2020). Dataset of Vietnamese teachers' perspectives and perceived support during the COVID-19 pandemic. *Data in Brief, 31,* 105788.

Yen, T.-F. (TF). (2020). The performance of online teaching for flipped classroom based on COVID-19 aspect. *Asian Journal of Education and Social Studies, 8*(3), 57–64.

Prof. Sibnath Deb Ph.D. & DSc, is Professor of the Department of Applied Psychology, Pondicherry University (A Central University), Puducherry. Prior to that, Prof. Deb acted as Director of the Rajiv Gandhi National Institute of Youth Development (An Institute of National Importance), Ministry of Youth Affairs and Sports, Government of India for three and half years (January 8, 2020–June 30, 2023). Professor Deb was acting as Director (I/C), Directorate of Distance Education, and Dean (I/C), School of Law, Pondicherry University. He also taught at the University of Calcutta. In 1994, Professor Deb did an intensive course on 'HIV/AIDS and Qualitative Research' from the University of Western Australia. From April 2009 to August 2009, Professor Deb visited the School of Public Health, Queensland University of Technology (QUT), Brisbane, Australia, as Visiting Faculty. Currently, he is also an Adjunct Professor at the School of Justice, QUT, Australia. During 2004–2008, he served the International Society for the Prevention of Child Abuse and Neglect (ISPCAN) as Council Member. In brief, he has 32 years of teaching, research and administrative experience and has produced 22 Ph.D.s in addition to publishing more than 100 research articles/book chapters in the leading national and international journals. Professor Deb has written nine books and edited 11 books. Some of his latest published books are (a) Child Safety, Welfare and Well-being: Issues and Challenges (2nd Edition, 2022, Springer Nature, Singapore); (b) School-based Family Counseling For Crisis and Disaster (Routledge, California, in press); (c) Health and Well-being: Challenges, Strategies and Future Trends (2022), Springer Nature, Singapore; (d) Youth Development in India: Future Generations in a Changing World (2021), New Delhi, Routledge. Professor Deb has received three national and three international awards in recognition of his contribution in the field of psychology including "Visitor's Award-2019" from the Hon'ble President of India Shri Ram Nath Kovind. His current areas of research interest include family dynamics, parenting styles, child safety, students' mental health, adolescent reproductive health and applied social psychology.

Dr. Tusharika Mukherjee is an industrial and organizational psychologist working in the area of diversity, performance, and personality relationship and creating sustainable work organizations. She obtained her Ph.D. in Applied Psychology from the University of Calcutta and pursued her postdoctoral research in the area of situation contingent performance variability in the Department of Work and Organizational Psychology, Justus Liebig University Giessen, Germany. At present, she is associated with the Centre for International Development and Environmental Research at Justus Leibig University Giessen, Germany, as an independent lecturer and trainer. She has over thirteen years of experience in University teaching, research, conducting skill development workshops, and consultation. Her other academic and research experiences include intercultural communication competence, work-life integration, team and leadership development, and didactics.

David Paul has 21 years of experience as Research Associate at National Institute of the Visually Handicapped—Regional Centre (Govt. of India) and served as Training and Placement Officer where he undertook research studies pertaining to jobs identification for the visually impaired and their performance evaluation. He previously taught Career Counseling and Counseling Psychology at RGNIYD, an apex organization of the Union Ministry of Youth Affairs and Sports. He is currently a Training Officer at RGNIYD. His passion areas include training, teaching, research, documentation, and dissemination on youth issues and specialize in applied psychology, career counseling and disability rehabilitation.

Part III
Youth, Adversities and Challenges

Chapter 17
Migration and Diaspora from a Young Adult Perspective: Reading Senzai's *Shooting Kabul* and Hidier's *Born Confused*

Kaustuv Chakraborti

Abstract Young Adult Fiction is a common nomenclature used in academia to distinguish works of literature which are meant for the consumption of teenagers and adolescents. Such literary works often work to bridge the gap between literary themes concerning children and adults and enable a smooth transition of the readership from one age group to the other. In other words, the themes, issues and motifs that pervade Young Adult literature are most often the centrepieces of literary works meant for the consumption of adults. Migration, Displacement and Diaspora are three poignant issues that pervade world literature in the contemporary era, where the movement and resettlement of a certain community from one geographical location to another becomes a major point of concern for the community in multiple ways. While most literary works prefer to provide the perspective of mature adults and their transition, the two literary works selected for this chapter place two members of the youth community at their centre. The two novels, written by award-winning authors, N. H. Senzai and Tanuja Desai Hidier, illustrate the predicament of two South Asian adolescents, who delineate their struggles in America and how they are in a state of continuous flux when it comes to their life in a new nation. This study will serve to illustrate how the global youth partakes in the challenge of adapting to a new and different culture and seeks to thrive in it and establish a renewed identity, all from the perspective of two young protagonists.

Keywords Young adult · Migration · Youth · Transition · Identity

K. Chakraborti (✉)
Department of English, Rajiv Gandhi National Institute of Youth Development, Sriperumbudur, Tamil Nadu, India
e-mail: kaustuv.2306@gmail.com

S. Deb and S. Deb (eds.), *Handbook of Youth Development*,
https://doi.org/10.1007/978-981-99-4969-4_17

Introduction

Defining the Genre

Young Adult Literature, popularly identified as YA Literature, deals with a body of writings which seeks to define its readership group through its nomenclature. This restriction does not hinder the process of reception or the perception of the literature in any way, especially if adult readership is considered for the said cause. The act of indulging in reading activities is not always governed by the individual(s) actively involved in it. The first choices in readership are often done for the readers by their guardians, which is ultimately shaped by society. The fact that the readership of these works is ultimately a culturally justified construct, is undeniable. Such constructions manifest on the basic premise of the exercise of power on the norms of age and experience. The elders in the family thus exercise their opinion about the selection/ rejection of a certain text, for the younger ones in the family. To understand the literature associated with this genre, it is very important to understand the term, "Young Adult."

Alice Trupe discusses the complexities in identifying the group of readers who can be classified as Young Adults.

> One of the issues involved in categorizing YA literature is the meaning of the term "young adult." Some children may be able to read young adult literature at age ten while others may not be ready for the more mature themes dealt with in many novels marketed to young adults. By some definitions, "young adults" include people in their early twenties. (viii)

Factors concerning readership and readability among young adults are socio-culturally governed. It is highly reliant upon their upbringing and their ability to be cognizant of the issues that are presented in the works. While dictionaries generally incorporate "young adults" as individuals in their "late teenage years or early twenties", a more clinical definition is offered by Elena Higley,

> Young adulthood is a unique developmental period that occurs between the ages of 18 and 25 years, during which there are key developmental tasks that allow the young adult to participate in self-exploration and identity formation. Currently, among various organizations there are differing definitions and age range inclusions for young adulthood, which cause confusion during program development, healthcare service delivery, and research.
>
> (*Qualifying Manuscripts* 17)

The issues and concerns that are presented by these works, most often, feature protagonists who are of the same age and who are undergoing a similar phase in their lives, which is quite similar to their intended readers. The books illustrate both the internal and external conflicts these characters face, while they transition from their teenage growth spurt to adulthood. The issue of authorship must also be discussed in this context. The individual involved in the process of writing is an adult in most scenarios. Hence, the issues and themes that are introduced by him/her in the text are often governed by their respective understanding of young adulthood. The greatest challenge for him/her is, how readable and poignant are the issues, which he/she presents through the works, for the readers. The preferences of the reader are important aspects that must be perceived and considered by the authors of Young Adult Literature. Unlike other generic divisions, wherein a piece of literature can be considered and analyzed based on certain structural and thematic similarities, YA Literature, specifically the YA Novel, adopts a different strategy and takes a significant detour.

> [...] the novel for young readers is a nexus—a core of connections and links. It is a nexus of other genres, including not only those more structurally-defined like science fiction or mystery but also the age-based genre categories of children's and young adult literatures. When a hierarchy is made of those categories, it changes what a book can be. (Cadden 303)

The focus of this particular study will center on YA Novels, so Cadden's classification aids the readers in understanding the subtle mechanisms that go into the making of the discursive site of the YA Novel. Another important aspect that necessitates a discussion here is the length of the book. Although YA Literature exists in the forms of both prose and verse, the attention span and the capability of the reader to comprehend the text needs to be accounted for. Social perceptions of a book also add to the understanding of the length of the book defining its readership.

> [...] the length of a book is for many people a determination of the age reader for which the book is meant[...]As picturebooks are not considered by many adults as advanced as novels, the length of the novel is sometimes erroneously assumed to be a measure of the relative precociousness of the middle elementary reader, and parents take greater pride in the length of the books their children read (and without pictures, of course) than in their literary merit. (Cadden 304)

Thus, any attempt to define YA Literature must consider all the complexities that have been mentioned here, in addition to catering to the ever-growing market of YA Literature. In the process of creation, the creator of such literature must remember that his/her primary target is to secure the attention of a wide audience of readers, who will invest a considerable amount of their leisure in reading the works. This is all the more pertinent for longer narratives, like novels, where the authors demand greater attention from the readers. To summarize any attempt towards defining YA Fiction, Karen Coats' statement seems to be the most suited,

> As a body of literature, YA fiction is organized around the same sorts of tensions that preoccupy the physical bodies and emotional lives of its intended audience: tensions between growth and stasis, between an ideal world we can imagine and the one we really inhabit, between earnestness and irony, between ordinary bodies and monstrous ones, and, perhaps most importantly, between an impulsive individualism and a generative ethics of interconnectedness. (316)

The themes and motifs need to be presented in a manner, which is both attractive and universally pertinent. Perhaps, the Harry Potter series, which was essentially a coming-of-age series of narratives, was able to achieve this objective and gain widespread acceptance. To understand this aspect in a better fashion, the current study necessitates delving into the genesis and evolution of Young Adult Narratives over the years.

A Brief History

The task of assimilating a historical narrative concerning YA Literature can never be assigned a state of assertion. Historiography is essentially selective and erroneous, as it is performed by individuals, who bring their ideologically shaped skillsets to the corpus of drawing out a historical narrative. It is essentially a narrative, like any other discourse, as it is subjective, selective and governed by human values. It is not, and can never be, an all-encompassing narrative that considers every aspect of the development of YA Literature. Deborah Stevenson notes,

> Literary historians always face decisions about what's worth noting and why, and what gets left out and why, and previous histories either mark their paths or provide a view they wish to counter. (179)

Stevenson, while elaborating upon the arduous task of drawing out a history of YA Literature, mentions the following about children's literature, which is very much applicable to YA Literature too,

> [...] it's the fictional prose narratives that receive the main focus; they have largely been the popular ambassadors of children's literature and the primary subject of the genre's historians, and as such they provide the most fruitful site for historiography. (179)

Within the scope of the same discussion, Stevenson further opines,

> It's also important to remember that literary historians are only human, and they bring their own subjectivity and biases, so that their judgments of historical significance are never objectively factual. Literary history is influenced by historians' views of the current literature and of class, by historians' field of study and home country, and by the needs of those who disseminate that history. Early historians of the literature were mostly male and mostly from the publishing industry, and for many decades publishers, librarians, and educators, each bringing the slant of their own discipline, chronicled the literature. (182)

Despite such impediments, it is necessary to draw out a historical sketch of the evolution of YA Literature and establish its legacy. This accentuates the preparation of a literary canon of YA Literature, thus aiding any attempt towards the literary analysis of texts which are classified within this genre. The creation of this canon will aid the process of literary and scholarly discussions within and outside classrooms and thus bring such works into the realms of critical discourses. They will be "...primarily, and quite rightly, concerned with engagement and response." (Coats 316) In a way, the creation of such 'histories' are "...convenient, allowing scholars and students to pick people and titles out of a considerable mass of past books." (Stevenson 183).

The earliest attempts towards drawing a history of Children's and YA Literature will take the reader to the days of the Roman rhetorician Quintilian, who,

> [...] argued for the importance of children's literary education, advocating the reading of Homer, classic drama, and the fables of Aesop in Greek as well as the Latin works of notables such as Virgil and Horace. (Stevenson 184)

The fables of Aesop, the *Jataka* Tales, and the *Panchtantras*, were immense contributions to world literature, in multiple ways. These works laid the foundation for the modern short story and, at the same time, they are some of the oldest surviving instances of Children's Literature, which shares certain attributes with YA Literature. Much of the early literature written for Children and Young Adults was educational and instructional. *Gesta Romanorum*, an anthology of Latin tales, was a favorite text among children and young adults, in Europe, during the 14th, 15th and 16th Centuries. What is quite notable about this work is, it was an important source for William Shakespeare, inspiring the plots of King Lear and The Merchant of Venice.

A momentous transition occurred with the invention of the printing press by Johann Gutenberg. The technology was brought to England by William Caxton. Caxton's invention paved the way for literature to flourish in Britain and be recorded for posterity. This study will restrict itself to the evolution of Children's and YA Literature in Great Britain. Extant texts from the 16th and 17th centuries have survived, which can be easily identified as the first instances of Children's and Young Adult Literature. This includes John Foxe's *Book of Martyrs* (1563) and Comenius' *Orbis Pictus* (1659). Charles Perrault's *Contes de Ma Mere l'Oye* (1697) was one significant text that emerged during the late 17th and early 18th centuries. The influence of folktales and folklores was felt for the first time beyond oral cultures, in this work. This collection was translated and published for the first time in Britain in 1729.

The 18th Century contributed two important books that shaped the scenario of Young Adult narratives. These were Daniel Defoe's *Robinson Crusoe* (1719) and Jonathan Swift's *Gulliver's Travels* (1726). Neither of the books was penned for the Young Adult readership, but these books sustain their popularity among the youth in terms of their sheer brilliance of narration. John Newbery was a major figure to have contributed significantly to the rise of Children's and YA Literature in the 19th and 20th Centuries. He was one of the first literary figures to have published non-educational books for children. Stevenson notes his significant contributions to children's literature along the following lines,

> Newbery paid attention not only to the content of his titles but also to their appearance, employing attractive engravings and flowered Dutch paper covers, creating a distinctive house style that foreshadowed contemporary tendencies for publishers to stamp their own individual design on their books. (189)

Attention to such minute details went a long way in establishing him as one of the founders of the publishing industry dedicated solely to children's titles.

The 19th Century witnessed finesse in the development of folklore and the fairy tale in Europe. Jakob and Wilhelm Grim, and Hans Christian Andersen played instrumental roles in the development of folklore during this period. English poet Edward Lear came out with his volume of nonsense poetry, *A Book of Nonsense*, in 1846. This work was a major inspiration for the Bengali poet Sukumar Ray, who also came out with his series of nonsense verses in the early twentieth century. Lewis Carroll's Alice's Adventures in Wonderland is considered a landmark work in the realm of YA Literature. The works of both Lear and Carroll were far removed from reality, yet, they wrote in a period when the trends of YA, as well as Children's writings, were shifting towards a realist trend. The evolution of technology and the movement of the masses from the suburban areas towards the city had already commenced, thus leading to the spurt of literary activities from the nineteenth century onwards. Reading was considered a prominent leisure activity and the readership consisted of representation from all ages. All of this contributed to the evolution of literature from the end of the nineteenth century. Children's and YA Literature were not left behind and they formed an important part of this growth. Just as all other literary genres, the YA Novel also explored various issues through its pages over the 20th and well into the twenty-first century. This study will focus on one of them.

Displacement, Migration and Diaspora

The gift of 20th-century technological advancements was accompanied by a series of negative implications too. The evolution of the printing press was able to cater to the demand of the reading industry and its requirements for cheap paperback editions. The evolution, though, was not limited to the publishing industry only. Advanced warfare was also facilitated by the advancement of technology. The result was witnessed through the two World Wars that were fought in the twentieth century and the continuous wars that are fought around the world even in the twenty-first century. While YA Literature of the period had mostly avoided narratives of the war and kept it consciously away from the readership, the youth population never ceased to exist and were some of the worst sufferers of the war. The trauma associated with the war was not restricted to the battlefield. The wars had a global impact and the population of the world suffered various atrocities. YA Literature, specifically YA Fiction, recorded some of these atrocities as narratives. Very often, these narratives provided a mediated or mellowed version of the aforementioned atrocities in their narrative. Literature associated with the Holocaust exemplifies this through Markus Zusak's The Book Thief and John Boyne's The Boy in Yellow Pyjamas. Adult Fiction often avoids the vagaries of circumlocution and addresses socio-political or economic issues with pronounced vehemence, an aspect that is consciously avoided in YA Fiction, keeping the readership in mind.

The problem associated with Diaspora Literature is quite similar and YA Literature associated with it treads carefully when it talks about the diaspora experience. Displacement and migration are fundamental aspects that are associated with the diaspora. Perceptions of porous geographical boundaries are represented in varied manners in world literature, depending upon authorial intentions. The modern world scenario of multiple countries prompts its citizens to readily act as globe trotters. Displacement, in this context, indicates movement from one geographical location to another. Very often, such acts are not done willingly and they ultimately lead to catastrophes. Under scenarios of displacement, the preservation of one's identity becomes a major concern. Migration is almost synonymous with displacement, but, a major difference between the two lies in their terminologies. While migration places the power to move in the hands of the displaced individual or family, displacement results from the activities of powers that are beyond the control of ordinary individuals. Migration is voluntary but displacement is not.

Diaspora Literature aims to study the condition and predicament of these migrated and displaced individuals, who have moved away from their homeland. This mode of literary practice is characterized by an overemphasis on the preservation of one's own culture in a foreign land and how identity is drawn from this endeavor. Adult novelists like Amitav Ghosh and Jhumpa Lahiri are pioneering figures of Diaspora Literature, who have often exhibited the strife of displaced and migrated individuals in their works. This predicament is accompanied by a constant longing for the almost Utopian homeland of the characters in the novel, which they are often unable to satiate.

Young Adults and Displacement

The years of adolescence and young adulthood are characterized by a growth spurt, along with the formation of a personality and identity. These years are quite tumultuous for the individual, as they undergo a period of transition, both physiological and mental. If such inner struggles are accompanied by outer tumults, in the form of geographical relocation and readjustment, the task becomes all the more difficult. What one reads and learns during such periods, shapes their personality and perspectives. Karen Coats rightly opines that,

> Young adult literature exerts a powerful influence over its readers at a particularly malleable time in their identity formation, and yet we still pay more critical scholarly attention to *Antigone* (Sophocles, c. 442) and *The Great Gatsby* (Fitzgerald, 1925) than we do to the potentially life-changing books our teens read on their own. It seems to me that if we believe that literature has something to say about what it means to be human, and if we further nuance that belief with the idea that national, ethnic, and women's literatures say something about the character and preoccupations of nations and the experience of being of a certain ethnicity or gender, then we ought to approach YA literature with the same careful scrutiny, even if it is written about and to young adults rather than by them. (315)

When fictional YA narratives take up issues of Displacement and Migration in their narratives, Lafuente opines that the following issues are often addressed,

> Many Young Adult novels focus on a disruption in the life of the protagonist and the subsequent personal growth that the character experiences. These disruptions often propel the main character forth on a journey—literal, metaphorical, or both—that leads to self-discovery, a higher level of emotional maturity, and, in general, a greater awareness of her identity. These disruptions serve to catalyse the emergence of a young adult from adolescence. (33)

The novels considered for this study are both YA Novels, addressing issues of Displacement as well as Migration in their narratives. The books also focus on the aspects of conflicts and identity formation and under what circumstances are they formed.

Textual Analysis

The Authors

Naheed Hasnat Senzai or N. H. Senzai is an American writer of Young Adult Fiction. She owes a part of her identity to her Afghan heritage. She can be truly identified as a global citizen based on her globe-trotting upbringing. Senzai claims,

> I grew up speaking two languages, balancing life lived on the edge of two cultures, and, happily, two cuisines—tandoori chicken and hot dogs, grilled side by side on the 4th of July. [...] I grew up in San Francisco, Jubail, Saudi Arabia, and attended boarding school in London, England where I was voted "most likely to lead a literary revolution" due to my ability to get away with reading comic books in class. I've hiked across the Alps, road-tripped through Mexico, swum with barracudas in the Red Sea, taken a train across the Soviet Union, floated down the Nile, eaten gumbo in New Orleans and sat in contemplation at the Taj Mahal. (Senzai *About*)

Senzai is primarily a writer of Young Adult Fiction and the novel taken for this study, *Shooting Kabul*, is her first book. This novel won the Youth Literature Award in 2010, awarded by the Asian/Pacific American Librarians Association. She wrote three other novels, out of which, *Saving Kabul Corner* is a sequel to *Shooting Kabul*. She has also contributed to a short story collection, which recounts tales narrated by contemporary Muslim voices. Senzai bases part of the narrative in *Shooting Kabul* on the lived experiences of her husband while escaping Soviet-controlled Afghanistan.

Tanuja Desai Hidier is an American author of Young Adult Novels. She spent a small part of her childhood in Bombay before permanently shifting to the US. She secured immediate fame with the publication of her first novel, Born Confused, which narrates the tale of an Indian-origin American girl. The book was published in 2002 and was the first narrative instance of the teenage experiences of a South Asian American girl. She has penned another novel titled, *Bombay Blues*. She is also an acclaimed singer cum songwriter in the US.

Shooting Kabul

Senzai's YA narrative places displacement, and the perils associated with it, as their core aspects. The novel is presented to the readers by employing the third-person perspective, but much of the narrative is centered around Fadi Nurzai and his exploits. The readers have also been informed that Fadi was on the verge of commencing middle school, an indication of his teenage years. Fadi and his family were fleeing from Kabul, when he loses his younger sister, Mariam, in the turmoil and scuffle of their escapade. What is very fascinating about *Shooting Kabul* is the complex web of discourses that is spun around the teenage protagonist Fadi, his two sisters, Noor and Mariam, and his parents, Habib and Zafoona.

The intentions of Habib and Zafoona are made very clear at the beginning of the novel before the reader gets too familiar with any of the characters. The family was intending to flee to America, to escape from the Taliban. The girls were the first to protest and Mariam rightly identifies the Taliban as the cause for their absconding. The perceptions and choices of Noor, the eldest sibling, cause an interesting exploration.

> "The Taliban is oppressing everyone, with a version of Islam that they've cooked up. They've banned everything! Music, movies, books, photography, and kite flying. Show me where it says that in the Qur'an. Show me!" (Senzai 12)

The mature assertions of Noor stand in stark contrast to the naivety of Mariam. For her, the only noticeable change is the length of her father's beard. The only hope that Habib could present for his younger daughter was the promise of Chocolates and Barbies in the US. The sudden arrival of the Taliban confused the fleeing group and Mariam was lost in the process. Fadi was the last one to hold her hand and he blamed losing Mariam upon himself. Neither of the girls wanted to leave Afghanistan, as presented through their protests, but the displacement had to take place, for the welfare of everyone. Even though the third person omniscient narrator focussed upon Fadi as the point of narration, there was nothing much that Fadi did throughout the narrative, other than blaming himself for the turn of events and grieving about it.

A visit to America though was nothing new for them. Habib had obtained his PhD in America and Mariam was born in America, but, Habib always wanted to move back to Afghanistan due to the moral obligation of contributing to the growth of his nation and freeing it from the Taliban reign. Fadi's ruminations of a past incident will go a long way to posit the stance of Habib and his family.

> While living in the United States, Zafoona had watched the news coming out in Afghanistan with growing concern. It had been in the spring of 1996, and Mariam had just been a year old. The Taliban had risen from eastern Afghanistan and had marched through the country, slowly gaining control. (Senzai 35)

The return to Afghanistan was always a cause of concern and the sudden displacement occurring in the narrative was not unexpected. The novel also reiterated how the Taliban were perceived as saviours by the Afghans and their moral corruption and method of governance came as an absolute shock to the Afghan citizens. Habib exclaims at a point in the narrative,

> "The Taliban came with so much hope," […] "Now fighting with the Northern Alliance has flared up. They are all the same—power-hungry and arrogant." (Senzai 51–52)

Shooting Kabul presents its readers with a striking picture of San Francisco. Fadi and his family were received by their relatives at the airport and were driven to a place named Fremont, which was a local community of Afghans.

> "Fremont has the largest population of Afghans in the United States," said Uncle Amin. "There are dozens of Afghan restaurants, cafes, and shops. You can drop by, get a cup of tea, and hear the latest news." (Senzai 56)

The presence of this small community in Fremont represented and manifested the diaspora experience. The home away from home for the displaced and migrated community. Uncle Amin even happened to call the place, little Kabul and the storefronts with Persian signboards excited Fadi.

Fadi's encounters at Brookhaven Middle School provided a further scope of discussion for the YA novel. The setting of the school premises, the presence of school bullies in Ike and Felix and Fadi vanquishing them contributed towards the physical and mental development of Fadi and prepared him to face challenging situations in his life. The presence of Ms Bethune also aided the development of the teenager Fadi. His love for photography was realized during the photography club meets.

The announcement of the photography competition was an important turn of events for Fadi. Even though the family had relocated to America, they were still unable to trace Mariam, till the end of the novel. Life continued with its usual ebb and flow, but the absence of Mariam was haunting, especially for Fadi and his mother, Zafoona. The winner of the photography competition would be able to visit India and Fadi wanted to use that opportunity to visit India, which was so close to Afghanistan. Once in India, he would be able to visit Afghanistan, which is so near. Fadi's innocent nature is well captured by Senzai in the narrative. He is presented as a character that is oblivious to the tensions between the South Asian nations. He might overhear his parents talking about the same, he understands very little about it. Like Miriam's relationship with her Barbie doll Gulmina, Fadi finds some solace behind the lens and occupies himself with finding the perfect image to be submitted to the judges. The camera serves a very similar role in Hidier's novel too. Fadi's ruminations with his favorite fictional character, Claudia, go to show his mental makeup in the novel. He is extremely fond of reading and whenever he is in trouble, he seeks the help of this imaginary friend. The novel ends on a happy note with news of Miriam and the parallel wish fulfilment of Fadi. Even though he is not able to win the photography competition, he gets to meet his idol, Clive Murray, during the exhibition.

Born Confused

The narrative scope and scale of Hidier's novel shares are quite dissimilar to Senzai's narrative. The narrative places the reader inside the topsy-turvy world of Dimple Rohitbhai Lala, the female protagonist of the novel. The novel is quite realistic in its portrayal of teenage and the gradual transition into adulthood. Fadi's elder sister, Noor, from *Shooting Kabul*, did face quite a few similar issues but central to that novel was the predicament of the natives residing in Afghanistan. The use of language in the novel is extremely interesting and unique, as is the portrayal of the characters. The first-person narrative technique adds to the joy of exploring the world of Dimple Lala, who is a teenager, undergoing various physiological changes.

A notable aspect of this novel is the assertion of the Oriental identity of Dimple Lala and her submission to the fact that it was the other identity in the US. The following quotation will justify the claim,

> In our twosome I was "the other one" —you know, the one the boy doesn't remember two seconds after delivering the pizza. The too-curvy, clumsy, camera-clacking wallflower with nothing but questions lately. (Hidier 2)

Her ruminations about Gwyn, her best friend, justify the claim even further.

> She had it all, Gwyn. And I had her, which by some sort of transitive theory gave me access to the allness she cupped in the palm of her hand. (Hidier 2)

The assertion of this identity and the problems rooted in this identity are deeply rooted in her birth and upbringing, which she elaborates upon in the novel.

> So, not quite Indian, and not quite American. Usually I felt more along the lines of Alien (however legal, as my Jersey birth certificate attests to). The only time I retreated to one or the other description were when my peers didn't understand me […] or when my family didn't get it […] Sometimes I was too Indian in America, yes, but in India, I was definitely not Indian enough. (Hidier 13)

The dichotomy and the assertion of this dichotomy with her identity are deeply rooted in her mixed upbringing in America, within an Indian household. The fact that the family had migrated and not been displaced, raises a very important question about their American-born children.

Tanuja Hidier faced similar issues in her childhood and growth years, as her upbringing was characterized by similar issues and predicaments. Physical appearance will hinder the mingling of the Indian culture with the American and the absence of family elders will impediment the incorporation of Indian values. What remains are faint memories, which confuse the creation of the identity to a far greater extent.

> India. I had few memories of the place, but the ones I held were dream clear: Bathing in a bucket as a little girl. The unnerving richness of buffalo milk drunk from a pewter cup. My dadaji pouring tea into a saucer so it would cool faster, sipping from the edge of the thin dish, never spilling a drop. […] Meera Maasi crouching on the floor to sift the stones from rice. Cows huddled in the middle of the vegetable market, sparrows nesting on their backs. A perpetual squint against sun and dust. The most delicious orange soda I'd ever drunk—the cap-split hiss, and then the bubbling Jetstream down a parched throat. […] But mainly all my memories of India were memories of Dadaji. (Hidier 13)

This further justifies the role of the elders in the household to transfer their values and ideologies to later generations, not as memories, but as teachings.

Amidst all of these flooding memories and questions over her identity, her concerns over her impending 17th birthday aggravate the issue even further for her. She was not very happy with the way her body had been shaping up, something which she had no control over, and she tried her best to hide it. Her futile attempts to wear dresses which are smaller than her ideal dress size leads to hilarious results. Dimple's mother chides her continuously to come to terms with her body.

> Dimple, she said.—You are a beautiful girl. You have hips. They're not going anywhere. This is the Indian body. We are not like these straight curveless Americans. [...] no matter how much you try you cannot change your bones. Your body is your temple; your body is your home. It tells you where you are from. (Hidier 25)

Dimple's interactions with her mother provide some of the most humorous situations in the novel. Dimple's greatest predicament, especially as a young adult, was her inability to fix herself to one particular identity. Perhaps, this was one of the major reasons why she hid behind the lens of her camera, Chica Tikka. The naming of the camera is also interestingly reflecting her confused identity of half-American, in Chica, and half-Indian, in Tikka. Her ever-endless emotional distress is further aggravated by her inability to date and go out with the boy of her choice, leading to further distress. Alice Trupe rightly observes that "...many teens experience stresses and traumas that trigger depression. It is not surprising, therefore, that emotional disturbance is a major theme of many young adult novels." (75) The emotional stress and trauma of Dimple is voiced by the first person narrative, wherein Dimple seems to be relieved to be able to vent out her distress and unease with the invisible reader. The use of language accentuates this claim, with the use of easygoing and contemporary slang, which seems to speak out of the pages.

Discussion

Both the novels about displacement and migration have brought out a very important aspect which is universal for any Diaspora narrative. They are family and familiarity. What they are left with are memories. Nancy Reynolds made the following observation about displaced citizens,

> Even for those driven by desperation, leaving home was a hard decision: family, tradition, language, food, everything familiar was left behind. The only way to keep the memory of home and cultural identity alive was to re-create them as closely as possible in the new land. Countless permutations of this journey have appeared as history, memoir, and fiction—including children's and young adult literature—detailing waves of immigration, the diasporas, what was lost and what gained in the struggle to adapt. Regardless of the cultures involved, YA fiction has focused most often on the cultural and generational gaps between the first and second generations of immigrants. [...] These narratives explore the gap between parents, who were shaped by the culture they left behind, and their children, who know only the new culture. The characters struggle to bridge the gap, not always successfully. (107)

The immigrant experience is not limited to the South Asian experience alone. The narratives explored in this study deal with the immigrant experience among homogenous communities. Problems associated with the mingling of different cultures and mixed heritage upbringing are well illustrated in various YA Novels. These include Hadley Irwin's *Kim* (1987), Sherry Garland's *Song of the Buffalo Boy* (1992), Sharon Flake's *Money Hungry* (2001), Anjali Banerjee's *Maya Running* (2005). These ultimately inform the reader/scholar about the multifarious issues and concerns with the immigrant and displaced experience. The study had consciously taken up two such narratives which offered a variation in terms of the displacement occurring within the scope of the text. A conscious attempt to reconstruct from memory is undeniable in these narratives. The problem is further aggravated for the youth, who are portrayed in these narratives, who will later go on to experience the atrocities that are depicted in adult narratives concerning migration and displacement. Although such YA narratives are mostly fictive, they are inspired often by real-life experiences. Hence, it may serve to sympathize with the reader of these books, who might have lived through such experiences but had no one to fall back and vent their frustration, like Dimple.

Conclusion

YA Literature in the twenty-first century had moved far beyond its didactic and instructive roots. More than modes of entertainment, they have been garnering a lot of recent critical attention through the recent interest in establishing a canon of YA Literature. To quote Karen Coats,

> Establishing a history of YA literature and even, dare we say it, a canon of significant texts, and showing those texts' ability to stand up to the rigors of critical scrutiny are all part of the process of legitimizing a marginalized literature in the field of literary studies. What remain rare in the critical discourse are studies that seek to theorize YA fiction as a type of literature that has its own constellation of concerns that mark it as distinctive from literature for either children or adults. (317)

While YA narratives tend to question established social norms to a great extent, at least greater than children's literature, it is by no means a literature of transition. YA narratives often delve into exploring the issues of adolescence, as found in Born Confused. A period of life that is "fraught with angst, drama, and change anxiety", adolescence is not a mere period of transition from childhood to adulthood. It is a period of life in itself, the period of Young Adulthood. The writers of YA narratives must keep this in this cognition when they set about the task of building YA narratives.

References

Primary Sources

Hidier, T. D. (2015). *Born Confused*. Scholastic.
Senzai, N. H. (2010). *Shooting Kabul*. Simon and Schuster.

Secondary Sources and References

About Naheed Hasnat Senzai. Retrieved from November 7, 2022, from http://www.nhsenzai.com/about/

Cadden, M. (2011). Genre as nexus: the novel for children and young adults. In: Shelby A. Wolf, et al. (Eds.), *Handbook of research on children's and young adult literature* (302–313). Routledge.

Coats, K. (2011). Young adult literature: growing up, in theory." Shelby A. Wolf, et al. (Eds.), *Handbook of research on children's and young adult literature* (315–329). Routledge.

Higley, E. (2019). Defining young adulthood. *DNP Qualifying Manuscripts* 17. Retrieved November 6, 2022, from https://repository.usfca.edu/dnp_qualifying/17.

Lafuente, E. M. (2016). Nationhood, Struggle, And Identity. In: M. Hilton and M. Nikolajeva (Eds.), *Contemporary Adolescent Literature and Culture* (33–45). Routledge.

Reynolds, N. T. (2009). *Mixed heritage in young adult literature*. The Scarecrow Press, INC.

Stevenson, D. (2011). History of children's and young adult literature. In: Shelby A. Wolf, et al. (Eds.), *Handbook of Research on Children's and Young Adult Literature* (179–194). Routledge.

Trupe, A. (2006). *Thematic guide to young adult literature*. Greenwood Press.

Dr. Kaustuv Chakraborti is currently working as Assistant Professor in the Department of English, Rajiv Gandhi National Institute of Youth Development, Sriperumbudur, Tamil Nadu. He completed his Postgraduate and Doctorate Degrees from Pondicherry University. His topic of Doctoral Research was 21st-century Spy Fiction. He was awarded the A. Lourdes Memorial Gold Medal in 2015, for being the best outgoing student of the M.A. English Batch, 2013–2015. He completed his Undergraduate Degree from the University of Calcutta. Dr Chakraborti's areas of Academic and Research interests include Literary Theory and Criticism, Popular Fiction, Digital Humanities, Children's and Young Adult Literature, and Cultural Studies. In addition to his academic endeavours, Dr Chakraborti has worked as a Summer Intern in the Department of Comparative Literature, Jadavpur University, in the capacity of a translator. Other than teaching English Literature at the Postgraduate level, he has also engaged lessons in Academic Writing and Functional English for Undergraduate students.

Chapter 18
Decolonizing Youth Development on Turtle Island (Canada): Research, Scholarship and Practice

Jemma Llewellyn and Nida Ansari

Abstract Today's youth bear witness to growing economic disparities, class inequalities, migrant otherings, and prejudicial thinking. Consequently, now more than ever, young people across Canada are calling adults into action, particularly those in positions of power, asking them to become allies and to create more spaces for youth voices to be heard (UNICEF Canada (2020a) Reimagine Playbook: UNICEF Canada, Toronto). This co-authored youth-adult chapter therefore not only acts as a direct answer to these calls to action but also exemplifies practices of adult allyship in a community-university partnership project, in Ontario, Canada and our decolonial practices in the scholarship of youth development. Using the theoretical framings of Popular Education (Arnold R (1991) Educating for a change. Between the Lines Press.), Pedagogy of the Oppressed (Freire (1996) Pedagogy of the Oppressed (1970) Translated by Myra Bergman Ramos), and the Integrated Youth Services model, this retrospective and reflective chapter will discuss the collaborative service-learning approach taken in the design and implementation of an online youth-led training program during the global pandemic. Created through a democratic process, with adult and youth stakeholders, the Youth Ambassador training program highlights the importance of a youth-centered approach to human rights within a youth mental health organization, while also giving an insight into long-term goals and commitments that are needed to decolonize this sector.

The authors are hopeful that the calls to action, promising practices, and provocations in this chapter for future adult allies and youth community development work can be maintained in all aspects of society.

Keywords Decolonizing · Youth development · Turtle Island · Canada · Research · Scholarship · Practice

---

J. Llewellyn (✉)
College of Arts, University of Guelph, Guelph, Canada
e-mail: jemma@uoguelph.ca

N. Ansari
College of Social and Applied Human Sciences, University of Guelph, Guelph, Canada

S. Deb and S. Deb (eds.), *Handbook of Youth Development*,
https://doi.org/10.1007/978-981-99-4969-4_18

An Ode To Turtle Island (Canada)

To the land, waterways, and multi-species inhabitants
That have been here since time immemorial
And continue to be here today
We give thanks

Mississaugas of the Credit Nation
Attiwonderonk
Anishnabewaki
Huron-Wendat
Haudenosaunee
Ojibway
Metis

We as settlers have the privilege of
Working
Studying
Playing
Learning
Unlearning
Growing
in what is colonially known as Guelph

Where are you joining us from today?
Who are you joining us as of today?

Introduction

Personal Historical Context

"Unsettling truths of settler colonialism involves messy processes that uncover not only new information, but also new questioning and understanding of who we are in the world. We are challenged to reflect on our collective histories and to reconsider the ways in which we relate to one another."

(*Research and Reconciliation: Unsettling Ways of Knowing Through Indigenous Relationships*, 2019, p.1)

Nida: I have always been a rule-follower. Specifically, my general understanding of the world as a young person was that I must follow the rules set out by the adults around me. Whether it was my parents, my teachers, or any other adults around me, the consensus was that I'd follow their lead, and seek out any information I wanted to know from them. I didn't necessarily question it, but the power dynamic was always there; it didn't feel right for me to think I had a say in decision-making or other "adult" things. This translated to my academic experiences as an undergraduate student, too. I've always felt a barrier between undergraduate students and professors, and an unnecessary block of knowledge and opportunity that is only accessible through age and experience.

The question is, how does one get to that position without the initial (in)experience? Who gets to decide who can break through that barrier? More importantly, why is the barrier there? It wasn't until working with The Grove, meeting Jemma and collaborating with her that I realized there was more to my own voice than I had initially thought.

Jemma: Growing up in Wales I always struggled with mainstream education as I did not like the way that the teachers would compare my abilities to my four older siblings. I didn't appreciate being spoken to as if I wasn't entitled to an opinion about the world and just had to sit and listen. I left formal education at sixteen and started a vocational course in Performing Arts where there was what felt like equal footing, I was asked for my opinions, and I was listened to. These two different interactions with teachers continue to shape the way in which I engage with children and young people, inside and outside of formal education. As a growing movement in children and youth studies, co-investigating, co-creating, and co-writing is an area I'm encouraged to continue to explore in my practice, research, and scholarship, and especially in this paper with Nida.

Colonialism and Youth Development

Research on children and young people's development continues to be a global phenomenon and their lives written through a colonial lens using colonial research practices of scholarship. Youth studies scholar Alyssa Richman highlights critical ethical concerns about insider/outsider adult-youth relationships, noting that there are many "… 'colonizing' aspects of adults researching youth…" (Richman, 2007, as cited in Best, 2007, p. 199), particularly concerning the ownership and dissemination of knowledge, which is presented from paternalistic thinking.

Furthermore, youth are presented more often as subjects, objects, and inferior beings, and less often as agents of change (Levison et al., 2021), also in the media and the oversight of this demographics agency is often political (Heath et al., 2007; Kay, 2019). Thus, impacting systemic decision-making in legislation and policies that are embedded within institutional and social structures, which impact young people's daily lives (LeFrançois & Coppock, 2014; Skelton & Aitken, 2019).

Even in the wake of COVID-19 youth were targeted and agency over their own education was stripped from them. The flip-flopping from adult decision-makers about when to transition back into in-person teaching has had a continued strain on young people's engagement with their formal learning. Premier Doug Ford, of Ontario, took to the media to publicly shame them about being irresponsible. In a press briefing, Ford said:

> Fifty per cent of the cases are in younger people now. And I've got a message to the young folks: guys, this party's not over. You've just got to make sure you follow the protocols and follow the guidelines, because what happens is you bring it home to one of your loved ones, your parents, your grandparents. It's unacceptable. (Robertson, 2021, paras. 2–3)

This comment by Ford only adds to the narrative about youth being a 'problem' for society that needs to be solved. In response, however, Ford received criticism for shaming them through the media (Robertson, 2021). Dr. Wendy Ellis highlighted that "shame tactic is probably not the most effective way to communicate with young people" (Mastroianni, 2020, para. 29). Dr. Joanna Henderson, director of the Margaret and Wallace McCain Centre for Child, Youth and Family Mental Health at the Centre for Addiction and Mental Health (CAMH) in Ontario noted that "[w]e're asking young people to make really complex decisions that weigh things like the health of their family and friends and themselves and public health against their mental health and the importance of social connection" (Mastroianni, 2020, para. 28).

Ford's somewhat paternalistic approach only amplifies the transhistorical representations and interpretations of youth culture and development, where power and biases are always in conflict with young people's agency (Petr, 2003), fueling the narrative of adultcentrism (Campbell, 2021). Add to this the feeling of that when they talk about issues that concern them "…they are not heard; their feelings are dismissed as unimportant, self-indulgent or [the issue is] just a passing phase" (United Nations Children's Fund, 2021, p. 5).

In response to the negative images of youth that transcend the media, there are growing calls to action from youth to adults across Canada, particularly those in positions of power, for allyship and solidarity (UNICEF Canada, 2020a, 2021):

> We should be in our classrooms learning lessons; instead, we are here to teach you some.
>
> Our home is on fire.
>
> The disabled are not disposable.
>
> Mental health matters.
>
> No justice, no peace.
>
> We are on stolen land.
>
> **Nothing about us, without us.** (p. 5)

In short, youth are asking for more spaces to be created for their voices to be heard. With such transhistorical prejudicial thinking, we turn our thinking to 'reconciliation'.

Borrowing from Indigenous scholars, Shawn Wilson (Opaskwayak Cree) and Lindsey Dupré (Métis), alongside Andrea Breen (settler), we are framing their question "what does reconciliation mean to you?" (2019, p. xiii), within the context of youth development. Performance scholar Ed Charlton (2021) notes that "reconciliation is now the principal language as well as the conceptual ideal through which post-conflict societies are conceived" (p. 1). In using this analogy to consider youth development, we recognize that conflict between youth and adults is deeply ingrained into societal thinking. Yet, it is an important concept for us to use, particularly as we are situated on Turtle Island Canada. We believe that reconciliation cannot be considered in our context without discussing the role of decolonization in the process.

While this chapter is not directly discussing engagement with Indigenous youth in the process of reconciliation and decolonization, we are communicating ideas about cross-cultural and generational dialogues that can and should be happening with non-Indigenous youth (widely defined) and communities on their own (4Rs Youth Movement, 2017). This chapter therefore acts as an intervention and response to calls for youth consultation and allyship (UNICEF Canada, 2020a, 2021). More importantly, it challenges readers to think about the colonial practices that are deeply embedded into the representation and interpretation of youth development through an adult lens in the academy.

We have, therefore, consciously embedded reflective interludes to make space for us to challenge such practices.

Hope

Pedagogy of the Oppressed principal visionary, Paulo Freire notes that "[i]t is imperative that we maintain hope even when the harshness of reality may suggest the opposite" (1996, p. ix). For youth, in what is colonially known as Canada the reality of youth mental health as a result of the pandemic were and continue to be adversely affected. Reports reveal that as one of the most affluent countries in the world, Canada ranks 30th out of 38 where children and young people under the age of 18 the worst mental health and wellbeing (Children First Canada, 2021; UNICEF Canada, 2020b), turning to substance abuse and in some cases suicide. With such a fragmented mental health system in Canada. The Mental Health Commission of Canada (2015) suggests that:

> In order to effectively address the needs of [emerging adults] transitioning to adult mental health and addiction services, an integrated, accessible, and responsive service system needs to be in place. We require a full continuum of services — from universal prevention and health promotion to the most intensive level of services for a small proportion of [emerging adults] with the most complex needs. (p. 7)

Additionally, the need for youth to be actively involved and engaged with the planning and implementation of such services is key for, as well as youth-friendly services, providing the ability for peers and families to be able to support youth with their mental health and recovery (Hawke et al., 2021; Mental Health Commission of Canada, 2015; Settipani et al., 2019). In June 2021, Children First Canada, in their report *Mitigating the Impacts of COVID-19 on Children and Youth: Policies and Programs*, highlighted specific recommendations for schools, government officials and parents, to assist with the long-term impact of children and youth being unable to attend school, clubs, or socialize with friends in person, because of the pivot to the online learning.

Hope for youth development during the harshness of the reality of the pandemic, for us appeared as a new relational experience through a mental health and wellness organization based in Guelph, Ontario, Canada, and its use of an Integrated Youth Service model (IYS). From its conception, they have focused on developing youth and their voices through multiply access points, including a seat at the partnership table, university partnerships, and youth working groups.

When Two Worlds Collide

Nida: Being a Psychology student at the University of Guelph, I had the opportunity of participating in a Co-op program, where I got to take part in work terms throughout my degree to gain meaningful professional experience, which then served as learning experiences to connect back to my degree. For my first work term, I was really interested in finding a job related to education or mental health in some way, to be able to deepen my understanding and work on my own transferable skills. Those two interests intertwined when I applied to the role of Peer Support Coordinator at The Grove (formerly the Integrated Youth Services Network) and was hired to research and develop content for their youth support training program. The Grove planned on hiring Youth Ambassadors to implement this support program but needed training resources to orient them to the hubs and the role. As a youth myself, I was able to spearhead the development of the training program, as well as work on other projects happening within the organization—one of which was to work alongside the instructors and students on a university course dedicated to creating informational allyship guides for the organization.

Through that collaboration I met Jemma, after which we started working together to put the content into functional workshops. Once the content and planning were completed, I was able to then co-facilitate the training workshops themselves with Jemma.

Jemma: It was almost serendipitous that I got involved in the organization. As I was coming to the end of reading a newsletter from the International Student Association at the University of Guelph, I spotted an undergraduate course called Civic Engagement and Service Learning: Exploring Allyship. I reached out to the course leader to see if I could join at a graduate level. The course immediately appealed to me as I had been searching for a framework that I resonated with in my research. After hearing The Grove's Director Cyndy Forsyth talk about her experience as a parent and her drive to help build an integrated mental health and wellbeing service for children and young people I knew straight away I wanted to get involved with the organization. The youth centered approach throughout the organization's infrastructure was something I hadn't seen since moving to Canada and I was intrigued to see what this looked like in practice. Upon meeting Nida, I was encouraged to see that she was playing an equal role and being supported in the creation of a training program together for her peers.

This chapter therefore aims to discuss youth development through the practice of decolonization in our co-authored writing approach, while noting the value of the

IYS model as a framework to support the development of an adult-youth co-created youth-led training program. We ask:

What promising practices does our adult-youth collaboration, inside and outside, of an Integrated Youth Service model and academia offer to youth development work in the practice of decolonization?

Using the principles of Popular Education and Pedagogy of the Oppressed, as a decolonial and emancipatory practice we discuss the training program. This includes notions of problem-posing education, critical consciousness, and the teacher-student paradigm. It is important to note that in continuing our commitment to decolonizing writing practices, this chapter consciously strays away from asserting that anyone involved in the training program, youth, or adult mentioned identifies as being oppressed, as the practice of labeling communities at a deficit is a colonial practice in and of itself.

We believe that the practice of decolonization must run through not only in the work we do in physical spaces but also in spaces that impact the mobilization of knowledge. In addition, the practices described in this chapter are deliberately not being presented as liberatory or emancipatory, for the participants, as only the participants involved in the training program can fully express if they identify with these concepts.

We therefore openly invite reflection from the reader when reading through this chapter and for them to consider (1) how they engage with young people in their local community, as an academic, decision-maker, educator and (2) if you see them as equal contributors to civic society.

Background

The Grove Hubs: An Integrated Youth Service Approach

The Grove Hubs, formerly known as the Integrated Youth Services Network, are seven sites located across Wellington County and Guelph in Ontario. This community-wide initiative consists of several service providers, which work together to deliver key services to children, youth, and their families across the county. As described in their business case, The Grove Hubs are a

> 'one-stop-shop' for youth aged 12 to 26, designed to meet needs for mental health, substance use, peer supports, and other community and social services. These hubs aim to answer to the need of quality services by focusing on rural youth, transitional-aged youth, and integrative technological practices. (Integrated Youth Services Network, 2020)

The Grove takes its inspiration from the Ontario wide framework of Youth Wellness Hubs Ontario (YWHO).

YWHO is a province-wide mental health initiative that aims to provide services to youth and their families "at the right time and in the right place" (Youth Wellness Hubs Ontario, 2022, para. 1). YWHO intends to have an active and crucial role when it comes to improving Ontario's mental health and addiction services for youth and young adults by:

- "Providing rapid access to easily identifiable mental health and substance use services with walk-in, low-barrier services and clear service pathways
- Providing evidence-based interventions matched to individuals' level of need, and supported transitions to specialized care services when the severity of [the] need is evident
- Integrating mental health, substance use, primary care, vocational, housing and other support services into a one-stop-shop model of care offered in a youth-friendly space
- Reducing transitions between services through co-location and shared services in a single place
- Establishing common evaluation across sites
- Co-creating services with youth & families" (Youth Wellness Hubs Ontario, 2022, para. 2)

YWHO builds on similar initiatives across the globe (Jigsaw in Ireland and Headspace in Australia) and other evidence-informed models already underway in Canada, such as Pan-Canadian ACCESS Open Minds, YouthCan IMPACT research hubs based in Scarborough, Toronto East, Central Toronto and the Foundry in British Columbia (Henderson et al., 2022; Youth Wellness Hubs Ontario, 2022). These service providers all come under an international knowledge sharing network called Frayme. In short, Frayme focuses on connecting a wide range of mental health and social services following an IYS model that is dedicated to working with youth and young adults (Frayme, 2022). This in turn, accelerates youth care integration and implementation strategies (Frayme, 2022).

As a recognized international model, the IYS approach takes a collaborative approach to the needs of health services, health care, educational support, housing services, and social services focusing on intervention and/or prevention (Youth Wellness Hubs Ontario, 2022). Included in the model is often a youth-friendly space with peer support services, youth and family engagement provisions. We believe that this leaves space for promising practices to occur in youth development.

Operating from and promoting dialogical spaces for youth came from The Grove's conception, where youth consultation and engagement remain at the heart of each of the service providers involved. Using a horizontal structure, wherever possible, projects, the design of the Hubs, and programming are created from a 'bottom up' grassroots approach. It aims to be adaptable to the needs of youth and promote a seamless transition into adulthood, from a mental health perspective (Halsall et al., 2019).

In addition to being connected to a large network of service providers, The Grove Hubs have developed a unique partnership with the University of Guelph that contributes to multiple aspects of youth development from multiple levels of engagement. One of these levels includes working with the Experiential Learning Hub to engage in service-learning and community-based learning opportunities with students. The Cooperative Education (Co-op) program at the University also offers hands-on experience, while the in-course application allows for reciprocity. The University of Guelph is also a member of The Grove's decision-making/governing committee and has their own hub site located on its campus, ensuring additional services are provided to not only youth in the community but also students (University of Guelph News, 2022).

Community-University Partnerships

Opportunities to engage with The Grove Hubs have also been offered through various service-learning programs, including students from computer engineering. Facilitated through the Experiential Learning Hub, service-learning programs are credit-bearing and where students engage in activities identified by community needs. This therefore gives them a practical understanding of the course content, while also broadening the students' perspective and appreciation for a discipline. In turn, this gives students an underlying sense of civic responsibility (Bringle & Hatcher, 1996; Jacoby, 1996).

However, Tania Mitchell (2008) notes that "[t]raditional interpretations of service-learning tend to emphasize students focusing on "pre professional" experiences…and the personal or social development of students (mostly attitudes toward leadership, altruism, and sometimes thoughts or feelings about the people served in the community)" (p. 51). Thus, many service-learning programs tend to not ask students to think about if there is an injustice that has created a need for the intervention in the first place.

In addition to the two programs, The Grove has access to the Community-Engaged Scholarship Institute. Community-Engaged Scholarship (CES) practices go beyond the "…canon of scholarship to define social problems worthy of analysis…" with professors acting as consultants with "…community organizations to develop topics for courses or research projects" (da Cruz, 2018, p. 155) for students (Morton et al., 2019). In the process of defining CES, Cynthia Gordon da Cruz (2017) lays out six core components of the practice:

> Component 1: Real-life social problems in our democracy are defined with or by the community
>
> Component 2: These real-life social problems are investigated in scholarly ways
>
> Component 3: Community-university partnerships are collaborative and mutually beneficial
>
> Component 4: Knowledge to address public issues is collaboratively developed with community and university members
>
> Component 5: Institutional resources are utilized to address these real-life public issues
>
> Component 6: Community research or projects are integrated with faculty members' research and teaching (p. 366)

The opportunities to decolonize the field of youth development practice, research, and scholarship are promising for the partnership between the University of Guelph and The Grove Hubs, potentially setting a precedent for the future of youth engagement. However, we take heed of Deborah Barndt's (2011) point that there is a "…deepening contradiction of increasingly neoliberal market-driven universities that at the same time promote community engagement and knowledge production for autonomy and social justice" (p. 132). Therefore, we must remind ourselves that "[i]t is in the spirit of popular education to continually reflect on these [political and economic] shifting forces, to respond to each new moment in fresh ways, and to be critically self-reflexive…" (Barndt, 2011, p. xv).

Our Youth Support Program and Pedagogy of the Oppressed

Popular Education in short "…has mainly been used as a tool to educate the poor, underprivileged groups, and the oppressed, thus operating as a form of social and political liberation, through "promoting education for all citizens" (Arnold, 1985, p. 1). Furthermore, at its root is "[w]orking partnership with communities and social movements, academics and community professionals" to develop "new approaches to community-based learning". The essence of this work is "knowledge democracy, promoting less socially divisive and more hopeful strategies for active citizenship" (Mayo, 2020, p. 2).

How the training program was created because of the IYS structure of The Grove Hubs speaks directly to these ideas. There was an identified need for The Grove to create a framework where youth could help support each other in a myriad of ways, in addition to the services offered by health and wellbeing professionals. Specifically, what was desired was a preliminary version of a peer support program that would be developed for youth, by youth, and with youth. To ensure the training program met the needs of the youth in the comment, a working group was established that consisted primarily of youth, mental health professionals, stakeholders, community members, and other adult allies. This working group thus led to the conception of the Youth Ambassador role at The Grove Hubs.

Critical for the development of this training program for youth is what Freire calls "problem-posing education" to present itself. Problem-posing education, for Freire (1996) responds "to the essence of consciousness—*intentionality*—rejects communiques and embodies communication" (p. 60). Furthermore, in "problem-posing education people develop their power to perceive critically *the way they exist* in the world *with which* and *in which* they find themselves; they come to see the world not as a static reality, but as a reality in process, in transformation" (Freire, 1996, p. 64). The way in which we put the training program together therefore needed to directly open up a space for dialogue about the spaces in which they work, live, and study in relation to how they and/ or their relatives came to be on Turtle Island. Here, we were able to rely on a co-created Indigenous allyship guide created by undergraduate students at the University of Guelph in consultation with the Indigenous Student Centre (see "Recommendations: Collaborative Provocations and a Call to Action").

Indigenous scholar Dylan Robinson (Stó:lō) notes that "[t]o read and repeat prescriptive acknowledgement without variance runs counter to the foundational values of acknowledgement" (Robinson et al., 2019, p. 21). Therefore, we were critically conscious about co-create a land acknowledgement practice that was not tokenistic and that could be used to direct Youth Ambassadors to consider their own positionality, while modeling a practice that could be passed on through peer education. At the beginning of each of the workshops the Youth Ambassadors were invited to share their own acknowledgement or participate in a moment of silent reflection with us.

The Train-the-Trainer model was used as a way for each cohort of Youth Ambassadors to have the necessary skills to facilitate future iterations of the training program, for them to train youth volunteers, and to run programs for youth attending the Hubs. In turn, this would mitigate the need for an adult facilitator there to train youth, instead their peers would act as role models alongside them. In this context we recognize the train-the trainer model as peer education. Inspired by Teen Talk Canada (2020a, 2020b), we felt that peer education breaks down the hierarchy of learning and the "banking model" of education that is present in traditional schooling. The "banking model" views students as receptacles that need to be filled with information to pass exams.

Instead, the peer education approach promotes equal status between the learner and the teacher, where each person plays these roles simultaneously. As a key idea in Pedagogy of the Oppressed, Freire (1996) notes that,

> [t]hrough dialogue, the teacher-of-the-students and the students-of-the-teacher cease to exist and a new term emerges; teacher-student with students-teachers. The teacher is no longer merely the-one-who-teaches, but one who is himself taught in dialogue with the students, who in turn while being taught also teach. (p.61)

Findings

Interlude: An Arts-Based Approach

Jemma: Being from a theatre background and familiar with working against the "banking model" through an arts-based approach I offered to bring my past experience of using applied theatre as a tool to co-develop and deliver a peer leader training program for youth. The difference here being that Nida and I needed to develop workshops suitable for an online context. Applied Theatre in short is an umbrella term used for drama and theatre practices, such as improvisation, role-playing, and devising in non-mainstream settings. It is often used for community engagement, social justice, and education and to facilitate collaborative approaches to participation.

Not knowing if the exercises would work in the time that we had and if they would translate online, I followed Nida's lead and we decided that the most important part for the Youth Ambassadors would be the role-playing activities on the last day and a few introductory drama games.

As a unidirectional method of teaching, Freire (1996) posits that "...banking education anesthetizes and inhibits creative power..." (p. 62). Using an arts-based approach for some of the training allowed for the Youth Ambassadors to investigate what Freire calls "thematics". He notes that "...the investigation of thematics involves the investigation of the people's thinking—thinking which occurs only in and among people together seeking out reality. I cannot think *for others* or *without others*, nor can others think *for me*" (p. 89). Here they were able to reflect together on what they thought the most pressing issues they might face in their roles and role-play possible situations.

Identifying as facilitator-participant, in this process, we recognized and understood that instead of transmitting our own knowledge about a topic or assuming that we knew what the issues are pertaining to a particular group of youth, we used our roles to support youths' development of reflective practice. This engagement of knowledge exchange, gave Youth Ambassadors the ability to mobilize their knowledge through cross-cultural dialogue, which "is rooted in respect, reciprocity, reconciliation, and relevance" (4Rs Youth Movement, 2017, p. 6).

This was also facilitated through the opening and closing circles, which are often associated with theatre workshops with youth, through check-ins and check-outs. The purpose of these circles, particularly because of young people feeling isolated and lonely, leading to further mental health concerns, was to create space and time for all of us to reflect in the moment.

A similar practice called 'Sharing Circles' have been used for generations and is a way of knowing and being for many Indigenous communities. Wright et al. (2016) share:

> Sharing Circle consists of members arranged in a circle, to which members may share their response one at-a-time without interruption. This design is intentional and a defining feature of Sharing Circles, as the emphasis is for every person to be heard.
>
> Among the many symbols that a circle represents for Indigenous Peoples, the Sharing Circle symbolizes continuity and equity, and these concepts mirror the qualities of a Sharing Circle; the inside of the Sharing Circle is a safe, inclusive, and non-judgmental space for members to express their beliefs, perceptions, and experiences. (p. 3)

These circles opened up opportunities for trust to develop and led to the change of the facilitator-participant paradigm and for knowledge exchanges to be possible. Going into the training program space online, we were both conscious of our positionalities inside and outside of the workshop and wanted to ensure that we were role-modeling the change in power dynamics at all levels of engagement was horizontal and not hierarchical.

Interlude: Impact on and Representation in Youth Development

Nida: For me, the development of a training program was quite an active learning process, and a direct impact on my own growth and evolution as a young person. Coming into this project, I was not fully aware of the concept of adult-youth allyship, and so I was consciously developing an awareness of it through the partnership I built with Jemma during the project's development. I went from assuming adults are the rule makers and youth are the rule followers, to understanding that there is potential for having a more dialogical relationship between adults and youth. Just becoming aware of the practice and seeing adults advocate for adult-youth allyship was enough to show me how important it is in any space where adults and youth are involved, and it has made me more confident to advocate for my own needs and goals as a young person, too.

While gathering feedback from youth that took the training program was a part of our process, we do not want to speak on behalf of those youth, as the ethical application process was not under the remit of this chapter. Therefore, what might be the various ways that knowledge could be mobilized from this project without removing the agency from youth? Here we take into consideration for the practice of knowledge mobilization in youth development through Fenwick and Farrell's (2011) notion that "knowledge mobilization in some formulations is portrayed as a linear and rational matter of designing more-targeted and appealing dissemination, but it is entangled in social processes and contradictory influences" (p. 2).

An example of the way in which youth mobilized their knowledge from this program has been through a podcast called "Get With The Grove" created and hosted by Youth Ambassadors (see "Recommendations: Collaborative Provocations and a Call to Action"). Furthermore, Youth Ambassadors have been able to represent themselves and their experience in this role in different forms of media online. Youth Ambassadors and attendees of The Grove alike have shared their approval of the youth-to-youth support model found in The Grove, with many reporting that they feel comfortable connecting with youth like them, finding a sense of community and relatability (Dowell, 2022). A Youth Ambassador commented:

> If you were to tell [a] 15-year-old me that a job would allow me to get over my fear of public speaking while also practicing pool skills, I would think you were joking [...] This role as a youth ambassador has highlighted many different qualities that I hold as a worker and an individual that I likely would have been too fearful of expressing in any other setting. To have a team of like-minded and kind-hearted individuals as co-workers who want to see you succeed in every aspect of your journey alters the way you view the risks you take. Being a youth ambassador is a role that allows you to be inspired by the youth in our community and allows you to be the most authentic version of yourself. (para. 9)

The Grove and its many stakeholders have shared positive feedback in media interviews that Youth Ambassadors are described as the "friendly faces" youth see when they walk into the hubs, often creating a safe space for youth to not only find community among peers, but also seek The Grove's mental health services and provide assistance in navigating the hubs' various resources and staff (Donaldson, 2022). In an interview with Dowell (2022), a Youth Ambassador shared:

> As youth ambassadors, we are in a unique position where we can allow our connections to grow in a very authentic way [...] There aren't many roles that allow for rapport building by playing pool and basketball or chatting about video games. Participating or chatting about these things may seem superficial to others, but it offers someone a sense of connection. It shows them directly that we are interested in what they are interested in, which can mean the world to someone who might not be open to talking about some of the things going on in their personal lives. Being a youth ambassador is being a peer that can offer a listening ear and some guidance as to what supports exist within The Grove or in the community. (para. 3)

We see this comment as evidence of the impact of using a peer education approach to the Youth Ambassador training program and in turn a promising practice for youth development.

Recommendations: Collaborative Provocations and Calls to Action

Jemma: With the global crisis that we are currently living in it is now more important than ever to build solidarity and allyship at whatever access point to young people adults in positions of power have. What I have learned and experienced through this process is that there is a real desire for young people to be involved in their education and access to civic engagement. If you are an adult, you must be willing to change your assumptions about the capability of youth to engage in civic education, and that they are the ones that can talk about their experiences. They too are resourceful in their own way and they know more about issues that concern them than adults do. In order to fulfill this, adults need to practice active listening, create platforms for young people to speak, and respect their points of view.

Nida: This entire process has shown me the potential of adult and youth collaboration that is not unilateral. Having a trusting partnership with adults first means that adults trust the youth to be knowledgeable in their own right. We bring different backgrounds, experiences and positionalities that have value and are necessary to acknowledge for there to be a genuine connection. Overall, having a mutual respect of both parties is crucial for there to be any significant collaboration or contribution to a greater cause.

Jemma: This work is like a muscle, it must be used consistently and carefully to have the desired mobility. This work has now started to make its way into the neoliberal make-up of universities, it is our collective responsibility, as people in positions of power to leverage these spaces. We must be critically conscious and reflexive about not perpetuating colonial narratives that are hidden within the historical concepts of these two practices.

Freire (1996) notes that, "[a] revolutionary leadership must accordingly practice co-intentional education" (p. 51). We therefore present to readers these Calls to

Action as an invitation to critically engage with the practice of decolonization in your own work through the participation in a movement towards creating more equitable spaces for youth and their social, emotional, and/or academic development.

Action 1: As a settler (widely defined), commit to the long-term practice and engagement of decolonization first with yourself, then you will be in a position to engage in conversation and practices in decolonization. If you are living and working in a country that has not directly been impacted by colonization it is still important to understand decolonization within the global scope of youth development. See 4Rs Youth Movement's (2017) *Seeding Reconciliation on Uneven Ground: The 4Rs Approach to Cross-Cultural Dialogue.*

Action 2: Identify potential arts-based approaches that can be used as reflective tools which make use of problem-posing education to explore youth concerns in the community. For more information about The Grove's training program and related tools, please contact the co-author at jemma@uoguelph.ca.

Action 3: As an academic (not discipline-dependent) that works in youth development, consider using a service-learning, a co-operative learning, or community-engaged approach to support and amplify youth voices in academic, research, practice, and scholarship. See Morton et al.'s (2019) "Graduate Students, Community Partner, and Faculty Reflect on Critical Community Engaged Scholarship and Gender Based Violence."

Action 4: As a community organization that works with youth, consider finding your local equivalent to an experiential learning or community-engaged institute at a university to help you develop resources for, with, and by youth. See work from the Experiential Learning Hub and the Community Engaged Scholarship Institute at the University of Guelph.

Action 5: Explore the possibility of alternative forms of knowledge mobilization (in your context) for supporting youth development and creative practices. See The Grove Hubs' resources provided on their website (www.thegrovehubs.ca).

Action 6: Investigate how you can (in your context) co-create dialogical spaces that allows for relational learning to happen. See Llewellyn and Ansari's (2022) "By, For, and With Youth: Transforming the Delivery of Training Programs".

Action 7: Investigated the promising practices that are used within an Integrated Youth Service model. See Lu et al.'s (2021) "The Grove Hubs Developmental Evaluation Final Report". See also Henderson et al.'s (2022) "Youth Wellness Hubs Ontario: Development and initial implementation of integrated youth services in Ontario, Canada".

Conclusion

It is cultural critic and scholar Raymond Williams (1976) who makes a note on key vocabulary in the modern world which we think seems apt to conclude our thinking and acknowledgements to future possibilities of this work. We assert that what we have offered in our retrospective pieces "...is not a neutral review of meanings. [It is] a vocabulary to use, to find [y]our own ways in, to change as we find it necessary to change it, as we go on making [y]our own language and history" (Williams, 1976, pp. 24–25).

In the Introduction chapter entitled, "The people, the poor, and the oppressed: the concept of popular education through time", in *A History of Popular Education: Educating the People of the World*, contributor Sjaak Braster (2014) notes that "[p]opular [e]ducation, like many social transformation concepts, develop their meaning over time" (p. 1).

In this retrospective and reflective paper, we have attempted to add our own contribution to the meaningful practices of Popular Education and Pedagogy of the Oppressed, through continuing our dialogical learning and challenging different colonial narratives within the academic, community, and personal spaces we inhabit.

By centering Freire's (1996) concept of dialogical teaching and communication whilst focusing on intersecting concepts including problem-posing education and critical consciousness, we hope we have given space for readers to consider the adult-youth paradigm beyond the walls of academia.

In turn, we hope to have inspired readers to reflect on the colonial narratives that continue to uphold adult centrism. Thus, we end with Black feminist thinker and activist bell hooks (2003) as a reminder that "[o]ne of the dangers we face in our educational systems is the loss of a feeling of community, not just a loss of closeness among those with whom we work … but also the loss of a feeling of connection and closeness with the world beyond the academy" (p. xv).

Epilogue: A Closing Dialogue

Nida: As an undergraduate student, this experience was so meaningful. Removing the barrier between higher education and my inexperience within it gave me a chance to learn so much that I was not aware of before, both in academia and in my own abilities. Not only have I been given many novel opportunities to branch out and network in different academic contexts (i.e., through papers, conference presentations, etc.*), I've also become more confident in my own knowledge and expertise as a young person, and that would not have happened without the chance to be inexperienced first.*

I think other youth in my position would want the same. There is so much that young people have to offer the world, and the world would be able to notice it if adults just gave those youth a chance to be part of the conversation. And based on how this process impacted me in a positive manner, it would only be appropriate that I continue this practice as I become older, so I too can make room for youth to speak on behalf of themselves.

Jemma: As an adult ally it is just as important for me to be able to recognize partnerships that are built on a foundation of trust. Working with other adults in this area requires a long-term commitment to community-engagement and not parachute practitioners. As a PhD student this process has been extremely humbling and confirming. All sections of society that offer spaces of learning to young people need to engage in different types of dialogical activities. Dimensions of Higher education do not currently value the voices of undergraduate students and continue to practice the "banking model" of education. Universities are perpetuating the notion that young people are just producers and consumers.

References

Arnold, R. (1985). *A new weave: popular education in Canada and Central America.*
Arnold, R. (1991). *Educating for a change.* Between the Lines Press.
Barndt, D. (Ed.). (2011). *¡Viva!: Community arts and popular education in the Americas.* SUNY Press.
Braster, S., Simon, F., & Grosvenor, I. (Eds.). (2014). *A history of popular education: educating the people of the world.* Routledge.
Best, A. L. (Ed.). (2007). *Representing youth: Methodological issues in critical youth studies.* NYU Press.
Bringle, R. G., & Hatcher, J. A. (1996). Implementing service learning in higher education. *The Journal of Higher Education, 67*(2), 221–239.
Campbell, S. (2021). The ethics of adultcentrism in the context of COVID-19: whose voice matters? *Journal of Bioethical Inquiry, 18*(4), 569–572.
Charlton, E. (2021). *Improvising reconciliation: Confession after the Truth Commission.* Liverpool University Press.
Children First Canada. (2021) *Mitigating the Impacts of COVID-19 on Children and Youth: Policies and Programs.* Children First Canada. Retrieved from https://childrenfirstcanada.org/wp-content/uploads/2021/06/CFC_PolicyReport_Final.pdf.
Community Engaged Scholarship Institute. College of Social & Applied Human Sciences. (n.d.). Retrieved from https://www.cesinstitute.ca/.
da Cruz, C. G. (2017). Critical community-engaged scholarship: Communities and universities striving for racial justice. *Peabody Journal of Education, 92*(3), 363–384.
da Cruz, C. G. (2018). Community-engaged scholarship: Toward a shared understanding of practice. *The Review of Higher Education, 41*(2), 147–167.
Donaldson, A. A. (2022). *The Grove officially opens U of G Hub just in time to address growing needs.* Guelph Politico. Retrieved August 2022, from https://guelphpolitico.ca/2022/06/21/the-grove-official-opens-u-of-g-hub-just-in-time-to-address-growing-need/.
Dowell, A. (2022). *Youth Ambassadors Helping The Grove Hub Combat Youth Mental Health Crisis.* Grand 101.1 FM. Retrieved August 2022, from https://thegrand101.com/2022/05/24/youth-ambassadors-helping-the-grove-hub-combat-youth-mental-health-crisis/.
Experiential Learning Hub. (n.d.). *Experiential learning.* University of Guelph. Retrieved from https://www.uoguelph.ca/experientiallearning/.
Fenwick, T., & Farrell, L. (Eds.). (2011). *Knowledge mobilization and educational research: politics, languages and responsibilities.* Routledge.
Frayme. (2022, June 13). *About Us.* Frayme. Retrieved August 2022, from https://frayme.ca/about-us
Freire, P. (1996). *Pedagogy of the Oppressed.* (1970) Translated by Myra Bergman Ramos.
Halsall, T., Manion, I., Iyer, S. N., Mathias, S., Purcell, R., & Henderson, J. (2019). Trends in mental health system transformation: Integrating youth services within the Canadian context. In *Healthcare management forum, 32*(2), 51–55. Sage CA: Los Angeles, CA: SAGE Publications.
Hawke, L. D., Sheikhan, N. Y., MacCon, K., & Henderson, J. (2021). Going virtual: Youth attitudes toward and experiences of virtual mental health and substance use services during the COVID-19 pandemic. *BMC Health Services Research, 21*(1), 1–10.
Heath, S., Charles, V., Crow, G., & Wiles, R. (2007). Informed consent, gatekeepers and go-betweens: Negotiating consent in child and youth-oriented institutions. *British Educational Research Journal, 33*(3), 403–417.
Henderson, J. L., Chiodo, D., Varatharasan, N., Andari, S., Luce, J., & Wolfe, J. (2022). Youth Wellness Hubs Ontario: Development and initial implementation of integrated youth services in Ontario, Canada. *Early Intervention in Psychiatry.*
hooks, b. (2013). *Teaching community: A pedagogy of hope.* Routledge.

Integrated Youth Services Network. (2020). *Business Case and Implementation Plan.* Retrieved from https://www.thegrovehubs.ca/_files/ugd/f4f390_ca879a21ce424fc297359e693e5e6fed.pdf

Jacoby, B. (1996). *Service-Learning in Higher Education: Concepts and Practices. The Jossey-Bass Higher and Adult Education Series.* Jossey-Bass Publishers, 350 Sansome St., San Francisco, CA 94104.

Kay, L. (2019). Guardians of research: Negotiating the strata of gatekeepers in research with vulnerable participants. *Practice, 1*(1), 37–52.

LeFrançois, B. A., & Coppock, V. (2014). Psychiatrist children and their rights: Starting the conversation. *Children & Society, 28*(3), 165–171. https://doi.org/10.1111/chso.12082

Levison, D., Maynes, M. J., & Vavrus, F. (Eds.). (2021). Children and Youth as Subjects, Objects, Agents. *Palgrave Macmillan, Cham.* https://doi.org/10.1007/978-3-030-63632-6

Llewellyn, J., & Ansari, N. (2022, March 31). *By, For, and With Youth: Transforming the Delivery of Training Programs.* Frayme. Retrieved from https://frayme.ca/learning-institute-shareback-2022/and-youth-transforming-delivery-training-programs

Lu, S., Varatharajan, T., Student, P. P., Costello, J., & Rush, B. (2021). *The Grove Hubs Developmental Evaluation Final Report.* Homewood Research Institute. Retrieved from https://hriresearch.s3.amazonaws.com/uploads/2021/11/The-Grove-Evaluation-Final-Report_-1.pdf.

Mastroianni, J. (2020). *Why shaming young people for breaking covid-19 rules won't work.* NOW Magazine. Retrieved June 2022, from https://nowtoronto.com/lifestyle/health/shaming-young-people-covid-19-rules-wont-work.

Mayo, M. (2020). *Community-based learning and social movements: Popular education in a populist age.* Policy Press.

Mental Health Commission of Canada. (2015). *Taking the Next Step Forward: Building a Responsive Mental Health and Addictions System for Emerging Adults.* Mental Health Commission of Canada.

Mitchell, T. D. (2008). Traditional vs. critical service-learning: Engaging the literature to differentiate two models. *Michigan Journal of Community Service Learning, 14*(2), 50–65.

Morton, M., Simpson, A., Smith, C., Westbere, A., Pogrebtsova, E., & Ham, M. (2019). Graduate students, community partner, and faculty reflect on critical community engaged scholarship and gender based violence. *Social Sciences, 8*(2), 71.

Youth Wellness Hubs Ontario. (2022, February 15). *What is Youth Wellness Hubs Ontario (YWHO)?* Youth Wellness Hubs Ontario. Retrieved August 2022, from https://youthhubs.ca/en/about/

Petr, C. G. (2003). *Social work with children and their families: Pragmatic foundations.* Oxford University Press.

Prentki, T., & Selman, J. (2003). *Popular theatre in political culture: Britain and Canada in focus.* Intellect Books.

Robertson, B. (2021, March 29). *Doug Ford blames young Ontarians for virus spread and people have a lot to say.* blogTO. Retrieved June 2022, from https://www.blogto.com/city/2021/03/doug-ford-blames-young-ontarians-virus-spread/.

Robinson, D., Hill, K. J. C., Ruffo, A. G., Couture, S., & Ravensbergen, L. C. (2019). Rethinking the practice and performance of Indigenous land acknowledgement. *Canadian Theatre Review, 177*(1), 20–30.

4Rs Youth Movement. (2017). *Seeding reconciliation on uneven ground: The 4Rs approach to cross-cultural dialogue.* 4Rs Youth Movement. Retrieved July 2022, from https://4rsyouth.ca/wp-content/uploads/2017/01/4Rs-Framework-Final.pdf.

Settipani, C. A., Hawke, L. D., Cleverley, K., Chaim, G., Cheung, A., Mehra, K., & Henderson, J. (2019). Key attributes of integrated community-based youth service hubs for mental health: a scoping review. *International Journal of Mental Health Systems, 13*(1), 1–26.

Skelton, T., & Aitken, S. C. (Eds.). (2019). *Establishing geographies of children and young people.* Springer.

Teen Talk Canada. (2020). *Peer Education.* Teen Talk. Retrieved June 2021, from https://teentalk.ca/peereducation/.

The Grove Hubs. (n.d.). *Resources*. The Grove Hubs. Retrieved from https://www.thegrovehubs.ca/resources.

The Grove Hubs. (n.d.). *New Podcast Feed*. The Grove Hubs. Retrieved from https://www.thegrovehubs.ca/podcast.

UNICEF Canada. (2020a). Reimagine Playbook: UNICEF Canada, Toronto.

UNICEF Canada. (2020b). Worlds Apart: Canadian Companion to UNICEF Report Card 16: UNICEF Canada, Toronto.

UNICEF Canada. (2021). Reimagine Playbook: UNICEF Canada, Toronto.

United Nations Children's Fund. (2021, October). The State of the World's Children. (2021). *On My Mind—Promoting, protecting and caring for children's mental health*. UNICEF.

University of Guelph News. (2022, June 22). *The Grove Hub—University of Guelph opens to address youth mental health needs*. U of G News. Retrieved July 2022, from https://news.uoguelph.ca/2022/06/the-grove-hub-university-of-guelph-opens-to-address-youth-mental-health-needs/

Williams, R. (1976). Keywords: A vocabulary of culture and society (London: Fontana). *Croom Helm*.

Wilson, S., Breen, A. V., & DuPré, L. (2019). *Research and reconciliation: Unsettling ways of knowing through indigenous relationships*. Canadian Scholars, an imprint of CSP Books Inc.

Wright, A. L., Wahoush, O., Ballantyne, M., Gabel, C., & Jack, S. M. (2016). Qualitative health research involving indigenous peoples: culturally appropriate data collection methods. *Qualitative Report, 21*(12).

Jemma Llewellyn is a Ph.D. student at the University of Guelph studying Critical Studies in Improvisation. As an applied theatre practitioner from Wales, UK, her research and practice focus on amplifying youth voices through adult allyship. Her research aims to disrupt and decolonize standard adult-youth paradigms in learning and identifies promising practices in multimodal approaches to local/global civic actions. She is a non-resident research associate at the Centre for Socially Engaged Theatre, University of Regina.

Nida Ansari is from Mississauga, Ontario, Canada. She completed a bachelor's degree in Psychology with a minor in French Studies at the University of Guelph. Nida took part in a co-operative education program as part of her degree. She completed two successful co-op work terms with The Grove-Youth Wellness Hubs Ontario, a youth mental health organization in Guelph, Ontario. As their Peer Training Coordinator, Nida spearheaded the development of their Youth Support Program. Nida's research interests currently focus on effective pedagogical practices for youth and adolescents, youth mental health, and overall leadership and engagement. Combining her love for education and psychology, Nida sees every opportunity as a meaningful learning experience, and strives to ensure that whatever she accomplishes has an impact on the community around her in some way.

Chapter 19
Suicide and Youth: Positive Psychology Perspective

Trina Banerjee and K. Jayasankara Reddy

Abstract Suicidality and self-harm among adolescents and young adults need immediate attention and support. This is often seen as a 'cry for help' where a feeling of entrapment experienced by individuals pushes them to see self-harm as a coping mechanism. Lack of social support and co-morbid emotional disorders influences suicidal ideation into planning and action. A general feeling of helplessness that gets triggered often leads to anguish. These emotions get internalized and directed inwards leading to self-directed anger which facilitates a suicidal act. Early detection and identification can prevent the loss of lives and help individuals to learn effective ways of coping. Gatekeeper Training for caregivers, teachers, and their peers will help in detecting the early signs of suicide risk. Intervention based on positive psychology will help not only in crisis management but also as preventive and maintenance therapy in holistic mental health. The concepts of hope, forgiveness, self-compassion, gratitude, and resilience can be incorporated into the intervention programs to build a better therapeutic system for youths dealing with suicidality. Practicing effective coping mechanisms every day and making it a ritual of one's daily life is the need of the hour. Integrating adaptive ways of emotional expression and learning matured means to deal with painful emotions and trauma is what needs to be incorporated into the intervention plan. The chapter focuses on these aspects and aims to make a connection between assessing and easy identification of youths in distress related to suicidality and providing a holistic intervention to help them cope with the situation.

Keywords Adolescents · Young adults · Suicide · Positive psychology · Suicide prevention · Crisis management · Preventive · Intervention

T. Banerjee (✉) · K. J. Reddy
Department of Psychology, CHRIST (Deemed to Be University), Bengaluru, India
e-mail: trina.banerjee@res.christuniversity.in

S. Deb and S. Deb (eds.), *Handbook of Youth Development*,
https://doi.org/10.1007/978-981-99-4969-4_19

Introduction

Suicide is defined as the act of killing oneself deliberately (Colman, 2009). Every year more than 700,000 people die due to Suicide (World Health Organization, 2022). Death by Suicide is a major concern among the youth. It is the fourth leading cause of death among 15–19-year-olds (World Health Organization, 2022). Suicide is mostly carried out by ingestion of pesticides, using firearms, and hanging self. Almost 77% of youth suicides take place in low and middle-income countries (World Health Organization, 2022). Suicide prevention and management is thus a matter of supreme importance worldwide and should be the priority of all countries.

Suicide leads to the loss of lives all across the globe. It leads to a loss of manpower and human resources. Sandler (2018), explains the effects of suicide in the form of "A Ripple Effect", where suicide is compared to a pebble in a pond and the waves that ripple outward are the effect of it. In suicide, the people closest to the individual have been affected the most: families, friends, colleagues, and confidants. There is sudden discontinuation of the relationship between the confidants and the person who died by Suicide which leads to physically missing the person. The physical absence also transcends to the psychological absence of the person which can be extremely painful for many and is often interpreted as a loss. Individuals grieve over the loss leading to an experience of bereavement.

However, this is the first wave of the initial effect of the ripple phenomenon. The loss of the person often leads to the ones surviving with survivor's guilt. If the acquaintances are aware of the mental health concerns the deceased was going through, the feeling of "what more could have been done" prevails, facilitating the guilt. Suicide thus becomes a trauma for many who experience the loss of their close connections.

Incidence of Suicide: International and National Scenario

Suicide is an important topic that requires undivided attention from healthcare professionals, as a significant percentage of the population dies by suicide every year. The Indian incidence rate of suicide is also not significantly different from global markers. In 2019, the suicide rate in India was 12.70, an almost 0.79% increase from 2018. There was a 5% increase in the suicide rate from 2017 and a 0.83% decline from 2016. In India, there was a 1.63% decline in the suicide rate from 2015 (World Suicide Rate 2000–2023). The male-to-female ratio of suicide has varied across the years between 2000 and 2023, with a reduction in the rate of suicide between females to males post-2018 (World Suicide Rate 2000–2023).

According to the World Health Organization and the Global Burden of Disease, almost 800,000 people die from suicide globally every year, amounting to one person every 40 s. (Ritchie et al., 2015) As of 2019, Suicide is the 15th most common cause of death among people, especially the youth (Amnesty International, 2019). Globally,

1.3% of deaths were from suicide reported in 2019 (Ritchie et al., 2015). Globally, suicide is more common in men than in women (Ritchie et al., 2015). In the methods chosen, as reported in 2019, the use of firearms was found in 60% of deaths by suicide in the US (Ritchie et al., 2015). Also, pesticide poisoning was found among 14 million people, or one in seven deaths, in the last 50 years to be a chosen method for suicide (Ritchie et al., 2015).

Suicidal Ideation

Suicidal Ideation is a precursor to a suicide attempt (Overholser & Spirito, 2003). All suicide attempts have a prelude of suicidal ideation, although all suicide ideation does not culminate in an attempt. Ideation of Suicide is explained as thoughts about reasons for death, specific plans to make an attempt, considering the availability of a method of suicide, and attitude toward accepting related thoughts (Beck & Steer, 1997). According to the Oxford Dictionary of Psychology, Ideation is defined as the act of forming ideas or mental images of things not at the time being experienced through sensation (Colman, 2009). Ideation involves translations of sensory inputs into conceptualization (Exner, 2003). It can be explained as a form of thinking which incorporates the organization of symbols or concepts by giving meaning to the same. Ideation indicates conceptualization which is a marker for reality testing and mediates decision-making and actions involving deliberate behaviors (Exner, 2003). Suicidal Ideation is often influenced by a depressive episode which is a major risk factor for suicide (Wakefield and Schmitz, 2016). Depression is often associated with ideas of worthlessness where the individual feels having no real value. There are feelings of self-inflicted guilt associated with reduced self-esteem and confidence (World Health Organisation, 2007). Self-harm can often begin in the form of suicidal ideation which are thoughts and actions of taking one's own life (Morrow et al., 2010). Passive suicidal ideation is a phenomenon where individuals report having a wish to die, although there is no involvement of active planning or steps (Morrow et al., 2010). It can also be active suicidal ideation which often may consist of planning, frequent thoughts of suicide, and mental rehearsals (Morrow et al., 2010). Suicidal ideation can progress toward suicidal attempts when the ideation proceeds into the individual's behavior. Hence it is essential to consider both for prevention of suicide and loss of life. It is important to understand and identify the factors which facilitate suicide ideation to become an attempt. Negative cognitions and painful emotions can be considered as factors that mediate the relationship between suicide ideation and attempt (Morrow et al., 2010). In a meta-synthesis review of literature conducted by Verrocchio et. al., (2016) it has been found that "mental pain" is a significant predictive factor of suicide irrespective of the presence of mental illness (Verrocchio et al., 2016). Psychological pain derived from a sense of loss can be a strong factor of vulnerability for suicide ideation (Morrow et al., 2010).

Suicide Attempt

A Suicide attempt is a self-inflicted, potentially injurious behavior with a non-fatal outcome for which there is evidence (either explicit or implicit) of intent to die. Suicide attempts may result in no injuries or non-fatal injuries. Suicide attempts that result in death are classified as 'suicide' (Morrow et al., 2010). Suicide attempts can involve a diverse set of suicidal behavior ranging from non-suicidal self-injuries, failed suicidal attempts, and actual death by suicide. Other suicidal behaviors may include deliberate self-harm, and parasuicide, which is characterized by a self-inflicted injury resembling a suicide attempt but not intended to be successful (Colman, 2009). Suicide attempts may also include other phenomena like suicidal behavior & self-harm gestures, which are collectively known as "suicidality" (Hausman et al., 2020). A Suicide attempt involves a lack of impulse control which is seen as a direct enactment of the ideation. Impulse control has a reverse relationship with suicide attempts, where lesser impulse control endorses a higher chance of a suicide attempt (Hausman et al., 2020).

Stigma and Myths About Suicide Among the Youth

Suicide has been an issue that has been stigmatized for decades. Stigma comes from a point of shaming the act. Shame is a socially constructed emotion (Barbalet, 2009) that aims at a self-punishing acknowledgment of something gone wrong (Niedenthal et al., 2017). Suicide leads to the loss of human lives or puts many lives at stake which leads society to create shame in an unconscious attempt to prevent the act from occurring. However, Suicide is often a culmination of mental health concerns and an extremely desperate "cry for help". An empathetic and validating stance is required instead of stigmatizing the phenomenon. Stigma leads to not addressing the issue which eventually facilitates misconceptions and myths, which could be detrimental to people. It is desirable that individuals communicate more about Suicide than withhold information.

Some of the common myths involve hesitation to ask individuals whether they are suicidal. This can be a strong deterrent to intervention and help-seeking behaviors. It is an absolute necessity for open communication to determine suicidality. Another common error is to assume that suicidal ideation will always lead to the act of suicide. All suicidal behavior is preceded by suicidal ideation; however, the reverse is not true. Both ideation and attempt should be taken seriously and the intervention and prevention plan must be considered with utmost importance. Suicidal ideation may not always lead to the act in itself. The ideation can be equally distressing and is often characterized by "death wishes" and a "lesser will to live".

A common myth about Suicide is that it happen "out of the blue" (Gomstyn, 2022). Many people fail to notice the soft signs which act as a precursor to suicide. Many ignore the signs, even when noticed, assuming it's a cognitive error on their part, or they are assuming the worst. An individual who is experiencing suicidal ideation may not communicate directly but their behavior will be in sync with their thoughts. The presence of a depressive mood, with hopelessness and helplessness is often a major indicator of suicide. Extreme guilt or feeling a burden to others are also among the crucial signs of suicide (NIMH, n.d.) A feeling of entrapment, with few to no reasons for living is also an indicator of suicidality which often follows withdrawal from friends and family, engaging in risky behaviors, giving away possessions or changes in appetite and sleep (NIMH, n.d.).

Understanding Suicide from a Neuropsychological and Social Perspective

Suicide is a topic that psychologists and researchers have tried to understand from different perspectives. Mainly understanding helps to explore the phenomenon and to help in prevention. The connection between mental health and suicide has been established long back and suicide is also considered a symptom of certain conditions worthy of diagnosis.

The Cry of Pain and Lack of Social Support

Williams (2001), explains Suicide as a "Cry of Pain". The theory revolves around the feeling of entrapment which is often triggered by traumatic life events. This pushes an individual to get into a state where there is no rescue, no escape, and a complete defeat ultimately leading to suicide (Williams, 2001). Negative emotions can also be triggered when there is a lack of social support. In a study by Tabaac, Perrin and Rabinovitch (2016), there is an inverse relationship between suicidal ideation and social support from family (Tabaac et al., 2016). Lack of social support leads to loneliness which can trigger a sense of isolation that may facilitate suicide (Lutzman et al., 2021). Negative emotions can lead to an inability to reach out or seek help. Studies reflect that a low help-seeking behavior among individuals with suicide ideation has often triggered a suicide attempt (Arria et al., 2011). This can also reflect a lack of verbal fluency at the neuropsychological level which contributes to making an attempt from ideation (Bartfai et al., 1990). Verbal fluency typically measures the number of words produced usually within a restricted category, or in response to a stimulus, and usually within a time limit (Lezak et al., 2004). A deficiency in this cognitive ability does indicate a deficiency in generating words meaningfully. Deficiency in verbal fluency has also been associated with depressive disorders and addictions (Nie et al., 2017). Depression and addiction related health issues also bring about social isolation and exclusion thus leading to poor social support. Hence the contribution of verbal fluency and lack of social support cannot be neglected.

Cognitive Deconstruction Affecting Planning

Negative emotions can instill negative automatic thoughts in an individual. A depressed affect can lead to low self-esteem and negative views about self (Montesano et al., 2017). A negative affective state can create cognitive distortions which facilitate suicidal ideation (Fazakas-DeHoog et al., 2017). Cognitive distortions are significantly more noticed among individuals with a history of suicide attempts compared to those with suicidal ideation (Yin et al., 2020). Baumeister (1990), proposed the concept of cognitive deconstruction for suicidal individuals. Cognitive deconstruction refers to the state which extracts the meaning from awareness, leaving a person with no sense of attribution, where threatening implications have no meaning (Baumeister, 1990). It involves a situation where there is no insight, and denial of implications or contexts. The individual experiencing suicidal ideation may experience a state of cognitive deconstruction due to the presence of cognitive distortions which are mediated by the negative effect created by the stressor. Cognitive distortions often facilitate an irrational way of looking at things and erroneous attributions to situations. This can influence suicidal ideation to become an attempt.

A state of cognitive deconstruction can influence the executive functions of suicidal individuals. Planning ability can be compromised with the negative affective state which prompts the suicidal attempt to be seen as the only possible way out. In a study by Moniz et al. (2017), depressed suicide attempters had performed poorly in tasks of planning as compared to non-depressed suicide attempters. This also explains how the state of cognitive deconstruction coupled with depressed affect tends to influence the behavior and facilitates a suicide attempt.

Response Inhibition and Impulsivity Leading to a Suicide Attempt

Impulsivity arises from an impulse which is described as a sudden spontaneous inclination or incitement to some usually unpremeditated action (Merriam-Webster, n.d). It can be seen as a propensity or natural tendency to perform an action. Response inhibition refers to the suppression of actions that are inappropriate in a given context and that interfere with goal-driven behavior (Mostofsky & Simmonds, 2008). There is a relationship between impulsivity and response inhibition as one is facilitated by the other. Impulsivity can be regarded as the emotional backup of response inhibition, where the latter is the neuropsychological correlate of the former. Response inhibition mediated by impulsivity also seems to play an important role in facilitating suicide attempts. In a study by Hausman et al. (2020) impulsivity was found to be a marker for suicide among military veterans. The influence of impulsivity in making a decision like suicide is also a product of the state of cognitive deconstruction. At the neuropsychological level, it can be attributed to deficits in response inhibition. Studies show suicide attempters perform worse in tasks of response inhibition as compared to individuals with suicide ideation (Yin et al., 2020). Suicidal Ideation is governed by the thoughts and ideas related to self-harm and killing oneself. It is often a result of severe depression or the personality characteristics of the individual (Morrow et al., 2010).

Suicide Planning Versus Action

Suicide planning is also different than the action itself. Suicidal behavior is a process that often starts with ideation, progresses to planning, and ends with action or attempt (Levinson et al., 2007). Assessing suicidal planning is important because it helps in the prevention of the same. It is noted that the odds of a suicide attempt with a plan are much higher than the odds of an impulsive attempt (Levinson et al., 2007). There are certain ways to determine suicidal risk. Aron Beck (1988), in his scale for assessing suicidal ideation, explores some of the factors used to determine the risk of suicide. Individuals with a risk of suicide have a lower wish to live with increased death wishes (Harmer et al., 2022). In suicidal planning, often the reasons for dying outweigh the reasons for living. Planning may either involve a desire for active suicidality or passive attempts to save or maintain life. This is often done by avoiding self-care and fostering risk-taking behavior (Ammerman et al., 2018). Usually an individual with suicidal planning has death wishes which emerge ranging from fleeting moments to longer periods of time. The death wishes are also intermittently appearing or quite persistent in the individual which pushes them to plan regarding the execution of the same. The attitude they may have towards the death wishes and ideation are often ambivalent or sometimes they accept and internalize the thought to believe that this is what they deserve. Thoughts related to "being a burden to others" is very common among people experiencing suicidal ideation and planning (Wilson et al., 2005).

Suicidal planning often involves a sense of "lack of control" that the individuals experience resulting in impulsivity (Smith et al., 2008). The suicidal ideation controls the planning and eventual execution of the act. Deterrents to suicide or phenomenon which hold individuals back from executing self-harm are often their reasons for living. The reasons for living are also associated with hope which often becomes a protective factor against suicide (Luo et al., 2016). Reasons for dying also similarly act as a motivational factor for suicide planning (Brüdern et al., 2018).

Suicide planning may involve the steps one contemplates for executing an attempt. Planning can be considered one step further than ideation, where individuals consider the methods of executing a suicide attempt. A suicide note is often found among individuals who attempt suicide. A study by Bhatia et al. (2006) suggests that 30% of suicide notes had a last wish mentioned.

Lack of Social Support, Depression and Hopelessness

The absence of support aggravates the feelings of loneliness which leads to suicidal ideation. The degree of social isolation also transforms suicidal ideation into suicidal planning. Loneliness is more experienced by older individuals and people who have retired from their professional life. The suicide rate among 65 years and above was estimated to be 6.5 times higher than younger people and significantly higher among rural residents (Zhong et al., 2016). Living alone is also seen as a bad prognostic factor for loneliness and suicide (Niu et al., 2020). Individuals living in a family setup are often a protective factor for suicidal planning. Their reasons for living often act as a deterrent to making a plan for suicide. Among the youth, living away from family, and staying in hostels for academic purposes can create a sense of isolation. An invalidating home atmosphere can also give rise to feelings of perceived isolation.

The lack of social support also gives rise to feelings of rejection which are highly correlated with suicide (Cawley et al., 2019). The rejection feelings can be real or perceived as well. The marginalized population, who are subject to feeling isolated from the mainstream, often experience a sense of rejection leading to increased suicidality (Cawley et al., 2019). Among adolescents particularly, a sense of rejection brings about a heightened risk of suicidality (Cheek et al., 2020).

Rejection brings about a sense of abandonment and neglect. It creates a sense of emptiness within and a hollow feeling leading to the need for affiliation and being loved (Ikpa, 2013). The failure to attain a sense of belonging and being loved increases suicidality. This also is correlated with the presence of depression. Depression is a strong risk factor for suicide and is often mediated by Hopelessness (Zhang & Li, 2014). Ideas or acts of self-harm are a diagnostic criterion of Depressive disorders in ICD-10 (World Health Organization, 2007). Depression and suicide are particularly risk factors for the youth and a concern for the college-going population. (Mackenzie, 2011). Depression is often associated with a sense of loss which is reflected in the loss of control of one's life (Weitkamp, Klein, & Midgley, 2016), perceived loss of identity with a loss of a job (Classen & Dunn, 2012) or financial loss (Pridmore & Reddy, 2012).

The loss brings about a sense of Helplessness, where the individual experiences a complete lack of control often leading to hopelessness and suicide (Lester, 1998). Helplessness is often correlated with depression, where an individual feels stuck or entrapped in a difficult situation, and any attempts taken to revive often result in failure (Miller et al., 1975). Helplessness often leads to suicidal ideation and an increase in the severity of depression can often transform into hopelessness and suicidal planning. Hopelessness, helplessness, and worthlessness are considered warning signs of suicidality, especially among the youth (Arora, 2020).

Internalized and Self-directed Anger

Suicide involves thoughts and actions which are aggressive in nature. It involves the thoughts or attempts related to the loss of life. Suicide or self-harm is self-directed aggression (De Leo & Krysinska, 2017). Aggression is the behavioral manifestation of the emotion of anger. Anger is an emotion that is used to fight off threats and is rooted in our brain's reward circuits (Devlin, 2019). It is a basic emotion that every human experiences, especially when one is triggered by a feeling of being wronged, injured, mistreated, opposed, or having obstacles in their path of progress (What is Anger?, n.d.). Aggression is thus, a self-preservative mechanism that helps us to deal with threatening situations. However, aggression can be harmful to others and the self particularly if it turns physically violent. With the years of evolution, hence some cultures consider aggression to be a negative quality and anger to be a negative emotion (Williams, 2017).

Repressed anger is anger that cannot be expressed, either due to a lack of validating space or due to a skill deficit on the part of the individual; and is pushed down into the unconscious. The repressed anger can also contribute to depression, where the aggression is rerouted towards the self (Sahu et al., 2014). Thus the severity of a suicide attempt merely reflects the intensity of anger one feels towards themselves.

Empowering Youth for Suicide Prevention

It is important that the youth be prepared for the prevention of suicide and the topic should be talked about and not kept under the wraps. Mental health has been a taboo for many years and Suicide particularly is a tabooed subject (Russel, 1968). This often prevents individuals from opening up and discussing suicidal thoughts and ideation. There is often a fear of judgment which inhibits open communication. However, by not bringing it up, suicide cannot be prevented.

Youth can be empowered to speak up about their mental health and the stress they go through by creating a non-judgmental and validating space. Validation doesn't involve agreeing with Suicide or self-harm as a way of coping. It is a sense of understanding and empathy to realize the emotional pain and trauma one goes through while they experience the same. One may be able to empathize more deeply when they psychologically put themselves in the other's position and try to understand the stressors they go through.

(i) **Gatekeeper Training**

Gatekeeper training is used as a Suicide preventive strategy. Gatekeeper refers to individuals who belong to a community and have face-to-face interactions with large numbers of people from that community as a part of their everyday life (Burnette et al., 2015). Gatekeepers in suicide prevention would be trained by mental health experts to identify or watch out for people at risk and to observe warning signs among the youth. Gatekeeping would mean that they execute these roles genuinely in protecting the youth from engaging in acts of self-harm (Burnette et al., 2015).

Gatekeepers need to be chosen carefully before getting involved in training. It's important that they have knowledge about Suicide which involves the etiological factors, co-morbid mental health concerns, and the stages of Suicide. It is also of utmost importance to determine their beliefs and attitudes about Suicide prevention. This involves whether the Gatekeeper considers suicide to be preventable, the appropriateness of intervention with at-risk individuals, and the concept of seeking help for mental health as a form of self-care (Burnette et al., 2015). The stigma and issues of gatekeeper reluctance to intervene must also be explored as that can be a serious deterrent to prevention. Also, the concept of Gatekeeper's self-efficacy is where they feel competent and comfortable identifying and facilitating referrals for at-risk individuals. With a statistic of 30% of college students reporting suicidal ideation (Ross et al., 2021) gatekeeper training becomes indispensable among the youth.

(ii) **Early Detection and Crisis Intervention**

Suicide originates from a space of genetic, biological, psycho-social, and cultural factors combined with an experience of trauma and loss (Anderson et al.,, 2017). Hence prevention and early detection strategies should be focused on a multifactorial approach. The approach should also be evidence-based so that the effectiveness is increased.

Early detection can be implemented by training primary care clinicians (Anderson et al., 2017). They are the ones who are majorly in contact with the general public and are involved with them from time to time. Psychoeducation about suicide and self-harm will be of utmost importance in such scenarios. A general practitioner has a significant role in early detection and prevention. The approach to a client reporting suicide is also treated with utmost importance. The clinicians should have a non-judgemental attitude and should be keen on providing hope, reassurance, and psychological support (Ryan et al., 2015). Early detection can involve being aware of certain signs like admitting to death wishes, buying or procuring firearms, having a history of suicidal attempts, or having the chance of overdosing on psychiatric medication like antidepressants.

Crisis intervention in suicide depends on the severity of suicidality. Hospitalization and close monitoring can be done for extremely serious situations. A careful risk assessment involving organized questioning can be done to determine the severity of suicidality (Large & Kapur, 2018). Crisis intervention is an action-oriented & family-based approach. It's important to build a rapport with the client to understand their strengths and weaknesses. A problem-focused approach in identifying the trigger often can be helpful. Targeting the problem can involve mobilizing and reorganizing the family. Making a plan of action, and reaching out for support to reduce the emotional pain and trauma is the goal of Crisis Intervention. However, it is important to remember that this is merely a bandage on the wound which pushes the client towards resolution.

Further in-depth steps are needed to intervene and make sure that the client does not resort to suicidality as a coping mechanism.

(iii) **Influence of Positive Psychology on Suicide Prevention and Intervention**

The concept of entrapment and suicidality is intricately intertwined (Teismann & Brailovskaia, 2020) which often becomes the trigger for low mood. Positive psychology is a study of optimal human functioning which aims to discover and promote the factors that allow individuals and communities to thrive (Seligman, 2017). Positive psychology-based interventions involve gratitude, kindness, happiness, hope, forgiveness, compassion, and resilience which are involved in the holistic wellbeing of the individual. Such interventions increase psychological and subjective well-being (Bolier et al., 2013).

Positive psychology-based interventions are not usually the first line of treatment for Suicidality. There are mixed opinions on whether they have a better treatment outcome over other cognitive therapies predominantly used in such scenarios. A study by Celano et al. (2017), suggests that cognitive focused intervention showed better treatment outcomes over positive psychology-based intervention among clients with suicidality. However, a study by Huffman et al., (2014) showed positive psychology-based interventions were associated with short-term improvements in treatment outcomes in an in-patient setting for clients with suicide. However, positive psychology can be used extensively in suicide prevention.

Interventions involving maintaining a gratitude journal, and practicing kindness and self-compassion can increase self-care and have a holistic impact on mental health. The focus shifts to what is valuable and important in their lives (Sansone & Sansone, 2010) and it influences the "reasons for leaving" in a person. Hope alleviates hopelessness and the willingness to live increases.

Conclusion

Suicide is an outcome of an extremely difficult state of mental health and it also affects the youth around the world. Awareness and addressing the issue instead of reinforcing the stigma is the appropriate way to deal with the situation. By involving positive psychological principles one can foster holistic well-being which will promote psychological growth among the youth. Incorporating adaptive habits can influence mental health and foster happiness.

Practicing Mindfulness-based techniques in everyday tasks and savoring daily chores help to maximize the sensory inputs and foster happiness. Maintaining a gratitude journal to be aware of things we are thankful for or conveying gratitude to others for their contributions to our lives can help us have better interpersonal relations and change our mindset about our own "victim"-positions. Implementing "Kindness Boosters" by showing compassion to others by helping the less fortunate facilitates prosocial behavior. Increasing self-empathy and validation to understand ourselves and others can make us calmer. Working on our strengths, improving communication, practicing assertiveness and other optimism based interventions can help one have enhanced wellbeing.

Incorporating positive psychology principles into our daily lives is equivalent to practicing physical exercises for maintaining fitness and physical health. Working on it and practicing it every day will help make us feel better and develop a better psychological health.

References

Ammerman, B. A., Steinberg, L., & McCloskey, M. S. (2018). Risk-taking behavior and suicidality: The unique role of adolescent drug use. *Journal of clinical child and adolescent psychology : the official journal for the Society of Clinical Child and Adolescent Psychology, American Psychological Association, Division 53, 47*(1), 131–141. https://doi.org/10.1080/15374416.2016.1220313.

Amnesty International. (2019). Retrieved from: https://www.amnesty.org/en/what-we-do/death-penalty/.

Anderson, J., Mitchell, P. B., & Brodaty, H. (2017). Suicidality: prevention, detection and intervention. *Australian prescriber, 40*(5), 162–166. https://doi.org/10.18773/austprescr.2017.058.

Arora, G. (2020, June 16). *Hopelessness, helplessness and worthlessness: know all the warning signs of depression from our expert.* NDTV. https://www.ndtv.com/health/hopelessness-helplessness-and-worthlessness-warning-signs-of-depression-from-expert-2247061.

Arria, A. M., Winick, E. R., Garnier-Dykstra, L. M., Vincent, K. B., Caldeira, K. M., Wilcox, H. C., & O'Grady, K. E. (2011). Help-seeking and mental health service utilization among college students with a history of suicide ideation. *Psychiatric Services, 62*(12), 1510–1513. https://doi.org/10.1176/appi.ps.005562010.

Barbalet, J.M. (2009). Conformity and Shame. In J.M. Barbalet (Ed.) *Emotion, social theory & social structure.*(pp. 103–125). Cambridge: Cambridge University Press. doi:https://doi.org/10.1017/CBO9780511488740.007.

Bartfai, A., Winborg, I. M., Nordström, P., & Asberg, M. (1990). Suicidal behavior and cognitive flexibility: Design and verbal fluency after attempted suicide. *Suicide and Life Threatening Behaviour., 20*(3), 254–266.

Baumeister, R. F. (1990). Suicide as escape from self. *Psychological Review., 97*(1), 90–113. https://doi.org/10.1037/0033-295x.97.1.90.

Beck, A. T., & Steer, R. A. (1993). *Beck scale for suicide ideation manual.* Psychological Corporation.

Beck, A. T., Steer, R. A., & Ranieri, W. F. (1988). Scale for suicide ideation: Psychometric properties of a self-report version. *Journal of Clinical Psychology, 44*(4), 499–505.

Bhatia, M. S., Verma, S. K., & Murty, O. P. (2006). Suicide notes: Psychological and clinical profile. *International Journal of Psychiatry in Medicine, 36*(2), 163–170. https://doi.org/10.2190/5690-CMGX-6A1C-Q28H.

Bolier, L., Haverman, M., Westerhof, G. J., Riper, H., Smit, F., & Bohlmeijer, E. (2013). Positive psychology interventions: A meta-analysis of randomized controlled studies. *BMC Public Health, 13,* 119. https://doi.org/10.1186/1471-2458-13-119.

Brüdern, J., Stähli, A., Gysin-Maillart, A., Michel, K., Reisch, T., Jobes, D. A., & Brodbeck, J. (2018). Reasons for living and dying in suicide attempters: A two-year prospective study. *BMC Psychiatry, 18*(1), 234. https://doi.org/10.1186/s12888-018-1814-8.

Burnette, C., Ramchand, R., & Ayer, L. (2015). Gatekeeper training for suicide prevention: A theoretical model and review of the empirical literature. *Rand Health Quarterly, 5*(1), 16.

Cawley, R., Pontin, E. E., Touhey, J., Sheehy, K., & Taylor, P. J. (2019). What is the relationship between rejection and self-harm or suicidality in adulthood? *Journal of Affective Disorders, 242*, 123–134. https://doi.org/10.1016/j.jad.2018.08.082.

Celano, C. M., Beale, E. E., Mastromauro, C. A., Stewart, J. G., Millstein, R. A., Auerbach, R. P., Bedoya, C. A., & Huffman, J. C. (2017). Psychological interventions to reduce suicidality in high-risk patients with major depression: A randomized controlled trial. *Psychological Medicine, 47*(5), 810–821. https://doi.org/10.1017/S0033291716002798.

Cheek, S. M., Goldston, D. B., Erkanli, A., Massing-Schaffer, M., & Liu, R. T. (2020). Social rejection and suicidal ideation and attempts among adolescents following hospitalization: A prospective study. *Journal of Abnormal Child Psychology, 48*(1), 123–133. https://doi.org/10.1007/s10802-019-00580-z.

Classen, T. J., & Dunn, R. A. (2012). The effect of job loss and unemployment duration on suicide risk in the United States: A new look using mass-layoffs and unemployment duration. *Health Economics, 21*(3), 338–350. https://doi.org/10.1002/hec.1719.

Colman, A. M. (2009). *Oxford Dictionary of Psychology*. Oxford University Press.

Devlin, H. (2019, May 12). *Science of anger: how gender, age and personality shape this emotion*. https://www.theguardian.com/lifeandstyle/2019/may/12/science-of-anger-gender-age-personality.

Exner, J. E. (2003). *The Rorschach: A Comprehensive System*. John Wiley & Sons.

Fazakas-DeHoog, L. L., Rnic, K., & Dozois, D. J. A. (2017). A cognitive distortions and deficits model of suicide ideation. *European Journal of Social Psychology., 13*(2), 178–198. https://doi.org/10.5964/ejop.v13i2.1238.

Gomstyn, A. (2022). *7 common suicide myths—debunked*. https://www.aetna.com/health-guide/suicide-myths-and-facts.html.

Harmer, B., Lee, S., Duong, T., & Saadabadi, A. (2022). *Suicidal ideation*. StatPearls Publishing.

Hausman, C., Meffert, B. N., Mosich, M. K., & Heinz, A. J. (2020). Impulsivity and cognitive flexibility as neuropsychological markers for suicidality: A multi-modal investigation among military veterans with alcohol use disorder and PTSD. *Archives of Suicide Research, 24*(3), 313–326. https://doi.org/10.1080/13811118.2019.1635930.

Huffman, J. C., DuBois, C. M., Healy, B. C., Boehm, J. K., Kashdan, T. B., Celano, C. M., Denninger, J. W., & Lyubomirsky, S. (2014). Feasibility and utility of positive psychology exercises for suicidal inpatients. *General Hospital Psychiatry, 36*(1), 88–94. https://doi.org/10.1016/j.genhosppsych.2013.10.006.

Ikpa, U. (2013, November, 14) *Consequences of child abandonment & neglect*. Cambridge Community Television. https://www.cctvcambridge.org/node/201904.

Large, M. M., & Kapur, N. (2018). Psychiatric hospitalisation and the risk of suicide. *The British Journal of Psychiatry: The Journal of Mental Science, 212*(5), 269–273. https://doi.org/10.1192/bjp.2018.22.

De Leo, D., & Krysinska, K. (2017). Suicide and self-directed violence. In S. R. Quah (Ed.), *International Encyclopedia of Public Health* (2nd ed., pp. 115–123). Academic Press. https://doi.org/10.1016/B978-0-12-803678-5.00438-0.

Lester, D. (1998). Helplessness, hopelessness, and haplessness and suicidality. *Psychological Reports, 82*(3 Pt 1), 946. https://doi.org/10.2466/pr0.1998.82.3.946.

Levinson, D., Haklai, Z., Stein, N., Polakiewicz, J., & Levav, I. (2007). Suicide ideation, planning and attempts: Results from the Israel National Health Survey. *Israel Journal of Psychiatry and Related Sciences, 44*, 136–143.

Lezak, M. D., Howieson, D. B., Loring, D. W., Hannay, H. J., & Fischer, J. S. (2004). *Neuropsychological Assessment*. Oxford University Press.

Luo, X., Wang, Q., Wang, X., & Cai, T. (2016). Reasons for living and hope as the protective factors against suicidality in Chinese patients with depression: A cross sectional study. *BMC Psychiatry, 16*, 252. https://doi.org/10.1186/s12888-016-0960-0.

Lutzman, M., Sommerfeld, E., & Ben-David, S. (2021). Loneliness and social integration as mediators between physical pain and suicidal ideation among elderly men. *International Psychogeriatrics, 33*(5), 453–459. https://doi.org/10.1017/S104161022000112X.

Mackenzie, S., Wiegel, J. R., Mundt, M., Brown, D., Saewyc, E., Heiligenstein, E., Harahan, B., & Fleming, M. (2011). Depression and suicide ideation among students accessing campus health care. *The American Journal of Orthopsychiatry, 81*(1), 101–107. https://doi.org/10.1111/j.1939-0025.2010.01077.x.

Miller, W. R., Seligman, M. E., & Kurlander, H. M. (1975). Learned helplessness, depression, and anxiety. *The Journal of Nervous and Mental Disease, 161*(5), 347–357.

Moniz, M., de Jesus, S.N., Pacheco, A., Gonçalves, E., Viseu, J., Bras, M., Silva, D. & Batista, S. (2017) The Influence of Planning and Response Inhibition on Cognitive Functioning of Non-Psychotic Unipolar Depressed Suicide Attempters. *Europe's Journal of Psychology. 13*(4). 717–732. doi: https://doi.org/10.5964/ejop.v13i4.1385.

Montesano, A., Feixas, G., Caspar, F., & Winter, D. (2017). Depression and identity: Are self-constructions negative or conflictual? *Frontiers in Psychology, 8*, 877.

Morrow, C.E., Bryan, C.J., & Apollonio, K.K.(2010). Empirically based assessment of suicide risk. In Kumar U. and Mandal MK.(Eds.) *Suicidal Behaviour: Assessment of People at Risk* (pp. 20–41) .New Delhi: Sage Publications.

National Institute of Mental Health. (n.d.). *Warning Signs of Suicide*. https://www.nimh.nih.gov/health/publications/warning-signs-of-suicide.

Nie, J., Zhang, W. & Liuc, Y. (2017). Exploring depression, self-esteem and verbal fluency with different degrees of internet addiction among Chinese college students. *Comprehensive Psychiatry. 72*(). 114–120. doi: https://doi.org/10.1016/j.comppsych.2016.10.006s.

Niedenthal, P. M., Krauth-Gruber, S., & Ric, F. (2017). *Psychology of emotion: Self-conscious emotions*. Taylor & Francis Group.

Niu, L., Jia, C., Ma, Z., Wang, G., Sun, B., Zhang, D., & Zhou, L. (2020). Loneliness, hopelessness and suicide in later life: A case-control psychological autopsy study in rural China. *Epidemiology and Psychiatric Sciences, 29*, e119. https://doi.org/10.1017/S2045796020000335.

Overholser, J & Spirito, A. (2003). Precursor to adolescent suicide attempt. In J. Overholser & A. Spirito (Eds.), *Evaluating and Treating Adolescent Suicide Attempters:From Research to Practice* (1st ed., pp. 19–40). Elsevier Science.

Pridmore, S., & Reddy, A. (2012). Financial loss and suicide. *The Malaysian Journal of Medical Sciences: MJMS, 19*(2), 74–76.

Ritchie, H., Roser, M. and Ortiz-Ospina, E. (2015) - "Suicide". Published online at OurWorldIn-Data.org. Retrieved from: 'https://ourworldindata.org/suicide'.

Ross, S. G., DeHay, T., & Deiling, M. (2021). The suicide prevention for college student gatekeepers program. *Crisis, 42*(1), 48–55. https://doi.org/10.1027/0227-5910/a000686.

Russell, N., Jr. (1968). The Taboo of Suicide. *Psychiatry, 31*(2), 173–183. https://doi.org/10.1080/00332747.1968.11023545.

Ryan, C. J., Large, M., Gribble, R., Macfarlane, M., Ilchef, R., & Tietze, T. (2015). Assessing and managing suicidal patients in the emergency department. *Australasian Psychiatry, 23*(5), 513–516.

Sahu, A., Gupta, P., & Chatterjee, B. (2014). Depression is more than just sadness: A case of excessive anger and its management in depression. *Indian Journal of Psychological Medicine, 36*(1), 77–79. https://doi.org/10.4103/0253-7176.127259.

Sandler, E.P. (2018). *The Ripple Effect of Suicide*. https://nami.org/Blogs/NAMI-Blog/September-2018/The-Ripple-Effect-of-Suicide.

Sansone, R. A., & Sansone, L. A. (2010). Gratitude and well-being: the benefits of appreciation. *Psychiatry (Edgmont (Pa. : Township)), 7*(11), 18–22.

Seligman, M. (2017). What is Positive Psychology? A Definition. *Positive psychology.org.uk*. http://positivepsychology.org.uk/what-is-positive-psychology/.

Smith, A. R., Witte, T. K., Teale, N. E., King, S. L., Bender, T. W., & Joiner, T. E. (2008). Revisiting impulsivity in suicide: Implications for civil liability of third parties. *Behavioral Sciences & the Law, 26*(6), 779–797. https://doi.org/10.1002/bsl.848.

Tabaac, A.R., Perrin, P.B., & Rabinovitch, A.E. (2016). The relationship between social support and suicide risk in a national sample of ethnically diverse sexual minority women. *Journal of Gay Lesbian Mental Health. 20*(). 116–126. doi: https://doi.org/10.1080/19359705.2015.1135842.

Teismann, T., & Brailovskaia, J. (2020). Entrapment, positive psychological functioning and suicide ideation: A moderation analysis. *Clinical Psychology & Psychotherapy, 27*(1), 34–41. https://doi.org/10.1002/cpp.2403.

Verrocchio, M. C., Carrozzino, D., Marchetti, D., Andreasson, K., Fulcheri, M. & Bech, P. (2016). Mental pain and suicide: A systematic review of the literature. *Front. Psychiatry. 7*(108). https://doi.org/10.3389/fpsyt.2016.0010.

Wakefield, J. C., & Schmitz, M. F. (2016). Feelings of worthlessness during a single complicated major depressive episode predict postremission suicide attempt. *Acta Psychiatrica Scandinavica, 133*(4), 257–265. https://doi.org/10.1111/acps.12521.

What is Anger? (n.d.). https://www.mentalhelp.net/anger/what-is-it/#:~:text=Anger%20is%20a%20basic%20human%20emotion%20that%20is,obstacles%20that%20keep%20us%20from%20attaining%20personal%20goals.

Williams, J. M. G. (2001). *The cry of pain.* Penguin.

Williams, R. (2017). Anger as a basic emotion and its role in personality building and pathological growth: The neuroscientific, developmental and clinical perspectives. *Frontiers in Psychology, 8*, 1950. https://doi.org/10.3389/fpsyg.2017.01950.

Wilson, K. G., Curran, D., & McPherson, C. J. (2005). A burden to others: A common source of distress for the terminally ill. *Cognitive Behaviour Therapy, 34*(2), 115–123. https://doi.org/10.1080/16506070510008461.

World Health Organization. (2022, June). *Suicide.* https://www.who.int/news-room/fact-sheets/detail/suicide.

World Health Organisation. (2007). *International Classification of Diseases-10 Mental and Behavioural Disorders.* AITBS Publishers.

World Suicide Rate 2000–2023. (n.d). https://www.macrotrends.net/countries/WLD/world/suicide-rate.

Yin, H., Xin, Q., Xue, X., & Li, E. (2020). Cognitive distortion in suicidal behavior. *Scholarly Jour0nal of Psychology and Behavioural Sciences. 38*(4). 369–374. https://doi.org/10.32474/SJPBS.2020.03.000168.

Zhang, J., & Li, Z. (2013). The association between depression and suicide when hopelessness is controlled for. *Comprehensive Psychiatry, 54*(7), 790–796. https://doi.org/10.1016/j.comppsych.2013.03.004.

Zhong, B. L., Chiu, H. F., & Conwell, Y. (2016). Elderly suicide trends in the context of transforming China, 1987–2014. *Scientific Reports, 6*, 37724.

Trina Banerjee is a Clinical Psychologist and Psychotherapist. She is currently pursuing a Ph.D. in Psychology from Christ (Deemed to be University), Bangalore, India. She has experience in teaching post-graduate Clinical Psychology and Research Methodology for the last 5 years and is a practicing Clinical Psychologist for the last 8 years. She received the best paper award in the National Conference of Indian Association of Clinical Psychologists in 2017 and has received the "Saugata Basu Memorial Award" from the University of Calcutta, for securing the highest marks in Clinical Psychology. Her research interests are Neuropsychology, Suicidology & Child and Adolescent Mental Health.

Prof. K. Jayasankara Reddy has M. Sc and Ph.D. in Psychology in the area of NeuroPsychology, also has a master degree in Clinical Neurophysiology and MBA in Higher Education Management. He has been an active teacher, researcher and practitioner in the field of Health, Cognitive

Neuropsychology and Neuroscience since then. Presently, working as Professor of Psychology and Co-ordinator for Center for Research at Christ University, Bangalore, Inda . He has guided and graduated 12 Ph Ds, 15 M. Phil by research and more than 90 postgraduate research project students in the area of Health, Neuropsychology and Cognitive Neuroscience. He has published more than 150 research articles in peer-reviewed journals, presented his research at more than 60 national and international conferences, and has also organized many conferences of national and international significance. Dr. Reddy is the recipient of Indian School Psychology Association (InSPA) – P K Subaraja Trust Best Performance Award – 2017 for his valuable services and contributions to the promotion of school psychology in India. Also received National Stress Management Research Award 2017 in recognition of positive contribution to the subject of Stress Management from the International Stress Management Association (ISMA). All through his career, he is identified for successful contribution as a teacher in the field of Cognitive Neuropsychology and Neuroscience, and as academic administrator at various capacities while maintaining a very high level of research output in terms of quality as well as quantity.

Chapter 20
COVID-19, Civil Society, and Youth Activism in India

Prabhat Kumar Datta and Badri Narayan Kar

Abstract COVID-19 virus has wreaked havoc on our planet. Caught unaware the state tried to rise up to the occasion and the civil society as the emerging third sector joined hands to respond to the unanticipated and multifaceted challenges either by working with the government or utilizing the services of the younger people in fighting against this challenge or by networking with similar organizations at the local level. India is currently credited with a demographic dividend. This article seeks to explore the impact of the pandemic on the youth in the sense of how they have been affected and how they have responded to this challenge against the wider context of the civil society and the local self -governing institutions The study will be based on the data to be collected from the different secondary sources across the country with special focus on two states, namely, Kerala and Odisha as these two states earned international reputation for their performance in the first phase of the COVID-19 pandemic. Broadly speaking, this article seeks to present an overview of how the civil society actors, young people and the local government institutions responded to the COVID-19 pandemic in India under the overall guidance by the state, to identify the challenges they have faced and what remains to be done to brave this kind of challenge in future.

Keywords COVID-19 · Civil society · Youth · India · Pandemic · Local bodies · Changeloomers · Blue brigade · Red volunteers

Introduction

COVID-19 has thrown a host of unanticipated challenges, and has caused different kinds of dismay and discontent in human society. Almost about 100 years ago, Sigmund Freud authored his monumental piece, titled *Civilisation and its Discontents* (1930). He penned the essay in the aftermath of World War 1, a time which witnessed a phase of radical and scientific transformation in the world of psychology

P. K. Datta (✉) · B. N. Kar
Department of Political Science, University of Calcutta, Kolkata, India
e-mail: dattaprabhat@gmail.com

S. Deb and S. Deb (eds.), *Handbook of Youth Development*,
https://doi.org/10.1007/978-981-99-4969-4_20

alongside the rise of authoritarian movements like Nazism. In this book, Freud tried to capture and analyze tensions between impulses driving human behavior and the constraints imposed by the structures of civilization. COVID-19 resembles to some extent that the historic phase of human society in the sense that this COVID-19 period has ushered in an era of despair and disappointments, coupled with dismay. It has brought the entire civilization to the brink of a grave challenge, the challenge of bringing about an effective balance between individual impulses and freedoms with collective responsibility. It has reminded the ideologues of growing neo-liberal state-centricity around the globe to re-think and accept that a developmental state has an indispensable role at least in times of turbulence and crisis in the society and that there is a need for curtailing individual freedom, of individuals as well as of states, in the larger interest of the collective. The pandemic has also called upon us to pay heed to the alarm that Stephen Hawking sounded in his BBC program captioned Stephen Hawking: Expedition New Earth on May 04, 2017 as follows:'As with climate change—epidemics and population growth, our own planet is increasingly precarious—.'

One may say that this precarity and the COVID-19 crisis engulfed human society like a tsunami. It has devastating effects on society, economy, polity, livelihood and psychological wellbeing of human beings irrespective of age, social status and gender. The sudden prolonged lockdowns in non-essential industries coupled with disruption in production and supply chains have shaken the world economy. This may directly contribute to social polarization and may undermine national safety and security. Some scholars have mentioned the political impact (Bonotti & Zech, 2021) and psychological consequences of the COVID-19 protocols including lockdowns (Passavanti, 2021) to contain the spread of the virus.

The virus with its highly infective capacity caught the entire human society unaware, and it was the first of its kind in 100 years. The state had to rise to the occasion in no time, and without considering the pros and cons of many of its steps, thus came prolonged lockdowns along with introduction of a series of protocols like social distancing, use of sanitizers and masks, and frequent handwashing. The civil society in many countries around the globe joined hands with states to help in the battle against COVID-19 (Bhargava, 2021).

The Indian state decided to tackle the situation by falling back on an obsolete colonial piece of legislation and by declaring a national lockdown. The Union and States worked together to put up a coordinated response largely on the basis of the Epidemic Diseases Act (EDA, 1897) and the National Disaster Management Act (NDMA, 2005) despite mild protests from some states that the central intervention was a stark violation of the basic framework of federalism. The NDMA is placed in Entry 23 of the Constitution's Concurrent List, whereby all tiers of the government including the third-tier institutions such as municipal and rural local bodies are authorized and expected to contribute to disaster management and mitigation activities. It can safely be said that the broad architecture and flexibility of the two Acts have allowed both Union and state governments to address the pandemic in diverse ways in keeping with local traditions but in pursuance of the national model.

Some states like Kerala, Punjab and Odisha were the first to make use of the EDA for the purpose of imposition of the partial lockdown before the central government appeared on the scene on March 24, 1919 to declare a nationwide lockdown which was done in phases. Once the nation-wide lockdown was imposed by the Union government, it directed all states to invoke responses as allowable under Sect. 2 of the EDA. The national government directed the citizens to strictly adhere to measures like wearing masks and maintaining physical distance to arrest the spread of the virus. The administration was geared to action through persuasion, and sometimes by imposing penalties. The administration was also tasked to focus their attention on tracing, testing, isolating and monitoring.

The Indian state decided to lay emphasis on three aspects, namely strict enforcement of lockdown norms, implementation of physical distancing norms and restrictions on economic and social activities (Ghosh, 2020). These norms and regulations were imposed without adequate preparedness and as expected, it created a number of problems on economic and social fronts, leading to unusual uncertainty in the market and 'panic buying', more particularly in cities. As Tandon and Ram (2020) have observed: 'Absence of clear directives from the government and the sharp digital divide exacerbated the chaos, which ended in massive migration of workers employed in urban areas to their villages'. The continuous lockdowns affected the society at large, more particularly the down-and–out, including a fairly large number of migrant workers who had neither any job security nor access to social protection resulting in joblessness, wagelessness and shelterlessness (Khanna, 2020).

This paper seeks to capture the role of the civil society as a backdrop for the study and to analyze the impact of this pandemic on the youth and their role in India in tackling the challenge either directly, or through civil society organizations or in association with local level government structures. This underscores the need for giving an overview of the civil society and the local government institutions to preface the core of the discussion. The issue will be posed in the context of the increasingly significant role of the civil society in the neo-liberal Indian state and the rise of the grassroots democratic structures created through two landmark constitutional amendments in 1992. It may be recalled that within a week of implementing lockdown provisions, the NITI Aayog (NA), a national planning body in Delhi, set up several coordination mechanisms to operationalize various relief, welfare and health measures (Tandon & Ram, 2020). One of these coordinating committees focused on NGOs included some civil society representatives as well. The NA initiated the process of creating a database of NGOs on its website under the label 'Darpan', and had listed about 92,000 NGOs before the pandemic began. An immediate appeal was sent to all these NGOs by the Chief Executive Officer of NA to provide support to affected households and to spread the messages widely for preventive health measures announced by the government (Tandon & Ram, 2020).

Currently, India has decentralized democratic structures at the local level both in rural and urban areas. Twin Constitutional amendments made in 1992 have paved the road for participatory governance and mandatory women's participation in local governance. In the villages, there are three-tiered structures at the three different administrative levels and at the lowest rung in the ladder there are villages where there are deliberative bodies called 'gram sabhas', to use the words from the constitutional amendment Acts (Datta, 2022). These are structures for participation of the villagers. At the urban level, there are also municipal bodies in the towns and cities. These bodies have down the line structures for citizens' participation institutionalized through ward committees. Significantly there is constitutionally mandated one third reservation of seats for women in both rural and urban local bodies (Datta, 2008).

Role of the Civil Society in the Containment of COVID-19

Civil society is understood in terms of a space outside the state, the market and the family which enables the citizens to pursue their common aspirations and participate in the overall development of the society (Clarke, 2016; Froissart, 2014). It is 'an intermediate associational realm between the state and family populated by organizations which are separate from the state and are formed voluntarily by members of society' (White, 1994: 379, Harriss, 2001). Regarded as the third sector, it has assumed special importance in the wake of the neo-liberal state around the globe (Clarke, 2016).

Conceptually speaking, civil society organizations are expected to engage themselves in the work and activities connected with the overall well-being of the masses at large. The CSOs can play a key role in designing strategies for development. They can deliver services to the doorsteps of the people through their networks as and when required. Besides, they act as a watchdog of the people to find out if the government is responding to the needs of the people, and is fulfilling the commitments made by the ruling parties at the time of elections. One of the most important functions of the CSOs is to carry on advocacy for the constituents and their causes. As it is situated between the state and the people they are supposed to promote democratic values in a number of ways, like bringing the voices of the marginalized (Almog-Bar & Schmid, 2014), monitoring public and corporate activities, providing the locus and opportunity for active citizenship (Van Til, 2000). As mediating institutions situated between the people and the state, this sector has an important role to play in enhancing and sustaining the representative character of democracy in myriad ways (Van Til, 2000; Alexander & Nank, 2009), and provide the locus and opportunity for active citizenship and function as change agents (Frumkin, 2002).

Civil society actors in many countries around the globe, no matter whether they are democratic or not, have always come forward to extend their support and cooperation to public institutions as well as members of the public at large to help the citizens during turbulent times. In many countries including India, they have responded positively to the COVID-19 pandemic challenge in myriad small and large ways either by networking with other civil society organizations or by extending support to the government at the local level or by both (Datta, 2022). In some places as in Kerala they partnered with businesses and public authorities to support local communities strapped for economic relief (Chathukulam & Tharamangalam, 2021; Biju, 2020).

Pandemic-related activism of civil society around the globe varies widely across contexts, but several common dimensions stand out prominently (Brechenmacher et al., 2020). First, across different cities and countries, citizens have come together in new voluntary associations and mutual aid societies. Second, they have been found raising money for emergency relief, collecting medical supplies and working as a sort of protective gear for the overburdened hospitals, by arranging oxygen cylinders for critical patients at home and delivering aid to those who lack other forms of social protection. Third, in a number of places, civic actors are collaborating closely with local government institutions and businesses.

A peep into the situation around the globe tends to show that some of the NGOs which are mandated to work for human rights changed their agenda to associate themselves with the work of the Pandemic. Reference may be made to Brazil's Community organization, Coletivo Rapo Reto (BBC, Brazil, 2022) which was set up to document police abuses in Rio de Janeiro. It used itself for denouncing fake news surrounding the pandemic. In addition to new mutual aid initiatives, many established civil society groups have shifted their work from longer-term projects to hands-on emergency relief. This flexibility is the inherent advantage of the CSOs.

In India, for example, civil society based organizations like self- help groups where women play a significant role, emerged as the frontline workers (Thomas & Prakash, 2020). But this third sector is still not very strong in India except in some states like Kerala, Uttar Pradesh, Madhya Pradesh. The recent attempt on the part of the state to bind the civil society in chains as is evident from the significant changes in the operating environment, has been a bone of contention between the civil society and the state. It has a disincentive effect on the civil society organizations in our country. To quote from a recent critique "This relates not only to changes in acts and regulation to control, such as Foreign Currency Regulation Act (which allows an organization to receive foreign funds), information technology laws, societies registration, but also in its inherent societal relationship" (Jayant, 2022). He continues that these changes speak of trust deficit between the state and a section of the civil society. What is important as underscored by the author is that this trust deficit creates confusion among the people about the civil society organizations.

The Impact of COVID-19 on the Youth: Global Perspective

Human beings are social species. They can grow and blossom themselves properly in an environment of meaningful social relationships. Everybody in the society irrespective of their age, social status, gender during pandemic has been experiencing unusual situations. One of the worst victims of COVID-19 is education. According to one UNICEF estimate made in 2021 schools for more than 168 million children around the globe remained closed almost entirely during lockdowns from March 2020 to February 2021 (UNICEF India, 2021).

The youth hold an important place in the civil society in view of their age, vibrancy and numbers They constitute a significant segment of our population who have to bear the heavy brunt of the socioeconomic impact of COVID The pandemic has disproportionate effects on the youth following exacerbation of inequalities and uncertainties which have caused reduction of the productive potential of the entire generation. The International Labour Organization (ILO) conducted a survey in 2020 to examine the immediate effects of the pandemic on the lives of youngsters in the age group 18–29. Globally speaking, following the outbreak of COVID-19 youth across the countries experienced three kinds of unpleasant situations in the domain of learning and employment, rights and social activism' (International Labour Organisation, 2020).

India has the largest youth population in the world today with half of its population below 25 years of age. Young persons in the age group 15–29 constitute nearly 27.5% of our population and the country will continue this pattern for another 20 years (Shivkumar, 2013). With imposition of prolonged lockdowns, youth started confronting challenges in almost all aspects of their life.

The prolonged closure of schools have had disastrous effects on them as they were forced to stay back home for a pretty long time. It caused irritation and loneliness. External support systems maintained by the society and the peer group outside the family broke apart. It brought in its wake a rapid transition from physical education to a new mode of online learning—a digital sphere of learning (Kapasia et al., 2020). According to one study in India, only 60% of students in schools were able to access remote-learning opportunities, while 80% of students were learning significantly less through digital education than in physical classes (UNICEF Press Release, 2021). Besides, transition to on-line mode has affected 'their learning and coping abilities, heightened pressures and mood disturbances impacting their sleep and concentration'. Another important aspect brought out by the report is that it may have impact on their problem solving and interpersonal skills which are primarily learnt and reinforced in schools and colleges through engagement in sports and recreational activities (Chauhan & Bhan, 2022) Inability to access by all equally increased the existing knowledge divide between the rich and the poor. The drop out risk is very high and this has another dimension on those who rely on mid-day meals in schools without which their nutrition levels remarkably come down.

According to a UN Women report, the dropout rate of girls is higher than that of boys in the pandemic. The report observes that 65 per cent of the parents are unwilling to continue education of girls to bring down costs. As per a poll conducted by UNICEF on International Women's Day 2022 in India, it was reported that at least 38% of respondents knew of a girl who had dropped out of school. While 33% respondents said that the girls who had dropped out of school were engaged in domestic work. About one-fourth (25%) of respondents also reported that the girls who had dropped out had got married (Yadav, 2022). Many of the young girls have been more badly affected as they were forced to revert to traditional roles in the families. This led to the increase in school drop outs. According to one estimate, nearly 10 million secondary school girls in India could drop out of school due to the pandemic (Trivedi, 2021). Their emotional turmoil is compounded by trauma caused by the increase in domestic violence and enhanced household responsibilities that give them little time to recuperate. An increase in unintended pregnancies and communicable disease-related adolescent mortality due to insufficient access to general healthcare services, especially for sexual and reproductive health can also lead to more anxiety (Yadav, 2022). There has been an increase in the numbers of child marriages during the pendency of the lockdown coupled with early pregnancy. The COVID-19 induced lockdowns encouraged many poor families to marry their daughters off as early as possible because the schools are closed (Banerjee, 2020).

The feeling of disconnection among the youth from communal life created a feeling of being left out and it was more intense for them than for older ones, according to a study on OECD countries (OECD, 2020). It might have eroded the basis of social capital. The younger ones could not learn community habits due to the loss of community interaction. Thus it disrupted the processes of inculcation of community values which act as a sort of safety valve in times of crisis. The core findings of a study in India (Suhail et al., 2021) bring this out.

A study on the mental impact of the COVID-19 on the youth in India has demonstrated that it causes mental issues like anxiety and depressive symptomatology. Students from less privileged backgrounds have experienced larger negative impacts due to the Covid-19 outbreak (Aucejo et al., 2020). Changes in daily routine including lack of outdoor activity disturbed sleeping patterns. Social distancing affected mental well-being of the students (Chaturvedi et al., 2021).

People who are young and looking forward to building a professional future are caught in the trap of various kinds of uncertainties. And one of the most important is definitely economics. The Centre for Monitoring Indian Economy showed that young workers were the most affected in terms of a fall in employment rate during the 2020 lockdown. Relative to the pre-pandemic level (January 2020) the employment rate during the lockdown fell the sharpest for the 15–18 age group followed by the 19–20 age group and 21–23 age group (Abraham, 2021). They have also been slower in recovery from the damaging legacies, as documented by State of Young Workers in India, 2021. These data help us make an assessment of the nature and extent of uncertainties in the livelihood sector experienced by youth in India.

The COVID-19 protocols have brought about a change in the consumption pattern of a section of the middle class youth. Dining out more particularly at the weekend, a widely prevailed western habit had started gaining good ground among the youth belonging to the middle class in the metropolitan cities of the country. But the outbreak of COVID-19 restrained the youth to opt for online food delivery chains, though initially there was some reluctance due to fear of getting infected by COVID-19 from the delivery staff. This has opened up a new channel of earning some money for the unemployed youth who are engaged in delivering food at the doorstep mostly on motorbikes But dining out with friends and members of the family used to strengthen social and family bonds. COVID-19 has weakened these bonds by taking away this opportunity.

Scholars have also drawn our attention to the political consequences of COVID-19 There is a view that the CORONA virus is disrupting democracy and governance worldwide (Brown et al., 2020). Of the 79 countries and territories that experienced a net decline in freedom in 2020, 35 of these declines—or nearly 45% were related to the pandemic (Slipowitz, 2021). Postponement of elections and rise of the omnipotent executive of the state are two distinguishing features. India experienced this situation in different states. All these might lead to erosion in the trust and legitimacy of the government. Youth who have an important role in democracy, are likely to develop political indolence which is dangerous for democracy. Youth are expected to bring in new ideas and churn the traditional society like ours. This process has faced a serious setback. This might pave the road for old values and superstitious beliefs coming back. The closure of schools will fuel this.

Some of the CSOs in India rose to the occasion and played remarkably significant roles by working with the youth and taking their support in joining hands with the state in tackling COVID-19. For example, PRAVAH, a Jharkhand-based NGO, has worked with the youth to run a program called leadership and entrepreneurship development program. Youth are called changeloomers. It was a year-long training program for the young people who would like to work as change agents and build social enterprises. For this purpose training programs were organized to help them learn skills. During the pandemic the changeloomers across more than 6 states are working for rebuilding India by supporting vulnerable communities gain livelihood and access healthcare.

The changeloomers rendered useful service during post-pandemic times, too. For example, they provided dry rations to women and daily wage laborers who have lost their jobs. They provided mental health support to children, adolescents and adults from marginalized communities. They initiated a programme of healing the sorrows and despairs by organizing street theaters etc. (Sarkar, 2021).

During the Pandemic the changeloom fellows who were working in different states realized the need for standing by the side of their communities. They demonstrated how they could communicate their actions to change the frustrated perception of the younger ones about their life into a positive one. They joined hands with the governments of six states to re-build India by supporting the vulnerable sections of the society.

Sudden lockdown has caused greater harm to the disadvantaged sections of the population in India. Mention may also be made of the tribal people in different parts of the country where access to the internet and availability of smart phones is extremely limited. The tribal children experienced another difficulty relating to language. This situation prompted one youth group called Dharamveer in a tribal panchayat in a Mayurbhanj district of Odisha to step in. The community mobilizers of Oxfam India facilitated the youth to conduct meetings and discuss the situation to find an effective solution. The local head teacher of the schools came forward and the local youth were allowed to take classes in open spaces and they had to wear masks. The classes for the children were conducted in their mother tongue and co-curricular activities without any fee were also organized to keep the kids happy and motivated during the harsh days of the pandemic (Noopur, 2021).

In a tribal district in Chhattisgarh, administration, youth and the UNICEF forged an alliance to fight against COVID, which resulted in creating a cadre over 6000 volunteers who were trained in social communication and community mobilization at the instance of UNICEF to enable them respond to the outbreak of the Pandemic. Significantly 60% of the volunteers were in the age group 18–25 and 40% of them were women. It was done through an initiative called *Yubadaya* launched in September, 2020. The primary objective was to channelize the local youth in such a manner as to ensure that they could reach out to marginalized groups and communities. They played a key role in sensitizing the community about the need for following COVID protocols including vaccination. They ran from door to door to ensure registration for vaccination. This partnership has brought certain lessons into the fore. First, it is important to involve the local administration and politicians to deal with a situation where the entire society is involved. Second, it is necessary to reward the youth for stimulating and sustaining their motivation (UNICEF India, 2021).

In Madhya Pradesh, the youth formed Blue Brigade Volunteers to support women and children in rural and urban areas. They were engaged in ensuring access to essential services and reducing adverse impact of COVID-19. They checked oxygen levels, distributed masks and were engaged in teaching people about proper hand washing techniques. They had also tried to deal with issues connected with vaccine hesitancy. And very significantly they operated a 'library on wheels' on a scooter to reach students with books (Sundarrajan, 2021). It was a great relief to students who got confined within the four walls of their houses.

Pandemic calls for spreading messages to the community as quickly as possible. And in this regard community radio played an important role. An important example is the use of community radio in Wayanad district in Kerala which is a home of 3000 tribal hamlets. The community radio worked wonders to break COVID-19 vaccine hesitancy in Kerala. One tribal girl named Ashwathy Murali from the Paniyar community produced community radio to remove misconceptions and myths about the vaccine and this initiative of a youth got spread like wildfire and resulted in total vaccination of the village in a remarkably short time. She received support from the National Health Mission and the Health Department of the Government of Kerala (Arivalan, 2021). It would have motivated her more if the state had taken the initiative to felicitate her in a public meeting after the normalcy was restored.

Young warrior movement launched by the Union Minister for Youth Affairs and Sports, UNICEF and its partner organization Generation Unlimited called *YuWaah* in India was founded in September 2018. The movement gathered momentum during the second phase of COVID-19. The primary objective of this movement is to engage young people across the country to work for the containment of COVID-19 and to extend help to the COVID-19 families and neighborhoods. About 3 million youth joined the movement and stood by the side of the migrants returning to their villages on foot. They collected money to stand by the side of the migrant workers. The total impact envisaged was to reach 50 million Indians since each young person was expected to enroll 10 and took pledges to take a specified action to protect themselves, their family and their neighborhood against COVID-19 (Generation Unlimited, 2021). The Ministry of Youth Affairs and Sports and the United Nations Development Programme (UNDP) joined hands to put in place a joint project strengthening Nehru Yuva Kendra Sangathan and National Social Service (NSS) in 58 districts across India. In this project the district youth volunteers were conceived as the main response pillars for COVID-19 to support local health authorities and deploy community level volunteers on the ground.

Significantly some of the political parties had also decided to mobilize their youth front to join the battle against COVID-19. *The Indian Express* reported on the eventful work organized by a team of 80 youth volunteers It was conducted at the behest of the Aam Aadmi Party helpline in Mumbai. This team worked in close unison with the Mumbai Municipal Corporation. The help line used to receive calls from COVID-19 patients and arranged beds in hospitals, and if it was found difficult the team used to escalate the calls to the senior leaders of the other political parties like Shiv Sena and Congress. Thus although the initiative was taken by a political party the young people were not hesitant to take support from other political parties to serve the interest of the COVID-19 patients (Thaver, 2021).

In West Bengal the younger members of the left parties led by Communist Party of India (Marxist) CPIM formed what is popularly known as the Red Volunteers. This group became prominent during the second phase of the COVID-19 in 2021. It was a time when the CORONA graph in West Bengal was rising alarmingly. The Red Volunteers played an important role in providing service delivery to the affected persons and strategizing their operations to local needs (The Telegraph, 2021). They engaged themselves actively in restarting sanitization drives, arranging masks for the people and hospitalization of the victims. They also contacted some doctors' associations seeking their help for providing telemedicine. They tried to reach COVID-19 affected people by using social media networks and their work received wide media coverage. And significantly left parties which have lost elections in recent times pinned hope on the Red Volunteers brigade during civic polls in urban areas (Business Standard, 2021) and the election data show that they have been able to make some inroads (The New Indian Express, 2021).

Young people are blessed with energy, intellect and desire to change the world for the better. What is required to set them on a correct path is the right set of skills, enlightened leadership, and the right kind of opportunities. Capacity building programs may be undertaken at the initiative of the CSOs and the state and they need to work in close unison. Young people need that their work is being appreciated for which society has to extend all support and the media has to play a proactive role. Thus to keep the younger ones energized and geared to action it is necessary to create what can be called a conducive ecosystem. They have rich potential which has to be harnessed to equip them with necessary skills to make them transform as agents of social change.

The dangerous tide of COVID-19 seems to be receding and the post-COVID world calls for immense creativity and resilience. And herein lies an important role of the younger people because it is they who are endowed with these qualities. They have excellent command over the new technology which can facilitate the process. Technology has done wonders during pandemic as the experience in Kerala tends to indicate (Datta, 2022). It has been widely used to sustain different facets of human life including education, remote work, virtual parties clogged by lockdowns. Its amazing role as an enabler can be utilized to reach more and more vulnerable groups. It is necessary to make sure that no one is left out in the recovery processes. The different kinds of skills of the youth such as interpersonal, emotional and technical need to be leveraged to quicken the process of recovery and instill faith and confidence in the minds of the people. The post-COVID society needs empathy, personal resilience, effective communication and the youth are blessed with all of them.

COVID has created fissures in the society. The marginalization of the marginalized has been enhanced through job loss, death of the earning hands, lack of access to education and the like. We need a transformative framework for development in the post-COVID era and the youth could be the principal harbinger of this transformation. For bringing about this transformation we need to launch new social movements, the core of which will be justice, participation and development of all. We have seen an upsurge of new social movements in India and now there is a need for another round of social movements with different orientations. In this movement the focus will be given on changing policies of the state in such a manner as to pay special attention to those who have been disproportionately affected by COVID-19 and to ensure that the state increases budgetary allocation on health. And there is a strong need for accessing them through technological tools. COVID-19 has exposed how insufficient our health infrastructure and the relatively successful state Kerala could meet this challenge during the first wave because of their better health infrastructures developed out of state budget (Isaac & Sadanandan, 2020).

Although there is no conclusive evidence that climate change is influencing the spread of COVID-19, the fact remains that some of the root causes of climate change such as deforestation has indirect effect on the rise and growth of this kind of virus. The loss of habitat forces the animals to migrate and come in contact with other animals and human beings and share germs. Scholars have examined the linkage of COVID-19 with climate change (Adil and Evgenia, 2022; Gupta et al., 2021).Youth has an important role to play in this regard. They can sensitize the society and work closely with the state and civil society groups to organize campaigns against, for example, deforestation by preparing leaflets and delivering lectures focusing on the negative effects of it with special mention of the CORONAvirus. It is believed that failure to act on issues connected with climate change and public health is likely to cut into development gains made in other sectors. It might affect the journey of our country towards the attainment of Sustainable development Goals (SDG). It has to be kept in mind that prolonged lockdowns have badly hit the financial safety net they might have had to fall back on.

Conclusion and Way Forward

The pandemic has taught us that we need to create a strong bridge between state and civil society where we have a huge youth population. In our country there is growing mutual distrust between the state and the civil society. While some of the civil society is partly responsible for this by maintaining indirect linkages with political parties, more particularly ruling political parties, it is high time for them to sustain their identity as the third space. Another current problem of civil society organizations in India is the growing fund crunch as the international funding agencies have started withdrawing from India because India is no longer an underdeveloped country. It has caused an unpleasant situation because even the leading NGOs are falling back on state support. It creates conditions for marriage of convenience between them and the state. In this way autonomy of these CSOs might get eroded. Broadly speaking this situation is very harmful for the healthy growth of our democracy as they are expected to work together to promote the cause of the people at large. This will have serious adverse consequences on the morale of the youth, many of whom look to civil society as their future work station. A strong civil society is now regarded as a necessary pre-condition for the successful blossoming of democracy and in our country where civil society has for long been relatively weak,new hopes have been generated because of the rise of the neo-liberal state which conceptually speaking, gives CSOs a prominent place. Sooner the irritation between the civil society and the state is resolved or at least reduced to a desirable level through dialogues the better it is for the entire society more particularly for our youth whose eyes are filled in with dreams and imaginations.

Civil society holds a place of great importance in a democratic society like ours because democracy cannot be realized without sustained engagement of the public with those who hold the reign of power. It may be mentioned that the last decades of the twentieth century are replete with examples of how the civil society worked against the authoritarian regimes. The mobilization of the civil society against 'undemocratic governments' after 1989 and the Velvet Revolutions in Eastern Europe amply demonstrated that the 'political public' can play an important role in politics. During the first decades of the present century large crowds gathered on the street and agitated in public spaces from Nepal to Libya to demand an end of the monarchies, dictatorships and tyrannies. In 2006, massive anti-monarchy agitation turned into what is popularly called pro-democracy movement, and could successfully bring an end to the monarchical rule. During 2007–08 lawyers in Pakistan led a democracy movement which forced the military government under General Parvez Musharraf to come to terms, and finally resulted in the return of electoral democracy. Strikingly, the protests that coalesced into the 'Arab Spring' following the self-immolation by a 26-year old vegetable vendor in protest against the public humiliation heaped on him by the police in the rural town of Tunisia, culminated in the demand for the resignation of the President Zina El Abidina who fled the country a month later (Chandhoke, 2020).

The role played by the youth in the handling of the epidemic has brought to the fore how important is this section of our population to brave these kinds of challenges. It is high time for the state and civil society to work together to clearly lay down the role of the youth in the activities undertaken at the instance of the state. This has to be integrated into the public policy for the youth. We should try our best to make the best use of demographic dividend by bringing in larger numbers of the youth in the processes of policy making There seems to be an urgent need for all the different political parties to give larger political space to the youth who constitute the backbone of the nation, and who are emotionally charged to make greater sacrifices, if required for the development of the country.

It cannot be denied that the present world is moving fast toward more digitalization. This factor has to be taken note of by the state and civil society for appropriate action. It calls for bringing about corresponding and necessary changes in the academic curricula with emphasis, for example, on life skills and social-emotional learning for the present century. It is a step forward towards building stronger and healthier post-pandemic social and economic systems.

As the Pandemic has demonstrated, the state holds a very important place in human life, more particularly in countries like ours, the state has to take all steps to rekindle hopes for a much brighter future and build and enhance trust of the youth on it. Trust deficit is regarded as one of the ailments of democracies in developing countries. Elections at regular intervals may legitimize the processes of governance but it assumes greater significance when it is coupled with trust. In this work youth can play an important role. Youth can engage themselves fruitfully with the activities of the state when they learn and realize from their personal experiences that the state is theirs. It calls for a truly welfare state with deep commitment for the protection of the interests of all in the society. A state which goes on increasing and demonstrating its teeth off and on and curtails individual freedom is disliked by the youth and if it is not arrested in time, they might rise in revolt against it as we know from the lessons from history. Thus our state is required to demonstrate its tolerance as far as possible in its dealings with the members of the civil society in general and youth in particular and to act proactively and expeditiously to address not only socio-economic problems the people are experiencing but also to promote democratic values like freedom and rights of the citizens which the youth value the most.

The state has to take initiative in capacity building of the youth for which the civil society organizations can be roped in. The state should support them in terms of giving funds for organizing appropriate skill development programs. In our country youth sometimes find it difficult to get suitable jobs because of the lack of required skill. In this high -tech world it is difficult and almost impossible to create more jobs by setting up factories. Besides this, the high-tech industrial sector calls for new skills. The state may work in close unison with the duly qualified research organizations including similar organizations in the third sector for making in-depth assessment of their skill needs and requirements of the market and organize skill development programs accordingly. The state should coordinate with the market to ensure employment of the duly skilled youth. This sort of training may help them looking for self-employment opportunities. In this regard some initial financial support from the state will be useful.

A good section of youth, more particularly from the marginalized sections of our society seem to be getting disillusioned as the neo-liberal state is moving away from the center-stage of developmental activities on economic and social front. Unemployment has turned out to be one of the serious critical challenges for the youth as the present development paradigm coupled with the use of modern technologies has led to the shrinking of the employment domain. This 'jobless growth' for countries like India with huge demographic dividend is likely to demoralize the youth more and more privatization in education is closing the doors of education for the weaker sections of our youth population. The state has to come forward to fund more educational institutions and build more health infrastructures at public cost with provision for easy access for them. The state has to create jobs for them to win back their trust and support. The crisis caused by the Pandemic has brought into light the need for a sort of social welfare state which has started rolling back following the aggressive rise of the neoliberal reforms.

References

Abraham, R. (2021). 'COVID-19 and India's Youth Force', *Hindustan Times*, December 16.

Adil, M. & Evgenia, P. (2022). Impact of COVID-19 on Attitudes to Climate Change and Support for Policies on https://www.imf.org/-/media/Files/Publications/WP/2022/English/wpiea2022023-print-pdf.ashx.

Alexander, N., & A. J., & Nank R. (2009). Public-non-profit partnership: Realizing the new public service. *Administration & Society, 41*(3), 364–386.

Almog-Bar, M., & Schmid, H. (2014). Advocacy activities of nonprofit human service organizations: A critical review. *Nonprofit and Voluntary Sector Quarterly, 43*(1), 11–35.

Arivalan, K. (2021). Kerala's Community Radio https://www.femina.in/trending/achievers/keralas-community-radio-rj-helped-an-entire-village-to-get-vaccinated-211270.html.

Aucejo, E.M. et al., (2020). The impact of COVID19 on student experiences and expectations: Evidence from a survey. *Journal of Public Economics*, 191. https://doi.org/10.1016/j.jpubeco.2020.104271.

Banerjee, B. (2020). "Child Marriages Surge during and after the Lockdown, Official Figure Tip of the Iceberg". *The National Herald.* 24 November.

BBC, Brazil (2022). https://witness.org/witness-partner-coletivo-papo-reto-featured-by-bbc-brazil/.

Bhargava, V. (2021). *Engaging Civil Society Organizations to enhance the effectiveness of COVID 19 Response in Asia and Pacific.* https://www.un.org/en/civil-society/csos-response-COVID-19, accessed on July 01, 2022.

Biju, T. (2020). Role of Kudumbashrees in COVID containment. *Purakala, 31*(28), 266–274.

Bonotti, M., & Zech, S. T. (2021). Recovering civility during COVID-19. *Palgrave Macmillan, Singpore.* https://doi.org/10.1007/978-981-33-6706-7_accessedonJuly01,2022

Brechenmacher, S. et al., (2020). Carnegie endowment for International Peace, April 2020).

Brown, F. et al., (2020). How will Corona- Virus Reshape democracy and Governance. https://carnegieendowment.org/2020/04/06/how-will-coronavirus-reshape-democracy-and-governance-globally-pub-81470 accessed on June 15, 2022).

Burrows, K. & Jessica, S. (2021). How Governments can Push toward a better tomorrow. https://www.pwc.com/gx/en/issues/reinventing-the-future/take-on-tomorrow/government-challenges.htmlaccessed on July 1, 2022.

Chandhoke, N. (2012). Whatever Has Happened to Civil Society? *Economic and Political Weekly* (EPW), June 6.

Chathukulam, J., & Tharamangalam, J. (2021). The Kerala model in time of COVID-19: Rethinking about state, society and democracy. *World Development*, 137.

Chaturvedi et al. (2021). COVID-19 and its impact on education, social life and mental health of students. *Children and Youth Services Review*, December. https://www.ncbi.nlm.nih.gov/pmc/articles/PMC7762625/

Chauhan, S. V., & Bhan, A. (2022). Mental Health in India; Well-being of youth during COVID-19, *Indian Express* March 19 https://indianexpress.com/article/lifestyle/health/mental-health-india-well-being-youth-covid-19-7826423/

Clarke, G. (2016). Governance and transnational civil society: The problem of transnational rent-seeking. *Journal of Civil Society, 12*(1), 82–100.

Datta, P. K. (2006). *Decentralisation, participation and governance*. Kalpaz Publications.

Datta, P. K. (2021). Public Service Delivery in Turbulent Times where Convergence Matters: Lessons from the Management of COVID -19 in Kerala, *Indian Journal of Public Administration,* Jan-March, 2022

Datta , P.K. (2022). Deliberative democracy in Indian villages in a book entitled *Deliberative Democracy in Asia* edited by Baogang He et al., Routledge , London and New york.

Fernandes, N (2020). Economic Effects of the CORONAvirus Outbreak on World Economy', IESE Business School Working paper no WP12 40 E, 2020, March 23).

Froissart, C. (2014). The ambiguities between contention and political participation: A study of civil society development in authoritarian regimes. *Journal of Civil Society, 10*(3), 219–222.

Frumkin, P. (2002). *On Being Nonprofit: A Conceptual and Policy Primer* (p. 2002). Harvard University Press.

Future of Jobs Report (2020).

Generation Unlimited. (2021). https://www.generationunlimited.org/stories/five-million-young-volunteers-help-break-chain-covid-19-transmissions-india accessed on June 13, 2022

Ghosh, J. (2020). A critique of the Indian Government's response to the COVID-19 Pandemic. *Journal of Industrial and Business Economics, 47*, 519–530.

Gupta, S. et al., (2021). Did climate change influence emergence, transmission and expression of COVID-19 Virus? *Frontiers in Medicine*, December

Harriss, J. (2000; 2001). Social capital construction and the consolidation of civil society in rural areas. Destin Working Paper No. 00–16, Development Studies Institute, London School of Economics.

Indian Express, 2021

International Labour Organisation. (2020). Youth and COVID-19: Impact on Jobs, Education, Rights and Mental Wellbeing, Survey Report https://www.ilo.org/global/topics/youth-employment/publications/WCMS_753026/lang--en/index.htm

Isaac, T. T. M., & Sadanandan, R. (2020). COVID-19, public health system and local governance in Kerala. *Economic and Political Weekly, 21*, 35–40.

Jayant, K. (2022). *Down to Earth*, April.

Jenkins, J. C. (2006). Nonprofit organizations and political advocacy." *In The Nonprofit Sector: A Research Handbook,* edited by W. W. Powell, and R. Steinberg, 307–32. New Haven, CT: Yale University Press).

Kapasia, et al., (2020). Impact of lockdown on learning status of undergraduate and postgraduate students during COVID-19 pandemic in West Bengal, India. *Children and Youth Services Review*, 116. https://doi.org/10.1016/j.childyouth.2020.105194).

Khanna, A. (2020). Impact of migration of labour force due to global COVID-19 pandemic with reference to India". *Journal of Health Management, 2*, 181–191.

Noopur (2021). Youth Volunteers as Teachers During Pandemic. (https://www.oxfamindia.org/featuredstories/youth-volunteer-teachers-during-pandemic accessed on June 13, 2022.

OECD (2020). Policy responses to Coronavirus: Youth and COVID 19, response, recovery and resilience, https://www.oecd.org/coronavirus/policy-responses/youth-and-covid-19-response-recovery-and-resilience-c40e61c6/

Passavanti et al., (2021b). The psychological impact of COVID-19 restrictive measures in the world. *Journal of Affective Disorders* January.

Sarkar, P. (2021). How young volunteers used art as an aid to rebuild post COVID India', https://www.youthkiawaaz.com/2021/09/art-aid-a-fundraiser-by-young-changeloomers-to-rebuild-post-covid-india/ accessed on June 13, 2022.

Shivkumar, G. (2013). India is going to become the youngest country by 2020, *The Hindu*, November 17.

Slipowitz, A. (2021). The devastating impact of COVID-19 on democracy' https://www.thinkglobalhealth.org/article/devastating-impact-covid-19-democracySuhail accessed on June 15, 2022.

Business Standard, December 10, 2021.

Suhail, A., Iqbal, N., & Smith, J. (2021). Lived experiences of Indian Youth amid COVID-19 crisis: An interpretative phenomenological analysis. *International Journal of Social Psychiatry, 67*(5), 559–566.

Sundarrajan, G. (2021).Youth and COVID-19: Stories of Creativity and Resiliencehttps://www.unicef.org/india/stories/youth-and-covid-19-stories-creativity-and-resilience

Tandon, R., & Ram, A. (2020). Source of life or kiss of death: Revisiting state-civil society dynamics in India during COVID-19 pandemic. *Nonprofit Policy Forum, 12*(1), 147–163.

Thaver. (2021). How a team of young volunteers is making a difference amid pandemic, *The Indian Express,* May 01, 2021 https://indianexpress.com/article/express-exclusive/ie100-the-most-powerful-indians-in-2022-7842489/.

The Telegraph, June 22, 2021.

The New Indian Express, November 28, 2021.

Thomas, J., & Prakash, P. (2020). Kudumbashree mission and COVID-19: A success story from the state of Kerala. *Int J Res Rev, 7*, 385–391.

Trivedi, D. (2021). 10 million girls at risk of dropping out of schools because of COVID pandemic, *Frontline,* January 25.

UNICEF, Press Release, March 10, 2021 https://www.unicef.org/india/press-releases/covid-19-schools-more-168-million-children-globally-have-been-completely-closed.

UNICEF India (2021). Youth volunteers fight COVID-19 pandemic in tribal districts in Chhattisgarh, https://www.unicef.org/india/stories/youth-volunteers-fight-covid-19-pandemic-tribal-districts-chhattisgarh.

Van Til, J. (2000). *Growing Civil Society: From Nonprofit Sector to Third Space.* Indiana University.

White, G. (1994). Civil Society, Democratization and Development (1): Clearing the Analytical Ground'. *Democratization, 1*(3), 378–389.

Yadav, D. (2022). Increase in school drop outs for girl child is alarming' *Times Now*,April 1, https://www.timesnownews.com/education/increase-in-school-dropout-rates-for-girl-child-is-alarming-states-unicef-india-article-90591261.

Dr. Prabhat Kumar Datta is the former Centenary Chair of Public Administration in the Department of Political Science, University of Calcutta, India and Adjunct Professor Institute of China Rural; Studies, Central China University, China. Currently he is a Senior Visiting Professor, Xavier Law School St. Xavier's University, Kolkata and member of the Mentor Group, Sadhu Ram Chand Murmu University of University of Jhargram, West Bengal.

Badri Narayan Kar is Special Secretary to the Government of West Bengal in the Department of Municipal Affairs. He is also holding the charge of the Additional Director, Institute of Local Government and Urban Studies .Besides, he is currently the Mission Director of Atal Mission for Rejuvenation and Urban Transformation (AMRUT) and Executive Officer, Nabadiganta Industrial Township Authority, West Bengal, India

Chapter 21
Youth Transition in the Digital Age: Balancing Digital Competency Demands and Preparing for the Future

Tusharika Mukherjee

Abstract The digital age has transformed our thoughts, actions, relationships, and work now more than ever before. It has necessitated increased engagement and participation on digital platforms for performing routine tasks of learning and social interactions. With the changing trends in the labor market, education, and training systems, the youth entering the workforce are now motivated to capitalize on their digital competencies (Osgerby, B. (2020). Youth culture and the media: Global perspectives. Routledge.). The knowledge, abilities, and skills that facilitate digital use have gained more prominence and appeal among employers and the youth competing for lucrative positions. In this transition from a non-digital to digital and now to a sustainable digital reliance, the youth finds itself at the juncture where it must prioritize building the competencies that can be future-proof, health facilitating, and give human beings more edge over automation. In this chapter, we explore the future of employability in a technology-driven world of work. The constant gap between what market demands and the skills youth can supply has insidiously led them to deal with the issues of underemployment and overeducation. We discuss the competencies that enable those entering the workforce to acquire the knowledge and attitude to succeed as an individual as well as a society. With the changing nature of work, individuals must find innovative ways of upskilling and reskilling themselves to thrive in the VUCA world. With the growing recognition of knowledge and lifelong learning as the key contributors for development in the digitalized workplace, skills like critical thinking, problem-solving, and self-regulation are drawing more attention. Finally, as a sustainable way forward in a digital world, we discuss the need for effective management of the digital skills at a community level. This includes embracing positive youth development to redress the impact of digitalization on the youth.

Keywords Digital transformation · Digital skills · Employability · Upskilling · Positive youth development

T. Mukherjee (✉)
Organizational Psychologist, Muenster, Germany
e-mail: tusharikamukherjee@gmail.com

S. Deb and S. Deb (eds.), *Handbook of Youth Development*,
https://doi.org/10.1007/978-981-99-4969-4_21

Introduction

About two decades ago the labor market witnessed a new trend of adding degree requirements to the job descriptions even for jobs that had no changes in the actual work. This trend of "degree inflation" peaked during the subsequent great recession of 2008–09 which in turn led businesses and labor corporations to move away from degree-based hiring and adopt skill-based hiring.

This recent reset of what the youth finds today as a vital value addition to their repertoire of knowledge and skills hints at three major types of changes. The first is a structural change in which employers are playing down the degrees primarily due to an imbalance between the supply and demand of skilled workers more significantly in the IT and management professions.

The second shift occurred as the pandemic hit the labor market in 2020 as job requirements for professions like nursing suddenly witnessed an overnight change, leading to a deprioritization of degrees. These shifts have rattled today's youth, who must now make a choice between acquiring professional qualifications and skills, to make a mark in the professional world.

In addition to these changes, the accelerated technological shift has led to the emergence of artificial intelligence in our professional (and personal) lives, and this rapid transformation has created a demand for professionals with new competencies.

Analytical reports about the future of the labor market make a distinction between the types of specialists who will be in demand (e.g., those skilled in disaster preparedness) and the ones that will soon reach redundancy primarily due to job automation and digitalization. At this juncture most organizations have moved to what is now popularly called skill-based hiring (Fuller et al., 2022). OECD (2017) reported that, "The dynamism of both skill demand and supply raises the question of how economies achieve a good match between the two…The perfectly competitive model relies on the assumption that perfect information on skill needs is available and that skills supply and demand can change instantaneously as well as the returns to skills."

In this chapter we address the question of how today's youth will not just remain relevant but flourish in the future, and describe it from the standpoint of how optimally they can balance the changing skill demands, altered work processes, and reinvented organizational structures. The developmental advantages of the digital transformation can be completely realized when societies ensure that everyone benefits from the digital transition and provides support for the existing and future workforce to develop the appropriate mix of skills. It is imperative to highlight that while digital competencies will enhance employability through increased self-efficacy and performance, there will also be the risk of the youth being exposed to digital malevolence. For example, the digital transformation has brought about digital disruption for many, leading to the marginalization of those who lack the resources to adapt to the technological transition. The proliferation of digital media usage via smartphones, computers, and other devices has escalated the use of social networking sites (Instagram, Facebook, TikTok) and instant messaging services (WhatsApp & Signal). Whether the engagement with digital technology is socially active (posting, liking, and sharing), socially passive (watching the content of others), or nonsocial (reading, watching videos, gaming, shopping, etc.), empirical research links all forms of digital usage with hedonic happiness and frequently with both mental and physical health issues (Berryman et al., 2018a, 2018b).

Changing Framework of Employability Skills in 2022

In 2020, OECD predicted that significant uncertainties and variations between educational programs, occupations, and sectors will accompany the transfer from higher education to the workforce. This makes it crucial for graduates to be prepared for this uncertainty because the labor market disruptions can potentially aggravate the impact of the uncertainties. A stark example of such disruption has been felt through the COVID-19 pandemic and the economic crises globally. Consequently, OECD (2020) recommends that interpersonal skills are more likely to be listed in the professional profiles of graduates with more erratic career paths. This demonstrates the need of higher education institutions continuing their work to create a broad skill set for its graduates that includes both technical and interpersonal skills.

Although there are other important reasons for attending college or university, for the majority of students the desire to find employment in a graduate position is a primary driver. In addition, there is generally a substantial average wage premium for tertiary graduates over those with less education, however, labor market disruptions have changed the requirements. In terms of educational requirements to enter and sustain in the labor market, the youth has to consider the uncertain trajectory of employability demands. Green and Henseke (2021) assert that the medium-term outlook for skilled jobs has grown notably obscure. The percentage of workers with post-secondary "tertiary education" has been steadily increasing worldwide. Green and Henseke (2021) posit that, "graduate underemployment—also termed 'overeducation'—has become a world-wide issue, especially in those many countries where governments in the 1990s and 2000s allowed higher education enrolments to expand rapidly, unconnected institutionally or economically to the more steady demands of their country's labour markets" (p. 2). According to the authors, one of the primary reasons is the divergence between what the market demands and what the graduates can supply. It seems reasonable to assume that the youth today must be competent in understanding the market and have the ability to meet the complex demands in order to have a successful life.

The globalized and modernized world of today is placing constant demands on the individuals to develop key competencies that can help them to contribute meaningfully to the society. Whether it is related to personal growth, interacting socially, balancing economic growth with environmental sustainability, participation in policymaking, or a skill as specific as using a computer language; youth needs to develop competencies that enable them to adapt to a fast-changing world. Competencies are defined as a combination of knowledge, skills, and attitudes, where knowledge is made up of facts, concepts, ideas, and theories that have been established and support understanding of a particular area or subject; skills are defined as the capacity to carry out processes and use the knowledge already known to achieve results; and attitudes are the disposition and mindsets to act or react to ideas, people, or situations. Basic employability skills are transferable core proficiencies that represent essential functional and knowledge skills and abilities required to succeed at all levels of employment in the twenty-first-century workplace (Overtoom, 2000). Eight dimensions of basic employability skills identified in 2000 included.

- basic literacy and numeracy skills
- critical thinking skills
- management skills
- leadership skills
- interpersonal skills
- information technology skills
- systems thinking skills
- work ethic disposition

In the past 20 years the requirements have become more well-defined and provide a clear direction for getting upgraded in terms of skills. The world economic forum forecasts that the youth will have to survive the double-disruption in the form of the pandemic aftermath and the increasing automation. Consequently the skills for 2025 will focus on the adoption of technology, critical thinking, problem-solving, and self-management. The Future of Jobs Report (2020) by the World Economic Forum suggests that at least 50% of the current workforce will require re-skilling as the core employability skills have to match with the changing times. The highest-rated skills for 2025 include:

- Analytical and innovative thinking
- Lifelong learning and active learning strategies
- Solving complex problems
- Critical reasoning and evaluation
- Creativity and initiative-taking
- Leading and social influence
- Digital presence, usage, control and monitoring
- Designing technology and creating programs
- Idea generation and reasoning

These skills, identified as the future skills, broadly cater to four major human functions of this era: problem-solving; self-management; people management; and technology usage and creation. These skills are relevant across existing as well as numerous emerging professions. The report also highlights three specialized skills, called the "cutting-edge skills," as "product marketing, digital marketing, and human–computer interaction" (Whiting, 2020).

The skills that will outshine others in the future have much to do with the composition of the workforce and how the organizations are going to approach their own repertoire of competencies, the competencies they need, and the expectancies that the skilled workers and organizations have from one another (Mugayar-Baldocchi et al., 2021). The authors assert that the pandemic has provided the organizations with the opportunity to reassess their talent pool and get a renewed perspective on the knowledge, skills, abilities, and other characteristics (KSAOs) for the current and future roles. This would also mean creating a larger and a more diverse talent pool for a competitive advantage.

Hancock et al. (2020) opine that, "by 2030, up to 30–40% of all workers in developed countries may need to move into new occupations or at least upgrade their skill sets significantly. Research further suggest that skilled workers in short supply will become even scarcer" (p. 63). They further state that organizations that will fail to adopt the changes and upskill its talent pool, will be left behind in the race of digital competence. The kind of skill transformation the workforce (both current and emerging) requires can be brought about through one or a combination of several processes, namely:

1. Redeploying: moving an individual to a new role within the company
2. Upskilling: strengthening the core of individuals' skills while assisting them in developing and advancing their competencies.
3. Reskilling: equipping employees with new capabilities.

Skills to Fit in the VUCA World

Events like the pandemic offer several examples that demonstrate how a crisis in one area of life—whether it be the economy, the environment, the health sector, politics, society, or technology—can be powerful enough to cause devastation in other areas of life. The immediate economic repercussions of a pandemic or any other geopolitical calamity that a generation or two must endure slow advancements made before the crisis and stifle future development. Surviving in a volatile, uncertain, complex, and ambiguous world (VUCA) will be based upon *reskilling* or *upskilling* and an evolving business strategy that can not only foresee unprecedented challenges but also turn them into unprecedented opportunities.

Individual agility is as crucial as organizational agility to function in a VUCA world. To succeed in this climate, organizations need creativity, empiricism, and agility. One of the key accelerators of organizational agility is discovering new ways to operate (2021). Thus, crises necessitate responses that are not only sufficient to restore order but also forceful enough to prevent additional damage to the development of youth. Agile working has provided a solution for surviving by focusing on providing (a) opportunities for organizations to reskill staff in preparation for the future, (b) innovative and people-centric organizations, (c) increased flexibility, (d) changed power structures (decentralization), and (e) equitable distribution of resources.

Professional learning done by a variety of workers and job seekers to acquire new abilities (also known as upskilling) is the new-age methodology for individual agility and resilience. People-centered training and reskilling/upskilling have the potential to boost individual engagement, retention, growth, and profitability. Organizations that put people at the center of the upskilling experience if they want to realize long-term benefit. The expectations that employees have of them are made clear via that lens, as are any potential obstacles in the way of any efforts to enable employees.

Tools like the Barney's (1991) VRIO Framework (the term VRIO is derived from the words value, rarity, imitability, and organization) can be used for assessing new abilities and devising effective programs for reskilling the workforce. The tool identifies valuable and rare resources that cannot be easily imitated and become a source of competitive advantage (Rothaermel, 2012). Secondly, such tools can enable identifying competencies that the youth can be trained in before they enter the workforce, thus reducing the gap between education and practice or demand and supply. For example, the VRIO framework addresses capabilities and talent requirement of firms by examining the following four questions:

- Which competencies will be valued by consumers and other stakeholders?
- Which industry-specific skills are difficult to find or rare?
- What abilities are unique or challenging to duplicate?
- Can the company deliver those abilities successfully? For instance, is their use ingrained in a culture that is suitable for handling VUCA issues?

Skills Mandate in the Digital Age

Digital competence has been globally identified as a key direction for development. Digital competence is essential for lifelong learning, as it involves "the confident and critical use of information technology for work, leisure, and communication" (The Council of the European Union, 2018). The United Nations declared in its 2018 report that over 90% of the jobs globally have a digital component. The European Union posited that competencies are defined as a combination of knowledge, skills, and attitudes, where knowledge is made up of facts, concepts, ideas, and theories that have been established and support understanding of a particular area or subject; skills are defined as the capacity to carry out processes and use the knowledge already known to achieve results; and attitudes are the disposition and mindsets to act or react to ideas, people, or situations.

With more employment being automated, technology playing a larger part in all aspects of work and life, and entrepreneurial, social, and civic competencies becoming increasingly important to ensuring resilience and ability to adapt to change, competence needs have altered. In today's *knowledge economy*, memorizing facts and procedures is essential but not insufficient for advancement and success. The knowledge economy largely depends on the creation, dissemination, and use of information and ideas. The knowledge economy encompasses a wide range of professions in various areas. These can include health professionals conducting study and data analysis as well as academic researchers, programmers, and software developers. These positions all involve using knowledge to help others in some way.

In a culture that is changing so quickly, abilities like problem-solving, critical thinking, cooperation, creativity, computational thinking, and self-regulation are more important than ever. They are the means by which what has been learnt is put to use in the present to produce fresh concepts, theories, innovations, and new body of knowledge. In addition, the creators of the Digital Skill Indicator commissioned by the European Union, Helsper et al. (2020) assert that the extant survey instruments have a tendency to focus more on technical, operational, and information processing skills than they do on communication, interaction, and content creation and production skills. The authors report that the cognitive interviews and performance evaluations revealed that many young individuals lacked a variety of skills, including essential abilities for processing and navigating information. Another knowledge gap existed in the process of producing and creating content. Testing individuals on these skills becomes even more challenging in a cross-national setup.

The Digital Skills Paradox

The current COVID-19 epidemic has sped up the broad digitalization of many under-resourced sectors. Secondary school children and students in the initial years of their higher/tertiary education have been among the most negatively impacted groups, with many of them being compelled to move to online learning. Rapid technological change has been difficult, and problems including poor digital literacy, lack of technology access, inequality, and institutional racism have made things much more difficult.

Like other social-economic-cultural-technological shifts the digitized world has had its unique set of outcomes and challenges, among which some are perceived as inevitable while others are preventable with effective management of the impact of digitalization, or the lack of it (digital gap), on the current and future youth development. For example: social networking sites (Facebook, Instagram, Twitter, Snapchat, & Tumblr) usage has skyrocketed in popularity and has emerged as a major area of influence on individual identity. Labels like "digital natives" and "net generation" (e.g., Prensky, 2001; Tapscott, 2008) indicate a generation that has a very close and continual interaction with digital technologies in ways that the digital space determines the attitude, expectation, behaviour, as well as qualification of the younger generation (Strohmeier, 2014).

The ramifications of the digital age can be understood by cataloging how the digital space has entered our general life. The first process in the digital change trajectory is the technical conversion of analogous information into automated information processing, known as digitization. On the other hand, digitalization is socio-technical in nature and refers to the adoption of digital processes into organizational or social functioning. Digital adoption can be viewed on a wide range extending from *digital transformation* (successful adoption) of digital processes to *digital disruption* which refers to the marginalization of specific entities (individuals, organizations, or communities) due to the digitalization of others operating in the same ecology (Strohmeier, 2020). While digital transformation has propagated innovation, collaboration, and flow of opportunities for those who have responded positively to this seismic shift, digital disruption has highlighted the vulnerabilities of some sections of the society.

According to Purdy (2021), the chief sales officer at one of the world's technological giants–Huawei Technologies, two things must occur for the digital transformation revolution to ensure that it is in everyone's favor: (a) digital education and training has to be made readily accessible in order to provide the undereducated and underskilled a greater opportunity at finding fulfilling employment; and, (b) nations ought to think about creating and implementing a national strategy for the future of work so that their citizens and businesses can compete in the development and application of technology. The declaration of the 2nd European Youth Work Convention (2015) states that; "Young people are increasingly engaging with new technologies and digital media. There is clearly a role for online youth work practice, in terms of exploiting a new space for youth work in a meaningful way, supporting digital literacy and enabling young people to deal with some of the associated risks."

With the proliferation of social media usage, there has been much debate on its impact on youth's mental health. Research in this field clearly indicates the presence of adaptive and maladaptive digital use and how they are linked with the proximate and distal contexts of the individual user (Stavropoulos et al., 2022). Digital usage has been seen to foster civic duty, electoral participation, and information seeking among youth socialized in a digital media environment (e.g., Ohme, 2019; Moeller et al., 2018). A correlation study by Berrymen et al. (2018a, 2018b) reported that a higher usage of social media increases the tendency to post vague and alarming content to draw more attention (e.g., intentionally posting highly personal and emotional matters anonymously). Such social media behavior is linked to mental health manifestations like suicidal ideation, lower empathy, social anxiety, and loneliness, and also acts as their warning sign (Berrymen et al., 2018a, 2018b).

Although scholarly opinions on the social effects of digital technologies on young people's lives are divided, it is generally acknowledged that keeping up with the most recent technology advancements has grown more difficult. While youth employees (sometimes referred to as digital immigrants) are required to learn to be "conscious of the always changing digital environment and the need to adjust material accordingly," youth in general (digital natives) are frequently capable of managing their digital environments alone (Pawluczuk et al., 2019; Livingstone et al., 2012). The digital world mirrors the physical world's gender imbalance. In comparison to males and boys, women and girls accept and use digital technology at a far lower rate. Along with this gender disparity in digital access, there is also a stark difference in meaningful digital use. Women's access to the full range of opportunities provided by digital is hampered by these usage discrepancies. Girls will have fewer employment possibilities and face more challenges to entering the economy without improved digital uptake and use (Unicef, 2021). Reports suggest that for women and girls, barriers such as using unintuitive mobile devices and content that is not available in their native tongue are far bigger than for men and boys (Unicef, 2021). In addition, more than half of the women digital users worldwide say that they have been harmed by technology in some way, and even a larger percentage believes that cyber security for women is becoming worse (including online sexual abuse, sharing of private photos and video without consent also known as revenge pornography). A major consequence of repetitive experience of online abuse not only impacts the psychological well-being of female users, but it also reduces their sense of efficacy in using digital services to their advantage like upskilling or job search (Web Foundation, 2020).

By 2025, 75% of the world's population is expected to have access to broadband internet through cable or wireless, according to an ambitious goal established by UNESCO and the International Telecommunications Union's (ITU) Broadband Commission for Sustainable Development (ITU, 2018). Thus, we urgently require a concerted international effort to assist the youth in developing the digital skills necessary to keep up with this rapidly evolving environment. In order to support students in participating and maximizing opportunities and limiting hazards in the digital world, it is crucial to foster *digital citizenship* along with a wider range of digital abilities. In a study on African youth, Oyedemi (2014) claims that despite majority of the youth can access internet, software for web page creation, blogging, and making content for social media, there is not much known about their *actual versus perceived skills,* which can be a major indicator of the socio-economic stratification and inequalities within the social system in terms of their digital skills.

Many young people lack advanced and occasionally even a fundamental digital ability, which limits their ability to participate in societies that are becoming more and more digital. Communities in general can vary in their digital skills due to "unlimited, good enough, or inadequate access" to informational technology (Steele, 2018). The hardest hit will be those with less education and undervalued job skills. Amidst the unequal distribution of digital skills, Helsper and colleagues (2020) report that those who are psychologically weak and have historically been marginalized may be less likely to be able to take advantage of the digital shift. Even more concerning is that they might also be less able to prevent its worse consequences.

Positive Youth Development

Positive youth development is a community-based initiative designed to promote specific psychological and behavioral functioning, which can be replicated in the area of professional growth and employability (Bowers et al., 2015). These functionalities are represented by "Five Cs": competence, confidence, character, connection, and caring (Geldhof et al., 2015; Lerner et al., 2005). The fundamentals focus of many educational systems currently as well as the need to develop information literacy, flexibility, and cooperative problem solving need to be prioritized in order to meet the increasing needs of the new digital era. The curriculum cannot be expanded to include more content or subjects in order to foster the development of a broad range of skills. Instead, it necessitates a different approach to teaching the academic disciplines that are already given priority in the curriculum of any particular nation. The youth can learn both the depth of the subject matter and the breadth of abilities concurrently valued in the labor market. A crucial aspect of youth development programs in this age is to shift the focus from deficit rectification (problem-reduction models) to strength building. From a developmental science perspective, positive youth development can be optimized by taking advantage of human plasticity and growing qualities among the youth that they value (Lerner, 2017).

Establishing best practices for better supporting educational staff in their tasks and improving their education, for updating assessment and validation methods and tools, and for introducing new and innovative forms of teaching and learning will support the development of key competences, their validation, and the provision of competence-oriented education, training, and learning (The Council of the European Union, 2018). At the community level, the Five Cs model (Geldhof et al., 2015; Lerner et al., 2005) recommends that the positive youth development must incorporate:

- Competence: Young people interact with a variety of complicated surroundings every day, including their schools, places of religion, families, peer groups, extracurricular activities, and jobs, among others. Youth who are progressing positively must be able to successfully traverse these environments and utilize the opportunities they offer.
- Confidence: When young people can successfully navigate their environments, they feel more confident. Confident youth think they can overcome challenges and make a significant difference in the world.
- Character: The youth when develops positively, it adopts the values reflected in the social norms and are more likely to manifest appropriate behavior based upon their moral judgment.
- Caring: Positive development goes beyond just looking out for oneself; thriving youth also demonstrate empathy and compassion for the thoughts, feelings, and experiences of others.
- Connection: Recognizing and promoting the youth as valuable and essential parts of their communities, forms the foundation of positive development. Investing in strong relationships within their communities and institutes has a two-way advantage of enhancing their own qualities and enabling positive living for others (Geldhof et al., 2015).

At the organizational level, the skill transformation via upskilling or reskilling must go hand in hand with strategic changes at the organizational level. According to Hancock et al., (2020), the continual shift in the workforce can be brought about by a three-stage process:

(i) Scouting—at this stage the organization creates a unified vision for its future in automation and digital, as well as the overall value of that future. Additionally, it pinpoints the most critical skill shortages by considering future requirements rather than just extrapolating from the past (the norm in much workforce planning). The organization's delivery readiness is then evaluated.
(ii) Shaping—at this stage the organization purports to develop upskilling programs, frequently in collaboration with employees, and to rethink work to meet the demands of a more digital future. In order to assist the deployment of talent

in the most significant upcoming jobs, this phase also entails building the infrastructure of what we refer to as a talent accelerator.

(iii) Shift—the third stage involves expanding the organization's range of talent-related initiatives. With this approach, it is acknowledged that institutional capacities for assisting workers in their transition to the workplace of the future are equally crucial to the short-term (and initially more pressing) talent objectives.

Research suggests that techniques like job crafting can be beneficial for those entering the workforce as well as the managers and the firms. Job crafting refers to reorganizing the components of the job to increase engagement and purpose (Lee, 2016). Three types of job crafting can yield favorable results when combined together viz., task crafting (reorganizing the tasks or actions in a job); relations crafting (remodeling the relations and interaction patterns in a job); and cognitive crafting (revamping how an individual perceives the tasks and the relationships in a job). In addition to ensuring autonomy and feedback in designing ones job, job crafting facilitates creativity and innovation in the jobs which would otherwise risk becoming redundant with time. Techniques like job crafting are prototypes of how old tasks and skills in a job can be blended with the new changes, similar to how individuals can be re-skilled or unskilled to find more relevance in the job market. In addition, job crafting interventions when used as a bottom-up approach by the individual to restructure one's own job, have been found to positively impact work engagement; improve the fit between the individual needs and job characteristics; enhancing social support among colleagues; elevating opportunities for self-development; fostering cautious risk-taking and embracing challenges; and reducing perceived job demands (Van Wingerden et al., 2017).

Personal Development Planning

Personal development planning (PDP) is more likely to be structured in work settings to coordinate self-improvement with organizational and corporate goals. The person can gain knowledge and experience to improve their performance in their work and/or advance their career. Personal development planning can be advantageous to both the individual and the organization. When employees expand and refresh their skill sets, the organization benefits. Additionally, it indicates that organizations would be better served by internal promotions rather than hiring fresh, unproven personnel. Organizations can benefit from PDP by connecting it to the annual employee review and assessment procedure. Companies prefer to use titles like employee development planning, professional development, and continuous professional development.

The general procedure of implementing a PDP in the workplace typically involves: establishing a vision or goal, assessing current strengths and developmental needs, setting SMART targets, determining when and how you will pursue training and development, maintaining records, and reflecting on learning (Cottrell, 2021).

The Council of the European Union (2018) upholds the value and applicability of informal and non-formal learning as demonstrated by the experiences gained through culture, youth work, volunteerism, and grassroots sports. It asserts that the development of critical thinking, analytical skills, creativity, problem-solving, resilience, and other critical interpersonal, communicative, and cognitive abilities that support young people's transition to adulthood, active citizenship, and working life is greatly supported by non-formal and informal learning. A range of learning styles and contexts are promoted by improving cooperation between various learning environments.

In addition to personal development, there needs to be support for infrastructure and connectivity especially in the developing countries where digital education can reach rural areas, unorganized work sectors, marginalized workers and migrants, as well as low-skilled individuals. The International Labour Organization recommends steps like infrastructure building, reducing red-tape and bureaucratic hurdles, supportive policies and legislations, creating opportunities for upskilling and reskilling, investing in calibrating the labor market right, facilitate acquisition of practical skills through effective apprenticeships and other work-based learning opportunities, address skill mismatch, and capacitate individuals and organizations to counter the hazards, in fostering a sustainable transition of youth in the digital age.

Conclusion and Way Forward

The ongoing digitalization and changing skills demand has implications for digital and non-digital skills that today's youth will invest in. The current and upcoming workforce can gain the skills necessary to engage in more meaningful employment and even profit from the digital transformation revolution by beginning to upskill. There is a risk that many people will be left behind as digitization is changing the future of work. Bridging the gap between the digital haves and have-nots is a necessity so that everyone can get an opportunity to be adequately informed and be able to showcase true talent. There is also a growing urgency to formalize norms or rules to safeguard people from digital harms. Developing digital literacy and addressing the knowledge gap can be transformational in terms of employability and bridging the digital divide. Companies and governments must coordinate on how to update present learning delivery systems or figure out how to develop new kinds of learning infrastructures for the benefit of both current and future workers as well as current students. With newer concerns surfacing with the pandemic and the volatility of the labor market, understanding the right balance of skills remains a recurrent task for the current and future generations.

References

Barney, J. (1991). Firm resources and sustained competitive advantage. *Journal of Management, 17*, 99–120.

Berryman, C., Ferguson, C. J., & Negy, C. (2018a). Social media use and mental health among young adults. *Psychiatric Quarterly, 89*(2), 307–314.

Berryman, C., Ferguson, C. J., & Negy, C. (2018b). Social media use and mental health among young adults. *Psychiatric Quarterly, 89*, 307–314. https://doi.org/10.1007/s11126-017-9535-6

Basic employability skills: A triangular design approach. http://internationalprofessor.com/documentation/JournalsArticles/18.journalrosenberg12.pdf

Cottrell, S. (2021). *Skills for success: Personal development and employability* (4th Edn). Macmillan International Higher Education.

Declaration of the 2nd European Youth Work Convention. (2015). https://pjp-eu.coe.int/documents/1017981/8529155/The%2B2nd%2BEuropean%2BYouth%2BWork%2BDeclaration_FINAL.pdf/cc602b1d-6efc-46d9-80ec-5ca57c35eb85

Fuller, J., Langer, C., & Sigelman, M. (2022). Skills-based hiring is on the rise. *Harward Business Review.* https://hbr.org/2022/02/skills-based-hiring-is-on-the-rise

Geldhof, G. J., Bowers, E. P., Mueller, M. K., Napolitano, C. M., Callina, K. S., Walsh, K. J., & Lerner, R. M. (2015). The Five Cs model of positive youth development (YD). *Promoting positive youth development Youth Development (YD). Lessons from the 4-H study Studies*, 161–186.

Green, F., & Henseke, G. (2021). Europe's evolving graduate labour markets: Supply, demand, underemployment and pay. *Journal for Labour Market Research, 55*(1), 1–13.

Hancock, B., Lazaroff-Puck, K., & Rutherford, S. (2020). Getting practical about the future of work. *McKinsey Quarterly, 1*, 65–73.

Helsper, E.J., Schneider, L.S., van Deursen, A.J.A.M., & van Laar, E. (2020). The youth digital skills indicator: Report on the conceptualisation and development of the ySKILLS digital skills measure. ySKILLS.

ITU. (2018). *UN Broadband commission sets global broadband targets to bring online the world's 3.8 billion not connected to the Internet.* International Telecommunications Union (ITU). https://www.itu.int/en/mediacentre/Pages/2018-PR01.aspx

Lee, L. (2016). *Should employees design their own jobs? Stanford Business.* https://www.gsb.stanford.edu/insights/should-employees-design-their-own-jobs

Lerner, R. M. (2017). Commentary: Studying and testing the positive youth development model: A tale of two approaches. *Child Development, 88*(4), 1183–1185.

Lerner, R. M., Lerner, J. V., Almerigi, J., Theokas, C., Phelps, E., Gestsdóttir, S., et al. (2005). Positive youth development, participation in community youth development programs, and community contributions of fifth-grade adolescents: Findings from the first wave of the 4-H Study of Positive Youth Development. *Journal of Early Adolescence, 25*(1), 17–71.

Livingstone, S., Hasebrink, U., & Görzig, A. (2012). Towards a general model of determinants of risk and safety. In Children, risk and safety on the internet (pp. 323–338). Policy Press

McClure, P. K. (2018). "You're fired", says the robot: The rise of automation in the workplace, technophobes, and fears of unemployment. *Social Science Computer Review, 36*(2), 139–156.

Moeller, J., Kühne, R., & De Vreese, C. (2018). Mobilizing youth in the 21st century: How digital media use fosters civic duty, information efficacy, and political participation. *Journal of Broadcasting & Electronic Media, 62*(3), 445–460.

Mueller, M. K., Phelps, E., Bowers, E. P., Agans, J. P., Urban, J. B., & Lerner, R. M. (2011). Youth development program participation and intentional self-regulation skills: Contextual and individual bases of pathways to positive youth development. *Journal of Adolescence, 34*(6), 1115–1125. https://doi.org/10.1016/j.adolescence.2011.07.010

Mugayar-Baldocchi,M., Schaninger, B., & Sharma, K. (2021). *The future of the workforce: Investing in talent to prepare for uncertainty.* McKinsey & Company. https://www.mckinsey.com/business-functions/people-and-organizational-performance/our-insights/the-organization-blog/the-future-of-work-the-now-the-how-and-the-why

OECD. (2017). *Getting skills right: skills for jobs indicators.* OECD Publishing.
OECD. (2020). *How are young graduates settling into the labour market?. Education Indicators in Focus, No. 76.* OECD Publishing, Paris. https://doi.org/10.1787/0cae6ba1-en
Ohme, J. (2019). Updating citizenship? The effects of digital media use on citizenship understanding and political participation. *Information, Communication & Society, 22*(13), 1903–1928.
Osgerby, B. (2020). *Youth culture and the media: Global perspectives.* Routledge.
Overtoom, C. (2000). Employability skills: An update. ERIC Clearinghouse
Oyedemi, T. (2014). Beyond access: Youth and digital skills. *Communicatio, 40*(2), 137–154.
Pawluczuk, A., Hall, H., Webster, G., & Smith, C. (2019). Digital youth work: youth workers' balancing act between digital innovation and digital literacy insecurity. In *Proceedings of ISIC: The Information Behaviour Conference.* http://informationr.net/ir/24-1/isic2018/isic1829.html
Prensky, M. (2001). Digital natives, digital immigrants. *On the Horizon, 9*(5), 1–6.
Purdy, A. (2021). *Why we need to bridge the digital divide and prepare for the future of work.* Forbes. https://www.forbes.com/sites/forbestechcouncil/2021/06/18/why-we-need-to-bridge-the-digital-divide-and-prepare-for-the-future-of-work/?sh=3aa375136117
Rothaermel, F. T. (2012). *Strategic management: Concepts and cases.* McGraw-Hill/Irwin, p. 91
Stavropoulos, V., Motti-Stefanidi, F., & Griffiths, M. D. (2022). Risks and opportunities for youth in the digital era: A cyber-developmental approach to mental health. *European Psychologist, 27*(2), 86–101. https://doi.org/10.1027/1016-9040/a000451
Steele, C. (2018). *How to bridge the digital divide.* Digital Divide Council. http://www.digitaldividecouncil.com/how-to-bridge-the-digital-divide/
Strohmeier, S. (2020). Digital human resource management: A conceptual clarification. *German Journal of Human Resource Management, 34*(3), 345–365.
Strohmeier, D.E.P.a.P.S. (2014). HRM in the digital age—digital changes and challenges of the HR profession. *Employee Relations, 36*, 4. https://doi.org/10.1108/ER-03-2014-0032
Tapscott, D. (2008). *Grown up digital: How the net generation is changing your world HC.* McGraw-Hill.
The Council of the European Union (2018). Council recommendation on key competences for lifelong learning. *Official Journal of the European Union.* https://eur-lex.europa.eu/legal-content/EN/TXT/PDF/?uri=CELEX:32018H0604(01)&from=LT
UNICEF. (2021). *Innovation and Technology for Gender Equality - What we know about the gender digital divide for girls: A literature review.* Unicef. https://www.unicef.org/eap/reports/innovation-and-technology-gender-equality-0
Van Wingerden, J., Bakker, A. B., & Derks, D. (2017). Fostering employee well-being via a job crafting intervention. *Journal of Vocational Behavior, 100*, 164–174.
Web Foundation. (2020). *The online crisis facing women and girls threatens global progress on gender equality.* https://webfoundation.org/2020/03/the-onlinecrisis-facing-women-and-girlsthreatens-global-progress-ongender-equality/
Whiting, K. (2020). *These are the top 10 job skills of tomorrow – and how long it takes to learn them.* World Economic Forum. https://www.weforum.org/agenda/2020/10/top-10-work-skills-of-tomorrow-how-long-it-takes-to-learn-them/

Dr. Tusharika Mukherjee is an industrial and organizational psychologist working in the area of diversity, performance, and personality relationship and creating sustainable work organizations. She obtained her Ph.D. in Applied Psychology from the University of Calcutta and pursued her postdoctoral research in the area of situation contingent performance variability in the Department of Work and Organizational Psychology, Justus Liebig University Giessen, Germany. She has over thirteen years of experience in University teaching, research, conducting skill development workshops, and consultation. Her other academic and research experiences include intercultural communication competence, work-life integration, team and leadership development, and didactics.

Chapter 22
Leaving No One Behind: Youth and Agenda 2030 for Sustainable Development

Durga P. Chhetri

Abstract The Agenda 2030 for Sustainable Development, agreed and endorsed by all member countries of the United Nations in 2015, promotes and enhances the Millennium Development Goals (MDGs). The set of 17 ambitious Sustainable Development Goals (SDGs) is based on the concept of "leave no one behind." The Agenda 2030 therefore calls for the overall development of the people including youth. Currently, 15-24 year olds make up 1.2 billion of the world's 7.5 billion population and 1.3 billion young people who will call the world home by 2030, the deadline for achieving the SDGs. This unparalleled proportion of youth is found mainly in 48 of the world's poorest countries. India has 231.9 million people between the ages of 15 and 24, which is 19.2% of the total population. The proportion of the young population is, therefore, very important from the point of view of sustainable development. They are considered as the "torchbearers" of the 2030 Agenda and play a key role both as beneficiaries of initiatives and policies and as partners and actors in the implementation of the Agenda. Against this broader background, this chapter focuses mainly on the three important areas viz., education, gender equality, and employment and all three areas are featured largely in the Agenda 2030 for the overall development of youth. Besides, this chapter also intends to offer policymakers and stakeholders information and analysis that can help them measure progress in addressing youth issues, assess policy gaps, and develop policy responses to achieve India's 2030 Agenda for sustainable development.

Keywords Youth · Sustainable development · Agenda

D. P. Chhetri (✉)
Department of Political Science, School of Social Sciences, Sikkim University, Gangtok, Sikkim, India
e-mail: dpchettri@cus.ac.in

S. Deb and S. Deb (eds.), *Handbook of Youth Development*,
https://doi.org/10.1007/978-981-99-4969-4_22

Introduction

The Agenda 2030 for Sustainable Development, agreed and endorsed by all member countries of the United Nations in 2015, promotes and enhances the Millennium Development Goals (MDGs). The Sustainable Development Goals (SDGs) serve as a global agreement between United Nations member States that have been widely adopted in "national development plans and academic research" (Rickels et al., 2016; UNDG, 2017; Cole et al., 2017; Cumming et al., 2017). The set of 17 ambitious Sustainable Development Goals is based on the concept of "leave no one behind." The Agenda 2030 therefore calls for the overall development of the people including youth. Currently, 15-24 year olds make up 1.2 billion of the world's 7.5 billion population and 1.3 billion young people who will call the world home by 2030, the deadline for achieving the SDGs. This unparalleled proportion of youth is found mainly in 48 of the world's poorest countries. India has 231.9 million people between the ages of 15 and 24, which is 19.2% of the total population. The proportion of the young population is, therefore, very important from the point of view of sustainable development. They are considered as the "torchbearers" of the 2030 Agenda and play a key role both as beneficiaries of initiatives and policies and as partners and actors in the implementation of the Agenda. Against this broader background, this chapter focuses mainly on the three important areas viz., education, gender equality, and employment and all three areas are featured largely in the Agenda 2030 for the overall development of youth. Besides, this chapter also intends to offer policymakers and stakeholders information and analysis that can help them measure progress in addressing youth issues, assess policy gaps, and develop policy responses to achieve India's 2030 Agenda for sustainable development.

The study is structured as follows. First, an overview of the global evolution of the SDGs and its comparison with MDGs is provided. Second, the meaning and definitions of leaving no one behind and youth are presented. Thereafter, three SDGs related to youth development viz., Education (SDG-4), Gender Equality (SDG-5), and Decent Work (SDG-8) were discussed and India's performance on these SDGs is also analysed. Finally, some recommendations are presented as a way forward for achieving SDGs.

What is SDGs 2030 Agenda?

The SDGs 2030 Agenda is an intergovernmental dedication and "a plan of action for people, planet and prosperity" (UN, 2015a). It contains 17 SDGs which are "integrated and indivisible and balance the three dimensions i.e. the economic, social and environmental" of sustainable development. The SDGs, which replace the Millennium Development Goals (MDGs), were announced by the UN General Assembly in September 2015 and entered into force on January 1, 2016. The UN General Assembly at its 70th session held on September 25-27, 2015, approved the 2030

Agenda for Sustainable Development which consists of 17 SDGs, 169 associated targets, and 244 indicators after "three years of multi-stakeholder consultations and intergovernmental negotiations" (UN, 2015a). In addition to the session of the UN General Assembly, the planning of Sustainable Development Goals was shaped by three high-level international meetings held in different places. Three meetings that influenced the formulation of the Sustainable Development Goals are (i) the International Conference on Financing for Development held in Addis Ababa in July 2015; (ii) Turkey's presidency of the G20 summit in Alanya in November 2015; and (iii) the 21st Conference of the Parties (COP21) held in December 2015 in Paris. The goals of sustainable development are more detailed compared to the Millennium Development Goals. These should be the goals of all countries and not just poor countries. The Sustainable Development Goals are more intrinsic, inseparable, and balance the three vital pillars viz.,— economic, social, and environmental—of sustainable development.

The UN's Sustainable Development Goals represent an unprecedented commitment to reducing global poverty and quality of life problems. After approval, all major bilateral and multilateral donors have included sustainable development goals in their humanitarian aid, development cooperation, and loan program. The 17 goals reflect a vision of the future based on four different pillars, i.e., people (human development), planet (environmental sustainability), prosperity (inclusive economic growth and change), and partnership (international cooperation). Based on the principle of universality, all members of the United Nations countries—whether they are OECD or developing countries—pledged to implement the Agenda 2030. Today, the goals of sustainable development have become a common reference point for governments, international development organizations, as well as civil society, and social movements. They are on the agenda of the most important forums, from G20 to the World Social Forum.

The purview of Agenda 2030 is more vast and expansive than that of the Millennium Development Goals that preceded the Sustainable Development Goals. The Millennium Development Goals included eight goals, 22 targets, and 60 indicators. Goals 1–7 focused on the Global South and include poverty, education, gender, health and environmental sustainability (UN, 2008). However, Goal 8 was applicable globally to "develop a global partnership for development" (UN, 2001) but had no quantitative targets (Hulme, 2007).

All member countries of the UN, including the State of India, subscribed to the SDGs and pledged to work toward the achievement of the SDGs. In his speech at the UN Sustainable Development Summit in September 2015, Prime Minister Narendra Modi said, "A large part of India's development agenda is reflected in the Sustainable Development Goals........Sustainable development of one-sixth of humanity will be of great consequence to the world and our beautiful planet." India, being a signatory to the declaration along with 193 countries, has welcomed the 2030 Agenda.

Defining "Leave No One Behind"

"Leave no one behind" is one of the essential principles of the 2030 Agenda. The principle is based on the consensus among the member countries that SDGs will not be achieved by 2030 unless all people including youth are put front and centre of planning, implementation, and monitoring. The UN documents define the term "leave no one behind within and between countries and population groups" (UN, 2015b). Para 4 of the documents says that:

> As we embark on this great collective journey, we pledge that no one will be left behind... We wish to see the Goals and targets met for all nations and peoples and for all segments of society. (UN, 2015b para 4)

The document also explains that "the left behind" refers to certain people whose identity— belonging to one or more groups—means that they face special discrimination and lack both voice and power. The SDG UN document states that:

> We emphasise the responsibilities of all States ... to respect, protect and promote human rights and fundamental freedoms for all, without distinction of any kind as to race, colour, sex, language, religion, political or other opinion, national or social origin, property, birth, disability or other status. (UN, 2015b)

The declaration also emphasizes how important "it is for everyone to be able to live a life of dignity" (UN, 2015b). The final document of the 2030 Agenda includes an indicative list of the remaining groups who are left behind: "...children, youth, disabled people, people living with HIV/AIDS, the elderly, indigenous peoples, refugees and internally displaced persons, and migrants" (UN, 2015b). The promise to leave no one behind is at the core of Agenda 2030 and one of its most unique attributes compared to the Millennium Development Goals. Although the MDGs have achieved significant progress in reducing overall poverty—both in terms of income and more broadly in health, education, and living standards—the poorest and most marginalized groups have often not benefited at all or sufficiently (Bhatkal et al., 2015; Ravallion, 2016). Stuart and Samman (2017) in their analysis of the 2030 Agenda's outcome document, define leave no one behind as:

- To end extreme poverty and reduce inequalities;
- To stop the group discrimination that has led to unequal outcomes for some disadvantaged or marginalized populations; and
- To reach the furthest behind first.

Youth Population and Sustainable Development in India

Agenda 2030 concerns all 1.2 billion young people in the world, who currently make up 16% of the world's population—and the 1.3 billion young people who will call the world home by 2030, the target date for achieving the Sustainable Development Goals (UN, 2017). An unprecedented proportion of the young population lives mainly in South Asian and African countries. India has the so-called youth boom, with the world's largest youth population of 356 million in the 10-24 age group, followed by China with 269 million youth (GoI, 2017). According to UNFPA's State of World Population report, Indonesia, the United States, Nigeria, Brazil, and Bangladesh are behind India and China in hosting large youth cohorts. Between 2001 and 2011, India increased the world's population by 161 million to become the world's largest contributor to global demographic change. India's 2011 Census showed that 65% of the total population is under the age of 35 and 50% is under the age of 25. Out of total 231 million young people, 121 are men and 110 million are women (Table 22.1). India is the youngest country in the world today with an average age of 29 years.

As far as the definition of youth is concerned, different definitions of the term are used in practice, and the same applies to different, mostly upper age limits for young people, which are related to local conditions, economic situation, and cultural characteristics of the country (Petković et al, 2019). Therefore, there is no single universally established definition of youth. The United Nations defines youth as between 15 and 24 years of age, while Article 1 of the Convention on the Rights of the Child (CRC) defines children as persons under the age of 18. The National Youth Policy of India 2003 covers all youth between the ages of 13-35 but is divided into two groups, viz. 13-19 and 20-35 (GoI, 2003). In the 2014 National Youth Policy, youth are defined as 15-29 years old, who are 27.5% of the population. The policy document says that youth is a more flexible category than a fixed age group. "Youth" is often defined as a person from the age at which they complete compulsory education to the age at which they find their first job (GoI, 2014). The study, Youth in India: Situation and Needs, defines youth as persons between the ages of 15 and 24, and this chapter follows the same definition.

According to UN statistics, out of 232 Sustainable Development Goal indicator frameworks, 68 focus on youth development. Of the 68 indicators, 53 directly provide information on the socio-demographic situation of young people and 15 on the environment that promotes the development of young people. In 2018, India ranked 112 out of 156 countries in the Sustainable Development Goals Index with a score of 59.1, while Sweden ranked first with a score of 85 (Sachs et al., 2018). As for South Asian countries, the average score for South Asian countries is 64.1 and India is fifth among seven countries in the world ranking (Table 22.2).

Education, SDG 4, and Youth

The 2030 Agenda for Sustainable Development is universal and indivisible and emphasizes above all that no one is left behind. The Goal 4 of the Agenda 2030 provides for all an inclusive and quality education for better society. In the comprehensive action plan 2030, education is essentially formulated as an independent goal (SDG 4) with its seven action targets. In the 2030 Agenda for Sustainable Development, education is not limited to SDG 4, but is linked in one way or another to almost all other SDGs (Table 22.3).

Table 22.1 Youth population in India

Youth (15-24)	Males	Females	Rural	Urban	Sex ratio among youth	SC youth population	% SC to total youth population	ST youth population	% ST to total youth	Percentage decadal growth of youth population
23,19,50,671	12,15,67,089	11,03,83,582	1,57,738171	74,212500	905	3,97,32,282	17.1	1,99,27,193	8.6	22.1

Source Census of India, (2011)

Table 22.2 India's SDGs scores among South Asian countries

SDGs	Afghanistan	Bangladesh	Bhutan	India	Nepal	Pakistan	Sri Lanka	India's Rank
SDG1	63.8	97	99.9	96.3	95.7	98.1	99.7	5
SDG2	40.3	46.8	49.3	39.6	48	37.6	44.5	6
SDG3	37.9	60.3	69.6	58.9	58.7	50.7	79.3	4
SDG4	6.9	63.9	47.6	64.8	59	42.5	90.9	2
SDG5	24.6	57	45.7	36.4	64.4	34.4	53.7	5
SDG6	49.3	77.3	74	70.2	78.4	50.2	82.3	5
SDG7	52	42.9	83.7	54	53.3	66.3	54.3	4
SDG8	31.2	63.1	64.2	61.1	59.4	40.4	78.6	4
SDG9	3.8	18	28.8	33.1	14	22	19.8	1
SDG10	65.4	76.5	68.3	49.1	83.3	58.1	36.5	6
SDG11	39.4	39.4	75.1	56.1	46.8	48.3	71.7	3
SDG12	82.1	77.5	74.5	81.6	84.5	79.2	67	3
SDG13	87.7	81.1	93.4	80.6	92.4	91.1	88	7
SDG14	48.4	51	45.2	53	45.2	51	53.9	2
SDG15	50.8	54.7	57.6	46.1	67.1	66.9	61.3	7
SDG16	47.6	60.7	78.6	71.9	53.5	54.2	69.3	2
SDG17	55	41.7	56.2	51.3	63.2	42.2	46.5	4
Score	46.2	59.3	65.4	59.1	62.8	54.9	64.6	5

Sources Sachs et al. (2018);Thampi, (2019)
Note Due to unavailability of score, Maldives is not included here

Education is one of the most important keys for the comprehensive participation of young people in society because it positively affects several dimensions of sustainable development including access to better employment, permanent escape from poverty, etc., and all of the above to achieve Agenda 2030. In addition, education helps prepare young people to work in the highly skilled jobs of the fourth industrial revolution. Education is a prerequisite for sustainable development. It will play a transformative role in solving all development challenges in the post-2015 era. In addition to being a focus of SDG 4, education directly contributes to achieving the goals of poverty and inequality reduction, health and nutrition, and national economic growth.

Significant gains in school enrolment and retention in India have made the current generation of youth the most educated in the region's history. India has the second largest school system in the world after China, with more than 1.5 million schools and approximately 280 million students. The provision of free public education for 6-14 year olds has grown enormously in recent years. In addition, several important programs and policies have been launched to ensure free and compulsory education for all children between the ages of 6 and 14 as a fundamental right. The Union government initiatives like Sarva Siksha Abhiyan (SSA) and the Right to Education (RTE) have given the Indian education system a much-needed boost. As a result

Table 22.3 Education and SDGs

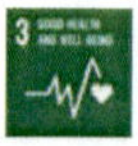	3.7: Provides access to better health services by 2030
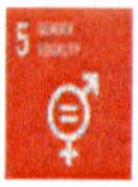	5.6: Ensure access to sexual and reproductive health, information and education for women aged 15-49
	8.6: Proportion of young people who are not working, studying must be significantly reduced.
	12.8: Ensure that people everywhere have the necessary knowledge and awareness of sustainable development.
	13.3: Improve education on climate change mitigation and adaptation.

Source Based on United Nations, (2015a)

of such initiatives, school enrolment is estimated at 95% of the school-age population, but participation rates and the quality of provision remain of concern. India's current literacy rate of 74% leaves considerable room for improvement in the education sector. Nine States/UTs have a literacy rate below 70%. The dropout rate in secondary education is close to 20%. Overall, India has made significant progress toward achieving education for all in achieving SDG4. According to NITI Aayog's SDG Index 2019, Himachal Pradesh and Chandigarh (scores between 65 and 99) are the top states and UTs in SDG 4 action. In the performer's category, there are 11 states and two UTs with an Index score of 51–65. However, seven states lagged behind in the aspirant category (index score below 50) (see Table 22.4). The statistics show that India has made progress in terms of educational coverage at various levels, but there are still gaps in progress, completion, and quality that affect young people and hinder the accomplishment of SDG4.

Gender Equality and SDGs: Leave No Woman and Girl Behind

Gender equality is one of the important goals laid out in the 2030 Agenda for sustainable development. The Agenda for Sustainable Development set the year 2030 a deadline to end all types of discrimination against women and girls and achieve gender equality and empower all women and girls. Gender equality and empowerment of women is a prerequisite for attaining all goals in the 2030 Agenda. Contrary to the

Table 22.4 Performance of states and UTs on select SDGs

States/UT	SDG 1	SDG 4	SDG 5	SDG 8	Composite SDG
	Index Score				
Andhra Pradesh	69	52	37	78	67
Arunachal Pradesh	34	58	33	52	53
Assam	48	44	33	62	55
Bihar	33	19	40	64	50
Chhattisgarh	49	52	43	67	56
Goa	53	71	46	71	65
Gujarat	47	47	36	75	64
Haryana	47	68	36	71	57
Himachal Pradesh	60	81	52	76	69
Jharkhand	28	42	34	70	53
Karnataka	49	67	42	78	66
Kerala	64	74	51	61	70
Madhya Pradesh	40	54	45	67	58
Maharashtra	47	65	41	70	64
Manipur	42	70	34	27	60
Meghalaya	68	55	34	65	54
Mizoram	67	61	37	42	56
Nagaland	56	47	42	28	57
Odisha	47	40	35	59	58
Punjab	48	67	46	65	62
Rajasthan	56	51	39	65	57
Sikkim	65	58	49	68	65
Tamil Nadu	72	70	40	74	67
Telangana	52	64	26	82	67
Tripura	70	55	32	63	58
Uttar Pradesh	40	48	41	64	55
Uttarakhand	64	66	38	73	64
West Bengal	52	50	38	72	60
A&N Island	48	61	48	55	61
Chandigarh	48	80	47	64	70
D&N Haveli	33	53	44	63	63
Daman & Diu	58	43	39	54	61
Delhi	54	64	27	60	61
J&K	58	54	53	46	59
Lakshadweep	56	62	37	43	63
Puducherry	56	67	35	58	66
India	50	58	42	64	60
Target	100	100	100	100	100

Source: NITI Aayog, 2019

Aspirant (0-49) Performer (50-64) Front Runner (65-99) Achiever (100)

Millennium Development Goals, the 2030 Agenda embraces gender equality and the empowerment of women and girls more holistically. According to the Sustainable Development Report, "Gender equality is a focus of stand-alone Goal 5 and except three, all SDGs contain specific goals that address the economic, social, political and cultural conditions that create gender inequality" (UN, 2017). The report also stated that Agenda 2030 sees equality as the foundation of its core principle: "No woman or girl is left behind."

Gender equality and women's empowerment have shown global recognition that both are important goals and preconditions for the success of all SDGs. The 2030 Agenda includes a particularly clear goal of addressing gender inequality, which remains widespread and persistent worldwide and places women disproportionately among the poorest and most marginalized. Gender equality under SDG 5 has also been prioritized in other goals through specific gender targets and indicators in areas such as poverty, health, and education. All goals of the 2030 Agenda will be accomplished when gender equality and empowerment of women are achieved. For example, women's access to decent work, better employment, and regular income not only contributes to poverty reduction but also supports better health, educational, and nutritional outcomes for women and girls. Therefore, the systematic introduction of the gender aspects is crucial both in the implementation and monitoring of sustainable development goals.

India has implemented gender-responsive public policies in a cross-sectoral manner to attain SDG 5. The Union Government is committed to developing effective measures for the promotion of gender equality. The government for the achievement of SDG 5 launched schemes like Beti Bachao Beti Padhao, Sukanya Samridhi Yojana, and Janani Suraksha Yojana. According to NITI Aayog SDG Index (2019), there is a gap in "gender-disaggregated information systems, declining participation of women in the workforce, persistent disparities in women's to and ownership of land, and women's entrepreneurship" (GoI, 2019). Himachal Pradesh and Kerala are the only two states that bagged a position in the category of performers in achieving the target of SDG5. All other states with an index score below 50 fell behind the aspirants category (see Table 22.4). Although the government of India has identified ending violence against women as a key national goal in line with Sustainable Development Goal 5, but violence against women is currently one of the biggest challenges that the Indian State currently faces. According to the National Crime Records Bureau (NCRB) 2022, "crimes against women increased from 56.5% in 2020 to 64.5% in 2021" (GoI, 2022). Of the total, the majority of crimes, i.e., 31.8% fall under the category of "cruelty by the husband or his relatives." Other categories of crimes against women include "assault on women with intent to outrage her modesty (20.8%), kidnapping and abduction (17.6%) and rape (7.4%)" (GoI, 2022). The state of Uttar Pradesh, as per NCRB, topped the list and Nagaland stood out as having the least number of crimes against women in 2022. According to the Global Gender Gap Report 2022, India ranked 135 globally in gender parity out of 146 countries. The report indicates the poor performance of India compared to neighboring countries like Bangladesh (71), Nepal (96), and Bhutan (126). The data clearly shows that a lot of work still needs to be done to achieve gender-related SDG commitments in India.

Decent Work, SDG 8, and Youth

SDG 8 with 17 indicators is an important goal dedicated to the promotion of sustainable and inclusive economic growth and decent work for all. This goal is strongly linked to many other SDGs like poverty eradication, health, education, etc., and therefore attainment of SDG8 is closely related to the other goals. In other words, failure to achieve other sustainable development goals would hinder the achievement of SDG8. Decent work for all is important for young people, as youth unemployment rates are very high in all regions of the world. As per the estimates of the International Labour Organisation (ILO), "around a fifth of 15-24 year olds worldwide were not in employment, education or training (NEET) and of these, 34% are young women and 10% are men" (ILO, 2017). The majority of youth (96.8%) in developing countries work in the informal sector. In contrast to formal work, "informal work is associated with low wages, leading to poverty, as it offers lower average wages than formal sector work" (Heintz et al., 2006; ILO, 2017). In developing countries, the majority of youth (70%) are in "working poverty" (ILO, 2017) and "more than 50% of youth are underemployed in low-income countries" (Ayele et al., 2018). According to the Periodic Labour Force Survey (PLFS 2020), the unemployment rate in India was 5.8% in 2019. The unemployment rate among the rural male youth (15-29 years) was 16.6% while the unemployment rate among the rural female youth was 13.8% during 2018-19. The unemployment rate among urban male and female youth was 18.7 and 25.7 percent respectively. According to the Global Employment Trends for Youth Report 2022, India lost large jobs in 2020 and 2021. Furthermore, the global pandemic caused by COVID-19 has exacerbated many labor market challenges for the people of the age group 15-24 years. As a result, young people in this age category have lost their employment at a much higher rate than adults.

India being a signatory to Agenda 2030 has started the journey to attain SDG 8. Several government programmes such as "Make in India, Start-up India, Skill India, and Digital India have been launched for the generation of employment opportunities to the youth in the country" (GoI, 2019). In addition, the federal government puts a lot of emphasis on creating a favorable business and trade environment in the country. The progress made so far has been attributed to the interventions of the government of India, particularly through its various flagship schemes for creating employment opportunities, promoting skill development and stimulating economic development for the masses. India aims at attaining SDGs by 2030 through various flagship programs by involving all citizens including youth. In order to accelerate economic growth, it is striving hard to generate decent employment opportunities and enhance the GDP of the country. According to NITI Aayog SDG Index 2019, seven states and six UTs are performers among the States and the UTs, respectively as far as SDG 8 is concerned. Eighteen states ranked in the category of Front Runners with Index scores of 65 and 99. However, three States and two UTs were behind in the category of Aspirants with an Index score below 50 (see Table 22.4).

Conclusion

With the growing youth population in India, it is an undoubted fact that education, gender equality, and employment sectors are keys to addressing youth challenges. Youth development is of high priority in all national and state policies. The government's youth policy can contribute to the success and achievement of Agenda 2030. Despite several government interventions aimed at addressing youth issues, there is a need to establish clear, responsive, and effective mechanisms to monitor the extent to which these interventions reach the wider youth population. In addition, global and national agendas emphasize the role of youth in the implementation and monitoring of the 2030 Agenda for sustainable development. According to the 2020 Sustainable Development Report (SDR), "India fared worse than Bhutan, Nepal, Sri Lanka, and Bangladesh. In 2020, India was ranked 117, two spots below 115 its rank in 2019 out of the 166 countries on the SDG Index" (SDR, 2020). The progress on the "leave no one behind" agenda is also failing to meet the needs of the young people. Eight years since the Agenda was agreed, this is extremely concerning. Thus, the attainment of Goal 4, Goal 5, and Goal 8 in India would require full involvement and inclusion of youth. The following recommendations are suggested to achieve the agenda of "leaving no youth behind" in India.

- It is recommended that all government policies, strategies, and programs promote inclusion and increase equality by putting "leave no youth behind" at the center of its work.
- Government should provide practical tools, guidance, and resources to all government staff and implementing partners to support the cross-government application of the "leave no one behind" principles and youth and gender-sensitive analysis across all policy and programming.
- Implement existing strategies and approaches including flagship government programs for youth development, Vision for Gender Equality, and the Youth Agenda, in collaboration with relevant civil society organizations.

References

Ayele, A., Oosterom, M., & Glover, D. (2018). Introduction: Youth employment and the private sector in Africa. In A. Ayele, M. Oosterom, & D. Glover (Eds.), *Youth Employment and the Private Sector in Africa* (pp. 1–15). IDS Bulletin.

Bhatkal, T., Samman, E. & Stuart, E. (2015). Leave no one behind: The real bottom billion. *Briefing Note*. Overseas Development Institute.

Census of India. (2011). Registrar General of India, Ministry of Home Affairs, Government of India.

Cole, M. J., Bailey, R. M., & New, M. G. (2017). Spatial variability in sustainable development trajectories in South Africa: Provincial level safe and just operating spaces. *Sustainability Science, 12*(5), 829–848.

Cumming, T. L., Shackleton, R. T., Förster, J., Dini, J., Khan, A., Gumula, M., & Kubiszewski, I. (2017). Achieving the national development agenda and the sustainable development goals (SDGs) through investment in ecological infrastructure: A case study of South Africa. *Ecosystem Services, Investing in Ecological Infrastructure in South Africa,* 27(Part B), 253-260.

Government of India. (2003). *National Youth Policy 2003*. Ministry of Youth Affairs and Sports, Government of India.

Government of India. (2014). *National youth policy 2014*. Ministry of Youth Affairs and Sports. Government of India.

Government of India. (2017). *India youth development index and report 2017*. Rajiv Gandhi National Institute of Youth Development, Ministry of Youth Affairs and Sports, Government of India.

Government of India. (2018). *NITI Aayog's SDG India index baseline report 2018*. Government of India.

Government of India. (2019). *NITI Aayog's SDG India index baseline report 2019*. Government of India.

Government of India. (2022). *National crime records Bureau*. Ministry of Home Affairs, Government of India, New Delhi.

Heintz, J., Vanek, J., & Chen, M. (2006). Informality, gender and poverty. *Economic and Political Weekly, 41*(21), 2131–9.

Hulme, D. (2007). *The making of the millennium development goals: Human development meets results-based management in an imperfect world*. Brooks World Poverty Institute.

ILO. (2017). *Global employment trends for youth 2017: Paths to a better working future*. ILO.

Periodic Labour Force Survey (PLFS). (2020). *Annual Report 2018-19*. Ministry of Statistics and Programme Implementation, Government of India.

Petković, J., Petrović, N., Dragović, I., Stanojević, K., Radaković, J. A., Borojević, T., et al. (2019). Youth and forecasting of sustainable development pillars: An adaptive neuro-fuzzy inference system approach. *PLoS ONE, 14*(6), 1–25.

Ravallion, M. (2016). Are the world's poorest being left behind? *Journal of Economic Growth, 21*(2), 139–164.

Rickels, W., Dovern, J., Hoffmann, J., Quaas, M. F., Schmidt, J. O., & Visbeck, M. (2016). Indicators for monitoring sustainable development goals: An application to oceanic development in the European Union. *Earth's Future, 4*(5), 252–267.

Sachs, J., Schmidt-Traub, G., Kroll, C., Lafortune, G., & Fuller, G. (2018). *SDG Index and dashboards report 2018*. Bertelsmann Stiftung and Sustainable Development Solutions Network.

Stuart, E., & Samman, E. (2017). Defining "leave no one behind". *Briefing Note*. Overseas Development Institute.

Thampi, A. (2019). Where does india stand on the sustainable development goals? progress and challenges. In Nitya Mohan Khemka & Suraj Kumar (eds.) *Social development and sustainable development goals in South Asia* (pp. 49-73). Routledge.

UN. (2001). *Road map towards the implementation of the United Nations Millennium Declaration: Report of the Secretary-General*. United Nations.

UN. (2015a). *Transforming our world: The 2030 Agenda for sustainable development*. United Nations.

UN. (2015b). *Resolution adopted by the General Assembly on 25 September 2015b [without reference to a Main Committee (A/70/L.1)] 70/1*. Transforming our world: the 2030 Agenda for Sustainable Development http://www.un.org/ga/search/view_doc.asp

UN. (2017). *The sustainable development goals report 2017*. Sales No. E.17.I.7. https://unstats.un.org/sdgs/report/2017.

UN. (2021). *Youth 2030: Working with and for young people*. UN Youth Strategy 2030. United Nations.

UNDG. (2017). *Mainstreaming the 2030 agenda for sustainable development: Reference guide to UN country teams*. United Nations Development Group.

Dr. Durga P. Chhetri is the Chairperson in the department of political science, Sikkim Central University, Sikkim, India. His research foci include governance, decentralization and federalism, gender studies, social justice, social theory and social exclusion/inclusion. He is the author or co-author of many scholarly articles and book chapters as well as five books, *including Gender, Power and Democracy in South Asia (2019), Divided Spaces: Discourse on Social Exclusion and Women in India (2014), Decentralised Governance and Development in India (2012), and Politics, Society and Development: Insights from Sikkim (2012)*. He was on the editorial board of the Indian Journal of Political Science, which publishes high quality, cutting-edge research in all areas of political science. He is a recipient of India's National Young Political Scientist Award 2017.

Chapter 23
Marginalized Youths and Inequalities: The Global Scenario and Way Forward

Subhasis Bhadra

Abstract The empowered youths are an important force for development and sustainable changes in any community and nation. Not just in the cross-section of time but rather in continuum toward sustainable development always, the youth population of a nation becomes the key driving force. Youths are the powerhouse, and they ideally fuel the nation's growth if used constructively. Youths are easy to mold and can easily be influenced; thus, they are often at the threshold of being misled, misused, and even pushed back from the arena of progressive thinking. Denial of rights and lack of access to social justice and welfare mechanisms led to persistent rejection to obtain the opportunities that are essential to attain a decent standard of living. Marginalization of youths is a systemic outcome of several factors, namely, socio-economic deprivation, political upheavals, prejudices stereotypes associated with sex, gender, race, caste, color, that compound the inabilities to cope with the challenges and further experience inequalities in the personal, professional, familial, or social sphere. Oppressed social situations negatively impact their potential and limit the availability, accessibility, and affordability of essential resources for development and well-being. Thus, inequalities grossly cripple their capabilities and aspirations. As a result, marginalized youths suffer from issues like emotional turmoil, substance abuse, addictions, suicidal tendencies and may develop delinquent behavior, and defy the social control mechanisms. Thus, marginalized youths are often used for rioting, and terrorist activities, inculcating hate and instigating violence by creating a fake sense of power and identity by the extremist political, religious, or separatist groups. Youths, the key role players to attend SDGs, need an empowering, barrier-free socio-economic-political environment for crafting a sustainable future and enduring peace.

Keywords Marginalized youths · Inequalities · Global scenario · Way forward

S. Bhadra (✉)
Department of Social Work, School of Social Sciences, Central University of Rajasthan, Bandarsindri, Kishangarh, Ajmer, Rajasthan, India
e-mail: bhadrasubhasis@gmail.com

S. Deb and S. Deb (eds.), *Handbook of Youth Development*,
https://doi.org/10.1007/978-981-99-4969-4_23

Introduction

Defining youths based on age is widely accepted as per the criteria determined by the United Nations. A person aged between 15 and 24 years is considered a youth, but the criteria of age are quite fluid, as few documents for practical purposes consider youth till the age of 32 or 35 years. Even understanding youths is closely associated with culture and societal norms and thus varies across regions. UNFPA defined youths under three categories, namely, adolescent (10–19 years), young (10–24), and youth (15–24 years) (UN, 2010a, 2010b). Comprehensively, "youth" is understood as a period of life full of potential but equally restricted with multiple challenges. Youths determine a basketful of dreams, tons of energy, and willpower to gain control and change the situation in accordance with their vision, ideas, motto, and aspirations. Adolescents and youth are always overarching terms and concepts that have both psychological and social correlates. Adolescence is the stage of change- physical, psychological, and corresponding social roles and expectations. The late adolescent stage is the youth and continues through the initial stage of adulthood. While childhood sets the foundation, the early youth stage is essential to building successful adulthood. At this stage, nurturing care, positive stimulation, exposure to a learning atmosphere, a healthy home and community environment, and effective peer relationships are very much pivotal for holistic growth and attaining successful adulthood. Thus, the youths aged between 15–25 need a wider spectrum of support and opportunities with resources and responsible stakeholders' engagements across the globe in every community. Often the local to global issues cause multiple limitations and challenges to facilitate a healthy environment for the youth that cause marginalization. The positive youth development models grossly stand on 5Cs (Lerner, 2009), which are competence, confidence, connection, caring, and character that are dealing with an individual's development and need to be supported with the social engagements and policies to reduce the inequality gaps in the society. If the inequality gaps widen, the availability, accessibility, and affordability become tough for some of the youth, who gradually become socially weak and vulnerable to many problems that limit their choices, and life chances to lead a successful life. In many societies, the marginalized youths are a special cohort with a number of associated socio-economic and political characteristics. These characteristics are certainly not independent of local and global realities that impact the life of the youths at the community and family levels.

Youths the Global Population

Every year, across the Globe 12th August is celebrated as International Youth Day (IYD) since 1999, as it was adopted by the UN (United Nations) World Conference of Ministers responsible for Youth, held between 8 and 12th August 1988 at Lisbon, Portugal. The key purpose was to bring the issues of youths to the forefront of the internal community and highlight the youths as the important partner in the development of global society. Further, the UN Security Council Resolution of 9th December 2015 underscored the urgent requirement to engage the youths as peace messengers, peacekeepers, or peace volunteers for promoting peace and counter extremist ideas and activities. Thereby, positing the youths all over the world as partners for promoting peace and security (UN, 2017). The Department of Economics and Social Affairs of the United Nations highlighted a few key messages based on the report World Population Prospect 2019. About 42% of the global population is below 25 years, i.e., four out of every ten people (Gray, 2018). The percentage of the youth population (15–24 years) reached its peak in 1985, while 19.3% of the global population were youth. Further, the number of youths (15–24 years) in 2019, was 1.2 billion, (16% of the global population), and it is projected to be 13% of the global population in 2065, with its peak in terms of the number of youths at 1.4 billion. A large number of youths are having homes in Central and Southern Aisa. It is very pertinent to note that the youth population in the poorest 47 countries will increase by 62% over the next three decades (UN, 2019). This critically calls for more investment in these countries and areas (sub-Saharan Africa, Oceania, Northern Africa, and Western Asia) to create opportunities for education, health care, to ensure effective engagement, productive employment, and decent work. In absence of special focus on youths, it may cause marginalization and exclusion causing a number of developmental issues and socio-economic problems. Essentially some areas will have a decreased youth population causing fewer new entries into the labor forces. According to the projection, the regions like Eastern and South-Eastern Asia, Latin America and Caribbean, Europe, and Northern America will have a decrease in the youth population. The greater access to sexual health helped the young women to decide about childbearing, still childbearing remains high in some developing regions (Latin America and Caribbean, Central and Southern Asia) that indicated higher exclusion of young women from access to sexual and maternal health care. Migration among the youths is another major feature that is impacting the demographic scenario of different nations and regions. In 2017, about 11% (258 million) of the global migrant population were between the age of 15–24 years who were living outside the country of their birth. The youths from the underdeveloped and developing regions have a higher trend of migration (UN, 2019).

The life of the youths is often full of turbulence, as there are a number of social, political, and climatic disturbances that keep impacting their choices, opportunities, life chances, and potentials. Such disturbances are often dragged over generations and spill over from local to regional and global context. Often the inability to focus on local solutions and not relying upon indigenous knowledge and practices are increasing the intensity of the problems. For instance, even after substantial efforts for peace-building, the number of children living in the conflict-affected zone in 2018 has increased by 75%, in comparison to 1990 (Gray, 2018). Syria, Somalia, and Afghanistan are the worst places where hospitals, schools, and educational institutions are targeted. The situation is equally true for the youths in war-affected countries in the Middle East, Africa, Asia, and Latin America. Severe atrocities are committed against the youths, like torture, abduction, sexual violence, and killing, that cause disability, orphanhood, and severe emotional and physical scars (UN Youths, 2019). The number of unschooled, droop-out children and youths has not significantly changed even after the implementation of SDGs, due to war, conflict, and refugee situations. The number of children, adolescents, and youths who were out of school in 2018 was 258.4 million, i.e., representing one-sixth of the global population of that age group. Gender disparity still exists and the girls are continually facing more problems in entering school and continuing schooling (UNESCO, 2019). Effective use of the internet among the youths is an important indicator of development. Access to the internet is also connected with poverty reduction, bringing development, and facilitating various job opportunities and extension of the business. Effective use of the internet influences positive youth development (Gómez-Baya et al., 2022). Internet use is more common among the youths who are more educated and living in more developed nations or regions. Thus, lack of access to the internet caused marginalization among the youths. All over the world the youths aged between 18–36 years of age use more internet than others (Gray, 2018). Shrinking of jobs has emerged as an issue causing serious marginalization of the unemployed and under-employed youths. Over two decades (1999–2019) the youth population (14–25 years) grew from 1 billion to 1.3 billion, but youth labor force participation declined from 568 to 497 million. This declining trend is connected with increasing enrolment in education, which would ensure a skilled labor force. But this also highlights that a large number of young people are in school, neither in training nor in gainful employment. The rate of unemployment was 13.6%, globally. About three fourth of the youths are in the informal job sector with low or unstable income (ILO, 2020). About 78.6% of youths all over the globe are of the opinion that technology access and up-gradation are essential for development and job creation. Youths also feel that "start-up ecosystem and entrepreneurship," are essential for youth development, at the same time climate change and conflicts are the most critical issues, challenging the life and opportunities of the youths across the world (Hewko, 2018).

Considering all the difficulties, and challenges, around the development of youths the global community is largely committed to working for youth development and building the future of the globe in a sustainable pattern with the motto of "no one leave behind"—the central principle of 2030 agenda of SDGs. The agenda of youth development by the United Nations is guided by the World Programme of Action for Youths (UN, 2010a, 2010b). This document has categorically mentioned fifteen priority areas for action to deal with problems of the youths, and facilitate inclusive development across the globe.

Issues Among Youths

Marginalization is a process and outcome of a number of unfavorable and restrictive factors, active in the socio-economic and political sphere. The marginalized youths suffer from a number of developmental issues and often have low achievements, and may have an unsuccessful or unsatisfactory adult life. The youths who are marginalized, are from the weaker sections of the society and often suffer from the lack of availability, accessibility, and affordability of the resources for growth. Marginalization often becomes a systemic default that undermines the rights, privilege, and social security of the weaker sections, and youths belonging to those social groups also face a similar situation. As fallout marginalization becomes deep-rooted and subsequent social issues start cropping up around the same. Similarly stereotyping happens regarding the status, role, and performance of these weaker sections of the society. The stereotypes based on gender, caste, class, creed, color of the skin, and places of origin are prominent all over the globe. Marginalization of the underprivileged section happens due to the imbalance of power in social situations that deeply impacts the outcome of development, and unequal distribution of resources gradually widen the gap between the dominant and subjugated sections of the society. Marginalization is a multi-dimensional process that has social, economic, political, cultural, and ecological references to the society and environment. Socially, the active interests of the powerful group tend to marginalize the submissive sections of the society which cause limitations of growth opportunities and life chances for the weaker sections of the society. The social exclusion process of marginalization influences the economic sphere that limits the availability and accessibility of financial resources like availability of loans, banking services from formal financial institutions, accessibility to profitable, fair-price markets, etc. As a result, the weaker sections become dependent on non-formal institutions and often become trapped in a vicious circle of loans and continue with exploitative experiences. The marginalization continues and the people become the victim of politics, where exercising their political rights and choice becomes irrelevant. Subsequently, within the social ecology the weaker, disadvantaged section becomes away from any decision-making power. Thus, the children, adolescents, and youths living in such families who are encompassed with layers of marginality, become victims of disempowering, dull environments that often strengthen the socially held stereotypes and further degrade, and dehumanize the situation. The nations and regions with low socio-economic development, disturbed political atmosphere, frequently affected by disasters, and ongoing conflict are having a higher number of marginalized youths. Within the developed nations too, there are numbers of marginalized youths due to various individual, and social factors that require special services and protection to establish equality, justice, fulfillment of rights, and ensure a sustainable future. Some of the important issues that cause the marginalization of the youths are discussed here.

- Increasing Stress And Inabilities To Cope

There are a number of factors that cause stress among the youths. The youths in academic institutions encounter stressful situations due to a number of academic demands and personal factors, while the youths out of school have stress to manage a livelihood and support the financial needs of the family.

Stress factors associated with academic engagement: Academic stressors among the youths are usually due to financial crisis, lack of career options, highly competitive job market, high parental or self-expectations, inability to cope with the demands of the academic courses, peer pressure, etc. (Hosseinkhani, et al., 2021). Academic stress is reduced with increased capacity for self-control, open communication (Jeong et al., 2019) with parents, peer support, a supportive student-centric learning environment, and additional support to the weaker section of the society, like, scholarship, supportive tutorials, provisions of free or subsidized hostel facilities, etc. Academics' success without stress is almost impossible, but, facilitating stress for the marginalized youths is essential for strengthening well-being, performance, motivation, and positive lifestyle toward the attainment of success. The lack of such consistent, special provisions, and supportive facilities with an adequate quality focus for the marginalized youths is evident all over the globe.

School dropout youths and associated factors: Many youths drop out of school at the primary and secondary levels. Dropping out is a major challenge for future developmental opportunities and to lead a successful life. There are a number of stress factors and reasons for the same. The domains of problems are related to personal, family, and community factors (Rumberger, 2013). On a personal level, abusive experience, rejection by peers, lack of ability to cope with mathematics, science, and language, inadequate academic support, and lack of motivation to continue studies cause a risk of dropping out of school at an early stage. In families, the financial crunch, demand to meet the family needs in family trade or agriculture, chronic illness or disability, death of the primary bread earner, and low value to academic attainment, often caused dropout. There are a number of community factors too that lead to dropout among the youths at the secondary level. Some of the important reasons are lack of secondary schools in the community, difficulty in transport and communication, community cultural practices and situations (e.g. early marriage, taking up a family profession like fishing, cultivation, low value toward academics, extensive addiction, higher rate of criminality, poor housing and social condition), extensive poverty, lack of welfare and social security measures. The youths who leave the school without completing graduation, or diploma, often face higher stress in subsequent life, which may cause addiction, social deviation, or earning a livelihood from menial jobs. These youths belong to marginalized families and communities and tend to be further excluded in the long term.

Mental health consequences of stressors among youths: Substance abuse, high-risk behavior, and suicidal tendencies are common mental health problems among adolescents and youths all over the globe. According to the WHO depression, anxiety and behavioral disorder are the most critical and leading causes of illness and disabilities (13% of the global burden of disease in the age group) among adolescents between 10 and 19 years. Thus, youths from the age of 15 onward are equally at a very high risk of having or developing mental health problems (WHO, 2021). In the absence of effective and efficient mechanisms to address the mental health issues, and promote positive mental health the youth encounter a number of limitations in development and often have a higher chance of mental health problems in adulthood with low achievements. Having optimal mental health is the most essential requirement for achieving the optimum level of functioning and productivity. But, the mental health problem among the youths is rising and becoming a serious concern. The National Mental Health Survey conducted in 2015–16 in India, reported the prevalence rate of mental health issues is 7.39% in the age group of 18–19 years. This figure excluded the addiction disorders (Gururaj et al., 2016). Globally it is reported that depression is the leading cause of disability among the youths and suicide is the fourth leading cause of death among the youths between 15 and 19 years. The poor mental health led to a lack of adjustment and substance abuse disorder. The onset of substance disorder happens mainly during the teenage years and it becomes dependent if continued without adequate interventions. Globally, there is a large gap in the epidemiological data, still, it is well established that 14% of the disease burden in the age group of 20–24 years, is due to alcohol and illicit substance use (Degenhardt et al., 2016). Thus, effective policy formulation and implementation of programs, rehabilitation, vocational training, stringing positive lifestyle, and coping are very much essential for the inclusion of these marginalized youths in the development program.

- Digital Dependency and Addiction

The internet, communication, and social networking are inseparable parts of the modern age. The revolution in communication technology has taken precedence over all other developments and innovations and took a central position in the life of the youths in schools and colleges across cultures and regions. The Internet is the new mode of learning, socialization, educational support, exposure, experiences, hobby, fun, attraction, entertainment, and addiction, further abuse, cause of illness, and suffering. The use of internet facilities is the need of the hour, as it opens the ocean of learning and virtually occupies a space larger than the real world that youth come across. For example, the internet has given exposure to libraries and ample reading materials, and sources of information, and given a wide space for finding new ideas, sharing hobbies, and developing friends across cultures, communities, and religions. The Internet truly made the global village where youths are active citizens, termed as "digital native and technology era" with an equal chance of positive and negative experiences and exposures. Dr. Ivan Goldberg in 1995 introduced the term "internet addiction" for pathological compulsive internet use. The DSM-V and ICD-11 mentioned the increasing problem of internet addiction and considered internet/online/video gaming as a disorder. The diagnostic criteria included the features like, preoccupation with internet games, withdrawal symptoms, increasing amount of engagement, unsuccessful attempt to control, loss of interest in other hobbies, use of internet games to escape from negative moods, and also the engagement with internet games can jeopardize other significant relationships, job, educational, and career opportunities (Goel et al., 2013). There is also substantial evidence on internet gaming transit to gambling disorder and substance abuse disorder. There are different patterns of addiction to the internet, such as gaming, gambling, chatting, being engaged in sexting, online shopping, or antisocial activity. Some traits commonly identified that increase the risk of digital addiction. There are low emotional stability, low agreeableness, and low extraversion (Kuss et al., 2013) (Öztürk et al., 2015). This also led to a number of general health issues (Floros & Ioannidis, 2021) among the younger generation particularly, that lead to further exclusion due to illness and sickness behavior. During the COVID-19 pandemic, the issue of internet addiction and dependency was reported to be a problem among many youths across different regions. Psychoeducational activities with a focus on a positive lifestyle, limit setting, engagement in physical activities, and household chores are essential (Potas et al., 2022). Digital addiction and dependency are causing a significant amount of exclusion and marginalization among the youths.

- Increasing Conflict, Unrest, and Disasters

Global warming, climate change, increasing number of hazards, and vulnerabilities are causing a greater number of disasters and conflicts over the last two decades. Human aggression and human consumption are the leading cause of an increasing number of conflicts and disasters that gravely affect the life of the youths across the nation and globe. The impact of climate change and global warming on human civilization is now absolutely evident which is threatening the coherent living of flora and fauna. Human aggression in all forms increased the number of wars, attacks, bombing, cross-border disturbances, insurgency, hate crimes, targeted attacks, and other aggressive, inhuman expressions and actions. The use of chemical weapons disasters and the threat of nuclear wars are always looming over civilization. Similarly, the unplanned consumerism, and prioritizing economic development over nature's protection are constantly increasing vulnerabilities and hazards with more occurrence of grave disasters. The degradation of the environment is also becoming a bigger threat for biological disasters, like, the spreading of pandemics. The affected region and survivors of conflicts and disasters fall back from the developmental growth for years, and they require adequate external support for revival. Youths within the survivors' community suffer due to a number of difficult issues like a broken home, threatening surroundings, halted educational engagement schooling, witnessing deaths, and personal experiences of trauma and loss (Fothergill, 2017). The youth survivors of disasters face a lot of crisis and marginalization for years and decades together. The nations and regions crippled with frequent insurgency, conflict, and war, the youths are largely used as warriors either as military or militant, while missing all their opportunities and potential for learning. The youths in the conflict-affected zone are very vulnerable to a number of abuses including severe forms of sexual violence. As the consequences of the armed conflict, the associated problems like poverty, unemployment, poor health facilities, lack of schooling, and poor governance are common issues that further marginalize the youths (UN Youths, 2019). Thus, every disaster and conflict marginalized a large number of youths in their most productive and formative age. In such situations, active measures of peacebuilding, disaster preparedness, and participation of youths in community rebuilding efforts are essential to facilitate rehabilitation and inclusion of the youth survivors of the conflict and disaster.

Alarming Facts and Figures:

- About 14 million youths were forcibly displaced due to disasters and conflict in 2011 and the number is increasing as unrest, conflict, and war are still spreading
- The Gross enrolment ratio in secondary education is 48% in the conflict-affected zone, which is 20% power from the global average. It is further less for the girls"
- The youths who became refugees due to the conflict have less than 1% enrolment in higher/tertiary education
- The quality of education in the conflict-affected areas and regions is a major challenge, as the teachers are often not trained and they are under threat too
- 90% of the casualties in the conflict related to direct conflict death are young adult males
- In case of homicide, 43% of the victims are aged between 15–29 years
- The rate of child marriage and partner violence is much higher in the fragile and conflict-affected states

Sources https://www.un.org/youthenvoy/armed-conflict/ (accessed on 6th June 2022)

- Economic Slowdown, Unemployment, and Unrest

It is about a lower rate of economic growth (GDP- Gross Domestic Product) than the previous year that often causes a decline in the productivity rate and increases in unemployment. The deepening economic crisis profoundly impacts the children, youths, and families, particularly the families belonging to different marginalized sections with poor socioeconomic backgrounds. While unemployment increases, a significant number of youths live without meaningful economic engagement and they feel left out leading to a lack of hope, frustration, anxiety, and social exclusion. The long-standing economic slowdown and the continuing problem of unemployment also give rise to other associated problems like crime, addiction, conflicts, gambling, etc. Often the mismatch between skills required in the job market and skills of the youths learned through academic courses, leads to increasing unemployment problems. Further, the lack of adequate employment for the educated youths is the major issue that is causing unrest among the youth. In developing countries, the problem of unemployment is more and it may also increase further. The cost of youth unemployment can be very high, from the social and economic development perspective. Youth unemployment causes conflict within the family situation and inter-generational poverty may rise high. Promoting safe, productive, decent working conditions, adequate wages, and a right-based framework has always been highlighted by ILO (ILO, 2018). Unless the engagement of youths in productive employment is considered at the center of social policies and programs and the aggregate demand for labor in the job market is expanding, it is not possible to include and integrate the disadvantaged youths into the labor market for gainful employment.

- Lack of Adequate Educational Facilities and Vocational Skill Building Opportunities

Education is the key to empowerment and dealing with the inclusion of marginalized youths. Empowerment deals with the ability to influence the surroundings positively and control the events in favor of self without compromising others' interests and well-being (Barker, 2003). Thus, an education that drives the empowerment with the inculcation of relevant knowledge and skills is essential for the youths to make them suitable for the employment market and live a satisfactory adult life. Education is also essential for the holistic growth that encourages life skills (e.g., analytical abilities, critical thinking, creative thinking, etc.) compassion, respect for others, tolerance, and pluralistic attitude, and makes them free from stereotypical thinking and prejudices. Thus, effective and efficient education is pivotal for nations' development and strengthening the foundation of the growth of the population. Education and learning in childhood influence the growth at the youth age and further help in successful adulthood. Developing employable, vocational skills need to be part of the education system, for enhancing youths' abilities to become suitably employable or become entrepreneurs. Unfortunately, the underdeveloped and developing nations always have a low focus on primary, secondary, or higher education, often spend less in the education sector, has poor infrastructure and support facilities like libraries, laboratories, qualified teachers, hostels, facilities for extra-curricular activities, and safe, secured learning environment. Without having such facilities, the youths belonging to poor families, live in remote villages, and belong to ostracized communities face the issues of marginalization.

The Dimensions of Marginalization

Marginalization is multi-dimensional. The social system operates within the power structure causing a number of conflicts among individuals, communities, and nations to dominate over resources and facilities. Such a social system is always active and throughout some people outside the mainstream cause marginalization. The marginalization of youths is thus analyzed here from multiple dimensions to explore the scenario and realities.

- **Regional Diversity**: The youths belonging to underdeveloped nations, and regions are more marginalized than those living in developed nations and regions. Regional disparity in youth development is quite evident from the lack of different facilities that youths need to have for their development, like educational opportunities, facilities for vocational training, internet access, job opportunities, and mobility. There are a number of restrictive socio-economic and political forces too. The low-developed region with a higher poverty rate often suffers from corruption, high crime rate, addiction, and insurgency. The youths of these nations or regions become the major victim of the situation and continue to face issues of marginalization.
- **Marginalization Based On Identities**: Individual identity is determined by a number of ascribed and achieved statuses. While the achieved status depends on the facilities and opportunities that someone receives, ascribed status is determined at the time of birth. There are a number of ascribed statuses that cause marginalization, like, ethnicity, skin color, religion, caste (in India), language,

community identities, nation or region of origin, etc. Particularly the migrants and refugee youths widely face marginalization in different situations. Like, in the USA the marginalization of African American youths often becomes a major issue that led to the social movement of "black lives matter" (Baskin-Sommers, et al., 2021). Marginalization of youths based on ethnic identity is a global issue in different regions. In Europe, the Roma community and itinerant travelers are quite marginalized and special interventions are made to ensure their betterment (European Commission, 2018). In India caste-based marginalization is quite common which leads to the subjugation of *dalit* and minority youths (Sinha, 2020).

- **Gender-Based Marginalization**: Gender discrimination is the root of gender-based marginalization across the globe. Discrimination against females exists in almost all patriarchal cultures, where women's rights, privileges, opportunities, and power are restricted and controlled, by family norms, religious practices, and even by state regulations. Such discrimination critically restricts the life chances of young women and the third gender. Masculine supremacy is often a cultural legacy that subjugates the young female more and the third gender too. Thus, the under-representation of young women in salaried jobs in the formal sector, in political leadership, and in administrative or entrepreneur positions is quite evident. Similarly, the provision of health services, education facilities, and economic opportunities are less for women and the third gender. "Feminization of poverty" crucially denoted the subjugation of women (Christensen, 2019). The concept of "missing women" propagated by Amartya Sen also pointed out the gender-based oppression from the time of birth (Croll, 2019). Though there are incidences, where men are discriminated against, but discrimination against women is comparatively much higher (Francesca, 2019). Youths of the society face the brunt of the problem and youths need to be effectively used for ending the discrimination.
- **Marginalization Based On Sexual Choices**: Marginalization based on sexual choices: Sexual orientation and identity are important aspects of youth development. Sexual choices to live as LGBTQ that are beyond the binary norms of gender are also a strong reason for discrimination. Often the LGBTQ youths face discrimination in family and public life in educational institutions and offices. The youths of LGBTQ communities report higher incidences of depression, anxiety, the tendency to self-harm, and suicidal attempt. These youths have higher perceived discrimination causing depression and self-harming tendencies (Almeida et al., 2009). In different critical situations like disasters, war, or during the COVID pandemic the LGBTQ youths faced disproportionately higher stressful situations (Bhadra, 2021).
- **Disabilities, Limitations in Physical Health Leading to Marginalization**: According to CRPD "people with disabilities as those who have long-term physical, mental, intellectual or sensory impairments, which when combined with negative attitudes or environmental barriers, prevent them from taking a full and active role in society." The youths with disabilities are the most marginalized groups, and face a number of social restrictions, lack of opportunities, discriminatory practices, social stigma, and neglect, at family and community levels.

Worldwide the number of youths with disabilities is about 180 to 220 million, and 80% of them are living in developing countries (UN, 2022). Such discrimination further becomes complicated with gender, ethnicity, and caste dimensions in addition to poverty-stricken life.

- **Low Educational Attainment and Vocational Skills**: Effective, quality education, learning, training, and vocational skill-building are the driving force of development. These are essential for maintaining a healthy living with adequate income. The youths without essential advanced knowledge and vocational skills as per the demand of the job market face exclusion and marginalization. Invariably, other social variables like poverty, lack of development, facilities for education, lack of safety and security, frequent disasters, political unrest, poor governance, and higher corruption decrease the opportunities for the youths to attain higher order skills. Such youths become unproductive economic youth (Bisht & Falguni, 2021). Often youths from poor families have a number of family responsibilities and many of them play the role of bread earner from an early age in their life. These youths continue to suffer from marginalization throughout their life cycle. They face a number of negative life events like injuries, illness, financial loss, forced displacement, frequent job loss, harassment, etc.
- **Victimization of Youths and Marginalization**: A large number of youths are victims of trafficking, violence, abuse, abduction, forced labor, forced marriage, and many inhuman treatments. Victimization of youths leads to a number of physical, psychological, and social disabilities that cripple their developmental potential within a restrictive environment. As discussed earlier, incidents like disaster, war, and displacement cause various types of victimization of the youths. In war, conflict, and disaster the sexual exploitation of young women is quite common. Similarly, young males face severe physical torture and sexual violence that absolutely jeopardize their capabilities. Further, in any society, the incidences like, peer violence, substance addiction, cyberbullying are major issues of victimization among youths. The youths suffering from such mal-treatment tend to have mental health problems and they become marginalized.

The dimensions of marginalization are multiple and the facts are correlated. The issues of marginalization are like a continuum and require designed, planned interventions with the engagement of multiple stakeholders to bring changes and facilitate well-being toward empowerment. Ending marginalization depends on the implementation of effective empowerment strategies.

Youth Empowerment and Well-Being

There are a number of essential prerequisites for the healthy, inclusive, sustainable development of youths. A supportive, safe, empowering learning environment is crucial for healthy living and maintaining positive lifestyle choices. The physical aspects include adequate nutrition, safe house, clean and hygienic sanitation facilities, medical facilities, adequate mobility, and communication services. Psychological development depends on learning opportunities, a safe nurturing atmosphere at home and community, educational opportunities, effective schooling, subsequent higher education, and engagement in sports and cultural activities. The social factors that contribute to the development of youths specifically include a cohesive atmosphere, opportunities for the development of life skills, leadership, freedom of choices and expression, and an atmosphere of mutual respect, acceptance, trust, and pluralistic values. There are multiple factors that are effective in combination to contribute toward the empowerment of youths.

- **Effective Participation**: Participation is one of the fundamental rights. Through active and effective participation youths can be an important source of innovation, change, and development. Participation of youths is a key agenda for the UN in various sustainable development initiatives. The development of youth organizations is an essential step to facilitating the emancipation of youths at various social and political dimensions. Youths' political participation is an essential aspect of strengthening the democratic structure of any society. Youths often played an important role in demanding, restoring, and strengthening the democratic structure of society. Their participation in economic (livelihood) activities is also important for development, as youths are the powerhouse of ideas, energy, and innovation and become the driving force for nations' development. Youths are a vital force for peace building, working together, technology revolutions, and bridging the gaps between communities and nations.
- **Supportive Community Structure for Healthy Living**: This included the facilities for effective physical, psychological, and social development. Further, a cohesive, politically and socially stable state of a nation is essential for successful development. A supportive environment ideally becomes stimulating for youths to flourish with their open ideas and creativity. A nation free from prejudices (religious, racial, linguistic, sexual, etc.), and with strong commitments toward human rights, and equality, can facilitate supportive developmental opportunities, better life chances, and open choices for the youths. Accountable governance, adequate budgeting, commitments to gender equality, and creating facilities for education, sports, and cultural development are essential for integrated youth development.
- **Promoting Peace Education and Community Cohesion**: Extensive damage is caused by conflicts in young minds. It is not just the war, rather the incidences of violence between the caste, class, ethnic, religious, linguistic, and regional groups cause severe unrest and trauma in the young mind. Peace education is an essential process for promoting knowledge, skills, attitude, and values that are crucial for behavior changes to enable children and youths to avoid conflict and violence thereby resolving conflicts peacefully and creating an environment of harmony and tranquillity to develop healthy relationships. This ensures social inclusion and integration of different groups in healthy social relationships. Schools help in shaping social norms, cultural values, and attitudes. Thus, peace education can bring a long-term change in society to end any form of violence and help in developing the value of pluralism, encouraging tolerance and acceptance, thereby

ending different forms of marginalization. Peace education should be framed according to the local, cultural, social, historical, and political context, and ensure an effective outcome. In this context youth's role in peacekeeping, peace-making, and peace-building is crucial (International Alert, 2020). Peacekeeping is about maintaining peace, thus there is no eruption of violence. Peace-making is about proactive measures for quick solutions to conflicts, restoration of discipline, and a non-threatening atmosphere for all. Peace-building focuses on the reduction of barriers, bridging the possibilities of conflicts, and achieving sustainable peace. Peace education in school is connected with achieving peace in society, and the political stability of the region or nation (Bhadra, 2022).

- **Promoting Life Skills, Embedded with Morals and Values**: "Life skills are abilities for adaptive and positive behaviour that enable individuals to deal effectively with the demands and challenges of everyday life" (Bharath & Kumar, 2010; WHO, 1997, 2005). Life skills development is one of the most effective interventions for building resiliency among youths. The pedagogical approach to life skills has enormous potential for developing positive coping abilities toward healthy living and maintaining well-being even during challenging times. The specific learning outcome and skill development for the participants are always the key focus for designing the LSE sessions. The youths are actively engaged through an activity during the session that may be role play, drawing, group game, group discussion, etc. The activities encourage the participants to resolve the given problem as a group through discussion, reflection, debate, sharing, exchanging views, and being psychically, psychologically active. Thereby, participatory learning takes place in a cooperative, supportive atmosphere and marginalized youths get equal chances to participate, voice their concerns and seek support (Bhadra, 2018). Such learning facilitates inclusive understanding and development in a sustainable pattern.
- **Sports and Games For Holistic Development**: Sports positively channelize the energy of the youths and are an important medium to learn self-regulation, group norms, controlling emotions, being focused, and being achievers. Group sports are an important medium to learn the role of an individual in a team and support the team for the best. Sports are inclusive in nature and bring the sports persons and athletes to the same space to work and evolve through gaining skills and by their performances. Sports events are equally important to bring the youths from different backgrounds to work together. Sports teach to accept defeat positively and again raise toward development. Biologically sports are pleasurable activities that facilitate the secretion of happy hormones for well-being and healthy development. Facilitating healthy sports spirits is an important dimension for youth development and ending marginalization, toward inclusive sustainable growth.
- **Facilitating Digital Competencies and Empowerment**: In twenty-first century digital capability become an important determinant of psychosocial well-being and adjustment as digital dependency of children and adolescents has increased over the last few years. Further, the pandemic situation has made digital capability relevant and visible to society (Iivari, 2020). Digital empowerment is about providing knowledge, skills, and abilities to use the digital device and access

relevant, appropriate, and useful information, and thereby, become a responsible citizen. Digital empowerment also encompasses the capacity of an user to be engaged in the virtual world without compromising real-life situations and maintaining a harmonious balance. Imparting knowledge about digital dependency and addiction is also essential to ensure the psychosocial well-being of children and adolescents. During the pandemic, schooling through online classes made the students highly dependent on digital devices and increased the risk of inappropriate use like gaming, sexting, chatting, or extensive use of social media. At this juncture, due to the stark digital divide, many students are away from school and many are addicted to surfing inappropriate content. Therefore, digital empowerment is most crucial for developing responsible online behavior and engagement, and also facilitating basic digital device to students who are unable to be part of the digital world.

- **Effective Youth Policy and Programme Implementation**: Policies are crucial to framing the program. Aligning with the UNFPA strategy for adolescents and youths (UNFPA, 2013), many countries have developed or redesigned their youth policies for effective action for the empowerment of youths and sustainable development. Youth policies are always futuristic to shape the future of the nation. Essentially the youth policies are having few important visions, like, sustainable development, holistic growth (physical, psychological, and sexual development), human rights protection (freedom of expression, protection from violence, abuse), social security (health, educational services), healthy living (adequate nutrition, safe environment, leadership development), strengthening possibilities for fulfilments of potentials, etc. Realization of policies requires substantial budget allocation, effective programming, a plan for implementation, development of supportive infrastructure (for health, education sports, training, etc.), training of manpower, continuous research, documentation, and tracking of the changes. Thus, youth development should always be a core agenda of any government.

Youths for Sustainable Development

Youths are considered the driving force for the achievements of the SDGs. They are the game changers as young people can drive the development with new energy, motivation, ideas, and heightened aspirations. The opportunities of the marginalized youths for securing a decent living are always a big challenge. A match between the education, training, skills development, and livelihood opportunities through seeking a job or by the start-up of an enterprise is most desirable. It is essential that youths drive the development, that they value their potential, and contribute to the sustainable development of their communities and nation. Youths as volunteers have often been engaged to bring many innovative local solutions to global problems. "Youths for SGDs" event of 2020 held in Bangkok focused on pandemic and environmental issues and discussed several innovative local solutions on "waste management and medical waste, energy conservation and accessibility and air quality" (UNDP, 2020). The following Diagram 23.1, adopted from a poster developed by the Ministry of Youth and Sports' National Youth Council, Nepal, and the United Nations Nepal in 2018, illustrated the role of youths as both beneficiaries and actors of SDGs and highlighted the importance of participation of youths in successful attainment of SDGs (UNDP, 2018). Diagram 23.1 explains the role of youths and inclusion of the marginalized youths for strengthening the inclusive approach to development.

Way Forward to End the Marginalization of Youths

Ending all forms of marginalization, and inequalities are a matter of commitment of the governments, and civil society organizations to implement the inclusive program from grassroots organizations to national, and international level. There are four important points for ending marginalization shown in Diagram 23.2 (Model for mainstreaming of the marginalized youths). These are (i) dimensions of the program for youth empowerment (ii) participation and engagement of youths at different levels (iii) domains of skill-building for marginalized youths (iv) essential documents for youth development.

- **Dimensions of the Program for Youth Empowerment**: The youth's empowerment program should be designed on four basic premises for the inclusion of the marginalized youths and strengthening grounds for empowerment. First, the promotion of social justice should be the primary focus that inculcates the value of equality, and equity and creates opportunities for everyone, thus no one is left behind. The ascribed status at birth should not limit the life chances to get facilities and services to raise and fulfill the potential. Second, the protection of human rights values and principles is an essential component for strengthening the democratic premises for the inclusion of the marginalized with their strong voices, opinions, and participation in social, economic, and political life. Human rights protection is also about strengthening the efforts toward inclusion, supporting the value of pluralism, and attitude of tolerance to differences of opinions with respect. Third, technological innovations and inclusions of the youths from the marginalized sections to adapt to the changing needs of the twenty-first century. Marginalization is marked by backwardness, inability, and inefficiencies. Any program for youths must be designed in line with the high technology innovation and adaptation for promoting positive coping, healthy lifestyle choices, and well-being. Fourth, strengthening the opportunities for decent work and livelihood promotions. Options for job or entrepreneurship are crucial for effective sustainable livelihood practice. A livelihood must ensure decent earning, and production of consumable quality-oriented goods or services and must gain adequate social recognition.

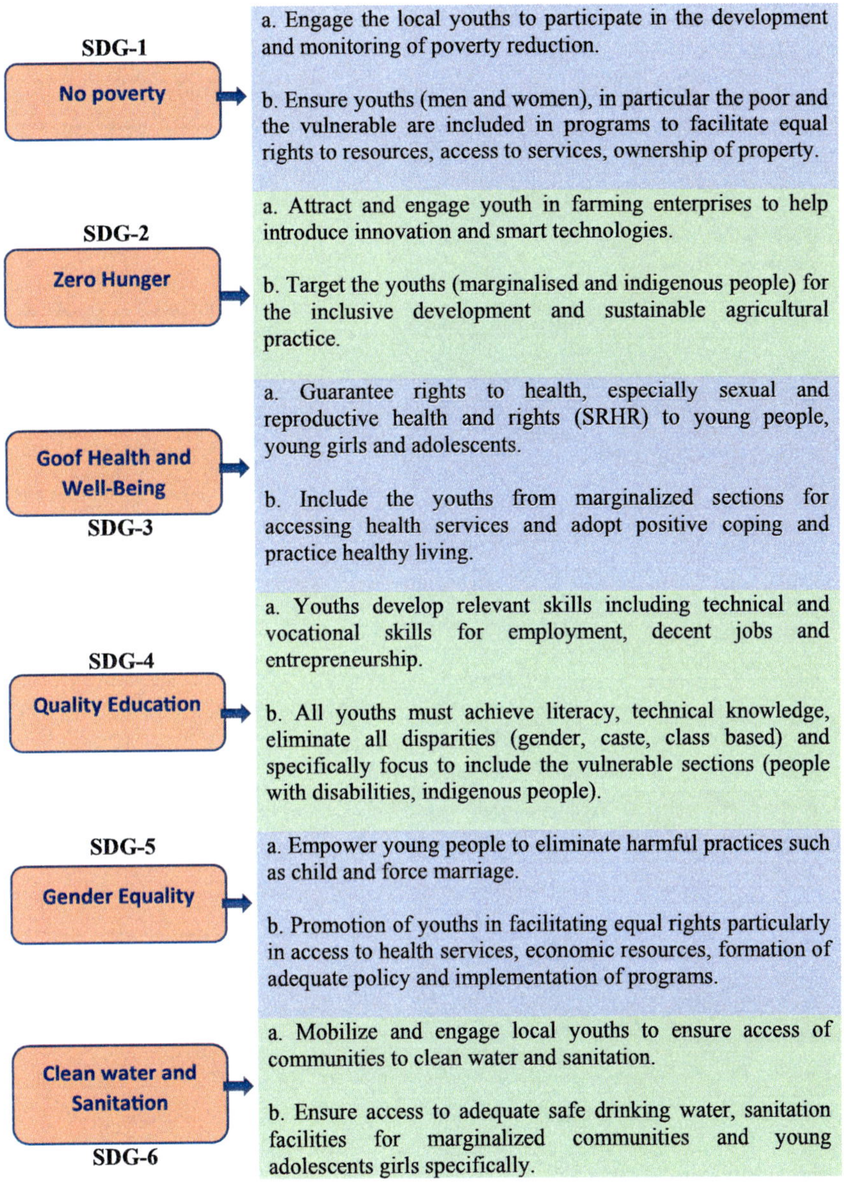

Diagram 23.1 Youth's Role toward SDGS, and Inclusion of marginalized sections

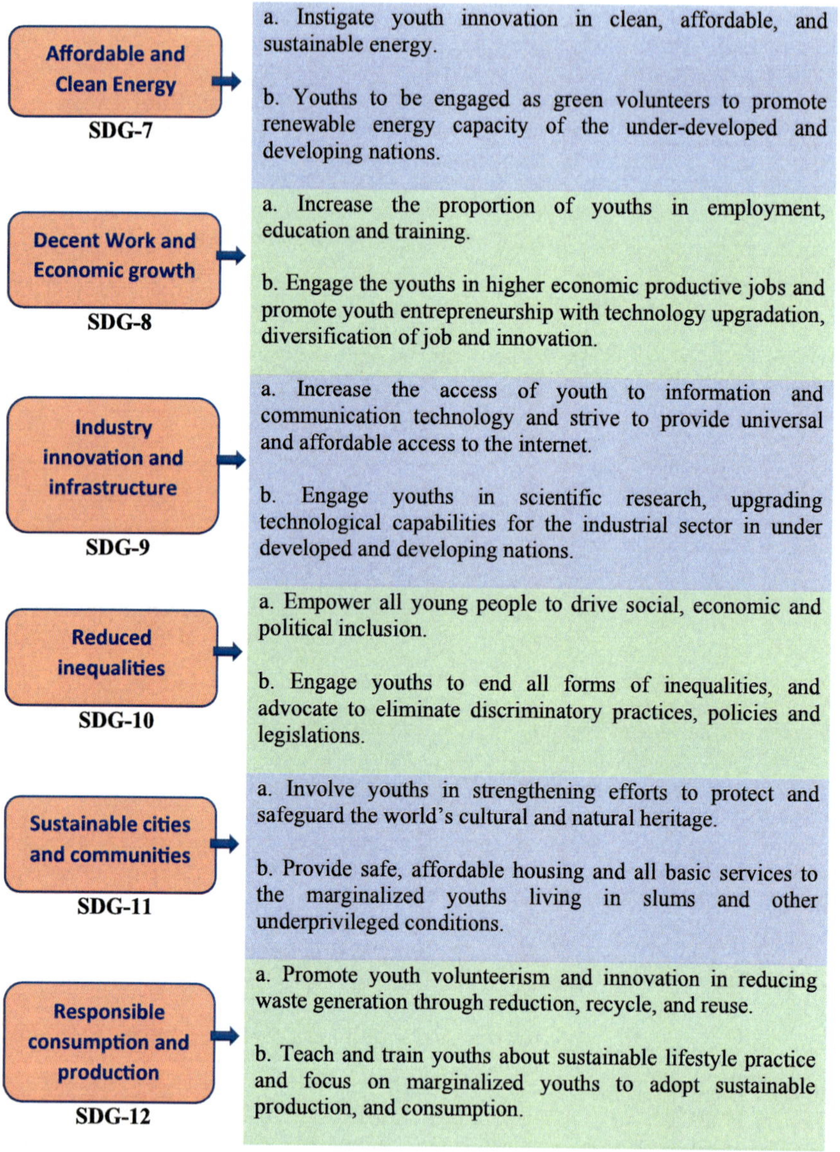

Diagram 23.1 (continued)

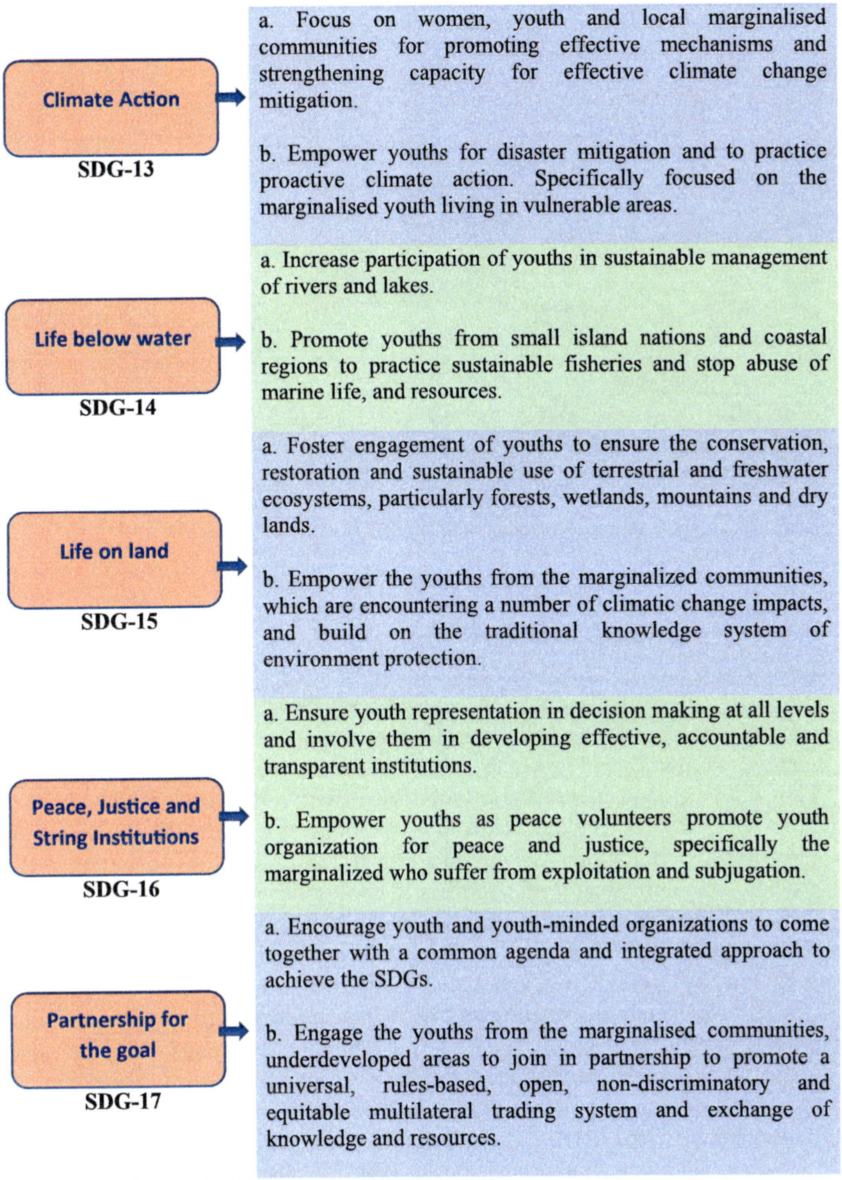

a. Role of youths towards SDGs.
b. Inclusion of marginalised youths for attaining SDGs

Diagram 23.1 (continued)

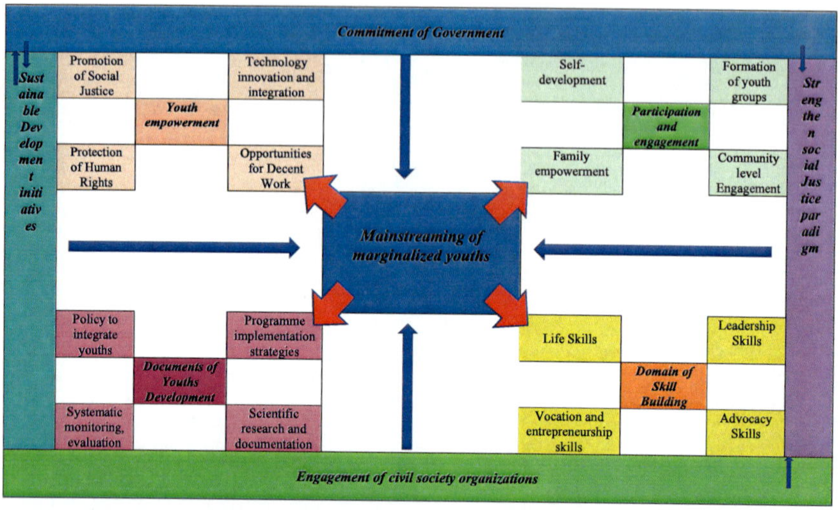

Diagram 23.2 Model for mainstreaming of the marginalized youths

- **Participation and Engagement of The Youths at Different Levels**: Effective, meaningful participation of youths determines the future of the nation. Participation of youth is related to democratic citizenship, personal & professional development, and active pro-social engagements. Similarly, engagement is about contribution for making a better world. There are four important aspects of participation and engagement for youth empowerment and to deal with marginalization. First, the development of self as an individual to have self-respect, confidence, and pro-social behavior. Having adequate education, skills, maintaining good health (physical, psychological, social, and spiritual), and ideas for better change are crucial at the individual level. Abilities to think independently and innovatively are crucial for taking part in decision-making or assuming the role of leader. Second, the formation of youth groups and their participation in social, cultural, economic, and political life are crucial for an inclusive approach. Development of youth organizations, engaging youths in different forums (in educational institutions, in economic activities, in political forums), and strengthening the voice of the youths are essential at the group level. Youths are important messengers of cultural exchange, promoting peace. Participation of youth groups, in social movements, is also essential and advocating the rights of the marginalized, for making a better equalitarian just society. Third, focus on family empowerment by extending endowment (the set of skills and resources owned by a family) and entitlement (provisions of receiving services from government, institutions, civil society organizations, and through market exchange) status. In any family, youths are important members who are expected to perform many roles and responsibilities. Thus, a focus on family strengthening and empowerment also facilitates the growth and inclusion of the marginalized sections. The marginalized families with poverty and multiple social exclusions often face various obstacles that hinder the youths to attain their full potential. Fourth, youths' participation and engagements at the community level are very crucial for promoting the youth volunteers for community development. Youths become an important force to organize community events, monitor development programs, provide support to vulnerable groups, and to ensure better accountability for the government and local authorities. Youths' participation in governance has a high potential to strengthen democracy.

- **Domains of Skill-Building for Marginalized Youths**: Skills are abilities to deal with problems and challenges, abilities to perform a task effectively, and the capacity to understand, interpret, and respond as per the demands of the situation and context. Skills are learned through experience and harnessed through repeated practice. Marginalized youths need various skills for enhancing their abilities to function effectively and perform complex tasks with efficiency. The marginalized youths, therefore, need to be supported with four important skill sets. First, life skills are essential for strengthening a set of ten mother skills, namely decision-making, problem-solving, creative thinking, critical, self-awareness, empathy, effective communication, interpersonal relationships, coping with stress, and coping with emotions (WHO, 1997). Life skills must be embedded in the education from the school and the focus should be maintained that the youths learn through a participatory process. Second, marginalized youths specifically should be trained to gain leadership skills. The leader must be able to communicate and influence others, engage his followers with commitments to a cause, and set goals to achieve promptly. A democratic value is always better for strengthening the grounds for leadership in the long term. Third, imparting vocational and entrepreneurship skills is essential for the marginalized youths to join in the livelihood and economic sector meaningfully. Vocational skills should be relevant to the time and context, as well as entrepreneurship initiatives should be supported with financial capital, marketing linkages, technological support, and expert guidance (according to the sector) opinion. Fourth, skill for advocacy among the marginalized youths is also very much essential for strengthening the voice of the marginalized at different forum that can facilitate adequate policy development, budget allocation, and program implementation. For social advocacy, generating data on the issue, documenting cases of oppression, and analyzing the same to influence and convince the masses and leaders is essential. Different mediums like media advocacy, political advocacy, use of power strategy, campaigns, and representation are crucial for raising the voice of marginalized youths.
- **Essential Documents for Youth Development**: Commitment toward development from all the stakeholders can bring a change in the status of the marginalized youths. Toward this direction, the framing of four basic documents that become pathways and milestones becomes crucial. First, a youth policy for sustainable development and engagement of the marginalized youths should focus on moral standards (inclusive, egalitarian, rights-based, empowering, etc.), normative values (inclusion of cultural values, indigenous knowledge,

gender equality, strengthening family and community engagements, etc.), welfare bureaucracy (including the offices, staff, budget, operational infrastructure, etc.), and promoting utilitarianism (strengthening social justice, democratic system, freedom, extending opportunities, etc.). Second, frame the program implementation strategy for the inclusion of the marginalized youths. The program should have short- and long-term action plans for achieving the visions set in the policy documents. The well-defined goal for inclusion of the marginalized youths and implementation of the program with SMART (specific, measurable, attainable, rational, time-bound) objectives are pivotal. Third, adequate data management to track the changes with a process of regular monitoring and evaluation would be the criteria for realizing the inclusion and empowerment of vulnerable youths. A program can be a response to a particular problem or for the holistic development of the youths in a state or nation. Thus, the fourth important set of documents comes from scientific research and continuous efforts of innovation (technological, economic, social, etc.). Research is needed to understand the emerging issues and also to forecast the problems in the forthcoming decades. Research brings innovations. Therefore, substantial scientific research and innovations are crucial with a focus on youths' empowerment. Similarly, opportunities for research for youths from the marginalized sections should be created as they become the innovators to design the future in various academic disciplines and could bring practical interphase in the field of practice.

Conclusion

Ending the issue of marginalization in any form among the youths is essential to reduce and end the inequality gap that exists in any society due to several systemic defaults that are driven by power politics, vested interests, corruption, lack of commitment of the government, and embedded discriminatory practices. Pertinent to mention that exclusion of youths is an outcome of various socio-economic and political realities. Ultimately, a safe, secured, healthy living that promises well-being for all is desirable to achieve the targets as visioned through the SDGs. Therefore, comprehensive measures are needed to end marginalization focusing on empowerment and well-being. Achieving and maintaining adequate holistic health (physical, psychological, social, and spiritual) is pivotal for well-being that contributes to maintaining a high level of functionality toward nation building, and sustainable development. Hence, effective measures toward the inclusion of marginalized youths are necessary for designing the way forward based on the principles of human rights and social justice.

References

Croll, E. J. (2019). Amartya Sen's 100 million missing women. *Oxford Development Studies*, 225-244. https://doi.org/10.1080/13600810120088840

Almeida, J., Johnson, R. M., Corliss, H. L., Molna, B. E., & Azrael, D. (2009). Emotional distress among LGBT youth: The influence of perceived discrimination based on sexual orientation. *Journal of Youth and Adolescence, 38*(7), 1001–1014. https://doi.org/10.1007/s10964-009-9397-9

Barker, R. L. (2003). *The Social Work Dictionary* (5th ed.). National Association of Social Worker.

Baskin-Sommers, A., Simmons, C., Conley, M., Chang, S.-A., Estrada, S., & Collins, M. (2021). Adolescent civic engagement: Lessons from black lives matter. *Proceedings of the National Academy of Sciences, 118*(41), 1–3. https://doi.org/10.1073/pnas.2109860118

Bhadra, S. (2018). Life Skills Education (LSE) in a volatile. In S. Deb (Ed.), *Positive Schooling and Child Development* (pp. 205–232). Springer.

Bhadra, S. (2021). Exploring dimensions of sexual issues in disasters and conflicts: Need to bridge the gaps between policy and practice. *Sexologies*, 1-7. https://doi.org/10.1016/j.sexol.2021.11.006.

Bhadra, S. (2022). Psychosocial support for protection of children in disasters. In S. Deb, *Child Safety, Welfare and Well-being: Issues and Challenges* (pp. 453- 484). Springer nature.

Bharath, S., & Kumar, K. K. (2010). Empowering adolescents with life skills education in schools-School mental health programme: Does it work? *Indian Journal of Psychiatry, 42*(4), 344–349.

Bisht, N., & Falguni, P. (2021). Exploring the magnitude of inclusion of Indian youth in the world of work based on choices of educational attainment. *Journal of Economics and Development, 23*(2), 128–143. https://doi.org/10.1108/JED-08-2020-0114

Christensen, M. (2019). Feminization of poverty: Causes and implications. In W. Leal Filho, A. Azul, L. Brandli, P. Özuyar, & T. Wall, *Gender Equality. Encyclopedia of the UN sustainable development goals*. Springer. https://doi.org/10.1007/978-3-319-70060-1_6-1

European Commission. (2018). *European social fund*. https://ec.europa.eu/esf/main.jsp?catId=63&langId=en

Degenhardt, L., Stockings, E., Patton, G., Hall, D., & Lynskey, M. (2016). The increasing global health priority of substance use in young people. *Lancet Psychiatry, 3*(3), 251–264. https://doi.org/10.1016/S2215-0366(15)00508-8

Floros, G. D., & Ioannidis, K. (2021). Editorial: The Impact of Online Addiction on General Health, Well-Being and Associated Societal Costs. *Frontiers in Public Health, 9*(676498), 1–2. https://doi.org/10.3389/fpubh.2021.676498

Fothergill, A. (2017). Children, youth, and disaster. *Oxford Research Encyclopedia of Natural Hazard Science*, 2–7. https://doi.org/10.1093/acrefore/9780199389407.013.23

Francesca, M. (2019). Are the processes underlying discrimination the same for women and men? A critical review of congruity models of gender discrimination. *Frontiers in Psychology, 10*(469), 1664–1078. https://doi.org/10.3389/fpsyg.2019.00469

Goel, D., Subramanyam, A., & Kamath, R. (2013). A study on the prevalence of internet addiction and its association with psychopathology in Indian adolescents. *Indian Journal of Psychiatry, 55*(2), 140-143. https://doi.org/10.4103/0019-5545.111451

Gómez-Baya, D., Grasmeijer, J. A., López-Bermúdez, E., Gaspar de Matos, M., & Mendoza, R. (2022). Positive youth development and internet use in a sample of Spanish adolescents. *Frontiers in Pediatrics, 10*(1), 2296–2360. https://doi.org/10.3389/fped.2022.842928

Gray, A. (2018). *What you need to know about the world's youth, in 7 charts*. https://www.weforum.org/agenda/2018/08/what-you-need-to-know-about-the-worlds-young-people-in-7-charts/

Gururaj, G., Varghese, V., & Benegal, V. (2016). *National mental health survey of India, 2015–16: Prevalence, patterns and outcomes*. National Institute of Mental Health and Neuro Sciences.

Hewko, J. (2018). *This is what millennials want in 2018*. World Economic Focrum. https://www.weforum.org/agenda/2018/01/this-is-what-millennials-want-in-2018/

Hosseinkhani, Z., Hassanabadi, H. R., Parsaeian, M., Osooli, M., Assari, S., & Nedjat, S. (2021). Sources of academic stress among Iranian adolescents: A multilevel study from Qazvin City. *Iran. Egyptian Pediatric Association Gazette, 69*(6), 2–9. https://doi.org/10.1186/s43054-021-00054-2

Iivari, N. (2020). Empowering children to make and shape our digital futures—from adults creating technologies to children transforming cultures. *The International Journal of Information and Learning Technology, 37*(5), 279–293. https://doi.org/10.1108/IJILT-03-2020-0023

ILO. (2018). *24. Youth employment*. https://www.ilo.org/global/topics/dw4sd/themes/youth-employment/lang--en/index.htm

ILO. (2020). *Global employment trends for youth 2020: Technology and the future of jobs*. International Labour Office. https://www.ilo.org/wcmsp5/groups/public/---dgreports/---dcomm/---publ/documents/publication/wcms_737648.pdf

International Alert. (2020). *Peace education in formal schools-Why is it important and how can it be done?* International Alert and British Council. https://www.international-alert.org/sites/default/files/Peace-Education-Schools-Formal-EN-2020.pdf

Jeong, E. J., Ferguson, C. J., & Lee, S. J. (2019). Pathological gaming in young adolescents: A longitudinal study focused on academic stress and self-control in South Korea. *Journal of Youth and Adolescence, 48*(12), 2333–2342. https://doi.org/10.1007/s10964-019-01065-4

Kuss, D. J., Griffiths, M. D., & Binder, J. F. (2013). Internet addiction in students: Prevalence and risk factors. *Computers in Human Behavior 29, 29*(3), 959–966.

Lerner, R. M. (2009). The positive youth development perspective: Theoretical and empirical bases of a strengths-based approach to adolescent development. In S. J. Lopez, & C. R. Snyder, *The Oxford Handbook of Positive Psychology* (pp. 149–163). Oxford: Oxford University Press.

Öztürk, C., Bektas, M., Ayar, D., Öztornacı, B. Ö., & Yağcı, D. (2015). Association of personality traits and risk of internet addiction in adolescents. *Asian Nursing Research, 9*(2), 120–124. https://doi.org/10.1016/j.anr.2015.01.001

Potas, N., Açıkalın, ŞN., Erçetin, ŞŞ, Koçtürk, N., Nilay, N., Çevik, M. S., & Görgülü, D. (2022). Technology addiction of adolescents in the COVID-19 era: Mediating effect of attitude on awareness and behavior. *Current Psychology, 41*(4), 1687–1703. https://doi.org/10.1007/s12144-021-01470-8

Rumberger, R. W. (2013). *Poverty and high school dropouts; The impact of family and community poverty on high school dropouts*. https://www.apa.org/pi/ses/resources/indicator/2013/05/poverty-dropouts

Sinha, C. (2020). Dalit leadership, collective pride and struggle for social change among educated dalits: Contesting the legitimacy of social class mobility approach. *Contemporary Voice of Dalit, 12*(1), 52–70. https://doi.org/10.1177/2455328X19898411

UN. (2010a). *Definition of youths*. https://www.un.org/esa/socdev/documents/youth/fact-sheets/youth-definition.pdf

UN. (2010b). *World programme of action for youths*. United Nations. https://www.un.org/esa/socdev/unyin/documents/wpay2010b.pdf

UN. (2017). *International Youth Day*. https://www.un.org/en/observances/youth-day/background#:~:text=In%201998%2C%20a%20resolution%20proclaiming,8%2D12%20August%201998).

UN. (2019). *International Youth Day, 12 August 2019*. Department of Economic and Social Affairs, Population Division, United Nations. https://www.un.org/development/desa/youth/wp-content/uploads/sites/21/2019/08/WYP2019_10-Key-Messages_GZ_8AUG19.pdf

UN. (2022). *Youth with disabilities*. https://www.un.org/development/desa/youth/youth-with-disabilities.html

UNDP. (2018). *UNDP, Nepal*. https://www.undp.org/nepal/publications/youth-and-sdgs

UNDP. (2020). *Youths for SDGs, Thailand*. https://www.undp.org/thailand/news/youths-sdgs?utm_source=EN&utm_medium=GSR&utm_content=US_UNDP_PaidSearch_Brand_English&utm_campaign=CENTRAL&c_src=CENTRAL&c_src2=GSR&gclid=Cj0KCQjwn4qWBhCvARIsAFNAMigkYKVO1LMn21SqNHRREMBL-tAzC1ergWZGOR_U7HHNVdbQqhyB3qUaAs

UNESCO. (2019). *New methodology shows that 258 million children, adolescents and youth are out of school.* UNESCO. http://uis.unesco.org/sites/default/files/documents/new-methodology-shows-258-million-children-adolescents-and-youth-are-out-school.pdf

UNFPA. (2013). *UNFPA Strategy on adolescents and youth towards realizing the full potential of adolescents and youth.* United Nations Population Fund. https://www.unfpa.org/sites/default/files/resource-pdf/UNFPA%20Adolescents%20and%20Youth%20Strategy.pdf

WHO. (1997). *Life skills education for children and adolescents in schools; Program on mental health.* World Health Organization, Mental Health Division.

WHO. (2005). *Child and adolescent mental health policies and plans. Mental health policy and service guidance package.* WHO.

WHO. (2021). *Adolescent mental health.* Retrieved May 31, 2022, from World Health Organization https://www.who.int/news-room/fact-sheets/detail/adolescent-mental-health.

UN Youths. (2019). *Youth and Armed conflict.* United Nations Department of Economic and Social Affairs. https://www.un.org/esa/socdev/documents/youth/fact-sheets/youth-armed-conflict.pdf

Dr. Subhasis Bhadra , is Associate Professor of the Department of Social Work, and Head of the Department of Sports Psychology, Central University of Rajasthan, India. Dr. Bhadra completed Masters of Social Work (Vidyasagar University), and holds M.Phil and Ph.D. in Psychiatric Social Work (NIMHANS, Bangalore). He started teaching from Assam Central University 2009 and then taught seven and half years in Gautam Buddha University, Greater NOIDA, Uttar Pradesh. Dr. Bhadra started his career in 2001 from intervention in Gujarat earthquake and subsequently worked in Gujarat conflict, Indian-Ocean Tsunami, Kashmir earthquake and ongoing conflict, Mumbai Train Blast, Uttarakhand flash flood, and in various disaster affected areas in India in other Asian countries like, China, Japan, Indonesia, Myanmar, through different organizations, namely, Care India, American Red Cross (India Delegation), International Federation of Red Cross, Oxfam India, Action Aid, International Medical Corps. During the ongoing pandemic, COVID-19, Dr Bhadra is actively engaged in providing psychosocial support to different groups through NGOs and Government Institutions. His research interests include peace building, youth empowerment, psychosocial support, disaster mental health, community & school mental health and sustainable development. In his credit there are a number of academic articles and book chapters, 2 books published by nationally and internationally reputed publishers.

Chapter 24
Risky Sexual Behaviors Among Unmarried Youth in India: Evidences from National Family Health Survey, 2019–21

Pragati Dattatraya Ubale and T. V. Sekher

Abstract Risky sexual behaviors such as engaging in paid sex, involving multiple sexual partners and unprotected sex enhance the risk of acquiring and transmitting STDs, including HIV/AIDS. Indian traditional norms value maintaining sexual abstinence before marriage. In contrast, over the last three decades, the growing body of literature has given corroborating evidences of the youth's increasing permissiveness and involvement in premarital sex. However, there is a dearth of data on the prevalence and safety of these behaviors. This study aims to analyze the risky premarital sexual behaviors and their influencing factors among 15–29 aged, unmarried, sexually active youth in India. The study used data of sexually active, unmarried youth (between age 15–29 years) from the 5th round of the National Family Health Survey (2019–21). Among the sexually active, unmarried women and men of age 15–29 years, 4.2% of women & 23.3% of men had more than one sexual partner and 17.24% of men had paid sex. When asked about ever use of the withdrawal method during intercourse, 7.68% of men and 9.91% of women reported its use. The likelihood of men's involvement in multiple sexual activities was higher than women and it was consistent across the socio-economic and demographic characteristics. No or less education, alcohol drinking, spending more time away from home, early age at the first sexual encounter and seeing fathers beat their mothers are the influencing circumstances that increase youth's risky sexual behaviors. Men who had paid sex and multiple sexual partners had higher use of withdrawal method, indicating multiple risk to STDs. The findings emphasize the urgent need to provide sex education and sexual and reproductive health services to unmarried youth in order to prevent risky sexual behaviors and its possible immediate consequences such as unwanted pregnancies, STDs, and HIV.

Keywords Premarital sex · Multiple sexual partners · Paid sex · Knowledge about HIV/AIDS · Indian youth

P. D. Ubale (✉) · T. V. Sekher
International Institute of Population Sciences, Mumbai, India
e-mail: madhavidattatrayadf@gmail.com

S. Deb and S. Deb (eds.), *Handbook of Youth Development*,
https://doi.org/10.1007/978-981-99-4969-4_24

Introduction

National Youth Policy of India defines youth as people in the age group of 15–29 years (Ministry of Youth Affairs and Sports, 2014) which contribute 27.2% of India's total population (RGI, TGPP 2021). That means every fourth individual in India is a youth. As it is considered that India's development is dependent on investment in youth, India's health also can be determined from the health of youth. A considerable burden of diseases, especially diseases related to sexual and reproductive health is on youth. According to the technical report of HIV estimates of NACO, youth between 15–24 years were estimated to account for 7% (1.70 lakhs) of the total PLHIV cases (NACO, 2022). According to NFHS-4 India, HIV prevalence is 0.02% among women and 0.10% among men who were unmarried and of age 15–24 (IIPS & ICF, 2017). This prevalence of HIV challenges the widely accepted assumption that Indian youth do not get involved in sex before marriage as traditional norms do not allow them. In Indian traditions, sexual intercourse is expected to be performed in marital relationships only; premarital sex is taboo and the chastity of unmarried youth, especially girls, is highly valued. The stigma on sex extends further up to the level that sex education, which comes under human rights, is not acceptable in India. Due to technological advancements and modernization, unmarried youth of India are increasingly engaging in sexual activities. However, there is a scarcity of research that assesses the safety of these sexual activities. Transmission of HIV in unmarried men and women is driven by their risky sexual behavior. Researchers define risky sexual behavior (RSB) as any sexual activity, which elevates the risk of contracting STIs/STDs including HIV/AIDS or becoming pregnant among unmarried youth. RSB includes early age of sexual debut, inconsistent use of condom, unprotected sexual activity, high-risk partners (sex workers, injection drug users and sex in exchange of money), or sex with multiple partners (Aral, 1994; Haffner, 1995; Taylor-Seehafer & Rew, 2000). In this study, we have used nationally representative data from the 5th round of National Family Health Survey (NFHS) of unmarried but sexually active 4,668 women and 4474 men aged 15–29. Weighted prevalence estimates of three risky sexual behaviors, including sex with multiple partners, paid sex, and use of the withdrawal method, were calculated. Bivariate differences in prevalence were examined by demographic characteristics (sex, education, caste, religion, residence, etc.) and covariates such as the age of sexual initiation, comprehensive knowledge of HIV, seeing the father beating mother, and alcohol drinking of respondents.

Traditionally, Indian youth are expected to follow celibacy till marriage. However, the mean age at marriage of Indian youth is increasing (IIPS & Macro International, 2007; IIPS & ICF, 2017; Das & Raut, 2023), the mean age at puberty is decreasing (Khadilkar et al., 2006; Pathak et al., 2014) and the age at which mature social roles are achieved is rising (Sawyer et al., 2012). In addition to these trends, technological advancements and availability of internet highways have spurred the youth's involvement in premarital sex. According to a review of the research on adolescent sexuality, up to 10% of unmarried females and 20–30% of unmarried males have engaged in sexual activity (Jejeebhoy, 1998). Nationally and sub-nationally representative data also shows the increasing trend of youth's involvement in premarital sex (IIPS & Macro International, 2007; IIPS & ICF, 2017; IIPS & ICF, 2021). Nevertheless, strong stigma and taboo surrounding sexual activities and unavailability of sex education programs give a conducive environment to risky premarital sexual activities. Though literature showing evidence of premarital sexual activities is increasing, the issue of risky premarital sexual activities remains poorly explored.

A study based on nationally representative, large-scale data of youth in India reported, among total sexually active men and women of age 15–24, 1.3 of men had sex with a sex worker, 0.2% of women had sex in exchange for money/favor, 29 percent of men and 25.5% of women reported having sex with multiple partners (IIPS & Population Council, 2010). Series of NFHS surveys shows percentage of unmarried men 15–49 aged, involving in paid sexual activities is higher than that of married men and the percentage is persistently increasing over the past 2 decades (1.0% in 2005–06; 2% in 2015–16 & 2.2% in 2019–21). Among never-married men who ever had sex, 2.2% of them had paid for sexual activity (IIPS & ICF, 2021). NFHS also provides information on multiple sexual activities of men and women. There is increase in mean number of lifetime sexual partners for never-married (15–49 aged) women but not for men (For women 1.11 in 2005–06, 1.4 in 2015–16 & 1.6 in 2019–21 and for men 2.49 in 2005–06, 1.9 in 2015–16 & 1.9 in 2019–21) (IIPS & Macro International, 2007; IIPS & ICF, 2017, IIPS & ICF, 2021). These findings show gender gap in multiple sexual partners is narrowed down from 2005 to 2021. Findings from NFHS also show that the percentage of unmarried men and women of age 15–24 years using a condom at their last sexual encounter is increasing (36.8% women in NFHS-4 versus 62.8% women in NFHS-5; 51.6% men in NFHS-4 versus 61.5% men in NFHS-5) (IIPS & ICF, 2017; IIPS & ICF, 2019). There are very few studies which explore RSB of unmarried youth, especially women.

Apart from nationally representative surveys, few small-scale studies always showed that the percentage of condom use was not high among unmarried youth (Santhya et al., 2011a, 2011b; Arora et al., 2014; Mathew et al., 2019; Sharma et al., 2022). Surveys often said that a significant proportion of unmarried adolescents are clients of commercial sex workers (Joshi & Chauhan, 2011; BSS, 2006; IBBS, 2015). According to a National report, 96.2% of FSWs reported using a condom at the last sex, which decreases to 87.8% when asked about consistent condom use (BSS-LITE, 2020). These findings indicate a significant number of clients exposed to the high risk of STDs, including HIV. Many studies on family planning have turned a blind eye toward withdrawal methods and focused on modern methods, especially condoms. However, when it concerns unmarried men and women, instead of considering condom use at the last sexual encounter, it is more important and valid to check the use of withdrawal method as it gives the percentage of men and women directly exposed to the risk of unwanted pregnancy as well as STIs/STDs. Coitus interruptus (withdrawal method) is not on the list of methods of contraception provided by the Center for Disease Control and Prevention (Miller, 2003).

There are very few small-scale studies, but they revealed that many unmarried youth engage in risky sexual activities. These studies are done in different settings with different samples (Arora et al., 2014; Dave et al., 2013; Dhapola et al., 2007; Mathew et al., 2019).

A study in Gujrat state of India of college-going students reported that 7.4% of women and 39.7% of men who are unmarried reported sexual involvement with multiple partners, 32% of men reported having paid sex, and nearly half of the respondents reported using withdrawal method (Sujay, 2009). The same study also reported that the withdrawal method was the second most used method after condoms among unmarried youth. In a study of male construction workers, nearly 30% of unmarried men reported multiple sexual partners, including commercial sex workers (Mathew et al., 2019). A survey reported 14.5% and 33.88% of sexually active men visited commercial sex workers and involved with multiple sexual partners respectively (Dave et al., 2013). This study also showed that 10% of men never used a condom during performing premarital sex. Like any other phenomenon, youth's entry into risky premarital sexual activities can be influenced heavily by social, demographic, and economic factors. Few studies tried to understand the factors influencing youth in risky sexual behavior.

Many studies linked migration for higher education and working status highly influences risky sexual behaviors and, ultimately it becomes a cause of HIV among youth (Wolffers and Fernandez, 1995; Saggurti et al., 2011; Mathew et al., 2019). A study based on NFHS found that older, less educated, early age at sexual debut, northeast men, and women from the south were more likely to go for multiple sexual partners (Singh et al., 2020). Also, men and women from the poor and rich wealth quintiles are more likely to have multiple partners than the middle wealth quintiles (Singh et al., 2020). Findings from the survey of youth in India reported older men and younger women, less educated, ever worked and the poorer were more likely to get involved in multiple sexual activities (IIPS & Population Council., 2010). Youth who are younger, uneducated or less educated, never worked, lived away from home, rural, and poor wealth quintile are less likely to be consistent about condom use (IIPS & Population Council., 2010; Dave et al., 2013; IIPS & ICF, 2021).

There are several consequences of risky premarital sexual activities, including contracting STIs, STDs, HIV, unwanted pregnancy, unsafe abortion, etc. The National Family Health Survey in its 4th round found that the prevalence of HIV was 0.27% in women (aged 15–49) with a one-lifetime sexual partner and 2.85% in those with five or more lifetime partners. Similar to women, it was 0.25% in men (aged 15–49) with a one-lifetime partner and rose to 1.6% in those with five or more lifetime partners (IIPs & ICF, 2017). A similar trend is observed for the youth of 15–25 years. Among men who had paid sex in the past year, HIV prevalence was 0.55% and 0.30% among those who did not have paid sex. Among youth aged 15–24, the prevalence of HIV was high among men and women who reported no condom use (0.22% of men who never used a condom versus 0.16% for men who ever used a condom & 0.17% of women whose partner/is never used condom versus 0.16% for women whose partner/s ever used condom) (IIPs & ICF, 2017). These findings give evidence that risky sexual behaviors increase the odds of acquiring HIV. A study based on 3,173 students in Gujrat reported that among the sexually active youth, 8.5% of women and 15.5% of men reported getting pregnant or making their partner pregnant, respectively (Sujay,

2009). In Key informant interviews with local gynecologists and pharmacists, they reported college students were among their leading clients for abortion (Sujay, 2009). A study by Dave and co-authors reported that 6.45% of men had a history of STDs and out of them, 50% never sought medical help (Dave et al., 2013). Many studies have confirmed through empirical research that most HIV transmission in India arises from male use of FSW (Kumar et al., 2005). The belief that youth, especially women, should protect their virginity until marriage prevents them from seeking treatment for consequences of risky sexual activities.

To fully understand the phenomenon of premarital sex in India, it is vital to comprehend risky premarital sexual activities and their influencing factors. Drawing on data of unmarried youth between the ages 15–29 from the 5th round of the National Family Health Survey, this paper examines the prevalence of risky premarital sexual activities across different social, economic, and demographic background characteristics.

In this study, the researcher used data from India's National Family Health Survey (NFHS-5), 2019–21. The NFHS survey has been conducted under the Ministry of Health and Family Welfare (MoHFW) and Government of India. NFHS collected information on demographic and health indicators, including sexual behaviors at the national, regional, state, and district levels. The NFHS survey asks the question of "have you ever had sexual intercourse" to all unmarried women (1,72,568) and men (33,397). The weighted percentage of premarital sex is 2.83% for women and 13.46% for men. We analyzed the data collected from sexually active 4,668 unmarried women and 4,474 unmarried men aged 15–29 at the national level.

Measures/Description of Variables

Following are the questions asked in the survey, which we considered as our dependent variables.

Multiple Sexual partners:

Q. In total, how many different people have you had sexual intercourse in your lifetime? And if the respondent has responded more than one, then he or she is counted as having multiple sexual partners.

Paid sex:

Q. Have you ever paid anyone in exchange for having sexual intercourse? If the person has reported yes, then he is considered as if he ever had paid sex. (This question is only asked to men.)

Use of withdrawal method:

Q. Have you ever used anything or tried in any way to delay or avoid getting pregnant? If yes, what have you used or done? And if the respondent reported the withdrawal method, that respondent is considered as he/she has ever used the withdrawal method. This study considers the withdrawal method as a risk for STI/STDs and unwanted pregnancy.

Independent Variables: Age, education, residence, caste, religion, region, wealth index and regular exposure to mass media, mobile use, internet use, ever worked, spent more than a month in a past year away from home, comprehensive knowledge of HIV, age at the first sexual encounter, and whether father ever beat mother.

Methods

We used univariate, bivariate, and multivariate analysis to come to the conclusions of the study.

Chi-Square Test (χ_c^2)

Common Bivariate statistics are used to test whether the distribution of the categorical variables is.

statistically different in two or more groups.

$$\chi_c^2 = \sum \frac{(O_i - E_i)^2}{E_i}$$

where O is the observed value, E is the expected value and 'i' is the ith position in the contingency table.

If the sample size is less than 1000, then Fisher's exact test is used to understand the associations.

Test for Multicollinearity: Pearson's R Correlation Coefficient Test

Collinearity occurs when two covariates in a multivariate model are highly related. If we take both of them into the model, it becomes unstable. Test for collinearity Pearson's r Correlation Coefficient is used to identify correlated binary, ordinal, and continuous covariates. A correlation of $r > 0.5$ is often considered collinear in social sciences. When two or more covariates appeared collinear, we kept the one variable most strongly associated with the outcome.

Logistic Regression

Post applying the above tests, we scrutinized the variables and multiple logistic regression was conducted between binary dependent variables of the study and categorical independent variables.

The logistic regression model is commonly estimated by the maximum likelihood function for dependent variables. The logistic model takes the following general form:

$$logit\ p = ln\, ln\left(\frac{p}{1-p}\right) = b_0 + b_1x_1 + b_2x_2 + \cdots b_ix_i + e_i$$

where $b_1, b_2, \ldots$ and bi represent the coefficient of each independent variable included in the model while e_i is an error term; ln [p/(1-p)] represents the natural logarithms of the odds of the outcomes.

Analysis of data is done by using Stata 16 software.

Results

Table 24.1 illustrates the significance of the association of respondents reporting multiple sexual partners and their background characteristics. Amongst the men and women who were sexually active, 4.2% of women and 23.3% of men were involved with more than one sexual partner. Since the number of women who answered for this question was less than 1000, we applied Fisher's exact test to analyze the significance of association and for men, Chi-square test was applied since they were more than 1000 in number. Age profiles suggested a positive association between age and multiple premarital sexual partnerships among young men (3.44% of 15–19, 3.97% of 20–24 versus 6.63% of 25–29 year-olds) and women (19.48% of 15–19, 22.48% of 20–24 versus 27.4% of 25–29 year-olds). Those with higher education were less likely than those with no education or primary or secondary education level to report multiple sexual relations (2.61% higher educated women versus 7.08% primary educated women; 23.% higher educated men versus 23.8% illiterate men). Middle-class youth (2.58% women and 18.91% men) were least likely to get involved with multiple sexual partners. When tested for the impact of drinking habit, both men and women showed drinking was positively associated with sexual involvement with multiple partners (3.92% of women who didn't drink versus 13.31% of women who drink; 20.73% of men who didn't drink versus 29.46% men who drink). Staying away from home for both men and women and working status of men were highly positively associated with their involvement in multiple sexual partners. Women mobile users reported higher involvement whereas women internet users reported lesser involvement with more than one sexual partner than their counterparts (4.8% mobile users versus 3.03% nonusers & 4% internet users versus 4.5% nonusers).

There was no significant association found between youth's comprehensive awareness on HIV/AIDS and their involvement with multiple sexual partners. For men, lesser age at first sexual debut was found to be associated with higher possibility of getting involved with multiple sexual partners (25% for 18 and below the age of sexual debut than 19% for 22–29 age of sexual debut). For the respondents who have seen their fathers beating mothers, their chances of getting involved with multiple partners were higher.

The results of the Chi-square test for the association between social, demographic, and economic characteristics and paid sex among sexually active men are shown in Table 24.2. On the whole, 17.24% of sexually active men reported that they ever had paid sex. Age profile showed that men in the age group 20–24 were less likely to have paid sex than their younger and older counterparts. The percentage of men involved in paid sexual activities decreased drastically from illiterate to highly educated men (33.39% illiterate versus 11.94% higher educated). Though findings were insignificant, men from urban areas (20.95%) were more likely to have paid sexual activities than rural men (15.05%). Least percentage of paid sexual activities was reported by the men in the middle wealth quintile than others. Men who reported alcohol drinking were more involved in paid sex than those who did not (15.61% who didn't drink versus 21.16% who drink). In addition, men who worked and who were away from home for more than one month had more chances of getting involved in paid sexual activity (18.82% & 22.02% resp.) than men who did not work or never been away from home (12.87% & 15.87% resp.). Exposure to mass media such as radio, TV, and newspapers, significantly increased youth's involvement in paid sex. However, mobile and internet use did not play any noteworthy role. Comprehensive knowledge of HIV/AIDS was positively associated with youth's nonparticipation in paid sexual activities (15% men who had comprehensive knowledge and 19% who had not). The percentage of men involved in paid sex was highest if their first sexual encounter was at or before 18 years of age. Men who had sex with multiple partners were higher (27.6%) to report paid sexual activities than men with one sexual partner (14.3%). There was a huge difference between reporting of men in paid sex if they had seen their fathers beating mothers (23.74% versus 14.47%).

Table 24.3 displayed the association between ever use of the withdrawal method and the social, demographic, and economic characteristics of the sexually active respondents. We used Chi-square test for women samples above 1000 and Fisher's exact test for samples less than 1000. For men, Chi-square test was applied. Reporting of ever use of withdrawal method among sexually active unmarried men and women was 7.68 and 9.91% respectively. Reporting the use of withdrawal methods was highest among women in the age group 15–19 and among men in age 20–24 years. When the education level changed from no education to higher education, the percentage of men and women reporting withdrawal methods was reduced almost by half. About 15% (14.99%) uneducated women and 7.41% higher educated women & 12.61% uneducated men and 6.56% higher educated men. There were 7.19% of women and 6.23% of men from the richest wealth quintile households, who reported the use of the withdrawal method, which was less than 10.27% of women and 7.57% of men from the poorest wealth quintiles. Women and men who reported drinking

Table 24.1 Involvement of unmarried youth (aged 15–29) in multiple sexual partners according to their background characteristics, India, 2019–21

	Women			Men		
Background characteristics	Percentage of Women who had more than one sexual partner	Number of sexually active women	Fisher's exact test (P-Value)	Percentage of Men who had more than one sexual partner	Number of sexually active men	Pearson Chi-square test
Age of the respondent						
15–19	3.44	311		19.48	970	59.76***
20–24	3.97	275	0.003***	22.48	2094	
25–29	6.63	122		27.4	1320	
Total	4.2	709		23.3	4385	
Level of education						
No education	3.27	36	0.96	23.8	174	0.929
Primary	7.08	38		23.01	288	0.818
Secondary	5.06	381		23.83	2493	
Higher	2.61	255		22.38	1431	
Residence						
Urban	3.26	680	0.787	21.98	1626	1.687
Rural	4.82	29		24.08	2759	0.194
Caste						
SC	2.78	156	0***	24.02	997	65.14***
ST	6.8	91		33.71	464	
OBC	5.23	262		19.62	1809	
Other	2.75	200		24.29	1114	
Religion						
Hindu	3.76	544	0***	22.86	3563	89.01***
Muslim	5.28	110		21.5	567	
Christian	11.73	29		22.28	96	
Others	0.6	26		40.37	158	
Wealth Index						
Poorest	3.75	120		26.09	711	7.90*
Poorer	5.82	134	0.255	20.86	884	
Middle	2.58	139		18.91	857	
Richer	7.11	134		21.9	962	
Richest	2.38	181		28.72	972	
Region						
North	4.03	112		23.99	487	85.96***

(continued)

Table 24.1 (continued)

	Women			Men		
Background characteristics	Percentage of Women who had more than one sexual partner	Number of sexually active women	Fisher's exact test (P-Value)	Percentage of Men who had more than one sexual partner	Number of sexually active men	Pearson Chi-square test
Central	4.66	323	0***	22.04	750	
East	1.43	155		22.67	1093	
Northeast	11.17	30		23.33	130	
West	4.47	71		27.49	1242	
South	8.25	18		17.56	682	
Alcohol consumption						
No	3.92	688	0.017**	20.73	3094	123.51***
Yes	13.31	21		29.46	1290	
Ever worked						
No	4.56	513	0.592	19.68	1167	19.71***
Yes	3.25	196		24.61	3218	
Away from home for more than one month in last 12 months	Fisher's exact and one sided					
No	3.99	606		22.43	3411	30.92***
Yes	5.41	103	0.084*	26.34	974	
Use of Mobile phone						
No	3.03	241	0.002***	34.86	152	0.015
Yes	4.8	468		23.16	3658	
Ever used internet						
No	4.5	282		21.88	703	0.201
Yes	4	427	0.031**	24.02	3107	
Mass media exposure						
No exposure	9.35	94	0.081*	23.67	328	4.027
Partial exposure	2.75	525		23.35	3249	
Full exposure	7.24	90		22.96	807	
Comprehensive Knowledge of HIV/AIDS						
No	4.23	450	0.888	23.22	578	2.2802
Yes	4.27	211		22.83	3664	

(continued)

Table 24.1 (continued)

	Women			Men		
Background characteristics	Percentage of Women who had more than one sexual partner	Number of sexually active women	Fisher's exact test (P-Value)	Percentage of Men who had more than one sexual partner	Number of sexually active men	Pearson Chi-square test
Seen father beat mother						
No	3.95	219	0.691	22.12	2973	21.60***
Yes	7.85	77		25.93	1272	
Don't know	1.84	7		24.56	139	
Age at first sex						
18 or less	3.97	394		24.9	1769	
19–21	4.84	211	0.692	24.22	1545	17.73***
22–29	3.75	104		19.32	1071	
Total	4.2	709		23.3	4385	

Note * $p < 0.10$; ** $p < 0.05$; *** $p < 0.01$
Source NFHS-5 (2019–2021)

of alcohol, their likelihood of reporting withdrawal methods increased drastically (9.62% women & 5.97% men who didn't drink versus 20.35% women & 11.76% men who drink). Exposure to mass media, mobile, and the internet did not influence youth's use of withdrawal methods significantly. For women, though insignificant, results show less usage of withdrawal methods among those who had comprehensive knowledge of HIV/AIDS. Though the association test is insignificant, men and women who had sex in later ages were the least when it comes to using the withdrawal method. Men who were involved in multiple sexual activities and paid sex were higher in percentage of using the withdrawal method (7.22 men with one partner versus 9.81% of men with multiple partners and 7.09 men who did not have paid sex versus 11.05% men who had paid sex).

Table 24.4 demonstrates the extent of association between background characteristics and youth's involvement in multiple sexual activities. Women of 25–29 years were twice likely to have multiple sexual partners than of age 15–19. Similarly, men of 25–29 ages were 82% more likely to have multiple sexual partners than that of 15–19 years. Men who drink were 82% and who stayed away from family were 39% more likely to have sexual encounters with multiple partners than their counterparts. Men had a 34% higher chance of involving themselves sexually with multiple partners if they observed their fathers beat their mothers.

Table 24.5 shows logistic regression for the association between two dependent characteristics; one is ever had paid sex and the other is ever use of withdrawal method and multiple independent background characteristics. Men from the richest wealth quintile were 25% less likely to have paid sex than the poorest. Among the

Table 24.2 Association between involvement in paid sex among sexually active and never married men (between 15–29 years), 2019–21, India

Background characteristics	Percentage of men involved in paid sex ever	Number of Sexually active men	Chi-square Test
Age of the respondent			
15–19	18.52	**951**	7.11**
20–24	16.06	2038	
25–29	18.14	1289	
Highest level of education			
No education	33.39	172	23.72***
Primary	23.76	279	
Secondary	18.4	2426	
Higher	11.94	1401	
Residence			
Urban	20.95	1584	1.5292
Rural	15.05	2693	
Caste			
SC	19.05	972	23.15***
ST	17.81	456	0
OBC	18.41	1766	
Other	13.45	1084	
Religion			
Hindu	17.46	3486	41.13***
Muslim	18.22	541	0
Christian	17.57	96	
Others	8.43	154	
Wealth Index			
Poorest	19.41	693	8.79*
Poorer	18.27	862	
Middle	14.54	839	
Richer	19.15	933	
Richest	15.21	951	
Region			
North	14.02	471	88.55***
Central	13.52	743	0
East	18.58	1066	
Northeast	7.44	129	
West	13.84	1211	
South	29.76	657	

(continued)

Table 24.2 (continued)

Background characteristics	Percentage of men involved in paid sex ever	Number of Sexually active men	Chi-square Test
Drink alcohol			
No	15.61	3027	6.33**
Yes	21.16	1251	
Ever worked			
No	12.87	1141	6.99***
Yes	18.82	3137	
Away from home for more than one month in last 12 months			
No	15.87	3,329	8.79***
Yes	22.02	948	
Owns a mobile			
No	20.1	149	2.6263
Yes	17.56	3572	
Ever used internet			
No	21.71	686	2.0129
Yes	16.75	3035	
Mass media exposure			
No exposure	14.19	320	6.68**
Partial exposure	16.57	3174	
Complete Exposure	21.16	783	
Comprehensive Knowledge of HIV/AIDS			
No	18.5	2687	10.28***
Yes	15.21	1450	
Seen father beat mother			
No	14.47	2926	31.24***
Yes	23.74	1215	
Don't know	18.54	136	
Age at first sex			
18 or less	20.49	1725	15.28***
19–21	13.05	1497	
22–29	17.85	1056	
Number of sexual partners			
One	14.3	3335	79.09***
More than one	27.6	943	
Total	17.24	4278	

Note * $p < 0.10$; ** $p < 0.05$; *** $p < 0.01$
Source NFHS-5 (2019–2021)

Table 24.3 Association between ever use of withdrawal method by sexually active unmarried women and men (aged 15–29) years in India and their background characteristics, 2019–21, India

Background characteristics	Percentage of women	Number of women	Chi-square / Fisher's exact Test	Percentage of men	Number of men	Chi-square Test
Age of the respondent						
15–19	10.57	1,985	18.30***	6.39	982	13.53***
20–24	9.27	1,926		8.44	2145	
25–29	9.82	757		7.41	1346	
Highest level of education						
No education	14.99	263	3.50	12.61	177	4.92
Primary	11.52	260		11.36	290	
Secondary	10.81	2,535		7.56	2546	
Higher	7.41	1,610		6.56	1461	
Residence						
Urban	8.69	1,787	14.81***	10.44	1663	4.37**
Rural	10.67	2,881		6.05	2811	
Caste						
SC	7.07	1,076	88.32***	9.71	1018	44.08***
ST	15.61	633		9.85	481	
OBC	10.06	1,769		6.75	1833	
Other	9.24	1,190		6.46	1142	
Religion						
Hindu	8.88	3,618	60.44***	7.4	3634	70***
Muslim	13.92	771		8.48	575	
Christian	13.29	172		20.41	100	
Others	10.29	106		3.22	165	
Wealth Index						
Poorest	10.27	785	28.68***	7.57	723	74.77***
Poorer	11.96	922		6.97	895	
Middle	10.23	828		5.54	884	
Richer	10.89	914		11.79	982	
Richest	7.19	1,219		6.23	989	
Region						
North	16.66	737	94.80***	11.03	495	102.39***
Central	7.74	2,198		6.92	761	
East	10.94	898		6.35	1111	
Northeast	11.52	189		16.06	140	
West	10.24	453		4.47	1269	
South	1.67	192		12.4	697	

(continued)

Table 24.3 (continued)

Background characteristics	Percentage of women	Number of women	Chi-square / Fisher's exact Test	Percentage of men	Number of men	Chi-square Test
Drinks alcohol						
No	9.62	4,541	40.35***	5.97	3153	17.47***
Yes	20.35	127		11.76	1320	
Ever worked			(Fisher's Exact)			
Never	9.63	523	0.070*	7.08	1183	0.308
Yes	8.95	204		7.9	3291	
Owns a mobile phone			(Fisher's Exact)			
No	9.7	249	0.255	8.39	158	0.021
Yes	9.31	478		8.32	3730	
Use internet			(Fisher's Exact)			
No	10.59	291	0.457	8.88	730	2.519
Yes	8.68	437		8.19	3158	
Mass exposure						
No exposure	10.21	710		3.73	337	2.996
Partial exposure	9.81	3,269	6.19**	7.74	3307	
Complete exposure	10.09	689		9.06	830	
Comprehensive knowledge of HIV/AIDS			*(Fisher's Exact)*			
No	10.57	467	0.349	7.12	2828	23.39***
Yes	8.01	212	0.19	9.48	1498	
Age at first sex						
18 or less	10.62	2600		7.44	1801	2.9406
19–21	9.75	1360	4.95*	8.67	1578	
22–29	7.61	708		6.65	1095	
Number of sexual partners			(Fisher's Exact)			
One	9.74	679	0.341	7.22	3363	7.48***
More than one	4.2	30		9.81	1022	
Have ever paid anyone in exchange of sex						
No	NA	NA	NA	7.09	3540	0.01
Yes	NA	NA	NA	11.05	737	
Total	9.91	4,668		7.68	344	4474

Note * $p < 0.10$; ** $p < 0.05$; *** $p < 0.01$
Source NFHS-5 (2019–2021)

Table 24.4 Logistic regression showing the association of unmarried youth's involvement in multiple sexual partners and background characteristics, 2019–21, India

Multiple sexual partners among women/ Background characteristics	OR	[95% Conf. interval]		Multiple sexual partners among men/Background characteristics	OR	[95% Conf. Interval]	
Age of the respondent				*Age of the respondent*			
15–19®				15–19®			
20–24	1.52	0.79	2.93	20–24	1.28***	1.06	1.53
25–29	2.02*	0.98	4.14	25–29	1.82***	1.49	2.22
Caste				*Caste*			
SC®				SC®			
ST	2.93*	0.85	10.16	ST	1.05	0.83	1.32
OBC	1.90	0.58	6.20	OBC	0.83*	0.69	1.01
Other	1.55	0.41	5.84	Other	0.92	0.74	1.14
Religion				*Religion*			
Hindu®				Hindu®			
Muslim	0.82	0.26	2.59	Muslim	1.06	0.82	1.35
Christian	1.40	0.53	3.70	Christian	1.39**	1.01	1.92
Others	0.57	0.17	1.89	Others	1.52***	1.17	2.00
Region				*Wealth quintile*			
North®				Poorest®			
Central	1.36	0.46	4.04	Poorer	0.90	0.73	1.11
East	0.47	0.10	2.14	Middle	0.84	0.67	1.04
Northeast	2.28	0.65	7.97	Richer	0.87	0.69	1.10
West	0.50	0.09	2.77	Richest	0.85	0.67	1.10
South	1.24	0.22	7.00	*Region*			
Alcohol drinking status				North®			
No®				Central	1.06	0.86	1.30
Yes	1.75	0.73	4.18	East	0.93	0.73	1.20
Spent at least one month away from home				Northeast	1.17	0.88	1.57
No®				West	0.94	0.73	1.21
Yes	1.79	0.89	3.61	South	0.58***	0.42	0.79
Mobile use				*Alcohol drinking status*			
No®				No®			
Yes	1.35	0.64	2.86	Yes	1.82***	1.57	2.11
Mass media exposure				*Ever worked*			

(continued)

Table 24.4 (continued)

Multiple sexual partners among women/ Background characteristics	OR	[95% Conf. interval]		Multiple sexual partners among men/Background characteristics	OR	[95% Conf. Interval]	
No exposure at all®				No®			
Partial exposure	0.35***	0.18	0.67	Yes	1.14	0.97	1.33
Full exposure	0.41**	0.17	1.00	*Spent at least one month away from home*			
				No®			
				Yes	1.39***	1.20	1.62
				Respondent's father ever beat mother			
				No®			
				Yes	1.34***	1.16	1.58
				Don't know	1.56***	1.13	2.14
_cons	0.03	0.01	0.13	_cons	0.17	0.12	0.23

Note * $p < 0.10$; ** $p < 0.05$; *** $p < 0.01$
Source NFHS-5 (2019–2021)

men who drink alcohol and who stayed away from home were 26% and 30% more likely to have paid sex than men who did not. Men with comprehensive knowledge of HIV were 16% less likely and men who have seen their fathers beating their mothers were 41% more likely to indulge in sex by paying, than their counterparts. Regarding the withdrawal method, men from the 25–29 age group, and who drink were 34%, and 32% more likely to use the withdrawal method than men 15–19 years age group, and who did not drink alcohol. Rural and richest men were 27% and 33% less likely to use the withdrawal method than their urban and poorest counterparts. Men with comprehensive knowledge of HIV were 51% more likely to use the withdrawal method during sexual intercourse.

Discussion

This study provides the most recent nationally representative estimates of risky sexual behaviors and associated influencing factors among India's unmarried and sexually active youth. This article draws inferences based on information collected from 4,668 women and 4,474 men aged 15–29. Though in India, marriage usually marks entry into sexual life, this study has clearly brought out that a significant percentage of youth are not only just getting involved in premarital sex, but also in risky sexual

Table 24.5 Logistic regression showing association of unmarried men's involvement in paid sexual activities and ever use of withdrawal method with background characteristics, 2019–21, India

Ever had paid sex/Background characteristics	OR	[95% Conf. Interval]		Ever used withdrawal method/ Background characteristics	OR	[95% Conf. Interval]	
Age of the respondent				*Age of the respondent*			
15–19®				15–19®			
20–24	0.86	0.69	1.07	20–24	1.21	0.92	1.59
25–29	0.90	0.70	1.16	25–29	1.34*	1.00	1.79
Level of education							
No education®							
Primary	1.09	0.65	1.83	*Place of residence*			
Secondary	0.96	0.63	1.47	Urban®			
Higher	0.79	0.50	1.27	Rural	0.73**	0.57	0.94
Caste				*Caste*			
SC®				SC®			
ST	0.79	0.59	1.07	ST	1.46**	1.02	2.08
OBC	0.87	0.70	1.10	OBC	1.08	0.80	1.46
Other	0.73**	0.56	0.97	Other	1.12	0.81	1.56
Religion				*Religion*			
Hindu®				Hindu®			
Muslim	1.71***	1.30	2.25	Muslim	1.13	0.79	1.62
Christian	0.44**	0.24	0.83	Christian	1.22	0.80	1.88
Others	1.01	0.69	1.49	Others	0.65*	0.42	1.00
Wealth Quintile				*Wealth Quintile*			
Poorest®				Poorest®			
Poorer	0.93	0.71	1.21	Poorer	0.98	0.72	1.34
Middle	0.87	0.65	1.17	Middle	0.90	0.64	1.25
Richer	0.85	0.63	1.15	Richer	0.73*	0.51	1.06
Richest	0.75*	0.53	1.05	Richest	0.67**	0.44	1.00
Region				*Region*			
North®				North®			
Central	0.73**	0.57	0.94	Central	0.59***	0.44	0.79
East	1.12	0.84	1.50	East	0.50***	0.34	0.74
Northeast	0.41***	0.26	0.66	Northeast	1.13	0.76	1.68
West	0.76*	0.55	1.05	West	0.47***	0.32	0.69
South	1.53***	1.11	2.11	South	0.44***	0.28	0.71
Alcohol drinking status				*Alcohol drinking status*			

(continued)

Table 24.5 (continued)

Ever had paid sex/Background characteristics	OR	[95% Conf. Interval]		Ever used withdrawal method/ Background characteristics	OR	[95% Conf. Interval]	
No®				No®			
Yes	1.26**	1.03	1.53	Yes	1.32**	1.07	1.64
Ever worked							
No®							
Yes	1.19	0.96	1.46				
Spent at least one month away from home							
No®							
Yes	1.30***	1.07	1.57				
Mass media exposure							
No exposure at all®							
Partial exposure	1.03	0.76	1.39				
Full exposure	1.29	0.91	1.82				
Respondent's father ever beat mother							
No®							
Yes	1.41***	1.17	1.71				
Don't know	1.18	0.76	1.83				
No®				No®			
Yes	0.84*	0.69	1.01	Yes	1.51***	1.24	1.85
_cons	0.19	0.11	0.33	_cons	0.12	−2.63	−1.65

Note * $p < 0.10$; ** $p < 0.05$; *** $p < 0.01$
Source NFHS-5 (2019–2021)

behaviors. This study discussed the three risky sexual behaviors—multiple sexual partners, paid sex, and use of withdrawal method during intercourse.

Among sexually active unmarried youth (aged 15–29), 4.2% of women and 23.3% of men reported they had more than one sexual partner. A study based on NFHS 4 showed among unmarried and sexually active participants of age 15–49, 31 percent of men and 14% of women reported more than one sexual partner (Singh et al., 2020). The sample of both the studies is same except the age. However, considering the majority of unmarried men and women belong to the 15–29 age group, if we compare the results, it is observable that both the percentage of men and women involved in multiple sexual partners decreased from 2015–16 to 2019–21. However, the mean number of lifetime sexual partners has increased for never married women but decreased for men (yet higher than women) from 2005–06 to 2019–21 (IIPS & Macro International, 2007; IIPS & ICF, 2017, IIPS & ICF, 2021).

The second risky sexual activity we considered was paid sex, and the question was asked to male respondents only. Nearly 17% of men with sexual history reported their involvement in paid sex. Consistent with previous literature, our study confirms that paid sexual partners are one of the leading sexual partners for unmarried men in India. In addition, the percentage of men involved in paid sexual activities is persistently increasing (IIPS & Macro International, 2007; IIPS & ICF, 2017, IIPS & ICF, 2021).

The third HIV-related risky sexual activity covered in present study is the practice of withdrawal method to avoid pregnancy of women. Our study documents about 9.91% of women and 7.68% of men have ever used the withdrawal method during premarital intercourse. Considering the least awareness about the modern contraception other than condom, uncomforting while accessing condoms, considerably higher awareness of withdrawal method than other traditional methods (IIPS & Population Council, 2010; Santhya et al., 2011a, 2011b), and unwanted pregnancy before marriage, many unmarried youth may opt for withdrawal method. However, many researchers criticize the use of withdrawal method by calling it "non-method" (Doherty & Stuart, 2011) or "better than nothing" (Miller, 2003) because of its consequences. Estimates obtained from the National Survey of Family Growth of the USA reveal, there is a predicted 18.8% chance of coitus interruptus failure (Kost et al., 2008). Additionally, within the first year of use, an estimated 27% of women who practice withdrawal methods had unwanted pregnancy (Trussell & Wynn, 2008). Moreover, a study showed respondents who reported inconsistent use of condom and withdrawal were 2.22 times more likely to acquire sexually transmitted infections than those who consistently used condoms (Sznitman et al., 2009). These findings indicate that there is a serious need to demotivate the use of withdrawal methods and promote the use of condoms among unmarried youth.

In this study we have tried to fill the gap in the literature by examining the associated factors of risky sexual behaviors and extent of those associations. The gender differences in youth's involvement with multiple sexual partners were crystal clear with men's participation was almost 6 times higher than women's, indicating men have more sexual laxity. These gender differences were consistent across all socioeconomic factors and they were persistent in all previous studies (Sujay, 2009; IIPS & Population Council, 2010; Arora et al., 2014; Singh et al., 2020). We could identify following reasons for this sexual double standard; firstly, women are less likely to be permissive of premarital sex hence they are less likely to get involved in premarital sex. Secondly, even if women involve in sex before marriage, they are more likely to prefer steadiness in sexual relations; they think about the safety of the act and value the feeling of love in those (Ghule et al., 2007).

We compared the findings within and between two types of ages, one was age of the respondents in completed years (three age groups: 15–19; 20–24, and 25–29 years) and age at the time of first sexual encounter (18 or less; 19–21 & 22–29). Our data revealed that, both men and women of older age and earlier age at sexual intercourse were more likely to get involved in multiple sexual partners than their counterparts. This result is consistent with previous study findings from the 4th round of NFHS (Singh et al., 2020). The plausible reason could be youth with older age and youth who entered in sexual activities in earlier age get more time for which they could be exposed to the risk of getting sexually involved with more than one partner than their counterparts. Women of age 15–19 years (teenagers) and women who had sex before or at 18 were more likely to report the use of the withdrawal method than their counterparts. These women may not be aware enough of modern contraception and may not be empowered enough to ask their partners to use a condom. Women tend to depend on men for contraception use (Ghule et al., 2007) mainly due to the patriarchal nature of Indian society. Also, men deny the use of condoms as it reduces their pleasure. In the youth in India study, only 30% of men and 20% of women agreed on a statement that condoms do not reduce sexual pleasure, meaning about 3/4th of unmarried youth believe that condoms reduce pleasure (IIPS & Population Council, 2010). This leads to an increase in the burden of contraceptive use on the shoulders of unmarried women. Previous studies showed earlier sexual initiation was found to be negatively correlated with condom use (Prata et al., 2006; Santhya et al., 2011a, 2011b; Štulhofer et al., 2007).

One of the interesting findings of this study is that men in the age group 15–19 and 25–29 were more likely to get involved in paid sexual activities than 20–24 years. In addition, men with age at first sex 18 or less and 22–29 were more likely to have paid sex than age 19–21. This could be because some younger (15–19 aged) men rush into sexual activities by paying at a younger age and some older (25–29 ages), not married and sexually inexperienced men, have to choose paid sex for sexual experience.

Our study revealed education played a paramount role in men and women's involvement in RSB. The risk of RSB was reduced to half if the respondent was highly educated as compared to uneducated. Though attaining higher education increases the age at marriage which may cause youth's involvement in sexual relations (Alexander et al., 2007; Xenos, 1993), our study demonstrates that sexual activities of higher educated youth were more likely to be safe than uneducated youth. Though statistically insignificant, it is important to note here that urban men were more likely to go for paid sex than rural men. The possible explanation for this could be that female sex workers are more easily accessible in urban areas than in rural areas.

Consistent with previous study based on NFHS 4 data (Singh et al., 2020), our study also showed men from the middle class were less likely to engage with multiple sexual partners. In addition, middle-class men were least likely to have paid sex. An explanation for this could be that middle-class people in India are the ones who keep themselves more tightly attached to Indian traditional norms than the rich and poor population. This results in more restrictions on men and women of the middle-class families by their parents, leading to fewer opportunities for them to get sexually involved with multiple partners and commercial sex.

The percentage of reporting of all types of risky premarital sexual behaviors was highest among those who reported drinking alcohol. Studies have shown that substance use is highly associated with risky sexual activities (Yadav et al., 2014; Chawla & Sarkar, 2019; Stoner et al., 2007). Sexual intercourse after consuming alcohol may lead to using condoms or the withdrawal method wrongly or not using any method at all and ultimately increasing the risks of STDs and unwanted pregnancy.

Working experience and staying away from home for at least a month in the past year were highly associated with men's involvement with multiple sexual partners and paid sex. Furthermore, women who stayed away from home showed higher likelihood of having sex with more than one partner. Best possible way to explain this association is that when youth start to work, they have to leave their parental house in most cases. If youth stay away from home, they are away from the direct supervision of parents (who are strict about following traditional norms of sexuality). Away from home environments offer greater privacy and may provide more opportunities to engage in RSB. A study by Saggurti et al. (2011) elicited the information that migrants were more likely to engage in sex with sex workers and have multiple (3 +) sex partners than non-migrants. Several studies documented that the spread of HIV/AIDS is associated with migration through risky sexual activities (Wolffers, 1995; Saggurti et al., 2011; Mathew et al., 2019).

Surprisingly, there was no consistent impact of traditional monological media such as newspapers, radio, and television as well as dialogical sources such as mobile and internet on youth's involvement in RSB. However, for women, the use of mobile was mildly associated with participation in sex with multiple partners and use of the internet was associated with less involvement with multiple sexual partners.

Unexpectedly, this study showed that comprehensive knowledge of HIV was not a significant predictor of youth's involvement in multiple partners or practice of withdrawal method. However, men's comprehensive knowledge of HIV/AIDS was positively associated with their less involvement in paid sex. Our study also found that men involved in paid sex and multiple sexual partners were more likely to use the withdrawal method.

Conclusion

This study illustrated that a considerable percentage of youth were involved in risky premarital sexual behaviors. Sexual double standards were evident as men were six times more likely to be involved in multiple sexual partners than women. Youth became more vulnerable to risky sexual activities when they were uneducated, younger in age, initiated sexual activities at younger age, drink alcohol, spend time away from home, and when they have seen their fathers beating their mothers. The risk of men getting involved in paid sex and with multiple sexual partners increases manifold when they are working and staying away from home. Comprehensive knowledge of HIV/AIDS reduced the risk of getting involved in paid sex among men. This study reiterates the need for comprehensive and age-appropriate sex education.

Recommendations

This study recommends efforts should be taken with the help of teachers and parents to improve SRH knowledge among youth to make them aware of the consequences of involvement in paid sex, withdrawal method use, and having sex with multiple partners. Youth, primarily women, should be provided their right to SRH care, irrespective of their marital status. Additionally, youth should be made aware of legality of abortion for unmarried women as per MTP Act, 2021. Age-appropriate and comprehensive sex education should be imparted. Sex education could be used to reduce the stigma surrounding sexuality and to minimize the underreporting of sexual activities, including risky ones. An earlier study demonstrated that youth who received sex education were relatively more aware about reproductive health issues than their counterparts, and majority among Indian youth, irrespective of their age and gender, favored introduction of sex education at school level, preferably from standard 8th onward (Tripathi & Sekher, 2013). Programs and policies should prioritize the ways for increasing age at first sex and making unmarried youth as part of family planning programs to reduce their vulnerability.

Limitations of the Study

Although widely accepted, NFHS data suffers from some limitations due to the cross-sectional nature of the survey. The causality of results cannot be determined with NFHS data but with associations. One concern about treating the withdrawal method as a risky premarital sexual behavior is that literature suggests that couples use the withdrawal method along with other methods of contraception as well. One apparent limitation is social desirability bias. The Youth in India Study revealed odds of disclosing premarital sexual activities are higher through anonymous sealed envelope format than face-to-face interviews (IIPS & Population Council, 2010). NFHS data was collected through face-to-face interviews. In India there exist a strong stigma on premarital sex which may result into serious underreporting of activities of premarital sex as well as risky sexual behaviors.

References

Alexander, M., Garda, L., Kanade, S., Jejeebhoy, S., & Ganatra, B. (2007). Correlates of premarital relationships among unmarried youth in Pune district, Maharashtra, India. *International Family Planning Perspectives*, 150–159. https://www.jstor.org/stable/pdf/30039237.pdf?casa_token=7aTzKlcO9tAAAAAA:JnqniqokYbxW7GuUVjzTvHE6yiNfPag2RcfNQd4c2j5s-nvEUNp5yNmysN9mECwb7NBVUjMk2oNHIs7DrArE2mKcy18FaiZjXNNUeG5n1Kli58pCH8M

Aral, S. O. (1994). Sexual behavior in sexually transmitted disease research: An overview. *Sexually transmitted diseases*, S59-S64. https://www.jstor.org/stable/44967059

Arora, V. K., Sharma, S., & Mahashabde, P. (2014). Sexual behavior among migrant construction workers in Indore. *Int J Med Sci Public Health.* 574–577. https://www.bibliomed.org/mnsfulltext/67/67-1392024180.pdf?1675935340

Behavioural Surveillance Survey-LITE. 2020. National AIDS control organization, Ministry of Health and Family Welfare, Governmnet of India and All India Institute of Medical Sciences, New Delhi. http://www.naco.gov.in/sites/default/files/BSS%20Lite%20Report.pdf

Chawla, N., & Sarkar, S. (2019). Defining high-risk sexual behavior in the context of substance use. *Journal of Psychosexual Health, 1*(1), 26–31. https://journals.sagepub.com/doi/pdf/10.1177/2631831818822015

Das, U., & Rout, S. (2023). Are delay ages at marriage increasing? Premarital sexual relation among youth people in the place of residence in India. *BMC Women's Health, 23*(1), 1-12. https://bmcwomenshealth.biomedcentral.com/articles/10.1186/s12905-022-02149-3

Dave, V. R., Makwana, N. R., Yadav, B. S., & Yadav, S. (2013). A study on high-risk premarital sexual behavior of college going male students in Jamnagar city of Gujarat, India. *International journal of high risk behaviors & addiction, 2*(3), 112. https://www.ncbi.nlm.nih.gov/pmc/articles/PMC4070158/

Dhapola, M., Sharan, M., & Shah, B. (2007). Migration, youth and HIV risk: a study of young men in rural Jharkhand. *Economic and Political Weekly*, 40–47. https://www.jstor.org/stable/pdf/40276716.pdf?casa_token=qlhqXkYxD1cAAAAA:UQTI9RAw0Er1zrFjq01EB3fF3p1nSwelcsDNl6TdXuV4mL_he2zVfHAGBKBg92xEqkRmTwprhYvYQOcwPsx3wYXflzmZxfSa8tD47JnnBpUswY8FZ18

Doherty, I. A., & Stuart, G. S. (2011). Coitus interruptus is not contraception. *Sexually transmitted diseases, 38*(4), 356. https://journals.lww.com/stdjournal/FullText/2011/04000/Coitus_Interruptus_Is_Not_Contraception.22.aspx

Ghule, M., Balaiah, D., & Joshi, B. (2007). Attitude towards premarital sex among rural college youth in Maharashtra, India. *Sexuality & Culture, 11*, 1–17. https://link.springer.com/article/10.1007/s12119-007-9006-6

Haffner, D. W. (1995). Report of the national commission on adolescent sexual health. *Facing Facts: Sexual health for America's adolescents: New York: Sexuality Information and Education Council of the United States.* https://pubmed.ncbi.nlm.nih.gov/12319704/

International Institute for Population Sciences (IIPS) and ICF. (2017). *National Family Health Survey (NFHS-4), 2015–16: India.* IIPS. http://rchiips.org/nfhs/NFHS-4Reports/India.pdf

International Institute for Population Sciences (IIPS) and ICF. (2021). National Family Health Survey (NFHS-5), 2019–21: India: Volume I. IIPS. http://rchiips.org/nfhs/NFHS-5Reports/NFHS-5_INDIA_REPORT.pdf

International Institute for Population Sciences (IIPS) and Macro International. (2007). *National Family Health Survey (NFHS-3), 2005–06: India: Volume I.* IIPS. http://rchiips.org/nfhs/NFHS-3%20Data/VOL-1/India_volume_I_corrected_17oct08.pdf

International Institute for Population Sciences (IIPS) and Population Council. (2010). *Youth in India: Situation and Needs 2006–2007*. IIPS. https://www.popcouncil.org/uploads/pdfs/2010PGY_YouthInIndiaReport.pdf

Jejeebhoy, S. J. (1998). Adolescent sexual and reproductive behavior: a review of the evidence from India. *Social science & medicine, 46*(10), 1275–1290. https://www.sciencedirect.com/science/article/pii/S0277953697100569?casa_token=roKsMjTWtyoAAAAA:XOCtTiCmd4ssEWScWe-38ANVI6KmhBcBLW6MxtB6sAi4Nrk10NKkDea_3-QdEA44aR-Xb551Y8H5

Joshi, B., & Chauhan, S. (2011). Determinants of youth sexual behaviour: program implications for India. *Eastern Journal of Medicine, 16*(2), 113. https://jag.journalagent.com/ejm/pdfs/EJM_16_2_113_121.pdf

Khadilkar, V. V., Stanhope, R. G., & Khadilkar, V. (2006). Secular trends in puberty. *Indian pediatrics, 43*(6), 475. https://www.indianpediatrics.net/june2006/june-475-478.htm

Kost, K., Singh, S., Vaughan, B., Trussell, J., & Bankole, A. (2008). Estimates of contraceptive failure from the 2002 National Survey of Family Growth. *Contraception, 77*(1), 10-21. https://www.ncbi.nlm.nih.gov/pmc/articles/PMC2811396/

Kumar, R., Jha, P., Arora, P., Dhingra, N., Rao, S. (2005). HIV-1 trends, risk factors and growth in India. In: Rao, S., (ed.) *National commission on macroeconomics and health background papers: burden of disease in India.* Ministry of Health and Family Welfare, Government of India. https://www.academia.edu/2867617/HIV_1_trends_risk_factors_and_growth_in_India

Mathew, G., Shanbhag, D., Subramanian, S., Lobo, C., Xavier, A., Dasari, P., & Goud, R. (2019). HIV-related high-risk behavior and awareness regarding HIV among the male workers at a construction site in Karnataka. *International Journal of Medical Science and Public Health, 8*(12). https://www.researchgate.net/profile/Prudhvi-Dasari/publication/335974790_HIV-related_high-risk_behavior_and_awareness_regarding_HIV_among_the_male_workers_at_a_construction_site_in_Karnataka/links/5ddab2f7299bf10c5a30ee9e/HIV-related-high-risk-behavior-and-awareness-regarding-HIV-among-the-male-workers-at-a-construction-site-in-Karnataka.pdf

Miller, R. (2003). Withdrawal: a very great deal better than nothing. *The Canadian Journal of Human Sexuality, 12*(3–4), 189–191. https://go.gale.com/ps/i.do?id=GALE%7CA120099103&sid=googleScholar&v=2.1&it=r&linkaccess=abs&issn=11884517&p=HRCA&sw=w&userGroupName=anon%7E2ab5dcb6

Ministry of Law and Justice, Legislative Department. (2021). *The medical termination of pregnancy amendment Act, 2021.* https://egazette.nic.in/WriteReadData/2021/226130.pdf

Ministry of Youth Affairs and Sports, Government of India. (2014). *National Youth Policy, 2021.* https://www.rgniyd.gov.in/sites/default/files/pdfs/scheme/nyp_2014.pdf

National AIDS Control Organization & Indian Council of Medical Research—National Institute of Medical Statistics (ICMR-NIMS), Ministry of Health and Family Welfare, Government of India. (2022). *Technical Report, India HIV Estimates 2021.* http://naco.gov.in/sites/default/files/India%20HIV%20Estimates.pdf

National AIDS Control Organization (2015). *National Integrated Biological and Behavioural Surveillance (IBBS), India 2014–15.* NACO, Ministry of Health and Family Welfare, Government of India. http://naco.gov.in/sites/default/files/IBBS%20Report%202014-15.pdf

National Behavioural Surveillance Survey (BSS). 2006. *Youth (15–24 Years).* NACO, Ministry of Health and Family Welfare, Government of India. http://naco.gov.in/sites/default/files/Youth_report_1.pdf

National Commission on Population, Ministry of Health & Family Welfare (2020). *Population projections for India and states 2011–2036: Reports of the Technical Group on Population Projections.* https://main.mohfw.gov.in/sites/default/files/Population%20Projection%20Report%202011-2036%20-%20upload_compressed_0.pdf

Pathak, P. K., Tripathi, N., & Subramanian, S. V. (2014). Secular trends in menarcheal age in India-evidence from the Indian human development survey. *PLoS One, 9*(11), e111027. https://journals.plos.org/plosone/article?id=10.1371/journal.pone.0111027

Prata, N., Morris, L., Mazive, E., Vahidnia, F., & Stehr, M. (2006). Relationship between HIV risk perception and condom use: evidence from a population-based survey in Mozambique. *International family planning perspectives*, 192–200. https://www.jstor.org/tc/accept?origin=%2Fstable%2Fpdf%2F4147639.pdf%3Fcasa_token%3DJbw6ENaD5BgAAAAA%3A6HVDVuEO6anJmNpT-msYYtDEgmmiTwchUZRykO5MnzpDKKzqpctTu0kCTfvJkBj9a_SVyLtqJWdPNaVSF7avwPjlfBOFY4ctWql-i1Xxb22Sk2n83Ns&is_image=False

Saggurti, N., Mahapatra, B., Swain, S. N., & Jain, A. K. (2011). Male migration and risky sexual behavior in rural India: is the place of origin critical for HIV prevention programs?. *BMC Public Health, 11*, 1–13. https://link.springer.com/article/10.1186/1471-2458-11-S6-S6

Santhya, K. G., & Jejeebhoy, S. J. (2012). *The sexual and reproductive health and rights of young people in India: A review of the situation.* https://knowledgecommons.popcouncil.org/cgi/viewcontent.cgi?article=1018&context=departments_sbsr-pgy

Santhya, K. G., Acharya, R., & Jejeebhoy, S. J. (2011a). Condom use before marriage and its correlates: Evidence from India. *International perspectives on sexual and reproductive health*, 170–180. Retrieved from: https://www.guttmacher.org/sites/default/files/article_files/3717011.pdf

Santhya, K. G., Acharya, R., Jejeebhoy, S. J., & Ram, U. (2011b). Timing of first sex before marriage and its correlates: evidence from India. *Culture, Health & Sexuality*, *13*(03), 327-341. https://www.tandfonline.com/doi/pdf/10.1080/13691058.2010.534819

Sawyer, S. M., Afifi, R. A., Bearinger, L. H., Blakemore, S. J., Dick, B., Ezeh, A. C., & Patton, G. C. (2012). Adolescence: a foundation for future health. *The lancet*, *379*(9826), 1630–1640. https://www.researchgate.net/profile/Susan-Sawyer/publication/258048400_First_paper_in_2012_Lancet_series_on_Adolescent_Health/links/00b7d526c65e9b6d01000000/First-paper-in-2012-Lancet-series-on-Adolescent-Health.pdf

Sharma, A., Goel, N. K., Prashar, S., & Choudhary, K. (2022). A cross-sectional study to assess the premarital sexual practices among Panjab University students, Chandigarh, India. *Journal of Family Medicine and Primary Care*, *11*(8), 4631–4634. https://journals.lww.com/jfmpc/Fulltext/2022/08000/A_cross_sectional_study_to_assess_the_pre_marital.80.aspx#:~:text=In%20students%20having%20a%20positive,were%20satisfied%20with%20sexual%20life.

Singh, S. K., Vishwakarma, D., & Sharma, S. K. (2020). An epidemiology of premarital sexual behaviour in India: exploring gender differences. *Journal of Health Management*, *22*(3), 389–412. https://www.researchgate.net/profile/Deepanjali-Vishwakarma/publication/344201014_An_Epidemiology_of_Premarital_Sexual_Behaviour_in_India_Exploring_Gender_Differences/links/5f80049392851c14bcb8f673/An-Epidemiology-of-Premarital-Sexual-Behaviour-in-India-Exploring-Gender-Differences.pdf

Stoner, S. A., George, W. H., Peters, L. M., & Norris, J. (2007). Liquid courage: Alcohol fosters risky sexual decision-making in individuals with sexual fears. *AIDS and Behavior*, *11*, 227-237. https://www.researchgate.net/publication/6982850_Liquid_Courage_Alcohol_Fosters_Risky_Sexual_Decision-Making_in_Individuals_with_Sexual_Fears

Štulhofer, A., Graham, C., Božičević, I., Kufrin, K., & Ajduković, D. (2007). HIV/AIDS-related knowledge, attitudes and sexual behaviors as predictors of condom use among young adults in Croatia. *International family planning perspectives*, 58–65. https://www.jstor.org/stable/pdf/30039204.pdf?casa_token=gYJwVOYXc-QAAAAA:B-N7W9uGreGHw5-DRr8AzA8f2zWuYwme2-guGcve3tXvjDs4HNWe8K-X6Tbhuxjry7mnd81feNy6L5G0e8KgWxKYlNf-AwuGBGYLzHBsm5BZ_OnbV3w

Sujay, R. (2009). *Premarital sexual behaviour among unmarried college students of Gujarat, India.* https://knowledgecommons.popcouncil.org/cgi/viewcontent.cgi?article=1510&context=departments_sbsr-rh

Sznitman, S. R., Romer, D., Brown, L. K., DiClemente, R. J., Valois, R. F., Vanable, P. A., & Stanton, B. (2009). Prevalence, correlates, and sexually transmitted infection risk related to coitus interruptus among African-American adolescents. *Sexually transmitted diseases*, *36*(4), 218. https://www.jstor.org/stable/pdf/44969265.pdf

Taylor-Seehafer, M., & Rew, L. (2000). Risky sexual behavior among adolescent women. *Journal for Specialists in Pediatric Nursing*, *5*(1), 15–25. https://doi.org/10.1111/j.1744-6155.2000.tb00082.x

Tripathi, N., & Sekher, T. V. (2013). Youth in India ready for sex education? emerging evidence from national surveys. *PLoS ONE*, *8*(8), e71584. https://doi.org/10.1371/journal.pone.0071584

Trussell, J., & Wynn, L. L. (2008). Reducing unintended pregnancy in the United States. *Contraception*, *77*(1), 1–5. https://www.contraceptionjournal.org/article/S0010-7824(07)00405-2/fulltext

Wolffers, I., & Fernandez, I. (1995). Migration and AIDS. *Lancet (London, England)*, *346*(8985), 1303–1303. https://europepmc.org/article/med/7475751

Xenos, P. (1993). *Extended adolescence and the sexuality of Asian youth: Observations on research and policy (No. 292).* East-West Center. https://books.google.co.in/books/about/Extended_Adolescence_and_the_Sexuality_o.html?id=6ypFAAAAYAAJ&redir_esc=y

Yadav, J., Bharati, K., & Singh, K. J. (2015). Pattern of substance abuse, sexual behavior and its determinants among unmarried youth in India. *Global Journal of Human Social Science*, *15*(8), 14-24. https://globaljournals.org/GJHSS_Volume15/3-Pattern-of-Substance.pdf

Pragati Dattatraya Ubale is currently a senior research scholar with a UGC doctoral fellowship at the International Institute for Population Sciences (IIPS), Deemed University, Mumbai, India. She has completed her M.Sc. and M.Phil degrees in Population Studies from IIPS and graduated in statistics from Pune University. She is currently exploring the issues related to dating, dating violence, premarital sexual activities, mate selection, and Sexual and Reproductive Health aspects by conducting a primary survey of college going unmarried youth of Mumbai city. Well trained in Statistics, Demography and Research Methods, her areas of research interests are gender, marriage, sexuality, sexual and reproductive health, intimate partner violence, and sex education. She has presented research papers in national and international conferences and seminars.

Dr. T.V. Sekher is Professor and Head of the Department of Family and Generations, and Head, Centre for Ageing Studies at the International Institute for Population Sciences (IIPS), Mumbai. He is the PI of the Longitudinal Ageing Study in India (LASI) and the Study on Global AGEing and Adult Health (SAGE-India). He was the National Coordinator of the District Level Household and Facility Surveys (DLHS-3&4) for the Ministry of Health and Family Welfare, Govt. of India. Dr. Sekher was Visiting Fellow at the Wellcome Trust Centre at UCL, London (2003), Maison de Sciences la Homme, Paris (2004), Lund University, Sweden (2005) and at Oxford Brooks University, UK (2009). He was Fulbright-Nehru Senior Fellow (2016-17) at Cornell University. He has authored and edited ten books, and has more than 100 research articles in national and international journals. He was consultant to Govt. of India, Planning Commission, UNFPA, UNICEF, Population Council and many other organizations.

Part IV
Role of Youth and Youth Development Index

Chapter 25
Youth Participation in Community Development: Issues and Implications

S. Lalitha

Abstract Youth is a dynamic category and a potential human resource for sustainable development and a resilient Society. Although they are numerically determined high but often seen less in terms of their participation in community development. Therefore, a few questions arise, while determining youth participation in Community Development viz., Why are youth neglected and not much discussed as a center of community development? Why is their least interest in community development critiqued rather than analyzed critically? Are the structural barriers hindering youth participation in community development? Are the youth disengaging themselves owing to the inter-generational conflicts? Do they possess a deep drive for individualization? Are they self-engaged? Are they afraid of accepting the responsibilities due to their commitment? Do they lack institutional support and guidance? which undermines youth participation in community development. Globally, the youth are a sizable population, and having realized that the United Nations emphasized the crucial role of youth explicitly in the 2030 Agenda especially for implementing the SDGs. Youth being a functional unit of any society, they can be made as social change agents for Community Development. They can play the roles of critical thinkers, change-makers, innovators, communicators, and leaders in achieving the SDGs by ensuring their active participation in the community development activities. This chapter focuses on the importance of socio-economic and political context of the youth and also the contextual factors that influence them in rendering their participation in community development. The strength-based approach in Social Work is suggested as a suitable intervention to work with youth, to enhance youth social capital for Community Development.

Keywords Community development · Participation · Strength-based approach · Sustainable development · Youth

S. Lalitha (✉)
Department of Social Work, RGNIYD, Sriperumbudur, India
e-mail: drlalitha.rgniyd@gmail.com

S. Deb and S. Deb (eds.), *Handbook of Youth Development*,
https://doi.org/10.1007/978-981-99-4969-4_25

Introduction

Youth is a matter of concern not because of their age but being a resourceful population. Although youth participation in civic engagement and community development have been emphasized by the governments at State and Central levels and at times emphasized by the International organizations such as United Nations and UNFPA, however youth participation in the community development activities is not significant especially in India, an aspiring country with a huge young population. This has become a point for discussion in any academic or political arena as to why youth participation is less or not seen in the community development activities. The country has National Youth Policy (2014) and the draft Youth Policy 2021; besides there are States that have their own State Youth policies and welfare programs despite the fact that youth participation is not seen overtly in community development activities. This chapter critically examines the reasons for disengagement of youth in community development, structural and systemic barriers to youth participation in community development, socio-economic and political contexts of youth in India, role of the youth as a critical change agent, and the need for explicit and sustainable participation of youth in community development to achieve the SDGs. This chapter also emphasizes the significance of strength-based approach in Social Work to devise a suitable intervention to promote youth participation in the community development activities.

Youth as a Heterogeneous Community: Characteristics and Trends

Youth is a concept, a category based on age, as well as an idealized and institutionalized group (Concept of youth., n.d.). Youth have certain attributes in general and they differ in needs and aspirations. Aspirations are created through social interactions and social existence by socializing. It is crucial to study young people in the contexts of their social lives (Ansell et al., 2020) in order to have a greater understanding of them. Though youth is a transitory stage (Andy, 2013), it is very important to understand them as their actions always determine their characteristics. Needs and aspirations of youth are diverse as youth being a heterogeneous population. So, location, time, gender, and context-specific strategies are imperative to gauge their needs and aspirations; and for devising suitable strategies for youth development. Over a period of time the term youth is constructed socially based on action and inaction. They are identified as contributors when their actions are rational, altruistic, and bring about positive results or constructive changes in the society. At the same time if their actions are irrational, destructive, and affects the society, they will be viewed as deviants are destructive forces. However, it should be noted that since youth are always interacting with the society through social relationships, it is not the youth that causes problems by their actions but rather the society. Youth demonstrate their resistance when they are under social pressure or are trying to gain approval from others. Adults commonly misinterpret youth resistance. Adults should attempt to identify the causes of youth resistance rather than finding fault with it. Also, youth are viewed by the society as being uncontrollable, although psychological theories emphasize that the youth go through a number of developmental stages that are prescribed by the society as well as endure stress and storm. Moreover, youth are generally brought into conflict as a result of their inactivity and lack of involvement in the community. Youth are consistently used by inter-generational conflict as problem-makers. Therefore, in order to better understand youth, the inter-generational power relationships should be examined (Jones, 2005).

The political factors also play a significant role in locating and constructing youth in the society. During pre-independence youth were viewed as change agents and as revolutionaries when they took part in the independence movement to fight against the colonial government. Later due to advancement of science and technology and globalization youth were connected globally and got access to global knowledge and expanded their global social connections. However, of late, volunteering for the social cause and exercising their political rights are seen very less since the youth detached themselves from the immediate society per se rather become more individualized. Lack of political awareness, political dis-engagement, and political divide are the reasons for youth not to have greater say in the community actions rather becoming victims of politics. Political awareness must be created in youth right from the school level. Issues related to politics and political matters must be discussed by youth freely at higher educational levels. Their affiliations to political movements and associations need to be encouraged (youth) and it is imperative to promote political leadership and political activism in them. Social norms become the barrier for youth not to engage in politics, especially it is evident among the female youth. Participatory structure and capacity building are the means for making youth a politically sound population for rendering participation in community development. Although the socio-political factors have greater influence for youth participation in community development, however, there are many more questions that remain unanswered and few among them are viz., Why the youth disassociate with community action? What makes them not to be a part of change? Also, why do the present youth possess a deep drive for individualization? Are they self-engaged? Are they afraid of accepting the responsibilities due to their commitment? Finding answers to these questions will be very helpful to engage youth productively in community development activities. The physiological and mental maturity must occur simultaneously for civilization in youth (Jones, 2005) otherwise it may be a threat to the society. The institutions such as family, school, neighborhood, and associations play crucial roles where the power conflict arises between the youth and adults. Young people must be allowed to experiment to achieve their own ethics. The morality (learned behavior) and the environment created by adults for the youth to experience and develop ethics matters during the developmental stages. When the development stages are not smooth the individual may encounter problems and challenges in later periods. Neuroscientists have also pointed out that experiences, well-being, and relationships have greater impact (Andy, 2013) on the development and the process of decision-making. So, they need adult support to search for positive experiences which will further enable them to fit into the social structures and as a contributor. When youth do not get opportunities for experiences they lack responsibilities. When youth lack adults' support they replace it with peers. So the self-identity is constructed during the youth stage with the influence of peer relations or peer bonding. Youth express themselves through culture and subculture means. They also express their resistance through culture and subculture. Sometimes their actions and expressions can be better understood through their music, dress, and drugs. Youth culture in the late modernity affects authenticity and transformative power (Jones, 2005). When young people are allowed to live autonomy they become independents. Persons nurtured with autonomy will have more sense of responsibility and function as a contributor. Those who were nurtured in a dependency culture will become reflexive and individualized. In order to promote development of individualization in youth they need to be connected with resources and support systems.

Community Development in India: An Overview

The term community development was identified as community participation by the United Nations in 1950s (Abbott, 1995) and it is viewed as a process designed to enhance socio-economic conditions of community by enlisting the people's participation (Murthy, 2013) and community collective efforts. It places a strong emphasis on the involvement of all those who are impacted, particularly local participation. It goes through several stages, including organising the community, identifying the needs of the community, designing programs by communities to answer the requirements, and carrying out the planned programs while making the best use of the resources at hand. Community development places a high value on self-help, independence, and altering one's viewpoint since it has great faith in people's inherent abilities.

In pre-independence times many experiments were made by the Indian government and the voluntary organizations with a view to promote people's participation in the developmental activities in rural areas (Maheswari, 1995). However, a great momentum happened only after independence when the community development program was launched on 2nd October, 1952. Although the Ministry of Community Development was established in 1956 to implement the rural development programs, later it was changed as the Ministry of Agriculture and Rural Development. But later it was further changed to the Ministry of Rural Development in 1969 and since then it has been promoting rural development through centrally and state-sponsored programs. When the community development program was launched its primary objectives were to bring about progress in the lives of people as a result people would be ensured with freedom, dignity, respect, security, self-reliance, and self-development. Social and economic development was viewed as key aspects of community development programs. Later the Urban development/community development programs were launched for enhancing the standard of living of people in the urban areas. Over a period of time and till date many programs have been launched and experimented for the socio-economic development of the people in the rural and urban areas. However, the development programs did not create a strong community forum or an active social movement at the grassroots to function as a change agent or active participants of the community development initiatives. Although the community development programs and schemes have inbuilt focus on the development of youth, however such programs have not yielded fullest participation of youth. So, it is necessary to understand why youth are disinterested toward community development? Also why are they neglected and not been much discussed as a center of community development? And why their least interest in community development is always critiqued rather than analyzed critically?

Youth in India: Role and Function as an Established Unit

India is the youngest country having 27.1% (Economy, 2022) of youth as per the Youth in India Report 2022. Youth is a primary course of discussion of the country since the country has a sizable proportion of youth. The youth policy of India (2014) emphasizes the holistic development and participation of youth in community development. It also illustrates the roles and responsibilities of youth to be active agents of change. Youth being a functional unit of a society, can be made as social change agents for Community Development. Youth social capital is significant for engaging them in community development. In order to make youth participate in community development activities they need to be better understood. Socio-economic and political contexts of the youth and the contextual factors influence the youth to render their participation in community development.

Firstly, understanding youth in their social context is prerequisite. Social context means social environment or the neighborhood in which the youth live in. Environmental factors influence youth and affect their characteristics. Youth cannot act in a vacuum. To make youth perform meaningful social action, their role and functions has to be well aware by youth and also a supportive social environment is essential to enable them to execute the intended action. Often the structural barriers are hindering the youth participation in community development. Social divisions form the basis of social structure (Wood & Hine, 2009). Social relationships, institutions, and groupings play a key role in determining power, status, and opportunities of the individuals. Also, the social systems like family, religion, geographical location, neighborhood, caste, power structure, etc., influence youth and control their actions. Youth actions are seen through behaviors and attitudes. Of course the behaviors and attitudes are shaped by the outcome of socialization and social interaction of youth when they encounter various social institutions. The self is developed through psychological and socio-political factors. Nature and nurture are the key essential aspects in the lives of a youth which reveals them as a burden or contributor to the society.

Secondly, the lack of adequate economic resources forces youth vehemently to take possessions of others and excludes them from formal production (Robert White, 2002) which supposedly gives legitimate identity. Denial of opportunities and non-participation in the formal economic sphere leads to youth idleness and exclusion; and has adverse impact on the lives of youth especially the marginalized youth in the society. Prolonged unemployment and gap in supply in demand for labor disintegrates youth in the society (Andy, 2013) and becomes reasons for risky behaviors in youth. So, it is imperative to capitalize the potential of youth (RGNIYD, 2017) in India for sustaining a stable growth in the global economy.

Thirdly, Young people's political opportunities are reduced by generational inequality, which stops them from using their creative abilities and energy to solve difficult problems that impact society as a whole. In the Indian context participation among youth is generally constrained based on systematic factors caste, religion, gender, education, location, and political divide. Also, the risky behaviors in youth, prolonged engagement in the social media, and individuation (consumer culture) lead them to have detached life and trouble them in establishing self-identity. A youth belonging to low socio-economic conditions, lives in a crime-prone area (Hall & Jefferson, 2006), will be having more chances to indulge in risky behaviors. It is not the youth who creates the problems rather the societal pressures create problems for the youth. So, to understand youth better it is imperative to understand their lifestyle, leisure time activities, needs, and aspirations and the factors that affect their lives. Further it is also necessary to know how youth relates with the adults? Whether adults are accepting the changes and trends? Are they showing an empathic approach toward youth? Whether the inter-generational conflict creates disengagement of youth in community actions?

Youth and SDGs: Agenda 2030

The Sustainable Development Goals are intended to combat the global issues of poverty and the social needs by promoting economic growth and environmental protections through different strategies (UN, 2022). Globally the youth population between 15 and 24 years are 16 percent. Although the 17 SDGs are directly and indirectly involving the youth, specifically the seven goals and 169 targets are youth focused. The UN views youth as the center of development and advocates that the youth development policies and programs should fulfill the needs and aspirations of youth. Further, youth are viewed as a key stakeholder in achieving the SDGs and for the sustainable future. It is emphasized that their knowledge of the triple bottom line of sustainability viz., economic, social, and environmental (Ismail et al., 2022) is an essential for achieving the SDGs. According to the World Youth Report (2020), young people in developing nations face significant social and economic problems and are frequently left out of choices that will affect their lives now and in the future.

Youth being a functional unit of any society, they can be made as social change agents for Community Development. They can be a dynamic force of political change and social transformation for which their participation in the decision-making process is essential (hand book youth). They can play the roles of critical thinkers, change-makers, innovators, communicators, entrepreneurs, and leaders in achieving the SDGs by ensuring their active participation in the community development activities.

Youth as Agents for Change in the Community

Community is a geographic territory bounded with a sense of belongingness and composed of various sub groups. Youth can function as an agent of change individually and as a collective. Youth need space for participation and contribution. Undermining youth potential by merely quoting their age, inexperience, culture, caste, and gender must be changed in the minds of adults, power structure in the community and in the policymakers. It is the youth who can better converse their issues that they encounter in their day-to-day lives. Today's youth are tomorrow's adults. If their opportunities are denied, how can they take up constructive roles in the later period? The community may have wider issues and needs. Since youth is also a part of the community, their voice should be heard in the community decision-making process. Trust, access to opportunity, social connections, and positive social relationships provide youth confidence and will inculcate the spirit of civic engagement. The International Labour Organization (ILO) (2020) says that globally the population of youth is increasing and at the same time the youth are experiencing structural barriers due to which they are prevented from entering into the labor market. Merely youth are in the informal sector globally and the working conditions are very dangerous and they are deprived of legal and social protection. Also, the youth face limited opportunities for training and career development. When it comes to India, youth face numerous problems especially the social exclusion, unemployment, lack of access to decent jobs, and lack of substantial skills for the labor market due to unstable political institutions and socio-political consequences. For youth to be productive members of society, the right skill sets, high-quality education, and training must be offered. In order for the young people to transition from an individualized space to a collective space. For this reason, youth ought to be seen as a partner in community development programs. Proactive policies that promote youth development will provide a way for youth participation in community actions. Youth development organizations must take a key role in creating awareness of the policies and programs in youth for their active engagement in community development.

Theoretical Framework for Youth Participation in Community Development

The transparency of the government, particularly in facilitating public engagement in the decision-making process, is the most important factor in community development. Youth development is a means of community development. A conducive and safe environment is a prerequisite for youth development. So a question arises whether youth have choices to share their lives? Do they make choices and take initiative in their own lives? Do they independently? But, in general, youth are seen as a dependent category, and this is also true in India. There is a notion that always persists in adults that youth are not engaged in community development activities. They are least engaged and busy with their personal commitments. Also youth are blamed for being more self-concerned and least concerned about community development. So the question arises that is it the youth are really not interested in community development activities or they were not given any opportunities for community engagement. But it has to be noted that the youth experience is dependent on the opportunities that they get. It is merely said that life with uncertainty and frequent being revised by youth affects their transition and makes them reflexive. The Bronfenbrenner (1979) theory of Ecological system depicts the individuals at the core of the system and illustrates the relationship between individuals and five major sub systems such as families, schools and peer groups, and external environments and broader socio-cultural contexts. Primarily the theory highlights the complex interaction between individuals and the subsystems and its impact on youth behavior and development (Fig. 25.1).

Also, it has to be noted that the youth in India lack institutional support and guidance. Although they extend their participation in various ways, what undermines youth participation in community development. Are they lacking technical knowledge and decision-making skills? If so, youth need to be provided essential training and capacity building. In fact, capacity building must be viewed as the objective of all community development programs and social welfare schemes. Youth can be involved in making community action plans and be made as the service delivery agent for which their rights are to be regarded. A proactive approach is imperative for community youth development for which young people need institutional support (Wood & Hine, 2009) and more particularly at the community level.

Promoting Youth Participation in Community Development Using Strength-Based Approach

Since youth is a transition period and a crucial stage their attitude and skills need to be sharpened to enable them to gain positive identity in self and in society. So any programs aimed for community development should be youth focused and must make youth a center for community development. For which the empathetic approach

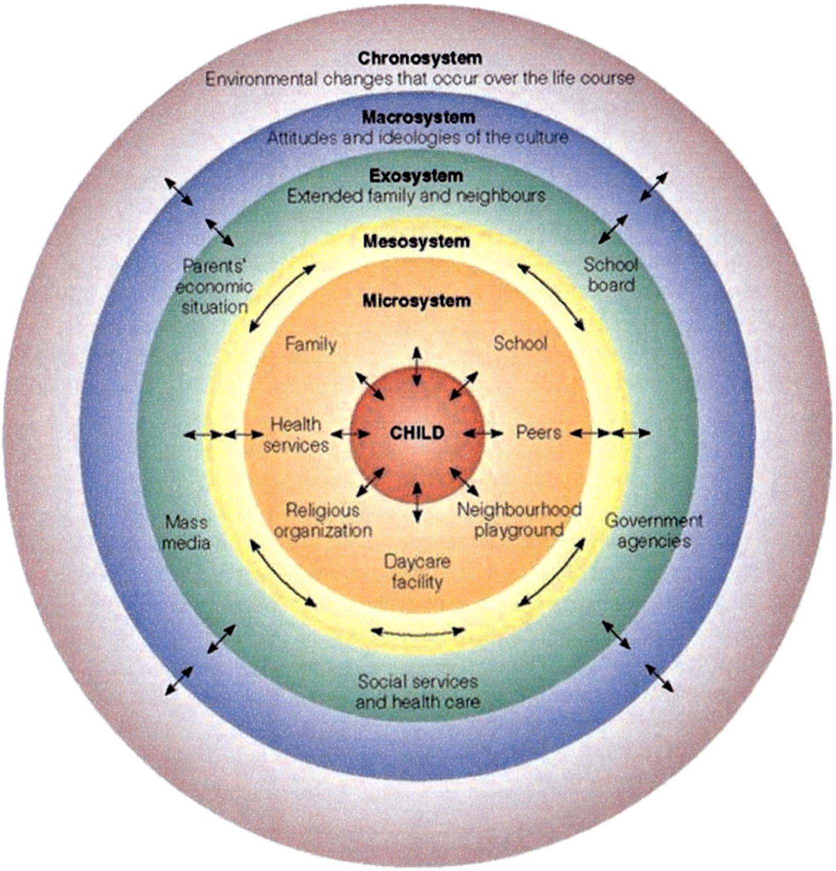

Fig. 25.1 Brofnfenbrenner's five ecological systems

is essential. Youth participation at different levels has to be meticulously planned and implemented. The fundamental problem of youth for non-participation in community development is that youth are never consulted nor approached by the authorities or the institutions which are responsible for policy formulation and implementation. It is always challenging for youth to identify the ways to participate in community development. The ways and means of participation are not widely told to the youth. To participate meaningfully in community development programs, they require the support of adults with the necessary skills and relationships. However, they are not given these things. The intergenerational conflicts, structural barriers, and systemic oppression also become a threat to participation of youth. Youth in India are pressurised for attainment of education and employment status and always it is not of their choice but of society. Although social interaction is viewed as a crucial element (Neal et al., 2013) in the development process the youth in late modernity are more individualized and less connected physically in the social interaction and socialization process. The less social interaction and less socialization results in a lack of sense of belongingness toward community development activities. Participation in community development requires a mere sense of responsibility which is in fact nurtured by the institutions such as family, school, religion, and neighborhood characteristics. If these institutions fulfilled their role by instilling the values, attitudes and skills in young people civic engagement and citizenship it would have certainly resulted in effective participation of youth in community development. Also, the citizenship opportunities should be contextual and must provide localized experience (Wood & Hine, 2009).

By realizing the youth potential, the 2030 Agenda emphasizes the youth participation in achieving the SDGs. Youth should be encouraged as active social agents and they must be made aware of different roles that they can perform in achieving community development. Youth always appreciate the innovative ways to engage themselves. Hence the channel of connecting and organizing youth for community development should be well thought and be often updated with the trends. Technology-enabled participation, real-time participation monitoring techniques, appreciation and acknowledging the youth in Social Media Platform, and peer-facilitated participation may be considered for youth participation in community development. Youth can be facilitated to extend their collective participation as an organized group such as youth club/forum or association (Lalitha et al., 2020). So, the local youth clubs/forums need to be digitally connected and audited for valuing their participation in community development activities. Community Youth Development model (Eccles & Gootman, 2002) can be encouraged to prevent risky behaviors and promote youth well-being; also the Youth-led development models (Ortega-Williams, 2020) can be encouraged to promote six Cs (competence, confidence, connection, character, caring/compassion and contribution). Also, a list of desirable competencies for young people was also developed by the Carnegie Council on Adolescent Development, and it encompasses academic, cognitive, civic, emotional, physical, social, cultural, and occupational competence.

The opportunity to contribute to one's self and community can be facilitated by youth workers, particularly professional social workers who have received training in youth work. For youth engaging in community development should give excitement, fun, and experience. They need friendly space, a safe environment, and mere acceptance for their engagement. In social work, a strength-based approach is widely used to help the client system to contribute for self and society. Strength-based approach focuses on the abilities and talents of the individuals and not on their short falls. To be an active social change agent the youth needs adequate support and opportunities. The youth need social connection inside and outside the communities to function as a social capital. If youth are given leadership responsibilities, they will contribute effectively to community development activities. Youth development (FCYO, 2000) is the process that all young people go through as they develop the personal qualities or skills required to participate in adolescence and adulthood. Youth leadership is a crucial part of the youth development process as it helps young people assess their own strengths, guide, direct, and influence others, and serve as role models (Wehmeyer et al., 1998).

Promoting developmental strengths includes resilience and youth development which will lead to creating and sustaining asset-building communities. The developmental assets framework can be used to analyze critically the life journey, hardship that they went through, and their reflective experiences (Silbereisen & Lerner, 2007) that they encountered in their community. Priorities and research findings form the foundation of social policy (Chopra et al., 2001). In light of the fact that government policies would undoubtedly have an impact on the country's youth, youth perception, aspirations, and priorities (Karnataka Jnana Aayoga, 2011) should be in line with those of the government. So, it is indispensable that youth should always be the focal point of policies and programs intended for community development because they are the active citizens with innovative thoughts; and can play a significant role in program planning and community mobilization.

Conclusion

If youth are regarded as a center of community development, then all the initiatives will be appropriated toward enabling youth to participate in community development. Instead of blaming the youth for non-participation it is the responsibility of the social, economic, and political institutions and especially the States to devise various ways and innovative strategies to encourage youth participation in community development. The conventional approach in community development programs needs to be altered with a youth friendly approach. Youth collective participation has to be appreciated in community development activities. Structure and the systems/institutions should provide favorable for youth to access and to participate in the community development activities. Youth-led initiatives have to be. The use of strength-based approach will help to increase youth social capital which is essential for successful participation of youth in community development activities.

References

Abbott, J. (1995). Community participation and its relationship to community development. *Community Development Journal, 30*(2), 158–168. https://doi.org/10.1093/cdj/30.2.158

Andy, F. (2013). *Youth studies: An introduction*. Routledge.

Ansell, N., Froerer, P., Huijsmans, R., Dungey, C., & Dost, A. (2020). Educating 'surplus population': Uses and abuses of aspiration in the rural peripheries of a globalising world.

Bronfenbrenner, U. (1979). *The ecology of human development: Experiments by nature and design*. Harvard University Press.

Chopra, J. K., Sen, S., & Manusukhani, G. S. (2001). *General sociology*. Unique Publishers.

Concept of Youth. (n.d.). http://sociologyaustralia.allenandunwin.com.s3-website-ap-southeast-2.amazonaws.com/files/RETHINK.PDF

Eccles, J., & Gootman, J. A. (2002). *Community programs to promote youth development*. National Academy Press.
Economy. (2022). Youth in India 2022 Report. https://journalsofindia.com/youth-in-india-2022-report/.
FCIO. (2000). *An emerging model of working with youth*. https://fcyo.org/uploads/resources/8141_Papers_no1_v4.qxd.pdf
Hall, S., & Jefforn, T. (2006). *Resistance through rituals, youth subcultures in post-war Britain* (2nd edn.). Routledge.
ILO. (2020). *Global trends for youth 2020: Technology and the future jobs*, Geneva. https://www.ilo.org/wcmsp5/groups/public/---dgreports/---dcomm/---publ/documents/publication/wcms_737648.pdf
Ismail, T. N. T., Yusof, M. I. M., Ab Rahman, F. A., & Harsono, D. (2022). Youth and their knowledge on the sustainable development goals (SDGs). *Environment-Behaviour Proceedings Journal, 7*(19), 329–335.
Jones, G. (2005). *Youth*. Polity.
Karnataka Jnana Aayoga. (2011). Study on youth perception, aspirations, expectations, and attitudes of youth in Karnataka. https://karunadu.karnataka.gov.in/jnanaayoga/Archives/Resources/Research%20Studies/Research%20Studies/Youth%20Study_full_report.pdf
Lalitha, S., Roseline, L. P., & Roul. (2020). SDGs and livelihood of slum youth in Chennai: A framework of implementation. *Perspectives in Social Work, XXXVI*(1).
Maheswari, S. R. (1995). Rural development in India: a public policy approach. *Asia-Pacific Journal of Rural Development, 2*. https://doi.org/10.1177/1018529119950208
Murthy, R. D. (2013). *Strategies for community organization*. New Delhi.
National Youth Policy. (2014). Testimony of RGNIYD & Ministry of Youth Affairs and Sports, Government of India.
Neal, J. W.,& Neal, Z. P. (2013). Nested or networked? Future directions for ecological systems theory. *Social Development*. https://doi.org/10.1111/sode.12018
Ortega-Williams, A., Wernick, L. J., DeBower, J., & Brathwaite, B. (2020). Finding relief in action: The intersection of youth-led community organizing and mental health in Brooklyn, New York City. *Youth & Society, 52*(4), 618–638.
RGNIYD. (2017). *Youth development index and Report*.
Silbereisen, R. K., & Lerner, R. M. (2007). *Approaches to positive youth development*. Sage. ISBN 978-1-4129-2288-3.
United Nations. (2022). The Sustainable Development Goals Report. https://unstats.un.org/sdgs/report/2022/The-Sustainable-Development-Goals-Report-2022.pdf
Wehmeyer, M. L., Agran, M., & Hughes, C. (1998). *Teaching self-determination to students with disabilities: Basic skills for successful transition*. Paul H. Brookes.
Wood, J., & Hine, J. (2009). *Work with young people*. Sage.
World Youth Report. (2020). *Youth development and participation*. United Nations. https://www.un.org/development/desa/youth/wp-content/uploads/sites/21/2020/10/WYR2020-Chapter2.pdf

S. Lalitha is currently an Assistant Professor of Social Work at the Rajiv Gandhi National Institute of Youth Development. A Visiting Fellow at King's College, London, UK, at the School of Education and Communication and Society in 2019. As an ICSSR Post-Doctoral Fellow, she worked at the Department of Humanities and Social Sciences, Indian Institute of Technology (IIT-Madras). She holds a Ph.D. (Social Work) from the University of Madras, a Master of Philosophy (Social Work) from Loyola College in Chennai, and a Master of Arts (Social Work) from Stella Maris College in Chennai. A PG Diploma in Human Resource Management was earned from Annamalai University, and she qualified for the UGC-NET in Social Work in 2000. She completed a certificate course in Administrative Management in Tokyo, Japan, in 2011. In Stockholm, she attended conferences funded by international grants, including World Water Week (2011) and Social Work and Social Development (2012). In the year 2015, she attended the Active Citizens

Social Enterprise Leadership Programme-A Global Master Facilitator Development Workshop in London, UK. She has presented papers at national and international conferences and published articles in national and international journals. As the Coordinator of the Centre for Dalit and Subaltern Studies at RGNIYD, she conducts training programmes for marginalized youth nationwide. Community development, water governance, youth studies, social inclusion, and social entrepreneurship are her areas of interest. Her memberships include Professional Social Workers Association, Chennai, Tamil Nadu, Indian Society for Professional Social Work, Chandigarh, India, and JICA Alumni Association of India. In 2022, she conducted a study on "Social Reality of Scheduled Caste Youth in Tamil Nadu with reference to Sustainable Development Goals".

Chapter 26
Youth Leadership and Participation in Political Processes

Bishakha Majumdar

Abstract Youth, the transition between childhood and early to middle adulthood, from a critical part of human existence, devoted to education, vocational skilling, career, marriage, and independent social participation. This makes the youth an interesting phase of encounter with institutions such as government, civil society, law, religion, and the economy. It also makes the youth an important stakeholder in the various policies and programs of the government of a nation. The political participation of the youth is, however, often subject to challenges such as apathy, misinformation, violence, anti-institutional sentiments, and lack of trust in the politics and institutional processes of the previous generations. Social media has also been a game-changer in youth politics—lending a platform to millions of youths to raise their voices but has been a major source of fake news and hate speech in youth politics. This chapter traces the recent trends in political participation of youth worldwide and in India, the factors influencing political participation of youth, and the policy interventions that encourage political activism among the youth in a way that is constructive and beneficial for the new generations. It also forwards interventions that may encourage youth participation in politics, train them in political processes, and ensure their active and informed participation in politics and policymaking.

Keywords Youth · Politics · Social media · Representation · Activism · Policy

Introduction

Why the Voice of the Youth Matters?

> No one is born a good citizen; no nation is born a democracy. Rather, both are processes that continue to evolve over a lifetime. Young people must be included from birth. A society that cuts itself off from its youth severs its lifeline; it is condemned to bleed to death.

B. Majumdar (✉)
Organizational Behavior and Human Resource Management, Indian Institute of Management Visakhapatnam, Visakhapatnam 530003, India
e-mail: majumdar.bishakha@gmail.com

S. Deb and S. Deb (eds.), *Handbook of Youth Development*,
https://doi.org/10.1007/978-981-99-4969-4_26

—Kofi Annan, Former Secretary-General of the United Nations

The post-pandemic world has seen unprecedented variabilities in lifestyles, economic behavior, social interactions, and geopolitics. As the world braves multiple waves of the COVID-19 pandemic, the threat of cross-border and transcontinental armed conflicts as well as of an economic downturn looms large. This is accompanied by changing climatic conditions and its impact on economies and livelihoods across the world. All these make the post-pandemic years of critical importance from the perspective of policymaking, more so for the future generations who are set to inherit this world order. The voice of the youth in policymaking and politics is assuming more importance today than ever before, as an increasingly dynamic world, marked by digital transformations, climate changes, and sustainability challenges is increasingly posing problems unfamiliar to the skills and experiences of the earlier generations.

Youth, the transition between childhood and early to middle adulthood from a critical part of human existence for its many flavors, possibilities as well as vulnerabilities. Early youth or adolescence encompasses the formative years of human existence, devoted to training, education, and vocational skilling, whereas late youth, beyond the teens, is marked by transition into the adult world and responsibilities, through career, marriage, and independent social participation, away from parental supervision. This makes the youth an interesting phase of encounter of the individual with important institutions of the human society such as government, civil society, law, religion, and the economy. It also makes the youth an important stakeholder in the various policies and programs of the government of a nation.

The importance of the voice of the youth in policymaking, however, goes beyond the simple strength of numbers. Youth inherit the nation designed by the choices of the citizens of today, and most policies and practices have impacts ranging beyond decades. It thus seems irrational to block the youth from a conversation that would concern them critically for the rest of their lives. Second, youth is a period of apprenticeship, and early induction into youth-friendly policy and social awareness projects helps the youth to learn the nuances of governance, politics, and public influence in a relatively safe and mentored environment. Such lessons prove critical for later plunge into lives as fully responsible citizens. Finally, across generations, the youth tend to bring in energy and willingness to challenge the status quo, owing to their early exposure to what is the disruptive technology of that time, and less likelihood of being habituated to do things the old way. Hence, the youth often bring in new thoughts and revolutionary ideas in policymaking, that may give the old, accepted praxis a reality check, and help the nation progress toward new avenues.

Political participation also brings in significant advantages for the youth. Political engagement is likely to make a youth feel empowered and optimistic and give him or her a sense of efficacy and optimism. Political engagement has also been associated with creativity among the youth as well as a sense of contribution toward the society (NDI, 2018).

However, despite its obvious advantages, youth participation in policy matters and community development is not very common. The 2020 World Youth Development Index found a global deterioration in the youth participation in political and civic matters since 2018 (The Commonwealth, 2020). The trend is worrying, as it might be indicative of a lacuna in implementing policy actions to encourage youth participation, or of a growing lack of interest and trust among the digital natives in the politics and institutional processes of the previous generations.

Youth and Politics: Different Forms

The youth, defined as the period between 13 and 29 by the United Nations (REF), is typically a period when a person takes an increased interest in the adult world and gradually takes up a more involved role in it. Early youth is usually a phase of relatively passive familiarization with politics, governance, and legal systems, whereas mid to later youth is marked by a more active induction into actual political processes. Paolillo and Gerbaudo (2022) classified political participation of youth as (a) low-intensity activities ("voting, consuming news, discussing politics in small circles"), (b) medium-intensity activities ("contact and interaction with politicians and political self-expression"), and (c) high-intensity activities ("campaigning and organization"). The different forms of youth participation in politics can be enumerated as below.

Youth as Influencers

The earliest possible induction of the youth in the political process is usually in the role of the influencer. Even before the youth can register as voters, they gain exposure to knowledge and opinions about political processes, governance, and policy-making. This knowledge is gained from educational curricula on national history, law, and general awareness. Also, from very early in life, one gets exposed to the political ideologies of one's parents and other significant adults in one's life. Political campaigns, and mainstream media coverage of political news, lives of politicians, further add to one's understanding of the political world and attitude toward it. All these help the youth form political opinions well before reaching the age of suffrage. A significant number of political opinions on social media come from youth, many of whom are not actively engaged in any form of politics. The youth also receive political insights from peers and teachers in schools and colleges. When shared with family, such political opinions may also serve to influence the political opinions of family members. The Indian scenario post-2018 reveals a significant trend toward the interest of youth in national and state-level politics, willingness to vote, and even actively campaigning for causes of one's interest on the roads or on social media.

Youth in Civic Engagement

Elrich (2000) defined civic engagement as "working to make a difference in the civic life of one's community and developing the combination of knowledge, skills, values, and motivation to make that difference. It means promoting the quality of life in a community, through both political and non-political processes." (p. vi) It involves civic action (volunteering in community activities), civic duty (willingness to make positive contribution to society), civic skills (ability to contribute to the society), and social cohesion (ability to trust and bond with others) (Elrich, 2000).

Civic engagement of the youth, political or apolitical, is not uncommon. Youth is a period of significant energy and openness to experience, making young people seek out ways in which they could bring about changes in the status quo. Further, lack of vested interests in the form of organizational affiliations, business interests, or other practical concerns of the adult world, often makes the youth particularly effective in pinning their interests in social upliftment activities that are not financially rewarding. Youth is also a time of heightened interest in socialization and group affiliations, making civic engagements in groups a particularly productive experience for the youth.

Outside government endeavors, multiple non-governmental organizations provide forums for civic participation of the youth. The most prominent among these are the United Nations Organizations and the UN Volunteers, which allow the youth to participate in national developmental activities. The Credit Suisse Youth Barometer 2020 survey revealed that environmental activism and gender equality remained among the top priorities of youth civic engagement across nations (Credit Suisse, 2020). Henn et al. (2022), in their study on the youth across ten European countries, found an increase in political action relating to environmental activism among the youth, with the youth environmental activists particularly likely to be women with considerable education.

Youth as Voters

The age of suffrage varies from country to country, but usually ranges between 18 and 21 years. Eligibility to suffrage provides the youth the opportunity to participate in the political process of the nation. In most nations of the world, youth form a significant part of the adult suffrage, and have the potential to influence political outcomes. As per 2019 electoral data, India had 900 million eligible voters of which 45 million are under the age of 25 (Somashwar & Owaga, 2020).

Voting patterns of youth have been of much interest for political scholars and politicians, as youth often play the kingmakers owing to the large number. Motivating the youth to register as voters and to vote has been of major concern for policymakers. Successive general and state elections have also seen a substantial number of campaigns targeted specifically at the youth and first-time voters of the electorate, marked by use of slogans mentioning the youth, increased focus on youth-centric policies on education, entrepreneurship, and digital empowerment, and use of social media and digital media for election campaigns (Somashwar & Owaga, 2020).

Youth in Student Politics

Student politics is a critical path of active exposure and participation of youth in the political process. In most countries, student politics starts with entry in higher education—where students elect their spokespersons from among themselves, to ensure that their interests are protected by the institutional authorities in curriculum design, hostel rules, placements and internships, and other academic concerns. Student unions may exist as independent associations without any extra-institutional affiliations or may exist as student wings of mainstream political parties. Student politics, at one end, allow the youth to actively participate in the process of voting in matters directly concerning their immediate interests. At the other end, it also enables students to hone their skills in influencing voters, seeking support, and securing a mandate.

Owing to their affiliation or alignment to mainstream political parties, student activists often raise their voices in support of or against different government policies or issues of national importance. This helps to raise in the youth awareness about the pressing issues of the day, different government policies, and international developments of diplomatic importance. Student politics has also lent India some of the most prominent political faces over the years, including national leadership for many mainstream political parties, cabinet ministers, and heads of states, attesting its importance as a training ground for the future leaders of the nation.

While the role of student unions in nurturing future politicians and building political acumen and awareness among the Indian youth is undisputed, the practice of student unions being largely aligned to mainstream politics often extends their activism to issues that are beyond the immediate concern of their electorate or their respective institutions. This has the advantage of making the youth aware of general electoral agendas and societal issues and is likely to make them responsible voters. However, the same often dilutes the sanctity of student politics and leads to animosity and impasse between student unions for issues beyond their control or concern.

Youth in Mainstream Politics as Political Cadres

The increased involvement of student leaders in issues of national politics has given rise to the representation of youth among the active members of mainstream political parties. Across the world, the youth from the grassroot level cadres for political parties. Youth are employed in a variety of tasks—such as demonstrations, activism, online and offline awareness campaigns, designing of campaign materials, and taking out marches and political rallies. In many cases, active youth political cadres receive stipends from their affiliated political parties since political activism could occupy substantial productive hours.

Mainstream party membership is available to young members of the society in most countries. For instance, the Labour Party of the United Kingdom allows an age of entry of 14 years. Most other political parties allow membership to teenagers and offer discounted membership rates to those in early youth.

Youth membership in mainstream political parties helps the youth connect with other people with similar political outlook in their neighborhoods or vicinity, receive member updates, influence party policies, and fulfill political ambitions going ahead. It provides groundwork in political activism and helps create new generations of political workers and leaders through opportunities of receiving mentorship, spotlight in the political arena, and building a political network that may assist in later political careers.

Youth in Mainstream Politics as Electoral Candidates and Policymakers

The direct participation of the youth in the law-making process starts with the youth contesting in public elections as candidates and getting elected for public offices. Roughly 2.6% of the world's elected lawmakers are aged below 30 (Inter-Parliamentary Union, 2021). Young, elected candidates play a significant role in heading the youth-related legislative exercises and youth committees.

Youth representation in mainstream political offices varies across nations. European nations are found to take the lead in this area, with roughly 5% of their legislators being aged below 30. However, the situation is not encouraging in the Americas and Asia, where participation as policymakers could come down below 2%. (Inter-Parliamentary Union, 2021).

Challenges of Youth and Political Participation in Modern Times

> There is no trust in the political process, in political parties. And they (young people) do not feel that they can change something by actively being involved in politics. A lot of young people have fought, been killed, and been wounded. But they still did not come to election and they still didn't want to elect a politician because they did not feel that somebody would represent them as they wanted.
>
> —Alona Shkrum, MP, Ukraine

Youth, across the ages, have been seen as a harbinger of new thoughts in political institutions and in society in general. The participation of the youth in politics is seen as critical for the survival of institutions, maintenance and upgrading of governance and societal orders, and transition of the nation into the future in a seamless way. Therefore, non-participation of the youth in politics has been a major concern for scholars and policymakers in recent times. For politicians and citizens alike, the challenge lies in making the youth interested in the existing political systems, so that the latter continue to thrive and gain from the inputs of the new stakeholders in the system.

Scholars have identified different factors as triggering the apparent apathy of the youth to political systems in the twenty-first century. Some of these are as follows:

Rise of Postmaterialist Values

Henn et al. (2022) attributed the lack of interest to the rise of what has been known as postmaterialist values, owing to greater prosperity and stability in the society and spread of awareness and education. Postmaterialist values have been defined to signify a shift from economic concerns to increased interest in self-expression and quality of life (Inglehart & Welzel, 2005; Norris & Inglehart, 2019). Rise of postmaterialist values in a society has been associated with decreased interest in existing political systems and structure and weakening attachment to political parties. The youth today, scholars opine, are likely to be critical of systems in general but highly engaged in specific causes that concern or interest them and less likely than the previous generations to vote out of habit (Dalton, 2015; Hay, 2007; Henn et al., 2022).

Lack of Institutional Trust

Paolillo and Gerbaudo (2022) found that even with the rise of social media activism among the youth in Europe and the USA, the numbers dwindle when it comes to high-intensity political participation among the Italian youth, such as taking up organizational membership, actively campaigning for political causes or attending protest events. The researchers attribute the phenomenon to "institutional suspicion"— or lack of trust in the intent or potency of mainstream political entities and see it as a failure of established political parties to overcome the political apathy of the youth and integrate them in politics of the nations. Again, in a study done by Institute of Politics, Harvard University, the American youth are losing their faith that politics and elections will be effective in improving their future (Milligan, 2022), and around 42% believed their votes make no real difference. On a similar note, the Youth in Development Policy: 2022 Update revealed that many youths across the world are turning their attention from institutional politics and over 83% of them believe that their governments are doing little to save the climate (USAID, 2022).

The COVID-19 pandemic has in many ways been a trigger for institutional distrust. The 2021 Edelman Trust Barometer reveals that while trust in governments increased at the start of the pandemic, over time, governments came to be perceived as the least trustworthy stakeholders in the fight against COVID-19 (Edelman, 2021). This might have been caused by inconsistent policies due to the unprecedented nature of the crisis, political infights, and blame games in combating COVID, and the questionable role of certain national governments in the origin and spread of COVID-19 infections across nations.

Political violence has also been seen as a major deterrence for the entry and interest of the youth in politics. Research in sub-Saharan Africa and the Middle East show increased disillusionment among the youth regarding politics, with a significant proportion believing that the system could not be effectively changed for the better with the current measures (e.g., Belschner, 2018; Mansouri, 2020).

The Democratic Divide

The democratic divide refers to a socio-political phenomenon, where educated, middle-class, male youth are found to be more likely to engage in politics and political discourses than their less educated or less privileged counterparts or than women (Chowdhury, 2016). The democratic divide significantly skews the political representation of the youth across different categories of engagement and makes the voice of the youth reflective of the interest of only a small minority of the youth.

The democratic divide may arise from a variety of causes that come with privilege or lack of it. Youth may not participate in politics because they feel less knowledgeable or confident about their opinions due to lack of information or poor grasp over language. They may also be lacking the resources needed for political engagement such as digital access, membership fee for political institutions, and time to attend meetings and demonstrations. In a research on Portuguese students, lack of time was cited as the most prevalent cause for non-participation in politics, followed by lack of opportunities for political participation, and lack of knowledge about institutions (Malafaia et al., 2021).

Political marginalization also creates differential political experiences for the youth, causing many youths to shun political participation and experience. Youths from marginalized sociocultural backgrounds face greater stress and conflicts than youths from non-marginalized backgrounds while engaging in politics—leading to a higher perception of costs over benefits. Oosterhoff (2022) revealed that this happens because laws and policies differentially affect youths from different backgrounds, leading to differences in the benefits drawn out of political participation. Again, researchers have reported that young women face “double discrimination,” in terms of age and of gender, while aspiring for public offices (Inter-Parliamentary Union, 2021).

The challenges for the democratic divide have become particularly prominent in recent times, with the COVID-19 pandemic and its aftermath. Widespread school dropouts have deprived children and youth of basic education, leading to a lifelong damage to their income prospects as well as a stifling of their political voices (The Economist, 2022). Another report states that global debt has risen to 303 billion US dollars in 2022, the burden of which will majorly fall on the children and the youth of today (Wilkes, 2022). Further, one in six youths lost their jobs during the pandemic, further aggravating the democratic divide leading to loss of political voices (Jabari, 2022).

Institutional Barriers for Entry of Youth into Policymaking

While representation of the youth in suffrage is encouraged, when it comes to political representation of the youth among policymakers, many nations of the world deter an early entry in policymaking. While the youth form 50% of the world's population, they form only 2.6% of the policymakers globally, and only 1.1% of them are women. Further, 24.6% of the countries of the world have no representation of people under 30 in the lower houses of the parliament and 73% of the nations have no participation in the Upper House (Inter-Parliamentary Union, 2021).

The poor representation is to a great extent driven by barriers such as age requirements for parliamentary houses. The minimum age limit for the Lower Houses of the Legislatures around the world ranges from 18 to 30, while the entry age for the Upper Houses ranges from 18 to as high as 45. (Inter-Parliamentary Union, 2021). Thus, there is a significant waiting time between the age of suffrage and age of contesting for office.

The legal and societal barriers to youth participation in political power operations have also seen multiple uprisings across the world, where there have been attempts to topple or significantly transform the existing political order led by the senior members of the society. Kagwanja (2005), for instance, describes the Mungiki Youth Movement in Kenya as a reaction to the violent political legacy of Kenya, characterized by the assassination of political opponents, ethnic militia, and vigilantism. Youth politics have thus often been seen as "politics from below"—the rise of the powerless against the overbearing rules and systems of the older generations (Cruise O'Brien, 1996).

Lack of Financing

> It's not cheap to run, and how big is a 25-year-old's salary?
>
> Irene Putri (MP, Indonesia)

Even when the age requirements are not highly prohibitive, the youth often lack the resources needed for political campaigning and running for office. Election campaign costs could run into several thousands of dollars for a single candidate, and parties are mostly not prepared to risk their funds on a relatively unknown face in the arena. This is also the reason why most youth candidates come from political families or from affluent households where the pressure for earning a living is not debilitating. The cost of running for the office may also be prohibitive for an early-career professional. For instance, in Nigeria, the cost of running for the President's post is as high as fifty thousand dollars—an amount most youths without a life of privilege can ill afford.

Lack of Stability

Youth is a time for building oneself—in terms of career, education, and family (McDonald et al., 2011). This makes full-time involvement in politics difficult for most youth, who need to divide their energy between education, career, and activism. Youth may also migrate for education or work to different regions from their home constituencies, making them feel alienated to the political contexts of their places of stay. Challenges also come from student loans, which may be considerable in many of the developed countries of the world. Pressure to pay off loans for education and to keep steady means of income make many youths lose interest in active politics until quite late.

Another challenge is lack of practical experience with national and regional issues owing to lower exposure. This makes the youth hesitate to take independent stands and also lower their credibility in the eyes of suffrage when compared to a senior politician.

Biases Against the Youth

While there is a lack of institutional trust on part of the youth toward established political systems and parties, the youth themselves face significant biases from the suffrage and fellow political workers. The IPU Youth Report identifies what has been called the "Old is Gold" syndrome, where the youth is often seen as less competent, inexperienced, and uninformed, and therefore not fit to hold responsible offices. The Report cites one case from Tunisia where the election of a young mayor led to resignation from older members who refused to work under a junior colleague. National culture also plays an important role in this regard particularly in countries that value age and experience and are driven by high power distance, collectivist sentiments, and rigid societal and family hierarchies based on age and seniority.

India and Youth in Politics: A Case Study of the Largest Democracy of the World

With a youth population of 464 million in 2011, India comes next only to China in terms of the youth potential of a country globally. However, utilization of the youth potential completely is often a challenge for nations. In 2020, India ranked 115 out of 181 nations when it came to political and civic participation, measured in terms of the voice of the youth in policymaking and community development, youth-centric policies, and perceived recognition for youth-led community activities (The Commonwealth, 2020). This reveals a considerable opportunity for progress when it comes to representation of the voice of the youth in forums that matter.

The youth (aged between 15 and 29) is projected to form over one-third of India's population post-2020, and more than 40% of the labor force of the country (MoSPI, 2017; UNICEF, EY India, & Viamo, 2020). It becomes essential therefore that the youth of India have a representative voice in the affairs and destiny of the nation.

When it comes to rights of the youth in India, the Fundamental Rights guaranteed by the Constitution of India to all citizens also enshrine access of the youth to equal treatment, means of livelihood, freedom of thought and action, and protection against exploitation. The Right to Education, incorporated in 2012, specifically guarantees universal education to youth of India, irrespective of financial or social privilege. Apart from these, there are multiple legal provisions specifically addressing the safety, security, and rights of adolescents and young adults.

Voice of the Youth in Policy Making

India has a universal adult suffrage, providing every individual aged above 18 a right to vote. The 2014 elections saw an impressive turnout of the 69% of the youth population voting. Independent India has had for long a culture of active student politics in major educational institutions. In a survey conducted in 2019 among the Indian youth, 39% opined that student politics is a natural part of student life (Statista Research Department, 2020). Almost all major national-level political parties and many regional political parties in India have their student wings, active across the country. Significant among these are the Akhil Bharatiya Vidyarthi Parishad (ABVP), a seventy-year-old institution affiliated to right-wing politics and among the largest student bodies of the world. Other major student unions are the National Student Union of India (NSUI), affiliated to the Indian National Congress, Student Federation of India (SFI), and All India Youth Federation (AIYF), aligned to the Communist Party of India and left-wing politics. In addition, there are student unions representing specific religious groups such as the Mor Gregorios Jacobite Students' Movement, All India Sikh Students Federation (AISSF), All India Muslim Students Federation or ethnic and social groups such as Chin Student Association, Birsa Ambedkar Phule Students' Association, Mizo Zirlai Pawl, and Twipra Students Federation. Student unions and student politics are highly active across many universities and colleges in India.

While it is not an entirely new trend, between 2017 and 2021, India has seen several instances of student activism on mainstream political issues spilling beyond campus walls and leading to major disruptions of educational schedules, sanctity, and peace. Such trends often lead to discouragement of youth from participation in political activism. For instance, 34% of the Indian respondents aged between 18 and 21 in a Statista survey felt that politics had no place in a student's life and at least 20% opined that big political parties must not interfere in student politics (Statista Research Department, 2020). The UN Volunteers, in collaboration with the Ministry of Youth Affairs and Sports, bring out the Youth Volunteering India, a newsletter documenting volunteering activities of the youth in India.

As in most other countries of the world, in India, too, constitutional provisions encourage late entry into the citadels of law-making. A study by India Today's Data Intelligence Unit (DIU) revealed that the average age of Indian parliamentarians has been above 50 since 1999, although it has shown a progressive decline since 2014, averaging at 55 years in 2021 (Rampal, 2019). The minimum age for becoming a member of the Rajya Sabha, the Upper House of the Indian Parliament is 30. While the minimum age of entry in the Lok Sabha is lower, at 25, as of 2021, only two members out of 543 in the Lok Sabha are aged below 30—both of whom are women. This again shows a considerable scope for improvement when it comes to representation of the youth voice in policymaking—involving legislative as well as social interventions.

The picture improves somewhat when it comes to rural self-governance. In terms of representation in the Panchayats, rural village-level elected governance systems, a relatively lower entry-age bracket resulted in a relatively higher representation of the youth in some states. For instance, over 60% of the Panchayat workers in Odisha, 44% of those in Chhattisgarh, and 40% of those in Bihar are aged between 21 and 35. However, the trends are not representative across the country, indicating a major scope for enhancing youth representation at the village level.

In 2021, India has multiple non-political organized youth forums flourishing across the country, providing the youth organized exposure to combat training, civic engagement, and social service. Some of the most well-known among these are the National Cadet Corps (NCC) and the National Service Scheme (NSS). The National Cadet Corps is governed by the Ministry of Defence and provides the youth of India exposure to social services, discipline, and adventure training, inculcating in them preparedness for serving the nation and encouraging military spirit and discipline among the youth. The NCC provides stipend, education training, and international exchange opportunities for the youth, and had around 1.15 million members progressing to the Indian Army, as per a 2016 estimate (Statista Research Department, 2021). The National Service Scheme, on the other hand, is governed by the Ministry of Youth Affairs & Sports, Government of India, and allows students from higher secondary to post-graduate levels to participate in government-led community service programs. NSS had a membership of 3.8 million Indian youths in 2018 and conducted multiple National Youth Festivals across the country every year, providing students forums to display their skills, network, and learn important skills in volunteering and social service. Other important youth forums include the Bharat Scouts and Guides (the Indian wing of the Boy Scouts movement, promoting teamwork, social service, and youth empowerment), and the Hindustan Scouts and Guides. The UN Volunteers, in collaboration with the Ministry of Youth Affairs and Sports, bring out the Youth Volunteering India, a newsletter documenting volunteering activities of the youth in India.

One forum specifically focused on the rural youth has been the Nehru Yuva Kendra Sansthan (NYKS), under the Ministry of Youth Affairs and Sports, which runs a nationwide network of youth clubs in rural areas, empowering the rural youth to participate in nation building activities. The significant contribution of the NYKS to the voice of the youth is the district, state, and national level youth parliaments, which provide the rural youth an exposure to democratic processes and policymaking.

Policies Encouraging the Voice of the Youth

To provide the youth an exposure to policymaking, the Ministry of Parliamentary Affairs, Government of India, has been hosting the Youth Parliament Program since 1966. The Youth Parliament simulates an actual parliamentary setting where adolescents in government schools may learn about laws and policymaking, debate on issues of national importance, and forward suggestions for policymakers of the country. The Youth Parliament had involved more than 0.4 million students till date (PHD Research Bureau, 2019).

Apart from prominent government institutions, several public-sector, corporate organizations, and non-governmental organizations also host forums to capture the voice of the youth. These include the various youth parliament programs by the National Youth Parliament Organization (The National Youth Parliament), Media Foundation (The Indian Youth Parliament), Swatantrata (Youth Parliament Program India), Navodaya Vidyalaya Samiti (Youth Parliament Program) to name a few. Such forums aim to provide the Indian youth with training in political debates and issues. It organizes several youth parliaments each year, where youths try to find solutions to policy problems through discussion and voting. Similarly, the India International Institute of Democracy and Election Management (IIIDEM), also runs Electoral Literacy Clubs for the youth in India.

With the adoption of the Digital India policy in the last decade, there has been a growing recognition of the power of the digital and social media in capturing the voices and concerns of the youth, and a tool to influence their political and policy opinions. To utilize this fruitfully, the biggest step till date has been the setting up of the www.MyGov.in portal, an official website of the Government of India providing regular updates on various policy decisions and outcomes, in multiple Indian languages, in a user-friendly and interactive way. www.MyGov.in accompanies this with various activities for the citizens, soliciting their views on draft policies, engaging them with quizzes, contests, and awareness campaigns, and crowdsourcing ideas for policy changes, designs of logos, or product innovations. Similar digital engagement platforms are provided by the Ministry of Youth Affairs, Ministry of Education, Ministry of Parliamentary Affairs, and other government bodies working for youth empowerment. Further, all institutes of higher education funded by the central government are now required to maintain an active official social media presence to showcase achievements of the institute, engage with youth stakeholders, and combat fake news about the institution.

There have been multiple initiatives in recent years to provide the youth an early exposure into governance and policymaking. Both houses of the Indian Parliament provide internship opportunities to undergraduate and postgraduate students under the Parliamentary Internship Programme (PIP), to work closely with members of the Parliament in their deliberation in the Houses and policy research. The Mahatma Gandhi National Fellowship is another major policy initiative to provide youth exposure in rural governance, and public policy management.

Social Media and Youth Politics

Social media has played a significant role in democratizing the platforms for the voice of the youth. Bennett and Segerberg (2013) opined that "digitally networked action" powered by social media promoted political engagement and action among the youth. Paolillo and Gerbaudo (2022) reported an upward trend in the political participation of youth in USA and Europe in recent times, in terms of political self-expression, contact with politicians, and voting, owing to the access to social media. The Credit Suisse Youth Barometer 2020 survey revealed that social media simplifies political action, by promoting quick exchange of views among peers, information sharing, and engaging in critical discussions (Credit Suisse, 2020).

Social media has been seen as a potent tool for the spread of postmaterialist forms of politics among the youth (Theocharis & Van Deth, 2017). Social media allows the youth to present individual opinions beyond party mandates and engage in nuanced political discourses and conversations that go beyond mere voting or mass demonstrations (Boulianne, 2020). Thus, it provides a forum for political engagements without political affiliations and allows the youth to have a gradual and controlled exposure to the world of politics without making significant commitment of time, money, and other resources.

Social media played a significant role in youth activism during the pandemic times. Cheng and Lam-Knott (2020) opine that the COVID-19 pandemic denied the youth access to campus and, with it, access to youth political forums. Many youths took activism to online media at this juncture—to protest government policies, generate civic action, and spread awareness. For instance, youth in China raised voices against the lack of transparency in the COVID-19 management policies in China and gathered funds online for medical workers (Wang & Hernandez, 2020). Again, youth in Africa have been found to make use of digital technology to assist frontline workers and spread awareness during the pandemic (Khadiagala, 2020).

India has one of the least expensive internet accesses in the world, and this, coupled with a growing network of high-speed connectivity boosted by public and private service providers, has made social media one of the most popular sources of entertainment and activism among the Indian youth. The popularity of social media in youth circles has made the platforms a powerful tool for political parties and social interest groups to target the youth and influence their opinions and choices. According to the 2019 report of UN Volunteers, 2 out of 3 Indian youth use social media for news and current events. Further, data shows that out of 190 million Indian youths active on social media, a substantial 30 million follow political pages and handle actively. Among non-political civic engagements, the Indian youths were found to show active interest in social media handles relating to Community Issues (19 million), sustainability (11 million), Volunteerism and Environmentalism (5 million), and charity (1.8 million). However, much of those participating in civic engagements in social media tend to be young adult males from urban areas, indicating a need for policy interventions for securing the voices of youths from more diverse backgrounds on social media.

Although hugely popular as a media of youth political discourses, social media has also been under the critical scanner for being a barrier to political engagement. One important barrier is the digital divide, which denies a significant proportion of youth across the world a voice in the political discourses of the new generation. Language barriers are also undeniable roadblocks, putting those not conversant with prevalent business languages at a disadvantage. Schlozman et al. (2010) opined that youth political discourses on social media present a lopsided voice of youths who are privileged to have access to quality education. Hence, while social media reflect, to a considerable extent, the prevalent trends among the youth, one must be cognizant of the fact that the voices may often be representing a miniscule minority, with the privilege of access, time, and language to be vocal on social networks (Sloam, 2014).

Policy Recommendations

Political apathy of the youth has important consequences for the future of a region (Resnick & Casale, 2014). Despite growing appreciation of the voice of the youth in policy matters and their increased dominance in policy conversations through orthodox or unorthodox channels, there remains considerable opportunity to promote political education, productive activism, and participation of the youth in the governance of the country, through direct or indirect means.

The Good Practice Guide from the United Nations Development Programme (UNDP, 2013) states that for effective youth participation in the political process, interventions need to happen at three levels:

(a) Legal interventions: including lowering the age of voting and of election, introducing youth quotas and reservations, and removing constraints such as political expenditure.

(b) Pre-electoral Period: focusing on civic education in schools and colleges, political incubators, small-scale youth projects, and providing access to internet and smartphones
(c) Electoral period: focusing on involvement of youth volunteers in campaigning and electoral processes, reaching out to the youth using social media, and including youth-centric agenda in the mandates.

Some possible interventions are enumerated below.

Youth Representation in Policy Making

One of the potent ways to make the youth gain trust and interest in the political systems is to enhance their representation in the political systems. Representation helps the youth to find role models among young political leaders, making politics immediately interesting. It also leads to the introduction of an agenda that represents the crises faced by the youth and is more likely to bring in solutions that are new-age and innovative.

Several countries of the world are presently exploring channels to lower the average age of policymakers and increase the representation of young adults in the legislature of the country. One avenue for this is amendment of constitutional provisions to lower the entry barriers for youth in the legislature. With a youth population that is progressing far beyond one-third of the nation's citizen strength, it may be essential for many nations to investigate the feasibility of easing the entry of youth into policymaking through constitutional amendments. For example, in Turkey, youth organizations have long campaigned for lower entry barriers and have successfully lowered the age for election to the Parliament from 30 to 25 (UNDP, 2013). Other solutions that have been suggested are youth quotas in the electoral offices—in the form of reserved seats in the parliament or legislated candidate quotas—where political parties must have a minimum proportion of the youth population in their list of prospective candidates. Very few countries of the world presently employ youth quotas in one form or the other, although their effects are expected to be positive in the long run (Belschner & Paredes, 2020).

Lowering the average age or introducing quotas alone however may not be sufficient to attract the youth in the roles of policymakers. Research showed that youth quotas are effective only when the young candidates have a strong chance of winning a seat (Belschner, 2018). Nations need to create support structures that help the youth deal with the demands of their ongoing life stages while dedicating their time to politics. For instance, the World Bank Group's program on Women, Business, and the Law survey (World Bank Group, 2016) revealed that early career childcare support may increase the representation of women in the parliament by more than 25%.

Role of Political Parties

Established political parties serve both as the royal road as well as the entry barrier for citizens in the political system. Political parties are instrumental in providing a structure that provides an interested citizen in finding articulation for one's voice, connect with like-minded citizens, and work for causes that interest oneself, in an effective manner. Political parties also provide funds for political activism to its members, security in case of backlash, and access to forums previously inaccessible to ordinary citizens. All these make political parties important players in the democratic political systems when it comes to participation of citizens in active politics.

Youth wings of political parties have been instrumental in inviting the youth into politics since ages, providing the needed mentorship, community, and backing (Malafaia, Menezes, & Neves, 2018; Rainsford, 2018). However, there are wide criticisms of political parties using youth members mostly as cannon fodder for active demonstrations and menial tasks, providing them little access to participatory management and decision-making. Party policies, actions, and agenda are set by senior members, who represent the voice of another generation. All these contribute to the institutional distrust among the youth. NDI (2022) reported that the growing economic crisis in Lebanon led to youth protests across the country, which ultimately culminated in the formation of youth-led political parties. Similar incidents are reported from Tunisia where the 3ich Tounsi work to provide support to independent candidates providing an alternative to established political ideologies.

While focusing on entry in terms of numbers, it also remains critical to find that the youth cohort working closely with the center of power are well-represented in terms of gender, social class, religion, ability, economic backgrounds, and access to privileges. Many youths who find a representation in policymaking come from political families themselves, making the representation an issue of privilege. With an expanding youth population, political parties need to be active in training and bringing to limelight able leaders representing this section of the suffrage. The youth wings of political parties can also play an important role in this regard.

The National Democratic Institute (2022), in their report focusing on strengthening linkages between the youth and political parties recommends a series of interventions by political parties that are needed to build trust and meaningful association between divergent political generations. These interventions, based on four key principles of "connect," "build," "serve," and "guide" include:

- Sustained dialogues and exchange of ideas between different generations of political workers
- Mentoring of new members by senior party members
- Participating in issues such as climate change activism that resonate with the youth
- Maintaining regular association with youth associations and civil society organizations that work for the causes of the youth.

- Involving youth members to create innovative content on social media pages of political parties—using short videos, live streams, memes, and other modern communication developments
- Enabling the youth to have flexible entry and exit systems in political parties, through the formation of youth wings, youth caucuses, and specific interest groups dedicated to the cause of gender, social justice, and climate.

Youth and the Political Voice

For a thriving democracy, it is essential that successive generations put their faith in the democratic machinery and actively participate in the election processes across the country. In India, the Election Commission of India, in collaboration with Facebook, has run a campaign since 2017, nudging young adults to register for the electoral roll on their birthdays. There are also several user-friendly IEC initiatives by the central and the state governments urging the youths to register as voters. Similar activities are carried on by political parties and non-governmental organizations. Here, again, the focus should be on ensuring representation of youths of diverse backgrounds and privileges in the electoral roll, along with developing a culture of making an informed choice as a voter (following issues relating to governance on a regular basis, knowing the candidates and their election manifesto, and knowing the policy concerns of the nation in general and the youth in particular).

Youth and Social Media

With the growing evolution of social media as a universal platform for showcasing political thoughts and preferences, and the popularity of social media among the youth, it is important that the youth is empowered to raise their voices on the social media in a constructive, informed, and productive manner. To this end, extensive educational programs on digital empowerment of adolescents and youths are needed, making them aware of the rules and best practices of being politically active on social media, detecting fake news, inciting, malicious, or seditious content, and fake profiles, knowing the cyber laws and responsibilities of the citizens in combating cybercrimes. Papaioannou (2022) recommended media literacy interventions to allow children and youth to make judicious use of social media for civic engagements and political activities.

Prominent institutions of the government and private sector, state persons, and government offices need to be active on different social media handles, to be the authorized sources of information on the concerned body. It may be useful, for instance, to identify youth volunteers to maintain the sanctity of political discussions on social media and train them to create valued content and flag malicious ones. Similarly, social media is also a potent tool to highlight the efforts of the youth in civic engagement and build networks among the youths interested in common civic agenda. The MyGov handles of the Government of India regularly highlight constructive achievements of youth volunteers and social champions. Similar efforts need to be escalated for private and public platforms for civic engagements.

While attracting the youth using social media, it is important for political parties to use means that resonate with the youth of today. Daly (2021) shares the case of Sinn Fein in Ireland that makes use of Tiktok and Instagram to connect with the youth and has a social media presence that overshadows that of rival political parties by about ten times (Holroyd, 2020). It is also important that such social media communication have an appropriate blend of facts, humor, and actionable inputs to interest the youth into politics.

Involvement of Youth in Policy Advisory

While incorporating the youth in legislative bodies is a long-drawn goal, a simpler exercise is to incorporate the youths in advisory bodies for policy formation and governance decisions. However, two-thirds of the countries of the world do not have any representation of the youth in national development planning or poverty reduction policymaking (GPY, 2015, 2014). While youth voices dominate the social media, in the absence of formal, methodical participation of the youth in policymaking, many opinions come across as uninformed or misinformed, and several brilliant ideas drown in the clutter of many conflicting voices. There needs to be concentrated effort in formalizing youth participation in policy advisory bodies, soliciting feedback on policy drafts from young professionals, civic rights champions, or subject-matter experts, and auditing the extent to which feedback from the youth was solicited, documented, and utilized in final policy decisions. Again, there need to be audits on the outcomes of the various youth parliaments and the extent to which such solutions or their refined versions influence policy decisions for the country.

Researchers have recommended initiatives led by civil society organizations such as youth town halls with policymakers, visits to legislatures, and internship opportunities with politicians who currently form a part of the government (NDI, 2022). One example of such initiatives is the Future Mentors program organized by Epsoo which allow youths from various European cities to mentor their city administration for sustainable development of the cities (Epsoo, 2022).

Political Education

Even when other interventions are present, for the youth to have a meaningful political impact, there must be attempts to build political awareness, sensitivity, and skills in the youth. This necessitates extensive and early political education through multiple channels. In their study on Portuguese youth, Malafaia et al. (2021) found that the school is widely perceived as a center of unbiased and structured political education. Thus, schools have a major role to play in educating children in politics and acting as a filter for propaganda, fake news, and biased opinions, that are widely prevalent as political news today (Elrich, 2000).

Educational institutions have a role in the political participation of the youth as well. Henn et al. (2005) found that youth with lower educational qualifications are more likely to turn to anti-institutionalism and authoritarian leadership as opposed to political participation and democratic, inclusive values. This phenomenon has been called the participation gap by Dalton (2017). Henn et al. (2022) also reported higher levels of environmental awareness and interest in environmentalism among youths who are highly educated, than those who are not. Thus, education in general and political education, in particular, is likely to create engaged citizens who do not hesitate in participating in political dialogues and who can make informed, knowledgeable contributions to the political transitions of the world.

While education in general enhances political participation, to be effective, there needs to be training in political processes, legacies, and methods. NDI (2022) recommends educational interventions in the forms of organized interviews and interaction of the youth with young political leaders and lawmakers, civic education, and community political education initiatives driven by the youths themselves.

Conclusion and Way Forward

Standing in a post-pandemic world where the doomsday clock is ticking more rapidly than ever before, it is not only desirable but also imperative to hear the voice of the youth and make them active stakeholders in policy designing, implementation, and assessment, and civic engagements. While the advent of digitalization has democratized platforms more than ever before, it has also given rise to disorganized activism, often drowning out knowledgeable opinions and constructive efforts from the youth. It is the need of the hour to audit the extent to which the voices of the youth from diverse backgrounds inform and influence policymaking, the extent to which the youth are empowered to make use of the resources available to them to participate in legislation and governance, and devise innovative methods to mentor, aid, and support the leadership of the youth in building the India of tomorrow.

References

Belschner, J., & Garcia de Paredes, M. (2020). Hierarchies of representation: The redistributive effects of gender and youth quotas. *Journal of Representative Democracy, 57*(1), 1–20.

Belschner, J. (2018). The adoption of youth quotas after the Arab uprisings. *Politics, Groups, and Identities*, 1–19. https://doi.org/10.1080/21565503.2018.1528163

Boulianne, S. (2020). Twenty years of digital media effects on civic and political participation. *Communication Research, 47*(7), 947–966.

Chowdhury, A. (2016). *Bridging the democratic divide in the UK*. https://fabians.org.uk/bridging-the-democratic-divide-in-the-uk/

Credit Suisse. (2020). Youth Barometer 2020: Equality, sustainability and social media. https://www.credit-suisse.com/about-us-news/en/articles/news-and-expertise/youth-barometer-2020-equality-sustainability-and-social-media-202009.html

Cruise O'Brien, D. B. (1996). A lost generation: Youth identity and state decay in West Africa'. In R. Werbner & T. Ranger (Eds.), *Post-colonial identities in Africa*. Zed Books.

Dalton, R. J. (2015). *The good citizen: How a younger generation is reshaping American politics*. CQ press.

Dalton, R. J. (2017). *The participation gap: Social status and political inequality*. Oxford University Press.

Daly, O. (2021). *Fit for purpose: How can the Irish political system adapt to meet the needs of young people*. TASC, University of Cambridge. https://www.tasc.ie/assets/files/pdf/tasc_policy_brief_on_irish_politics_youth_020321_f.pdf

Edelman. (2021). *Edelman trust barometer*. https://www.edelman.com/sites/g/files/aatuss191/files/2021-03/2021%20Edelman%20Trust%20Barometer.pdf

Erlich, T. (2000). *Civic responsibility and higher education*. Greenwood Publishing Group.

Espoo. (2022). Young people from across Europe are mentoring decision-makers this spring. https://www.espoo.fi/en/news/2022/03/young-people-across-europe-mentoring-decision-makers-spring

GPY2015. (2014). *The global youth call: Prioritizing youth in the post-2015 development agenda*. https://www.un.org/youthenvoy/wp-content/uploads/2014/09/The_Global_Youth_Call.pdf

Hay, C. (2007). *Why we hate politics*. Polity Press.

Henn, M., Weinstein, M., & Forrest, S. (2005). Uninterested youth? Young people's attitudes towards party politics in Britain. *Political Studies, 53*(3), 556–578.

Henn, M., Sloam, J., & Nunes, A. (2022). Young cosmopolitans and environmental politics: How postmaterialist values inform and shape youth engagement in environmental politics. *Journal of Youth Studies, 25*(6), 709–729.

Holroyd, M. (2020). *Ireland election: How Sinn Féin dominated the social media campaign*. https://www.euronews.com/2020/02/10/ireland-election-how-sinn-fein-dominated-the-social-media-campaign

Inglehart, R., & Welzel, C. (2005). *Modernization, cultural change, and democracy: The human development sequence*. Cambridge University Press.

Jabari, M. (2022). How to give the world's youth a voice in shaping global challenges. The World Economic Forum. https://www.weforum.org/agenda/2022/08/how-to-give-the-worlds-youth-a-voice-in-shaping-global-challenges/

Kagwanja, P. M. (2005). Clash of generations? Youth identity, violence and the politics of transition in Kenya, 1997–2002. In *Vanguard or vandals* (pp. 81–109). Brill.

Khadiagala, G. M. (2020). The role of youth in governance and leadership in a post-COVID-19 world. https://www.africaportal.org/features/role-youth-governance-and-leadership-post-covid-19-world/

Lam-Knott, S., & Cheng, Y. (2020). Youth politics in the time of pandemic: A view from Asian cities. National University of Singapore. https://ari.nus.edu.sg/youth-politics/

Malafaia, C., Neves, T., & Menezes, I. (2021). The gap between youth and politics: Youngsters outside the regular school system assessing the conditions for being (com) ing political subjects. *Young, 29*(5), 437–455.

Malafaia, C., Menezes, I., & Neves, T. (2018). Living, doing, and learning from politics in a youth wing of a political party. *Qualitative Report, 23*(1).

Mansouri, F. (2020). Youth and political engagement in post revolution Tunisia. *British Journal of Middle Eastern Studies*, 1–17.

McDonald, P., Pini, B., Bailey, J., & Price, R. (2011). Young people's aspirations for education, work, family and leisure. *Work, Employment and Society, 25*(1), 68–84.

Milligan, S. (2022). Youth Losing Faith in Politics: Poll. US News. https://www.usnews.com/news/politics/articles/2022-04-25/youth-losing-faith-in-politics-poll

MoSPI. (2017). Youth in India. Central Statistics Office: Ministry of Statistics and Programme Implementation, Government of India. http://mospi.nic.in/sites/default/files/publication_reports/Youth_in_India-2017.pdf

National Democratic Institute. (2022). Bridging the divide: Strengthening partnerships between young people and political parties. https://www.ndi.org/sites/default/files/NDI_BridgingTheDivide_Report_Final.pdf

NDI. (2018). *Youth political participation programming guide*. https://youthguide.ndi.org/

Norris, P., & Inglehart, R. (2019). *Cultural backlash: Trump, Brexit, and authoritarian populism*. Cambridge University Press.

Oosterhoff, B., Poppler, A., Hill, R. M., Fitzgerald, H., & Shook, N. J. (2022). Understanding the costs and benefits of politics among adolescents within a sociocultural context. *Infant and Child Development, 31*(2), e2280.

Paolillo, M., & Gerbaudo, P. (2022). Mobilised yet unaffiliated: Italian youth and the uneven return to political participation. *Journal of Youth Studies*, 1–17.

Papaioannou, T. (2022). Youth and participatory politics: enhancing digital engagement through media literacy education. In *The Routledge international handbook of children, adolescents, and media* (pp. 403–411). Routledge.

Rainsford, E. (2018). UK political parties' youth factions: A glance at the future of political parties. *Parliamentary Affairs, 71*(4), 783–803.

Rampal, N. (2019). India is young, its leaders aren't. India Today. https://www.indiatoday.in/diu/story/india-young-voters-old-mps-lok-sabha-1538175-2019-05-30

Resnick, D., & Casale, D. (2014). Young populations in young democracies: Generational voting behaviour in sub-Saharan Africa. *Democratization, 21*(6), 1172–1194.

Schlozman, K. L., Verba, S., & Brady, H. E. (2010). Weapon of the strong? Participatory inequality and the internet. *Perspectives on Politics, 8*(2), 487–509.

Sloam, J. (2014). The outraged young': Young Europeans, civic engagement and the new media in a time of crisis". *Information, Communication & Society, 17*(2), 217–231.

Somashwar, A., & Owaga, T. (2020). Do the youth of the country actually value their vote? Young India Foundation. https://youngindiafdn.medium.com/do-the-youth-of-the-country-actually-value-their-vote-6c2e01db0093

The Commonwealth. (2020). Global Youth Development Index and Report 2020. https://thecommonwealth.org/sites/default/files/inline/5023_V3_Book_lores_smaller.pdf

The Economist. (2022). Governments are ignoring the pandemic's disastrous effect on education. https://www.economist.com/leaders/2022/07/07/governments-are-ignoring-the-pandemics-disastrous-effect-on-education

Theocharis, Y., & Van Deth, J. W. (2017). *Political participation in a changing world: Conceptual and empirical challenges in the study of citizen engagement*. Routledge.

UNDP. (2013). Enhancing youth political participation throughout the electoral cycle. https://www.undp.org/sites/g/files/zskgke326/files/publications/ENG_UN-Youth_Guide-LR.pdf

UNICEF, EY India, & Viamo. (2020). Voices of youth: South Asian perspectives on education, skills and employment. https://www.unicef.org/rosa/media/4556/file/Voices%20of%20Youth%20-%20South%20Asian%20Perspectives%20on%20Education,%20Skills%20and%20Employment_June%202020.pdf

Inter-Parliamentary Union. (2021). Youth participation in national parliaments. https://www.ipu.org/youth2021

USAID. (2022). Youth in development policy: 2022 update. https://www.usaid.gov/sites/default/files/documents/USAID-Youth-in-Development-Policy-2022-Update-508.pdf

Wang, V., & Hernandez, J. C. (2020). Coronavirus crisis awakens a sleeping giant: China's youth. The New York Times. https://www.nytimes.com/2020/03/28/world/asia/coronavirus-china-youth.html

Wilkes, T. (2022). Emerging markets drive global debt to record $303 trillion—IIF. https://www.reuters.com/markets/europe/emerging-markets-drive-global-debt-record-303-trillion-iif-2022-02-23/

World Bank Group. (2016). Women, business and the law: Getting to equal. http://pubdocs.worldbank.org/en/458191519943376087/4pager-WBL2017-ChildCare.pdf

B. Majumdar a fellow of the Indian Institute of Management Indore, Bishakha Majumdar is presently a faculty of Organizational Behavior and Human Resource Management at the Indian Institute of Management Visakhapatnam. She has co-authored the books *Youth Development in India: Future Generations in a Changing World and Disadvantaged Children in India: Empirical Evidence, Policies and Actions*. She has also authored several case studies and research papers in human resource management and public policy and has been an Associate Editor of the journal South Asian Survey by Sage.

Chapter 27
The Critical Value of Global, Regional, National, and Subnational Youth Development Indices in Developing Inclusive and Evidence-Based Youth Policy and Programs

Gemma Wood

Abstract The primary goal of a Youth Development Index (YDI) is to enable action in youth development. The objective of this chapter is to highlight the advantages of bringing out the YDI. YDIs are powerful tools for expanding access to relevant and inclusive data about young people. Because of their composite nature, YDIs can build on statistical data assets on a global scale. By compiling data from youth-related datasets at global, regional, national, and sub-national levels into a small set of comprehensive and harmonized measures, YDIs enable users to take complex, multi-dimensional quantitative data and make it easier to interpret. Global, regional, national, and sub-national data sets allow for different interventions at all levels, and so, maximize potential impact on youth development. Using sub-national data in YDIs provides context-specific indicators that measure local challenges and identify areas with opportunities for growth. Sub-national data is crucial because of the large spatial variations in development at this level, and the differing policies and programmatic actions that occur. The practice of publishing and broadly disseminating YDI data and reports encourages and enables youth advocacy efforts and facilitates communication and engagement with influential stakeholders, the media, and the general public. By attracting public interest and stimulating open discourse, the Global and harmonized national YDIs can advance collective knowledge and attitudes toward young people and the social, structural, and policy issues that impede or enable their development.

Keywords Youth development index · Critical value · Global · Regional · National · Youth policy · Programs

G. Wood (✉)
Numbers and People Synergy, Canberra, Australia
e-mail: gemma@numbersandpeople.com

S. Deb and S. Deb (eds.), *Handbook of Youth Development*,
https://doi.org/10.1007/978-981-99-4969-4_27

Introduction

Today, the world has the largest youth population that has ever existed (Christian, 2020). Close to two billion people in the world today are between 15 and 29 years of age (Commonwealth Secretariat, 2020). During this period of life, individuals begin to make a substantial contribution to the economic and social development of a country as they join the workforce, pursue further training and education, and engage in civic and political participation. Young people may also assume new responsibilities, such as the rearing of children, the care of older relatives, and managing their own health and wellbeing.

Youth Development Indices (YDIs) are a collection of composite indicators that provide a quantitative snapshot of the current state of young people within a given geographical region. YDIs use multivariate analysis to combine data from a broad range of youth-related indicators and generate simple, quantitative representations of complex and multi-dimensional youth development concepts. These representations are comprehensive while also being easier to analyze, interpret, share, and apply.

The development of a YDI is guided by a theoretical framework that defines the aspects of youth development being measured and provides a clear understanding of how indicators and variables should be selected and grouped for analysis to yield a composite indicator or set of indicators that are meaningful and fit-for-purpose (Organization for Economic Co-operation & Development, 2016). YDIs provide an evidence base that can be used to assess and compare progress in youth development both over time and between populations of interest.

The use of composite indices using demographic data to quantify performance in key areas of interest at the country level has become increasingly popular as a useful tool in public policy analysis, decision-making, communication, and accountability (Organization for Economic Co-operation & Development, 2016). In the youth development space, early adopters of composite indicators began producing country-level YDIs in the early 2000s, including the *United States Child Well-Being Index* (2003), the *Brazilian Youth Well-Being Index* (2007), the *Malaysian Youth Index* (2011), and the *India Youth Development Report* (2010), Commonwealth Secretariat (2016b).

The first large-scale YDI was the Global Youth Development Index (GYDI), which was produced in 2013 for the Commonwealth Youth Programme (CYP) using data from across 170 countries. The GYDI was composed of 15 key indicators grouped into five thematic areas, called domains (Fig. 27.1 refers), that represented key priorities for global youth development at the time (Commonwealth Secretariat, 2013). The development of the GYDI domains was informed by the foundational principles of the Universal Declaration of Human Rights, the UN Sustainable Development Goals (SDGs), youth development strategies such as the Commonwealth Plan of Action for Youth Empowerment (PAYE) and the UNDESA World Programme of Action for Youth (WPAY), and the expert input of researchers, youth development specialists, senior government officials, and youth representatives (Commonwealth Secretariat, 2013).

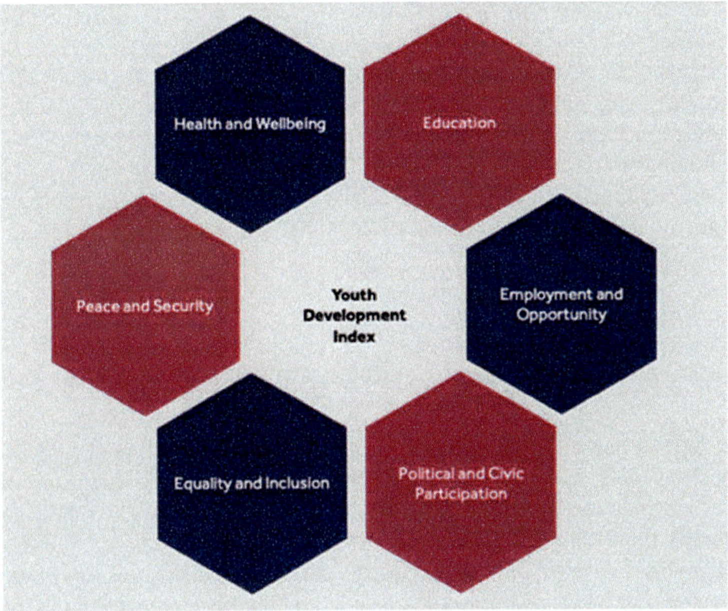

Fig. 27.1 2020 global youth development index domains

When the GYDI was reproduced in 2016, the Commonwealth partnered with UNDESA, UNDP, UN-HABITAT, UNESCO, CARICOM, the African Union, the Pacific Community (SPC), and the Institute for Economics and Peace (IEP) to undertake an extensive, expert, consultation process to identify strategies that would strengthen the global impact of YDIs. The result of this engagement process was the development of the *Commonwealth Youth Development Index National and Regional Toolkit: A Guide for Developing Regional and National Youth Development Indices* in 2016. The central objective of the *Toolkit* is to guide and encourage the development of robust regional and national YDIs with harmonized measures that can support more informed youth policy and program design processes, and strengthen efforts for more transparent and accountable decision-making at the local (sub-national), national, regional, and global levels (Commonwealth Secretariat, 2016a, 2016b).

Since then, government groups and humanitarian agencies such as the UN Population Fund (UNFPA), the Institute for Economics and Peace (IEP), the International Labour Organization (ILO), the World Health Organisation (WHO), the World Banks, and the Association of Southeast Asian Nations (ASEAN) have partnered with young people, youth development experts, and social development specialists, such as Numbers and People Synergy (NAPS), to create and deploy an ever expanding repository of harmonized national and regional YDIs. These YDIs have been developed using the *Toolkit* approach, and include the *Bangladesh YDI*, the *Indonesia YDI*, the *Cambodian YDI*, the *Namibian YDI*, the *Pakistan YDI*, the *Association of Southeast Asian Nations YDI*, The African YDI, the *Australian YDI*, and the *2020*

Global Youth Development Index (Commonwealth Secretariat, 2020; Numbers & People Synergy, 2023).

This work has demonstrated that country-level YDIs can be highly effective, relevant, versatile, inclusive, and accessible tools in advancing youth development when created using: (1) a strongly participatory, end-to-end approach; (2) a theoretical framework that is anchored in the Global Youth Development Index (GYDI) domains; and (3) sub-national data that can be disaggregated by geography, age, sex, and as many other population characteristics that are associated with inequity and variation in youth development, wherever possible.

Recommended Approach for Developing Effective YDIs

To facilitate systematic, impactful, and inclusive YDI development processes, it is critical to apply an analytical framework that is rooted in participatory design with key stakeholders and aligned with broadly relevant priorities. The framework provided by the *Commonwealth Youth Development Index National and Regional Toolkit* provides an excellent roadmap that can be adapted as necessary to meet the analytical requirements as needed. As detailed by the Commonwealth (2016b), the key steps to successful YDI development are as shown in Fig. 27.2.

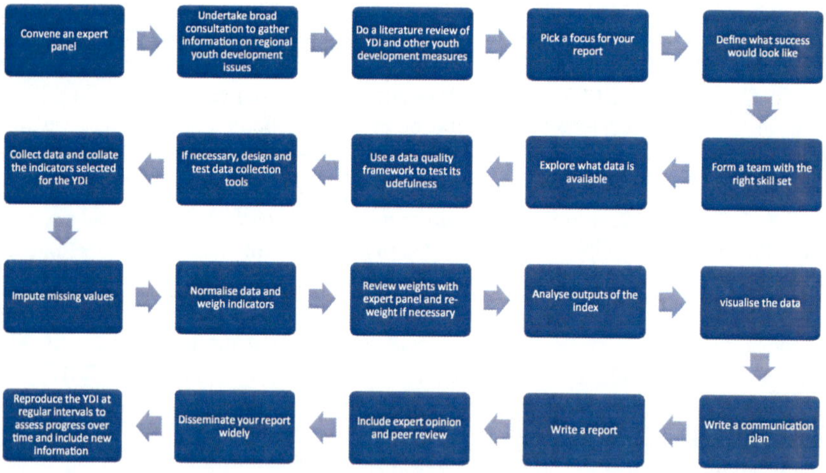

Fig. 27.2 Recommended approach for developing effective YDIs

Key Advantages of Harmonised Global, Regional, National, and Sub-national YDIs

The primary goal of the YDI is to enable action in youth development. YDIs are powerful tools for expanding access to inclusive, relevant, and easy to interpret measures that meaningfully represent young people.

Because of their composite nature, meaningful YDIs can be created using readily available statistical data assets, thereby leveraging decade's worth of investment in data collection and data quality improvement processes on a global scale, at relatively low cost.

Another key advantage of using composite indicators in youth development is that they can easily be adapted or scaled to reflect evolving priorities, to incorporate process improvements and changes to best practice, and to include novel data sources. Examples of continuous improvement in the GYDI and harmonized national YDIs are described in the next section, and examples of the demonstrated impact of these indices are contained in the highlighted boxes throughout this Section.

YDIs that are created using data aggregated at the national level can be used effectively to provide an absolute assessment of youth development at the country level and to form the basis for comparison of performance in youth development domains relative to other jurisdictions. However, YDIs built using nationally aggregated data can mask sub-national variations in youth development.

By leveraging in-country data assets and modeling the analytical framework on the GYDI and its domains, country-level YDIs that are constructed using sub-national data can provide insights into inequalities or variations across sub-groups of young people within a nation, while also enabling meaningful comparison with young people in other regions. YDIs that use sub-national data can be adapted to include indicators that are of specific importance in the local context and cannot be captured at the national level, as well as indicators that address gaps in data coverage or quality in GYDI data that might otherwise exclude groups of young people from having their needs and priorities included in decisions that will impact their ability to realize their potential. The use of sub-national data can also help measure short-, medium-, and long-term issues for planning and policy design. See Box 1 for an example of data shaping policy and funding decisions.

Box 1: Suicide Prevention Funding and Focus, Particularly For Aboriginal and Torres Strait Islander Young Men Following the release of the first Australian YDI in 2016 media coverage picked up on the fact that the report revealed suicide rates for Aboriginal and Torres Strait Islander men aged from 25 to 29 were higher than those reported by any other nation at https://www.abc.net.au/news/2016-08-12/indigenous-youth-suicide-rate-highest-in-world-report-shows/7722112 and https://vimeo.com/178837585. While not necessarily caused by the YDI release conversations definitely increased around this time with policy and programme interventions along with funding becoming more of a priority for both jurisdictional and Federal Governments as can be seen at https://www.mediastatements.wa.gov.au/Pages/Barnett/2016/08/150000-dollar-grant-for-Aboriginal-suicide-prevention.aspx.

Since effective, evidence-based youth policies and programs increasingly rely on high-quality, timely, and relevant data to develop an accurate and comprehensive understanding of the current situation, to highlight population sub-groups that most need support, and to identify priorities for action, creating harmonized YDIs with sub-national data enables the development of targeted youth development interventions at all levels of government, helping to maximize the potential impact of investments in youth development. The Global YDIs and harmonized national YDIs support the strategic use of data to create value and realize the full potential of global data assets and analytical capabilities. This results in sounder decision-making and provides thought leadership in youth development that is problem-driven and integrated across domains (United Nations, 2020).

By design, the Global YDIs and harmonized national YDIs align closely with the United Nations' priorities for the responsible and impactful use of data in supporting priorities for action in youth development (United Nations, 2020). The UN Secretary-General's 2020–2021 Priorities for People and Planet can be seen in Box 2.

Box 2: UN Secretary-General's 2020–2021 Priorities for People and Planet

1. Decade of Action to Deliver the SDGs by 2030
2. Climate Action
3. Gender Equality
4. Human Right and the Rule of Law
5. Peace and Security
6. Governance and Ethics for the Future
7. Delivering UN Reform
8. Data Protection and Privacy

"Recognizing that we have not fully unlocked our data and analytics potential, this Strategy will guide us through a long-term transformation: So that everyone, everywhere nurtures data as a strategic asset for insight, impact and integrity—to better deliver on our mandates for people and planet."—António Guterres, Secretary-General (United Nations, 2020).

The UN Secretary-General's Envoy on Youth, with young people themselves, suggested the following as important data traits which YDIs provide:

- Creating spaces and opportunities for meaningful participatory engagement with young people in decision-making, monitoring, and accountability processes;
- Capturing diverse voices and experiences at all levels from municipal to local to ensure that youth development activities do not "leave the furthest behind";
- Giving young people access to data that is relevant to them in a way that is easy to understand; and
- Exposing areas where data collection about young people needs to be strengthened or expanded and driving efforts to address issues in youth data quality or availability (ActionAid, 2020).

This last point has been of particular note in more recent YDIs with data gaps being identified and primary data collections designed to fill them. Box 3 highlights examples where National Youth Surveys have been designed for this purpose.

Box 3: National Youth Surveys and Youth-Specific Agenda to National Statistical Instruments (Pakistan and Namibia) Through the YDI design phase in Pakistan it was found that many indicators deemed important through the consultation phase were not adequately captured in existing data sets. UNDP funded a National Youth Survey, designed by NAPS in consultation with the Pakistan Bureau of Statistics, capturing Mental Health, COVID-19 and YDI specific indicators. This was published separately to the YDI with the YDI report and dashboard at https://www.numbersandpeople.com/projects and Youth Survey at http://youthpolicypk.com/.

As similar National Youth Survey has been designed for Namibia and will go out to the field in 2023.

The practice of publishing and broadly disseminating YDI data and reports encourages and enables youth advocacy efforts and facilitates communication and engagement with influential stakeholders, the media, and the general public. By attracting public interest and stimulating open discourse, the Global and harmonized national YDIs can advance collective knowledge and attitudes toward young people and the social, structural, and policy issues that impede or enable their development.

By ensuring wide dissemination of the YDI reports and, more recently, data dashboards, there is increased accountability and transparency while creating pathways for young people to directly impact the decisions that have an impact on them (United Nations, 2020). YDIs can empower young people and decision-makers with information about social and economic issues impacting youth for advocacy (Commonwealth Secretariat, 2016a). By involving young people in the design, showcasing how their data is used and respecting data sovereignty YDIs have the power to creating data advocates in young people. This in turn encourages the strengthening of the role of young people in monitoring and evaluation, another UN goal (ActionAid, 2020). Box 4 showcases the importance of data in youth mainstreaming and youth policy.

Box 4: Data for Youth Mainstreaming Youth Mainstreaming is becoming more common place globally (Youthpolicy.org, 2008) and data is becoming increasingly seen important in the monitoring and evaluation space. A free course on Youth Mainstreaming, including a module on Evidence-Based Youth Policy and Programming at https://cwlearn.commonwealth.int/course/.

The Global and harmonized national YDIs support further research in youth development and provide a framework for a common research agenda that is forward-looking and addresses challenges impacting youth that are newly emerging, under-recognized, or poorly understood (United Nations, 2020).

Youth Consultation Findings

The different YDIs that have been produced have had varying levels of youth consultation. Indonesia and Australia, for example, had quite extensive youth consultation, particularly with respect to which domains and indicators were to be included. Young people were also on the expert panel with government, academia, NGOs, and civil society guiding the entire project. Other countries and regions have relied more heavily on stakeholders who work with or for young people, with only a few young people engaged in the entire process. There are many reasons for these variations, including funding and time constraints. Nevertheless, no matter how large or small the youth representation, there have been consistent themes received from young people regarding the issues they deem as important to deal with in their own and their peers' lives. A summary of some of the youth voices NAPS has heard over the past 7 years is below. Box 5 highlights the importance of youth in the creation of YDIs.

Box 5: Youth Leadership, Engagement, and Co-design Consultation with youth is an indispensable part of developing priorities for YDIs. Youth consultations are conducted across various countries as part of the development of the YDI for country, regional and global reports. Apart from the youth, these consultative workshops include key government and non-government stakeholders to inform the development of country-specific YDIs that are appropriately structured for comparability with other countries whilst reflecting local priorities. The scope of the consultations varies from multiple youth consultation workshops per sub-national geographical territory to singular national youth representative forums. Recent NAPS authored YDI reports provide a summary of youth priorities from the reports for the Global, ASEAN, African

Union, Barbados, Indonesia, Cambodia, Bangladesh, Namibia, Pakistan and Australian YDIs. See below for more details.

Stakeholders, both youth and others, consistently consider the opportunity for employment and quality of education to be a priority. Youth link these two priorities as the quality of education is directly related to the ability to secure suitable and available employment. Good government and economic management are priorities that youth associate with employment.

Another priority from all stakeholders is the importance of access to quality education and employment, with remote locations, the demands and expectations of family, poverty and living with a disability identified as issues of vulnerability.

Additionally, youth place importance on the impact of drug and alcohol abuse on wellbeing, vulnerability to mental health stressors and suicidal tendencies, and a need for the voice of youth to be welcomed and incorporated into policy development. Youth describe feeling deeply affected by disruptions to family and community networks caused by lack of safety in the home, gender-based violence and other forms of gender inequality, suppressed political freedoms, and having to leave for the city or overseas to find employment. The desire for greater social connection is evident in both developed and developing countries. Other priorities include living pressures expressed during both education and youth employment as well as fairer policing, judicial, and sentencing processes.

Improved access to the internet and accurate information is important to youth along with greater freedom of movement and opportunity for female youth, particularly in rural areas. Youth wish to see an end to the practice of child marriage and all family violence.

In addition to the youth-specific priorities for the main domains noted above, youth consultation has also identified a set of other priorities. These include Safety, Community and Culture, Racism, Housing, Social and Family Network and Poverty. For Safety youth want to see greater justice in the policing, judiciary and detention, reduced rates of sexual and other violence particularly in the family home and greater equality between genders. Equality also includes fair access to public spaces for youth. Youth believe that greater participation and involvement in the community will increase a feeling of safety.

Youth identify housing as a priority that relates to various domains, including safety, connectedness to community, relationship to family, and wellbeing. Youth describe Poverty in terms of the need for social inclusion, housing, transport, and equality of opportunity. Youth seek Gender Equality particularly in relation to child marriage, access to education, leadership in the community, and freedom from violence. The vulnerability of youth with disabilities is identified by youth in accessing transport, education, and opportunity.

The results of youth consultation compared to broader stakeholder consultation differ in that there is a greater emphasis on mental health, including suicide, drug and alcohol issues, cost of living pressures, the impacts of racism, the need for real life practical skills for living, and managing personal finances and a need for greater connection to culture and community. Youth articulate a unique perspective on the priorities required to foster development.

Ongoing Development of YDIs

Since their initial introduction, the content, process, and application of YDIs has been adapted and enhanced to continuously improve its quality and relevance, its inclusivity, and its potential impact as a decision-making tool. Box 5 summarizes the improvements made in the Global YDI (GYDI) while Box 6 looks at improvements beyond the GYDI.

Box 6: Continuous Improvement of the Global YDI By its 2020 iteration, the GYDI had been expanded to include 27 indicators measuring youth development in 181 countries. The five original GYDI domains of health and wellbeing, education, employment and opportunity, civic participation, and political participation had been revised and expanded into include concepts of peace, security, equality, and inclusion, including a greater emphasis on gender equality, across 6 re-defined domains (see Fig. 27.1). Domain weightings were also redistributed to account for newly available research evidence and limitations in data availability (Commonwealth Secretariat, 2020).

Feedback from National YDIs conducted between 2016 and 2023 has suggested a need to widen the domains to include safety, gender, culture, and climate. The indicators in the YDIs are strategically developed to track progress on critical goals. However, previous YDIs have faced data availability and conceptual limitations.

While much data collection from and about youth has been carried out, there are some youth cohorts who have remained poorly represented. Data improvements could mean amplifying the important voices of the following under-represented cohorts:

- Females
- LGBTQIA+
- Migrants
- Humanitarian Refugees
- Climate Refugees
- Sex workers
- Child slaves
- Child soldiers
- Child Wives/Husbands
- Disabled

- Mentally Ill
- Drug abusers
- Homeless

Gender has routinely become an issue that needs better capture in YDIs, but the definition of gender changes across contexts. For this reason, most YDIs have sex disaggregation, where possible in the data, and use that for gender analysis. Many countries include "transgender" as well as "male" and "female" and some include "other" in collections, although it is common for this to be used to identify one's sexuality, not necessarily gender. LGBTQI+, where legal and disaggregated in data, have been identified as a vulnerable group that many focus groups with young people have brought up as deserving of a strong voice to government through YDIs.

There has also been a lack of focus on disability access in previous indexes, which potentially could fall under the domain of participation and across many other domains.

Many discussions have also taken place around potential additional Domains for future YDIs, Including:

- Climate Change
- Digital Citizenship
- Peacebuilding
- Freedom of expression/media

Box 7: Improvements to YDIs since 2016

- Global YDI—Inclusion of new Domains Equality & Inclusion and Peace & Security
- ASEAN—Discussion on Environment (Climate Change) and Media and Digital Citizen and inclusion of Equity and Inclusion and Safety and Security
- Codesign with youth (leading to inclusion of Culture and Community Domain in Australia)
- More youth on the expert panels from design through to launch of YDIs
- Primary data collection to fill data gaps
- Greater focus on mental health not just physical health
- Inclusion of text boxes from a diverse set of experts (NGOs, academics, advocates, young people, politicians, public servants and more)
- Youth as peacebuilders included in the consultations on peace and security
- Inclusion of Skills in Education Domain
- Data dashboard publication (transparency of data e.g. Australian at https://www.numbersandpeople.com/aydi2020).

What the YDI is not

The YDI is not an exhaustive measure of youth development but it does provide a holistic snapshot using indicators split into domains. It should not be seen as the means to an end but rather a "conversation starter" based on a high-level overview of youth development. The lived experience of young people is far too varied to be captured in an index and so the YDI should be partnered with other data, research, and consultation prior to use in informing policy and program changes.

More generally, the main limitation of the YDIs and measurement indexes is the challenge of localized application versus scalability. Scaling aggregate data provides substantial benefits for policymakers wanting to ensure that outcomes are balanced and equitable across geographical territories. However, the drawback is that this inhibits the ability of the YDI, as a tool, to find appropriate and comparable data. What is possible, however, is for data and results to be captured and reported at a local scale. There is also scope for developing additional local measures that may reflect priorities, as a complement to YDI results. Where data sets may be too small to be meaningful or missing altogether, imputations can be used to incorporate averages from larger population sizes.

"The YDI attempts to give a number which can be utilised in evidence-based policy and monitoring and evaluation. However, it is important to acknowledge what it does not do:

- The YDI does not cover all aspects of youth development in their fullness; it is limited by the number and quality of indicators that can be included in it.
- The YDI is dynamic and changes over time; however, progress within youth development is slow moving and certain policy impacts can take generations to measure. As such, slow or lagged movement can be expected from policy change, as opposed to immediate, large-score changes.
- Composite indicators are a way to measure complex ideas simply, which can lead to important fluctuations, inequalities and localised issues being hidden in the overall scores.
- Disaggregation of the YDI into cohorts of interest—whether cultural, geographical, gender or ethnic—could lead to better-informed policy than using the YDI as a whole.
- Many datasets used to compare countries and regions are calculated differently, making direct comparisons impossible. An understanding of the differences in the data will help in avoiding incorrect comparisons and in harmonising the data for inclusion in an index" (Commonwealth 2016b).

Conclusion

The primary goal of the YDI is to enable action in youth development. YDIs are powerful tools for expanding access to relevant and inclusive data about young people.

Because of their composite nature, YDIs can build on statistical data assets on a global scale. By analyzing data from youth-related datasets at global, regional, national, and sub-national levels using a small set of comprehensive and harmonized measures, YDIs enable users to take complex, multi-dimensional quantitative data and make it easier to interpret.

Global, regional, national, and sub-national analyses allow for different interventions at different levels and so maximize their potential impact on youth development.

Using sub-national data in YDIs provides context-specific indicators measuring local challenges and areas with opportunities for growth. Sub-national data is crucial because of the large spatial variations in development, and the differing policies and programmatic actions that occur.

The practice of publishing and broadly disseminating YDI data and reports encourages and enables youth advocacy efforts and facilitates communication and engagement with influential stakeholders, the media, and the general public. By attracting public interest and stimulating open discourse, the Global and harmonized national YDIs can advance collective knowledge and attitudes toward young people and the social, structural, and policy issues that impede or enable their development.

References

ASEAN. (2022). *The 2nd ASEAN youth development index*. https://asean.org/the-2nd-asean-youth-development-index/

Christian, T. (2020). Forward. In C. Secretariat (Ed.), *Global youth developmet index and report*. Commonwealth Secretariat.

Commonwealth Secretariat. (2007). *The commonwealth plan of action for youth empowerment 2007–2015*. Commonwealth Secretariat.

Commonwealth Secretariat. (2013). *Youth development index results report*. Commonwealth Secretariat.

Commonwealth Secretariat. (2016a). *Global youth development index and report 2016*. Commonwealth Secretariat.

Commonwealth Secretariat. (2016b). *Commonwealth youth development index national and regional toolkit: A guide for developing regional and national youth development indices*. Commonwealth Secretariat. https://www.thecommonwealth.io/wp-content/uploads/2020/02/National-YDI-Toolkit.pdf

Commonwealth Secretariat. (2020). *Global youth development index and report 2020*. Commonwealth Secretariat.

ILO. (2019). *Skills for youth employment*. https://www.ilo.org/skills/areas/skills-for-youth-employment/WCMS_672181/lang--en/index.htm

NAPS. (2020). *Australian youth development index*. NAPS.

Numbers and People Synergy. (2023). *Numbers and people synergy: Our Projects.* https://www.numbersandpeople.com/projects

Organization for Economic Co-Operation and Development. (2016). *Handbook on constructing composite indicators: Methodology and user guide.* OECD.

The, Rt, Hon. Patricia Scotland QC. (2021, August 10). Launch of the. (2021). *Global youth development index report.* Mariborough House, United Kingdom.

United Nations. (2020). *United nations secretary-general's data strategy.* https://www.un.org/en/content/datastrategy/index.shtml

United Nations Department of Economic and Social Affairs. (2010). *World programme of action for youth.* United Nations.

Youthpolicy.org. (2008). *Youth mainstreaming as a strategic tool for youth development.*

G. Wood is a statistician and community development researcher with over 20 years of experience in research and consulting roles in the private, public and NGO sectors. She has maintained a focus on increased equity and opportunity for all social groups and particularly marginalised and vulnerable people. Gemma has partnered with the United Nations Population Fund (UNFPA) and the Commonwealth Secretariat to prepare frameworks for National and Regional Youth Development Indexes (YDIs). She has been a keynote speaker at forums focusing on evidence-based policy through the Commonwealth Secretariat and United Nations Department of Economic and Social Affairs (UNDESA). YDIs Gemma has worked on include Global, ASEAN, African, Indonesian, Cambodian, Barbados, Namibia, Bangladesh, Pakistan and Australian YDIs. She has led stakeholder engagement with disadvantaged groups, youth, youth organisations, government and NGOs across Africa, South-East Asia and the Pacific. These consultations have been to develop a better understanding of specific local issues and to find out what development measurement data is available now and what might be available in the future.

Part V
Youth and Mental Health

Chapter 28
Conditions for Young People's Mental Health: COVID-19, Tiktok, and Relational Space

Marianne Billington and Tom Billington

Abstract This chapter draws on conversations between the two authors (daughter and father) that arose initially during family meals, walks, and coffees in our home city of Liverpool. The conversations took place as, like many across the world, we emerged from our experiences of COVID, Marianne having now completed her first year at University and Tom having stepped down from his own formal academic responsibilities. While acknowledging the relative privilege of her vantage point, Marianne reflects on the impact of COVID on her life. In particular, she focuses on the ways in which social media, especially TikTok, filled the spaces vacated by in-person human interactions with friends in previously familiar places in the local community such as schools and clubs. She reflects on the combined impact that COVID and TikTok have had, both on the modes of communication now being shared with previously unknown young people of her age, but also on her exposure to unforeseen and often unregulated influences and values from across the world in new *relational* spaces. The conversations traverse culture, economics, gender and politics as new imperatives, standards and values begin to shape and define young people's sense of identity and mental health. The chapter utilizes mixed methods. It is a response to contemporary calls to involve young people in research that affects their lives (Efuribe et al., 2020) and is driven by Marianne's own experiences and narratives (White, 1989; Billington, 2000). It accords with social constructionist principles (Gergen, 2015) in providing the space for Marianne to develop her ideas while at the same time incorporating quantitative data and research.

Keywords Youth · Mental Health · COVID-19 · Tiktok · Space

M. Billington
University of Manchester, Manchester, UK

T. Billington (✉)
University of Sheffield, Sheffield, UK
e-mail: t.billington@sheffield.ac.uk

S. Deb and S. Deb (eds.), *Handbook of Youth Development*,
https://doi.org/10.1007/978-981-99-4969-4_28

Introduction

> [There are] acute mental health impacts (loneliness, isolation, anxiety) as well as longer-term repercussions from disrupted education (missed parts of curriculum, home schooling, canceled exams, periods of isolation) on young people…as a result of the COVID-19 pandemic (Scott et al., 2021).

This chapter draws on conversations between the two authors (daughter and father) that arose during family meals, walks, and coffees in our home city of Liverpool (UK). The conversations took place as, like many across the world, we both emerged from our experiences of COVID, Marianne having finally engaged in her first year of studies at University and Tom having stepped down from his own formal academic duties in one UK University setting for the last twenty years.

While acknowledging the relative privilege of her own individual vantage point (white, middle class, higher educated), Marianne reflects on the ways that COVID has affected all aspects of her own life but the lives of all those with whom she began to share new social spaces. COVID-19 had caused the cessation of direct human interactions with friends in previously familiar places in the local community such as schools and clubs and, in particular, she considers the ways in which social media, but especially TikTok, filled the (*relational*) spaces that had to be vacated during the pandemic. She reflects on the combined impact that COVID and TikTok have had on the modes of communication now being shared with previously unknown young people of her age, but also on her exposure to unforeseen and often unrestricted and unregulated influences and values from across the world.

It is important to incorporate young people's voices relating to COVID (Efuribe et al, 2020) and this chapter was driven primarily by Marianne's thoughts and feelings as she struggled to re-adjust to life after COVID. Her thoughts and feelings were drafted initially by Tom before being subject again to Marianne's scrutiny, comments, and amendments. Methodologically too, the chapter is a hybrid, driven initially by personal experiences in the form of narratives (White, 1989; Billington, 2000; Efuribe et al., 2020) but also other forms of qualitative research (Gergen, 2015) as well as quantitative data and research.

Our initial conversations did not arise in a vacuum, however, and were triggered in part by family discussions occurring over the period of COVID and its lockdowns and in which Marianne found her voice on issues concerning culture, economics, gender, and politics. Specifically in respect of this chapter, however, Marianne developed her thinking around issues relating to body image, humor, self-esteem, and the values and imperatives that are shaping and defining young people's identity and sense of wellbeing in a post-pandemic world.

Young People, Mental Health, and The Concept of Relational Space

Well before COVID-19, concerns had been growing globally in respect of mental health (WHO, 2015). In recent years, these concerns have been directed increasingly toward the mental health of children and young people, manifest in a raft of publications from governments and institutions, for example, the World Health Organization (WHO, 2010), the Australian Government (2019), the Department of Health and National Health Service England (DoH & NHS, 2015), the National Institute for Mental Health, USA (NIMH, 2018) and in New Zealand the Youth Parliament (2016). Research into the emotional wellbeing and mental health of children and young people is being conducted across many different cultural and national contexts, for example, China (Zhang & Du, 2018), India (Lai et al., 2016), Iran (Salimi et al., 2017), Japan (Sekizaki et al., 2017), Mexico (Bravo-Sanzana et al., 2015), South Africa (Mfidi, 2017) and the UK (Billington, 2022).

While there is debate around the intensity and demographic reach of mental ill health among young people, policy and research point to a sustained increase in the prevalence of mental ill health among young people, suggesting a wider, and growing, public health issue (Patalay & Gage, 2019). This view is reinforced by a worldwide growth in specific diagnoses such as attention deficit hyperactivity disorder (ADHD), attachment disorder, autism spectrum condition (ASC), depression, eating disorders as well as early-onset dementia and psychosis (WHO, 2010, 2019). Young people, of course, are victims to forms of harm and abuse that are themselves associated with mental health problems (Kisely et al., 2018), for example, bullying (Mehta et al., 2013), domestic violence (Holt et al., 2008), exposure to war and civil conflict (Pritchard & Choonara, 2017) and drug and gang culture (Gulliver et al., 2010). There is evidence to suggest that more young people are experiencing anxiety, trauma and attempting suicide (O'Connor et al., 2018) while in the UK the rise in the rate of young women reporting self-harm, for example, is a matter for public concern (Morgan et al., 2017). Outcomes can be serious for the young people affected, in some instances tragic, and each individual sufferer warrants clinical or service responses.

There is some research, however, which questions that acceptance of a massive pre-COVID rise in young people's mental health problems (Pitchforth et al., 2018) while there is also research which challenges the blurring of the boundaries between a holistic approach to human wellbeing and a more sharply delineated medical/psychiatric arena of mental illness (Patalay & Fitzsimmons, 2016). There are other critical voices who suggest that the rise of concern is allowing a therapeutic language and culture to be inserted inappropriately into schools (Ecclestone & Hayes, 2009). There are also educational researchers, however, who are just as concerned to ensure that mental illness shakes off the stigma to which it has long been attached (Allan, 2018) while others illuminate the ways in which mental health intersects with a range of human differences, not only in our schools but across our communities, for example, disability (Liddiard, 2017), ethnicity (Rosen et al., 2017), gender (Ussher,

2011), sexual orientation (Burton et al., 2013) and young people in public care (Luke et al., 2014).

While mental health issues affect people at the level of individual experience, there is gathering evidence that the root causes and manifestation of the majority of mental health-related problems are affected by circumstances that lie beyond both the individual and the arena of medical or clinical health (Cromby et al., 2013; Thomas et al., 2020; WHO, 2016). In this chapter, therefore, we consider the ways in which COVID-19 and social media, in particular, TikTok, have created what William James would have regarded as new specific "conditions" for young people's wellbeing and mental health (James, 2010 [orig.1890]).

Like James, we too have sought to evade traditional boundary disputes between the psychological and the social. We have used the term *relational* as a means of encouraging more dynamic understandings of persons that represent more realistically the fast-changing and interconnected global, environmental, and technological circumstances.

The *relational* is an emerging paradigm which acknowledges that human lives are experienced in the dynamic multi-dimensional conditions of time–space that have been well understood in the physical sciences for decades. The *relational* can be found in education, for example, professional expertise (Edwards, 2011), power (Billington, 1996, 2006), learning (Hersted & Gergen, 2013), and evaluation (Gergen & Gill, 2020) but also in psychoanalysis too (Mitchell, 2014; Son, 2006) where the term can tend to invoke narrower conceptualizations of individual "selves." The *relational* in this chapter moves beyond dyadic inter-subjectivities and links to uncertainties that have stubbornly persisted from the nineteenth-century scientific interest in association (Blackman, 2008) through to contemporary social constructionism as "…a process of coordination that precedes the very concept of the self" (Gergen, 2009: xv).

For many young people, COVID-19 and the expansion of social media, in particular, TikTok, has been creating new *relational* spaces (after Winnicott, 1971). These spaces are the conditions for living in which young people are defining their identities and in which their wellbeing and mental health are being negotiated. COVID-19 has triggered the emergence of new *relationalities*, in our environments and in our socially interactive worlds.

COVID-19 and Young People's Mental Health

When asked what mattered most after the outbreak has been reduced, the singular response from youth can be surmised in one quote, "If possible, getting back all/or most of my missed opportunities" (Efuribe et al., 2020).

As parents we had become acutely aware of the increasing pressures upon our children as they grew older through the education system but these were exacerbated dramatically by the onset of COVID in February 2020. As for many people across the globe, our family life changed, as by now young adult offspring (and ourselves as their parents) had to adjust to new daily routines and create new ways of being in the world enforced by a global disease. The pressures upon young people, however, became particularly acute, whether in respect of their family relationships, friendships, or in terms of their re-shaping identities.

Our children had always been active in the local community, whether in sports clubs, youth clubs, or in the case of Marianne, dancing schools and choirs. All of a sudden, however, like many young people across the world, Marianne found herself physically isolated from her friends and struggling to adjust to school closure. Young people can have mixed feelings about schools and their education but for many who may have fantasized about an occasional day off school due to severe weather or some other misfortune, their dream of a day away from school suddenly became a reality without any foreseeable end (Lee, 2021).

Having constructed ideas about herself, her family, and friends over the course of her childhood, Marianne and whole cohorts of young people who were fortunate to be contemplating higher/further education or employment, found themselves in situations in which the nature of what life was, or was going to be like, was suddenly thrown into disarray. In Marianne's case she had grown up with the expectation that if she worked hard at school, she would pass her examinations and progress to University. There she would increasingly develop the means by which she could exercise some control over her life. While acutely aware that she has always been fortunate in this respect, that certainty of a life path had suddenly been disrupted. What she had worked for over the years was now under threat and what had presented as a certainty was now at risk from a physical disease, the full extent and trajectory of which was unknown.

Different countries dealt with the pandemic in different ways but in the UK "lockdowns" for many young people were implemented nationally, lasting several months and repeated over the course of 18 months. Shortly after the onset of the first lockdown it soon became clear to young people such as Marianne and her friends that they had experienced their last day in school. While that might have presented for some young people in the past as a welcome prospect, the circumstances of this enforced cessation of her education were such that she was thrust into the uncertainty of not knowing what was to happen in respect of her examinations and thus her whole future.

The uncertainties of lockdown affected everyone, and for us as parents we were unable to provide the reassurance that all would be fine. The lottery of life, and the ill-fortune experienced by many young people across the globe had perhaps for the first time affected young people who had realistic expectations of following a predictable path to a relative success known to previous cohorts and generations. What was "normal" had to be re-thought and re-negotiated as the statistics for daily infection rates came to dominate the national mood, perhaps for two years, while in some countries consideration of those rates is still impacting on young people's prospects and expectations.

During lockdowns, lessons were canceled and then schools closed. There was uncertainty about the actual examinations too and new arrangements were eventually made for our children's futures which we had worked as parents for years assiduously to protect and which were under threat. While coping with the uncertainties of unknown endings and the prospect of seismic life-course changes, at the same time learning materials were hurriedly placed online by teachers, no doubt similarly fearful for their own futures. The whole nature and structure of "learning" itself became a completely different process, not something that happened in the social context of schools, classrooms, and shared peer experiences, but in a technological space from which direct contact with other humans became extremely limited.

At the outset of COVID-19, Marianne and her friends had been gearing themselves up for the last final push toward life-affecting A-Level examinations while at the same time preparing for the usual accompanying end-of-year rituals. The school "prom," for example, is a tradition that enables young people and their teachers to mark the end of a phase of their lives and to come to terms with change, loss, and potential futures. The hopes, expectations, fears, and joy associated with such rituals were suddenly denied and ripped away from Marianne and her friends as "normal" daily life came to an abrupt halt. As a family we are just beginning to realize the impact of these losses and that we had become aware that the pandemic had not only posed a threat physically but to our mental health and wellbeing.

We found that the percentage of individuals with anxiety was almost double during the COVID-19 assessments compared to pre-pandemic levels…our findings suggest that anxiety in response to COVID-19 is not just an initial reaction but potentially the start of a persistent problem that extends beyond the pandemic (Kwong et al., 2020).

There were glimmers of hope when the pandemic seemed to be abating only for the infection statistics to rise again to dampen any hopes of a return to normal:

> Around three-quarters of young people who responded to our survey said that the current lockdown has been harder to cope with than the first one, for a variety of reasons: a growing sense of isolation; a loss of faith in their prospects for the future; freezing weather that disrupts basic routines; and for those in school or university, the pressures of home learning (Young Minds, 2021).

Phrases such as "unprecedented" and "new normal" entered the vocabulary and as families we began to devise ways of surviving, not just physically but psychologically and emotionally. We went in search of new daily routines for work and play as we sought to retain some sense of purpose. We sought forms of exercise, mental and physical, but all forms of direct human interaction and contact had somehow overnight become dangerous. The close physical proximity to other people was suddenly a matter of alarm and fear.

Governments frantically sought ways of protecting businesses and livelihoods as the very fabric of society seemed to be in danger. People's jobs and financial security came under threat in a way not even experienced during the 2008 financial crash while the chain of goods, services, and provisions for daily living in shops came under severe pressure. We all had to queue for food for the first time in decades and there were major shortages of what many in the world have for many years been sufficiently fortunate to regard as basic goods.

It was not only the damage to our mental health that was caused by the disruption of our daily routines but it was the breakdown of the familiar, and the desperate search for new daily rhythms. There were restrictions on physical touch and even proximity to other human beings became subject to regulation in a manner previously unknown. We began to fear, not only the future but one another as all other people became a potential threat to our very existence, even in our own families. Messages from the government indicated that the state was intervening with the very nature of human interaction itself. The changing rules about human closeness, distance, and physical touch and all the uncertainties ushered in by the pandemic, induced for many what was a heightened fear and imminent sense of mortality.

Many of us have been fortunate to live our lives, confident in the knowledge of the statistical probability that a good education together with family security plus hard work would lead to all kinds of social, financial, and positive life benefits. These beliefs were challenged and were in danger of being overwhelmed by the anxieties and fears that began to afflict across the generations. Scott, McGowan, and Visram (2021) suggested in their research that the impact of COVID-19 on young people could be understood as having.

> Three central themes: (1) impacts upon mental health and emotional wellbeing; (2) disruptions and changes to education and school life; and (3) frustration, burden and responsibility.

Marianne's ideas as to the person she was, and her expectations as to the person she might come to be were in turmoil, but she was just one out of a whole cohort of young people whose very identities were being challenged in a manner not experienced on a global scale for generations. At the very moment that research had, for several years, been illuminating the pressures on young people and the associated risks to their mental health, COVID created a devastating change in conditions and we are now beginning to count the cost of the extent to which young people's mental health and wellbeing were impacted by the upheavals of the pandemic. The impact was not only on young people in the UK, however, or on one particular stratum of society, but on young people from across the globe and across many diverse populations:

> Children and adolescents experienced adverse mental health effects, including feelings of social isolation, depression, anxiety, and increases in maladaptive behavior. The findings highlight the impact of severe restrictions on vulnerable populations' wellbeing and mental health outcomes, including children, adolescents, and those with autism spectrum disorder (ASD) (O'Sullivan et al., 2021).

A whole raft of specific mental health issues have been studied with overall results suggesting an increase in mental health problems in young people since the start of the pandemic with those from disadvantaged communities suffering perhaps even more than most:

Since the lockdown, 30.3% had poor mental health, and 10.8% had self-harmed. Young people identifying as Black/Black British ethnicity had the highest increased odds of experiencing poor mental health...behaviorual disengagement...self-blame...and substance use...negative affect...sleep problems' (Dewa et al., 2021).

Not only have there been increases in symptoms indicative of anxiety and depression, but there have been reported increases in rates of sleep problems and self-harm. Young people have spoken of themselves in respect of the burden they present to their families while others give testimony to a range of negative effects such as depression, sense of frustration, and a sense of responsibility for others that is difficult to manage.

There are some studies that point toward the benefit experienced by young people during the lockdown, for example, in terms of family closeness. While this is true in our family, these studies would seem to be in the minority, however, and in the main the research reiterates the negative impact of COVID and, for many what was an increasing sense of loneliness and isolation (Fancourt et al., 2021; McKinlay et al., 2022).

Loneliness increased…and changes in loneliness were greater for females, those with higher perceived social support…and those with greater concerns about the pandemic's social impacts. Depression (but not anxiety) increased during this time with changes in loneliness accounting for much of the increase in depression (Lee et al., 2020).

The conversations of daily life pre-COVID, the casual arrangements to meet with friends, had disappeared overnight and many young people retreated to their bedrooms. Young people between 16 and 25 have in the past been more susceptible than most to suffer mental health issues and the newly enforced isolation experienced during the pandemic was especially bewildering for many. The changes to social life wrought by COVID increased the chances that the sense of loneliness experienced by many young people for the first time, would develop into full-blown mental health symptoms:

> Social isolation and loneliness increased the risk of depression, and possibly anxiety at the time at which loneliness was measured…Duration of loneliness was more strongly correlated with mental health symptoms than intensity of loneliness…Children and adolescents are probably more likely to experience high rates of depression and most likely anxiety during and after enforced isolation ends. This may increase as enforced isolation continues (Loades et al., 2021).

The whole nature of young people's social worlds had changed during COVID and it was at just this moment of the potential isolation and despair encountered in their particular *relational* spaces, that millions of young people across the world turned increasingly to social media and, in particular, found TikTok.

Social Media and the Phenomenon that is TikTok

> Tik Tok is a new platform that young people love…has both positive and negative sides like any other medium (Serli et al., 2022).

"Generation Z" refers to those young people born after 1996 who have never known of a world without social media (Pew Research Centre, 2019). Marianne had been just one of the millions of young people across the globe who have not known a world without smartphones, the internet, Instagram, Facebook, and many more technologies and "apps" which have burgeoned as part of the latest socio-technological revolution. We have been living through a digital revolution that has changed the conditions for human existence and has been affecting the kinds of lives young people might live and influence the kinds of people they might become.

TikTok was launched in China as recently as 2016 and the following year ByteDance launched an international version focusing on videos, in particular dance videos and lip-syncing. Its success has been exponential and by the end of 2021 TikTok could boast '3 billion downloads…one third of all social media users in less than four years' and by August 2021 ByteDance had a reported valuation of $280 billion (Dean, 2022).

TikTok has been described as the "most popular app of 2020 and 2021" (Curry, 2022) and its most popular categories are "entertainment, dance, pranks, fitness/ sports" (Dean, 2022). Having been a dancer from five years old it was quite natural for Marianne to be attracted to TikTok which, even pre-COVID, had provided a vibrant new space in which she and her friends had begun to augment their usual daily interactions. While previous generations had shared significant events from listening to the radio, watching the television, or attending the cinema, materials appearing on TikTok would become those significant events for her generation, occurring almost on a daily basis. TikTok became the source of conversation with her friends such that it became difficult for young people if they could not keep up with the latest videos. Social pressure built as young people spent more and more time on TikTok for fear of being excluded and Marianne and her friends were exposed to a world of "influencers" who can "have up to 100 million followers and earn up to $5 million a year…" (Dean, 2022).

TikTok filled a particular niche in the market and interestingly it has had a predominantly female demographic which has been celebrated by many women although the gap [between females and males] has declined each year' (Curry, 2022). But how did TikTok manage to attract the legions of young people, initially, primarily young women and how did specific areas of content come to dominate?

The success of TikTok has partially been attributed to the algorithms that were built into its design, luring and then capturing the interests of young people, for example, by analyzing an individual's choices and search preferences. "TikTok's algorithms have proved especially adept at plugging creators into niche communities that share interests, hobbies" (Ohlheiser, 2021). It is the algorithms that determine how any specific is either perpetuated, modified, or ignored. One adult dance teacher described something of the scale of the phenomenon to which Marianne became increasingly drawn during the course of the pandemic:

> …during a rehearsal break, a teenage girl told me that her 'favourite dancer ever' was Charli D'Amelio…I soon discovered that Charli is a sixteen-year- old American girl, who, with her 15-30 seconds performances (most of them entirely choreographed and showed only from the hips up), has attracted 80 million followers worldwide (Cervi, 2021).

While the attention of generations of Western female dancers might in the previous century have been influenced by Anna Pavlova or Ginger Rogers, or perhaps more recent celebrities from the stage or screen such as Jennifer Lopez, Charli D'Amelio is a product of the TikTok generation. She is someone who started out posting videos of herself dancing in her own home and who has now evidently achieved an audience of over 100 hundred million "followers." Charli would evidently seem to be the eponymous "girl next door" and someone with whom young women might identify. Previously unknown young people, and still perhaps unknown to adults, have become household names to younger generations as "trends" would emerge, popping up on phones as part of the algorithm that was constantly working out the kinds of videos that would be of interest, for example, to young people such as Marianne. In her case, it has been BTS, a South Korean "boy band" who has provided her, not only with a kind of sanctuary, but a source of energy, life, and hope.

New digital technologies led to a new vocabulary, for example, of memes, duetting, and stitches, each of which would perform a unique function in determining the kinds of *relational* spaces to which Marianne might be invited. Increasingly, however, it was not just young women who were being drawn to the power of TikTok but, increasingly, men and even governments:

Social media...delivering healthcare education and communication with citizens. Provincial Health Committees (PHCs) in China have begun to adopt the micro-video sharing platform, Tik Tok, to engage with local residents and communicate health-related information' (Zhu et al., 2020).

The potential implications for our young people caused by social media platforms such as TikTok are vast. Just what are the collective cultural symbols to which our young people are being exposed, however, and what are the precise effects on their wellbeing and mental health?

Young People, TikTok, and COVID

The power and impact of the internet has become a research focus and at its most extreme there have been concerns and claims that internet use might even result in a "brain structure that is different" (Rothman, 2016). While neuroscience invites all kinds of frequently misleading headlines (Billington, 2017), the impact of the TikTok phenomenon on young people has become of concern to governments and it has been banned at times in certain countries, for example, India and Pakistan. There, the opposition has not been on account of any physiological or neurological concerns but it has been thought "necessary to limit access to various media, including TikTok, so as not to be carried away by immoral behaviour" (Serli et al., 2022).

COVID-19 and the various social control measures implemented by governments occurred at a moment in time when the despair and loneliness being experienced by young people saw them turn to TikTok in their hundreds of millions. As a family, like many across the world, we were confined to our homes for weeks and months other than for essential shopping and exercise. Our particular home situation is not extravagant, but we were sufficiently fortunate both to live in a house in which each of our children had their own space, and to dwell in an area of the city blessed with two wonderful public parks. While we were able to enjoy the parks and the streets in the community as perhaps never before, back in the home, for many hours of the day, Marianne and her brothers would retreat to their own respective bedroom spaces which were fast becoming no mere place for sleep but a gateway to a *relational* world of which we, as parents, were largely unaware and from which we were excluded.

For Marianne, TikTok was a source of enjoyment, fun, and connection with her friends and other young people. It was a source of social contact, and exposed her to new interests and opportunities that replaced those that would have been offered in the fast diminishing prospect of University. She would initially spend hours looking at the various videos selected by her developing individual algorithm. Unquestionably, Marianne continues to see TikTok as a positive social phenomenon and a massive contribution to her own sense of wellbeing but it did raise issues of concern and she had to make choices.

The new algorithms, while gathering knowledge as to Marianne's individual preferences, would for some reason occasionally place in front of her unusual content. These surprising offers would seemingly appear at random and occasionally contain materials that might be seen as tempting in some way to new areas of thought or activity. Marianne has spoken of TikTok's "dark side," the *relational* spaces for social interaction of which she thankfully has only a vague awareness. Marianne has had antennae for potential dangers, however, and these "dark" spaces are perhaps the ones that had prompted government concerns and led to banning orders. The seemingly random and unsought content occasionally presented to Marianne would seem to have been heavily "male" in orientation and contain material that Marianne found offensive, for example, whether politically or in terms of the values being represented. The basis upon which such material should appear merely by chance (i.e. the algorithm) is not clear.

It could be said that these spaces merely presented dangers equivalent to the kind many young people might typically have faced pre-COVID, for example, on the streets. It could also be argued positively that the choices Marianne has learned to make have provided her with valuable lessons as to the kinds of interests and influences to which she wishes to be subjected. A more vulnerable and less highly educated young person than Marianne, however, might presumably have stumbled unwittingly into areas from which it might be difficult to escape unscathed.

While she believes that there are sites that might entice young people into situations in which they might be susceptible to potential exploitation, Marianne believes that the vast majority of contributors to TikTok that she encounters have sought to remain in the more socially acceptable spaces. She continues to see much of the content she accesses as spaces in which she can share what might be regarded as innocent pleasure, fun, or enjoyment (especially those involving BTS!).

She also acknowledges, however, that some young people have taken advantage of the new technologies being offered to blur various boundaries, for example, presenting images of themselves that represent only what could be described as their "ideal side." These are the kinds of images now being circulated by young people that have been edited to exaggerate positive qualities or conceal negative ones, for example, in respect of physical features.

The new technologies have been enabling young people not only to choreograph or compose, but to manufacture positive, perhaps not wholly accurate versions of themselves. Some young people have sought to represent themselves favorably, for example, in ways that could be considered physically attractive. Body image became a huge concern as young people such as Marianne were presented with images and choices made by the algorithm that would have caused her to reflect on her own image and ultimately perhaps even identity. In the process, a young person would inevitably compare themselves with other peers of her age with implications for self-esteem. While Marianne was able to follow trends to which she was well-suited, she was nevertheless being invited to consider her "ideal self."

As a parent, I am skeptical that the TikTok algorithm is value-free since presumably it has been created, initially, by an adult human. At the very least, TikTok seems to be the latest, ultimate product of an unregulated market that could not be assumed to be an innocent bystander in the cultivation of social choices, identities, and values. TikTok is in the business of commodifying young people's lives. Clearly, as a site for the negotiation of social values, TikTok's effect could be both positive and negative and Marianne's description of its contents suggests that it is a platform that is populated by the core currencies of music, dance, and fashion.

Western young people have increasingly been targeted in recent years by businesses who have realized the market potential and many young women across the globe have, for example, long been acculturated into focusing on body image. The materials on TikTok have consequences since they offer the potential for either affirmation or self-disavowal. At its worst, TikTok could be said to have played a key role in a wholly inappropriate sexualization and fetishization of young women and their bodies, with significant ramifications for feelings of self-worth. Many young women will have been lured into comparing their own physical features with contributors and, in the absence of adult regulation and guidance might have drawn negative conclusions about themselves, with implications for self-esteem. No doubt the choices Marianne has been having to make are similar to those faced by generations of young people in the past, for example, in television or at the movies, but social media platforms, in this case, TikTok was intervening in young people's lives in ways over which parents and national governments had little control.

TikTok's algorithm was successful in attracting young people's attention and was able to achieve longer contact times than its social media competitors (Iqbal, 2022). While Marianne has clearly enjoyed the opportunity to engage and share preferences and opinions with "like-minded people," the challenges she has faced suggest that TikTok cannot claim to be an entirely benign or neutral presence. She was 18 years of age at the beginning of lockdown and was able to make her own decisions. Under "normal" conditions, we would as parents have had some control, for example, as to the time she would be expected back in the house after being with friends. During lockdowns, however, the bedroom door could be shut and she would be distant from us, making her own choices and decisions on TikTok, and exposed to influences over which we as parents would have no control.

Social Media, COVID, and Parenting

Many houses have become quieter during recent years as direct forms of social interaction have been affected by social media use. Should the young person be interested in music, there is no longer even any need for them to have the external speakers at full volume for whenever they feel the urge for pounding rhythms, we as parents can just tell them to put on their headphones. On the other hand, however, since the spread of social media it has sometimes been difficult to speak with our children, oblivious as they can become to all life outside their head once headphones are on. Previous generations of young people had quite naturally sought to exclude their parents from many aspects of their lives but for Generation Z, social media has created *relational* spaces in which they can roam without parental knowledge, oversight, or direction.

Many families during COVID, however, were thrown more closely together as parents worked from home and young people who were still in compulsory education began to face the demands of online learning. Both employment and education found their way into homes in new ways and the emergent *relational* spaces threw up new hybrid forms of work and learning. Many parents will have had to juggle their online work commitments with overseeing their children's home learning. This additional pressure on parenting was especially difficult for parents of young people with some form of disability or special learning need since many will have become accustomed to managing their lives and responsibilities with various forms of additional support. Those adults looking after young people in public care were also under massive pressure as they too were deprived of the resources and respite provided by school attendance.

For some families, however, COVID-19 provided opportunities to create a different and more rewarding family life. Some families were able to adapt to a slower pace with greater personal choice, for example, and managed to create *relational* spaces in which the enforced closeness did not overwhelm but provided welcome opportunities to re-create intimacies perhaps lost since early childhood.

Invariably, however, the young person could return to the default position of their smartphone. The connection between some people and their mobile devices has assumed an intimacy suggesting that the bond has become psychological/emotional. The relationship between user and technology can assume something of the quality that an infant has with their earliest infantile "transitional object" (Winnicott, 1971), i.e. an object that served as a proxy for the intimacy of the infant's primary attachment. This is evidenced on those occasions when one happens to glance at the child's screen. People can be secretive about what they are viewing, not necessarily on account of any covert activity, but as an indication of the primary (i.e. attachment) relationship with the technology.

Such behavior may have arisen as a result of the need for separation or privacy, as family members had been thrown physically together in a way not known for many years. Nonetheless, the nature of the relationships and the *relational* spaces shared between young people and their parents have changed on account of social media and then either exaggerated or re-enforced by COVID-19. Marianne is in many respects a different person now than she was prior to COVID-19. She has encountered loneliness and anxieties in ways that just could not have been foreseen prior to the pandemic. She has even continued to struggle since emerging from lockdowns and she has found it difficult to adjust to her first year at University.

Many University campuses too have struggled to rekindle the vibrancy of pre-COVID times. Attendance at lectures has been lower in many instances as it became difficult to entice young people away from the bedroom cocoons that they had created for themselves during the pandemic. Having had to become accustomed to seeing close physical proximity as potentially dangerous, we have assumed that we can all revert easily to pre-pandemic behavior. For some, stepping outside the family home and once again beginning to make direct in-person human relationships has been difficult and for some, such relationships can still be problematic, even potentially dangerous.

University staff have also struggled, since we too had to adapt to the pandemic and can only now begin to assess the impact of the technological solutions that were devised. It seems likely that there will always be some young people who benefit from online learning but we are just beginning to realize the consequences of a purely online learning model. Universities are striving to find a different balance in hybrid models comprising online and face-to-face delivery while individual members of staff are attempting to evaluate our own preferences, i.e. whether best to continue working from home or resume in-person back on campus.

In respect of the young people, however, there continue to be many like Marianne who found it difficult to adjust to their studies after the pandemic. Some young people may even have lost trust in both the conditions for living and in themselves both as learners and as young adults facing the world. Deprived of the joy prior to the original aborted transition to full University life, we are hoping that the coming semester might see young people becoming more relaxed about social contact again. As a family, we are hoping that University campuses can once more become those *relational* spaces that stimulate the energetic striving for new knowledge and experience in which young people such as Marianne can finally begin wholeheartedly to enjoy the next phase of their lives.

As a family, we had as good a lockdown as we could possibly have expected. We have not so far lost any family member to the pandemic and up to this point have been lucky in avoiding any serious financial problems. On reflection though we too as parents have been mourning the loss of that sense of hope, excitement, and optimism that was such a feature of our children's youth and that was brought to such an abrupt end by COVID-19.

We have been fortunate, however, in that we have been able to use lockdowns as an opportunity to discuss important issues, the kinds of conversations that will hopefully enable our children to emerge more politically attuned and resilient in the face of continuing uncertainties regarding their future world. It is out of those conversations that Marianne and I were drawn to write this chapter and make sense of what has been happening in our lives. We hope now that she and her generation can finally begin again to re-create their own dreams and opportunities that we feared had been lost forever.

References

Allan, C. (2018). The mental health crisis is down to government policy, not stigma, *The Guardian*, 16th. October, https://www.theguardian.com/society/2018/oct/16/mental-health-crisis-government-policy-not-stigma accessed 20th. February 2019.

Australian Government (2019). The social and economic benefits of improving mental health, *Productivity Commission Issues paper: Mental Health Inquiry.*

Billington, T. (1996). Pathologizing children: Psychology in education and acts of government, in E. Burman, G. Aitken, P.Alldred, R. Allwood, T. Billington, B. Goldberg, A.J. Gordo Lopez, C. Heenan, D. Marks & S. Warner (Eds) *Psychology discourse practice: Regulation and resistance* (pp. 37–54). London: Taylor & Francis.

Billington, T. (2000). *Separating, losing and excluding children: Narratives of difference.* London: Routledge Falmer.

Billington, T. (2006). *Working with children: Assessment, representation and intervention.* London: Sage.

Billington, T. (2017). Educational inclusion and critical neuroscience: Friends or foes, *International Journal of Inclusive Education, 21*(8), 866–880. https://doi.org/10.1080/13603116.2017.1283717

Billington, T., Gibson, S., Fogg, P., Lahmar, J., & Cameron, H. (2022). Conditions for mental health in education: Towards relational practice. *British Educational Research Journal, 48*(1), 95–119. https://doi.org/10.1002/berj.3755

Blackman, L. (2008). Affect, relationality as the 'problem of personality': Theory and psychology. *Theory, Culture & Society, 25*(1), 27–51.

Bravo-Sanzana, M., Salvo, S. & Mieres-Chacaltana, M. (2015). The importance of emotional health in schools, a factor for improving mental health and learning achievement, *Salud Publica De Mexico*, 57(2), 111–112, ISSN: 0036–3634 accessed 20th. February 2019.

British Academy (2021). THE COVID DECADE Understanding the long-term societal impacts of COVID-19 [Internet]. https://www.thebritishacademy.ac.uk/documents/3238/COVID-decade-understanding-long-term-societal-impacts-COVID-19.pdf

Burton, C. M., Marshal, M. P., Chisolm, D. J., Sucato, G. S., & Freidman, M. S. (2013). Sexual minority-related victimization as a mediator of mental health disparities in sexual-minority youth: A longitudinal analysis. *Journal of Youth and Adolescence, 42*(3), 394–402.

Cervi, L. (2021). Tik Tok and generation Z. *Theatre, Dance and Performance Training, 12*(2), 198–204. https://doi.org/10.1080/19443927.2021.1915617

Cromby, J., Harper, D., & Reavey, P. (Eds.). (2013). *Psychology, mental health and distress.* Basingstoke: Palgrave Macmillan.

Curry, D. (2022). TikTok app report 2022: Holistic overview of the most popular app of 202 and 2021. *Businessofapps.com* (24th. August) accessed 25th. August.

Dean, B. (2022). TikTok user statistics. *Backlinko.com* (5th. January) accessed 25th. August.

Dewa, L. H., Crandell, C., Choong, E., Jaques, J., Bottle, A., Kilkenny, C., Lawrence-Jones, A., di Simplicio, M., Nicholls, D., & Aylin, P. (2021). CCopeY: A mixed-methods Coproduced study on the mental health status and coping strategies of young people during COVID-19 UK Lockdown. *Journal of Adolescent Health, 68*, 666–675. https://doi.org/10.1016/j.jadohealth.2021.01.009

DoH & NHS England (2015). *Future in mind: promoting, protecting and improving our children and young people's mental health.* Retrieved 06.06.18 from https://assets.publishing.service.gov.uk/government/uploads/system/uploads/attachment_data/file/414024/Childrens_Mental_Health.pdf.

Ecclestone, K., & Hayes, D. (2009). *The dangerous rise of therapeutic education.* London: Routledge.

Edwards, A. (2011). Building common knowledge at the boundaries between professional practices: Relational agency and relational expertise in systems of distributed expertise. *International Journal of Educational Research, 50*, 33–39.

Efuribe, C., Barre-Hemingway, M., Vaghefi, E., & Suileman, A. B. (2020). Coping with the COVID-19 crisis: A call for youth engagement and the inclusion of young people in matters that affect their lives. *Journal of Adolescent Health, 67*, 16–17. https://doi.org/10.1016/j.jadohealth

Fancourt, D., Steptoe, A., & Bu, F. (2021). Trajectories of anxiety and depressive symptoms during enforced isolation due to COVID-19 in England: A longitudinal observational study. *Lancet Psychiatry, 8*, 141–149. https://doi.org/10.1016/S2215-0366(20)30482-X

Fisher, H., Lambert, H., Hickman, M., Yardley, L., & Audrey, S. (2021). Experiences of the coronavirus disease-19 (COVID-19) pandemic from the perspectives of young people: Rapid qualitative study. *Public Health in Practice, 2*, 100162. https://doi.org/10.1016/j.puhip

Gergen, K. J. (2009). *Relational being.* New York: Oxford University Press.

Gergen, K. J. (2015). *Invitation to social constructionism* (3rd ed.). London: Sage.

Gergen, K., & Gill, S. R. (2020). *Beyond the tyranny of testing: Relational evaluation in education.* New York: Oxford University Press.

Gulliver, A., Griffiths, K. M., & Christensen, H. (2010). Perceived barriers and facilitators to mental health help-seeking in young people: A systematic review. *BMC Psychiatry, 10*, 113. https://doi.org/10.1186/1471-244X-10-113

Hersted, L. & Gergen, K.J. (2013) *Relational learning: Practices for dialogically-based collaboration.* Chagrin Falls, Ohio: TAOS Institute.

Holt, S., Buckley, H., & Whelan, S. (2008). The impact of exposure to domestic violence on children and young people: A review of the literature. *Child Abuse & Neglect, 32*(8), 797–810.

Iqbal, M. (2022) TikTok Revenue and Usage Statistics (2022). *BusinessofApps.com.* Updated 19th. August

James, W. (2010 [orig. 1890]) *Principles of psychology*, Vols. 1 & 2. Mineola, NY: Dover Publications.

Kisely, S., Abajobir, A., Mills, R., Strathearn, L., Clavarino, A., & Najman, J. (2018). Child maltreatment and mental health problems in adulthood: Birth cohort study, *The British Journal of Psychiatry, 213*(6), 698–703.

Kwong A.S.F., Pearson, R.M., Smith, D., Northstone, K., Lawlor D.A., & Timpson N.J. (2020). Longitudinal evidence for persistent anxiety in young adults through COVID-19 restrictions. *Wellcome Open Research, 5*, 195. https://doi.org/10.12688/wellcomeopenres.16206.1

Lai, K., Guo, S., Ijadi-Maghsoodi, R., Puffer, M., & Kataoka, S. H. (2016). Bringing wellness to schools: Opportunities for and challenges to mental health integration and school-based health centers. *Psychiatric Services, 67*(12), 1328–1333.

Lee, J. (2020). Mental health effects of school closures during COVID-19. *Lancet Child Adolescent Health, 4*, 421. https://doi.org/10.1016/S2352-4642(20)30109-7

Lee, C. M., Cadigan, J. M., & Rhew, I. C. (2020). Increases in loneliness among young adults during the COVID-19 pandemic and association with increases in mental health problems. *Journal of Adolescent Health, 67*, 714–717. https://doi.org/10.1016/j.jadohealth.2020.08.009

Liddiard, K. (2017). *The intimate lives of disabled people.* London: Routledge.

Loades, M. E., Chatburn, E., Higson-Sweeney, N., McManus, M. N., Borwick, C., & Crawley, E. (2020). Rapid systematic review: The impact of social isolation and loneliness on the mental health of children and adolescents in the context of COVID-19. *Journal of American Academy of Child Adolescent Psychiatry, 59*, 1218–1239. https://doi.org/10.1016/j.jaac.2020.05.009

Luke, N., Sinclair, I., Woolgar, M. & Sebba, J. (2014). *What works in preventing and treating poor mental health in looked after children?*. London, NSPCC/Oxford: Rees Centre.

Mehta, S. B., Cornell, D., Fan, X., & Gregory, A. (2013). Bullying climate and school engagement in ninth-grade students. *Journal of School Health, 83*(1), 45–52.

McKinlay A.R., May, T., Dawes, J., Fancourt, D., & Bu, A. (2022). 'You're just there, alone in your room with your thoughts': a qualitative study about the psychosocial impact of the COVID-19 pandemic among young people living in the UK' *British Medical Journal Open, 12*(2), https://bmjopen.bmj.com/content/12/2/e053676

Mitchell, S. A. (2014). *Relationality: From attachment to inter-subjectivity*. New York: Psychology Press.

Mfidi, F. H. (2017). Mental health issues of school-going adolescents in high schools in the Eastern Cape. *South Africa, Africa Journal of Nursing and Midwifery, 19*(3), 2219–2232.

Morgan, C., Webb, R. T., Carr, M. J., Kontopantelis, E., Green, J., Chew-Graham, C. A., Kapur, N., & Ashcroft, D. M. (2017). Incidence, clinical management, and mortality risk following self harm among children and adolescents: Cohort study in primary care. *British Medical Journal*. https://doi.org/10.1136/bmj.j4351

NiMH (2018). Children and mental health, *National Institute of Mental Health*, https://www.nimh.nih.gov/health/publications/children-and-mental-health/index.shtml retrieved 20th. February 2019.

O'Connor, R., Wetherall, K., Cleare, S., Eschle, S., Drummond, J., Ferguson, E., & O'Carroll, R. (2018). Suicide attempts and non-suicidal self-harm: National prevalence study of young adults. *Bjpsych Open, 4*(3), 142–148.

Ohlheiser, A. (2021). TikTok recommendation algorithms. *MIT Technology Review, 124*(2), (Mar/April) 52–53.

Omnicore (2020). TikTok by the numbers: Stats, demographics & fun facts. *Omnicore*. 12th. February. Available at: https://www.omnicoreagency.com/tiktokstatistics/ (accessed 22 September 2020)

O'Sullivan, K., Clark, S., McGrane, A., Rock, N., Burke, L., Boyle, N., Joksimovic, N., & Marshall, K. (2021). A qualitative study of child and adolescent mental health during the COVID-19 pandemic in Ireland. *International Journal of Environmental Research in Public Health, 18*, 1062. https://doi.org/10.3390/ijerph18031062

Patalay, P., & Fitzsimons, E. (2016). Correlates of mental illness and wellbeing in children: Are they the same? Results from the UK Millennium Cohort Study. *Journal of the American Academy of Child & Adolescent Psychiatry, 55*(9), 771–783.

Patalay, P., & Gage, S. H. (2019). Changes in millennial adolescent mental health and health-related behaviours over 10 years: A population cohort comparison study. *International Journal of Epidemiology, 48*(5), 1650–1664.

Pew Research Center. (2019). Defining generations: Where millennials end and generation Z begins. https://www.pewresearch.org/fact-tank/2019/01/17/wheremillennials-end-and-generation-z-begins/

Pitchforth, J., Fahy, K., Wolpert, M., Viner, R.M. & Hargreaves, D.S. (2018). Mental health and wellbeing trends among children and young people in the UK 1995-2014: Analyses of repeated cross-sectional national health surveys, *Psychological Medicine*, 1–11, https://doi.org/10.1017/S0033291718001757

Pritchard, E. & Choonara, I. (2017). Armed conflict and mental health, *BMJ Paediatrics Open*. 1:e000087. https://doi.org/10.1136/bmjpo-2017-000087

Rosen, C., Jones, N., Longden, E., Chase, K.A., Shattell, M., Melbourne, J.K., Keedy, S.K. & Sharma, R.P. (2017). Exploring the intersections of trauma, structural adversity, and psychosis among a primarily African-American sample: A mixed-methods analysis, *Frontier Psychiatry, 8*(57). https://doi.org/10.3389/fpsyt.2017.00057.

Rothman, D.A. (2016). Tsunami of learners called Generation Z. https://www mdle.net/Journal/A Tsunami_of_Learners_Called_Generation_Z.pdf

Salimi, M., Jafarkhani, F., & Jamebozorg, Z. (2017). Designing a happy learning environment in schools and investigating its relationships with stress and mental health, *Muṭāli'āt-i Ravān/ Shināsī-i Bālīnī. Clinical Psychology Studies, 7*(28), 111–124.

Sekizaki, R., Nemoto, T., Tsujino, N., Takano, C., Yoshida, C., Yamaguchi, T., Katagiri, N., Ono, Y., & Mizuno, M. (2017). School mental healthcare services using internet-based cognitive behaviour therapy for young male athletes in Japan. *Early Intervention in Psychiatry, 13*(1), 79–85.

Serli R., Abdul, M. & Ependi P. (2022). The Behavior of TikTok users in Palopo City and responses to the Qur'an. *Jurnal Studi Al-Quran, 18*(2), 257–282 https://doi.org/10.21009/JSQ.018.2.05

Scott, S., McGowan V.J., & Visram, S. (2021). 'I'm Gonna Tell You about How Mrs Rona has affected me'. Exploring young people's experiences of the COVID-19 pandemic in north east England: A qualitative diary-based study. *International Journal of Environmental Research in Public Health 18*:3837. https://doi.org/10.3390/ijerph18073837

Son, A. (2006). Relationality in Kohut's psychology of the self. *Pastoral Psychology, 55*, 81–92.

Thomas, F., Hansford, L., Wyatt, K., Byng, R., Coombes, K., Finch, J., Finnerty, K., Ford, J., Guppy, K., Guppy, R., Hughes, S., McCabe, R., Richardson, H., Roche, D., & Stuteley, H. (2020). An engaged approach to exploring issues around poverty and mental health: A reflective evaluation of the research process from researchers and community partners involved in the DeStress study. *Health Expectations.* https://doi.org/10.1111/hex.13065

Ussher, J.M. (2011). *The madness of women: Myth and experience.* Abingdon, Oxon: Routledge.

White, M. & Epston, D. (1990). *Narrative means to therapeutic ends.* Adelaide, Dulwich: Centre.

WHO (2010).*Mental health and development: Targeting people with mental health conditions as a vulnerable group* (Geneva, World Health Organization) Retrieved 02.09.18 from http://apps.who.int/iris/bitstream/handle/10665/44257/9789241563949_eng.pdf;jsessionid=6D0B06365FF45AA7078F11A0FB211E5C?sequence=1

WHO (2015). Mental health atlas 2014 (Geneva, *World Health Organisation*). http://apps.who.int/iris/bitstream/10665/178879/1/9789241565011_eng.pd

WHO (2016). Growing up unequal: gender and socioeconomic differences in young people' s health and well-being, ISBN 987 92 890 1423 6 [13].

WHO (2019). Child and adolescent mental health, https://www.who.int/mental_health/maternal-child/child_adolescent/en/ accessed 20th. February 2019

Winnicott, D. W. (1971). *Playing and reality.* London: Penguin.

Young Minds (2021). Coronavirus: Impact on young people with mental health needs. [Internet]. Available: https://youngminds.org.uk/media/4350/coronavirus-report-winter.pdf

Youth Parliament (2016). Inquiry into how can we better deal with mental health issues and suicide prevention in schools, Health Select Committee (NZ), http://www.myd.govt.nz/documents/youth-parliament-/health-sc-background-paper.pdf accessed 21st. February 2019.

Zhang, H. & Du, Y. (2018). Chinese school curricula should include mental health education, *The Lancet Psychiatry, 5*(8), PE18, 1st. August https://doi.org/10.1016/S2215-0366(18)30217-7 accessed 21st. February 2019.

Zhu, C. Xu, X. Zhang, W. Chen, J. & Evans, R. (2020). How health communication via Tik Tok makes a difference: A content analysis of Tik Tok accounts run by Chinese provincial health committees. *International Journal of Environmental Research and Public Health, 17*(1), 192.

Chapter 29
Mitigating Mental Health Burden of Youth During COVID-19 Through Resilience and Hope: Evidences from India and Germany

Tusharika Mukherjee, Sibnath Deb, and Shayana Deb

Abstract In the global crisis caused by the COVID-19 pandemic, young professionals and graduating students experience considerable psychological adversity due to the uncertainty surrounding their futures. Given the positive psychological outcomes and the potential to alleviate stress, we examine the role of resilience and hope in causing a substantial variance in the stress response to anticipation of crisis among Indians living in India and Germany. Resilience, hope, crisis apprehension, and the psychological response to the COVID-19 pandemic were measured among participants from India and Germany (*n* = *650*) via an online survey using non-probability convenient sampling. Parallel mediation and conditional indirect effects showcase the differential roles of resilience and hope among socio-culturally similar but geographically divergent groups. Hope mediates the effect of pandemic-led crisis apprehension on perceived stress among those residing in India; resilience operates to mitigate stress among those from Germany. Findings highlight the contradistinctive role of resilience and hope in reducing stress and imply an urgent need for promotion of ameliorative practices. Resilience effectively mitigates the psychological burden of the COVID-19 crisis and can be promoted to reskill individuals; however, elevating hope in a crisis obligates prudence.

Keywords COVID-19 · Stress · Anticipatory Crisis · Resilience · Hope · Mental Health

T. Mukherjee (✉)
Work and Organizational Psychologist, Muenster, Germany
e-mail: tusharikamukherjee@gmail.com

S. Deb
Ministry of Youth Affairs and Sports (MYAS), Government of India (GOI), Tamil Nadu, Pennalur, Sriperumbudur 602 105, India

S. Deb
Department of Psychology, CHRIST (Deemed to Be University), Bengaluru, India

S. Deb and S. Deb (eds.), *Handbook of Youth Development*,
https://doi.org/10.1007/978-981-99-4969-4_29

Introduction

In March 2020, the World Health Organization (Zhou et al., 2020) declared COVID-19 as a global pandemic causing serious psychological fear and dismay among people of all demographic sections. A sense of panic was triggered by continuous reporting of deaths of people affected by COVID-19 and lack of adequate health facilities. Psychological distress, anxiety, and depression have been observed among people diagnosed with COVID-19, those under quarantine, and even those not physically affected by COVID-19 (Qiu et al., 2020; Zhang et al., 2020). India reported one of the highest shares of confirmed COVID-19 cases in the world as reported by the end of the year 2020 (World Health Organization, 2020). Similarly, despite an effective curb in the rising cases during the initial phases of the pandemic in mainland Europe, Germany witnessed a rapid surge in cases necessitating the furtherance of restrictive measures (Robert Koch Institute, 2020).

Evidence of psychological distress related to COVID-19 started appearing approximately after the initial recognition of its physical damages. During January–February 2020, a study in China revealed that concerns about the disease coupled with precautionary measures led to moderate to severe psychological impact in more than 50% of the population, with about 16 percent of the general population experiencing severe depressive symptoms, 30% reporting severe anxiety, and about 8% reporting severe stress as an immediate psychological response to COVID-19 (Wang et al., 2020). A March–April 2020 study in Germany showed that individuals spent about 4–5 h a day thinking about COVID-19, with about 10% indulging in more than 10 h of contemplating about the disease; largely outweighing the average worrying time of healthy individuals of 28–55 min (Petzold et al., 2020). An Indian study reported about 74% people with moderate levels of psychological stress due to COVID-19 with about 25% reporting pessimism and hopelessness (Grover et al., 2020). Likewise, in Germany, incidence of depression, symptoms of anxiety, and distress were reported to have significantly increased since the outbreak (Bäuerle et al., 2020), with about 25% of the population experiencing subjective deterioration of psychological symptoms (Knolle et al., 2020). The psychological impact of the pandemic on the student population in Germany reveals increasingly worsening mental health conditions including depression, sleep disorders, and anxiety, especially among female respondents (Schlichtiger et al., 2020). Various factors, including gender, marital status, social support, specific experience with COVID-19 infection, length of isolation, have contributed to the vulnerability to psychological distress across populations during the pandemic (Brooks et al., 2020).

The thread of commonality across demographic divisions has been a sense of crisis, either perceived and/ or experienced by those who have been directly impacted by the pandemic, or the apprehension of an impending crisis that has gained validity and strength over time due to the recurrence of the pandemic as well as its impact on public health policies, economic stability, and its future mitigation, as communicated by the decision-makers (Crayne & Medeiros, 2020). Drawing from the model of crisis perception (Billings et al., 1980), the anticipated crisis due to the current pandemic can be characterized by the uncertainty associated with its management, a sense of urgency in making decisions to ensure security, and a perception of spillover onto areas that are valued by an individual. The appraisal of the COVID-19 situation as a current threat and the future expectancies of the extent of personal damage (Folkman, 2010), point at our capacities as individuals, communities, or nations, to deal with questions like *'What will happen?' 'When will it happen?', 'What can we do about it?'* and, *'how will our actions impact us?'*.

Resilience and hope act as strengths for human beings in dealing with any adversity in life and in interpreting the situation positively (Avey et al., 2008; Dar et al., 2021; Duggal et al., 2016; Munoz et al., 2020). Resilience is an attributional, behavioral, and emotional response, leading toward positive outcomes in the face of challenges and risks (Yeager & Dweck, 2012). In the face of a crisis, this adaptive coping mechanism of resilience performs the dual function of mediating the effects of stress on both the brain and the behavior, and also developing protection against neuropsychological impairment (Russo et al., 2012). Hope is goal-directed thinking based on two interrelated cognitive components—one's perceived capacity to find alternative ways of reaching the goals (pathway thinking) and the necessary motivation (agency thinking) to use those pathways (Lopez et al., 2018). This goal pursuit behavior is associated with positive emotions operating in a feedback loop of positive reinforcements. On the contrary, failure in attaining the desired goals can continually reinforce negative emotions and consequently block goal pursuit (Lopez et al., 2018). Hope bears a strong relationship with stress, both creating contextual upsurge and downturn of emotions (Folkman, 2010). In the face of uncertainties or sudden changes, hope enables counterbalance of discomforting information with opposing and calming expectations (Folkman, 2010). Linking crisis apprehension in personal development and the capacity to withstand the resulting stress through resilience and hope can provide necessary insights in mental health studies.

Given the detrimental effect of COVID-19 pandemic on mental health, the present study was carried out to investigate the role of resilience and hope as ameliorative mechanisms in dealing with stress when the pandemic-contingent situation is appraised as a likely crisis. We further explore whether this relation of resilience and hope with stress is incidental to the country of residence, particularly when the respondents share similar socio-cultural background (Fig. 29.1). This is the first study to investigate the psychological response to the COVID-19 crisis among Indians residing in socio-politically and economically different setups. The findings of the present study would benefit the community and youth leaders, policymakers, and healthcare professionals, particularly psychologists, to focus on the mental health needs of adversity-affected people through promotion of strategies that alleviate the psychological burden during the pandemic and thereafter.

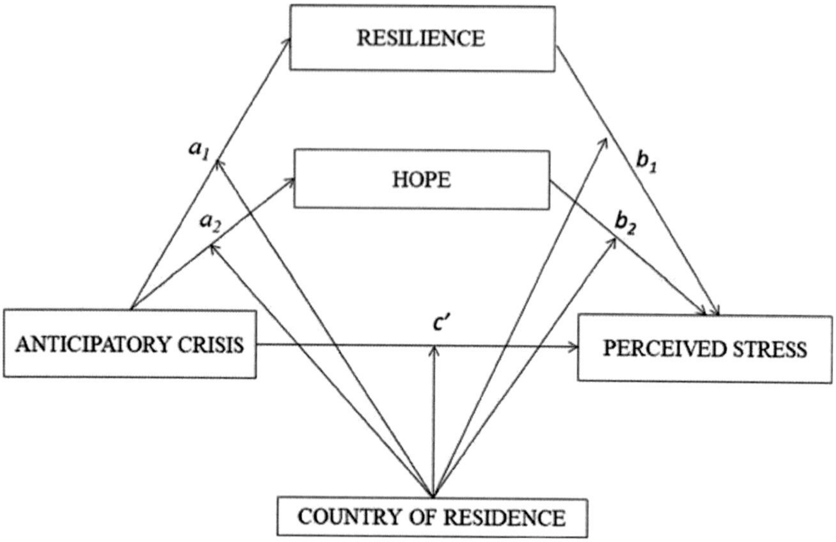

Fig. 29.1 Conceptual model of the study. a_1, a_2, b_1, b_2, c' are paths of the statistical model

Method

Participants

The data for this study was obtained via a cross-sectional study employing a self-administered online survey from respondents based in India and Germany between June and October 2020, during the outbreak of the COVID-19 pandemic and amidst precautionary activity restrictions imposed in both the countries. Data collection occurred during the nationwide lockdown in India between June and August, and during the resurgence of cases after the initial phase restrictions in Germany, between September and October, 2020. A group of 316 India-based and 334 Germany-based respondents (aged 18–36 years) participated from different states of both countries, in the online survey using non-probability convenient sampling.

Measures

Background Information Schedule: A structured information schedule was developed to collect demographic and socio-economic information of the study subjects. Nine questions pertain to demographic and socio-economic background, and six questions are related to personal feelings resulting from the pandemic answerable on a five point scale. The anticipatory crisis measure consisted of questions from the BIS that reflected feelings of restlessness due to COVID-19, activity restrictions and precautionary measures, as well as the worry associated with prospective performance evaluation or job insecurity. The items included are: (i) Are you feeling restless because of the COVID-19 pandemic and lockdown? (ii) Are you worried about the examination and future career? The scores on these items were accumulated to derive a composite score for anticipatory crisis. Cronbach's *a for* the scale was 0.517, despite the correlation between the items being statistically significant (0.01 level), which can be attributed to the low number of items (Tavakol & Dennick, 2011).

The Perceived Stress Scale (PSS; Cohen et al., 1983*):* Ten items measure the degree to which various situations in one's life are labeled as stressful, specifically during the past month. Items tap how unpredictable, uncontrollable, and overloaded the respondents find their lives. The scale also includes a number of direct queries about current levels of experienced stress. Psychometric properties of PSS have been ascertained by a number of previous studies (Lengacher et al., 2011; Mimura & Griffiths, 2008). A high score indicates high stress. In our study the Cronbach's *a* for the PSS was 0.77 (India) and 0.86 (Germany).

Adult Hope Scale (AHS; Snyder et al., 1991*):* The AHS intends to measure Snyder's cognitive model of hope based on an interactively derived sense of successful (a) agency (goal-directed energy), and (b) pathways (planning to meet goals). The AHS is a measure of 12 items for adults of the age 15 years and above. It has two sub-scales: agency sub-scale, consisting of 4 items and pathway sub-scale, also with 4 questions. There are 4 filler items in the scale as well. The AHS gives us the two independent scores of agency subscale and pathway subscale by summing up the 4 items of each subscale. It also gives us the overall hope scale by adding both agency and pathways subscales. High scores on agency and pathway subscales and total hope are indicative of high levels of hope which show that the person is highly hopeful and motivated to achieve his/her goals, and highly capable of designing means to achieve his/her goals. Cronbach's *a* in this study was 0.707 (India), 0.86 (Germany).

Brief Resilience Scale (BRS) (Smith et al., 2008)*:* The BRS wishes to assess the ability to bounce back or recover from stress. There are 6 items in BRS. Of these 6 items, 3 are reverse scored. The responses of the items are added/ summed up for all six items that gives a total score ranging from 6 to 30, which is divided by the total number of items answered, giving the resilience score. The higher the total score on BRS, the greater will be the resilience. The Cronbach's *a* of the BRS with the present sample was 0.626 (India), 0.803 (Germany).

Ethics

The present study was subjected to ethical approval and obtained the requisite clearance (Ref. No. RGNIYD/ADMIN/20–21/SEC/001). All procedures performed in collecting data from the participants were following the ethical standards of the institutional and/or national research committee and with the 1964 Helsinki declaration and data protection protocol. Participation in the study was voluntary and participants were ensured anonymity, confidentiality of information, and data protection, through an informed consent form prior to the survey.

Results

The preliminary descriptive analysis and mediation analysis were performed independently for the two samples. We hypothesized that the anticipatory crisis during COVID-19 is negatively related to resilience (H1a), negatively related to hope (H1b), and positively related to perceived stress (H1c). All hypotheses were tested using a conditional process modeling program, PROCESS macro (IBM SPSS software), that utilizes an ordinary least-squares or logistic-based path analytical framework to test for both direct and indirect effects (Hayes, 2013). Prior to conducting the main analyses, the data was screened for univariate and multivariate outliers, with none found in the two samples. Correlation analyses were conducted to examine the bivariate associations among the study variables (Table 29.1).

We employed parallel mediation for our first set of analyses. Here we hypothesized that anticipatory crisis is associated with perceived stress through a causal chain of linkages with resilience (H2a) and hope (H2b). Precisely, anticipatory crisis predicts stress and that is mediated by resilience and hope (H2). All indirect effects were subjected to follow–up bootstrap analyses with 5000 bootstrap samples and 95% bias-corrected confidence intervals. Results indicated that in the Germany-based sample anticipatory crisis is indirectly related to perceived stress through its relationship with resilience. Figure 29.2 shows that higher anticipatory crisis has a positive link with resilience, which significantly mediates the relation with perceived stress ($b = 5.755$, SE = 0.379, 95% bootstrap confidence interval (CI): 5.0102, 6.4997: $b =$ 0.998, SE = 0.005, 95% CI: 0.9881, 1.0088). The total effect obtained by regressing perceived stress on anticipatory crisis without consideration of the mediator ($b =$ 3.717, SE = 0.379, 95% CI: 2.9705, 4.4633) and the direct effect (b = −2.0288, SE = 0.0432, 95% CI: −2.1138, −1.9439) reveals partial mediation. In contrast, respondents in India showed a decrease in resilience as the anticipatory crisis increased (b = −1.765, SE = 0.308, 95% CI: −2.3706, −1.1600). The indirect effect of anticipatory crisis on perceived stress is significantly mediated by resilience ($b = -0.4808$, SE = 0.0849, 95% CI: −0.6478, −0.3138) and hope ($b = -0.1602$, SE = 0.0329, 95% CI: −0.2249, −0.0954), unlike the Germany-based sample, where resilience singularly mediated the link between anticipatory crisis and perceived stress. Partial mediation by resilience and hope is revealed by the lower direct effect of anticipatory crisis on perceived stress ($b = 3.0564$, SE = 0.4757, 95% CI: 2.1204, 3.9924) as compared to the total effect ($b = 4.5785$, SE = 0.4931, 95% CI: 3.6083, 5.5488). Due to the abundance of factors that influence psychological variables, Judd and Kenny

Table 29.1 Correlations, means, and standard deviations (SD) in the Germany-based (n = 334) and the India-based sample (n = 316). The correlations below the diagonal are for the Germany-based sample, and those above the diagonal are for the India-based sample

Variables	1	2	3	4	5	6	7	8	9	Mean	SD	Mean	SD
										Germany		India	
Anticipatory Crisis	–	−0.311**	−0.286**	−0.207**	−0.304**	0.465**	0.035	0.027	0.015	1.1677	0.78769	1.3671	0.67003
Resilience	0.655**	–	0.340**	0.268**	0.337**	−0.456**	−0.073	0.019	0.033	24.7066	7.22093	18.8291	3.83251
Hope	−0.291**	−0.465**	–	0.897**	0.869**	−0.408**	−0.004	0.057	0.063	48.1946	8.46798	47.4715	9.80261
Agency^{h}	−0.262**	−0.458**	0.919**	–	0.562**	−0.392**	0.001	−0.002	0.035	23.7246	4.77124	23.2722	5.85719
Pathway^{h}	−0.270**	−0.391**	0.909**	0.671**	–	−0.327**	−0.007	0.109	0.079	24.4701	4.49197	24.1994	5.22887
Perceived Stress	0.497**	0.976**	−0.456**	−0.454**	−0.377**	–	0.170**	0.076	0.088	19.1018	6.24296	20.2152	6.70308
Gender	0.134*	0.209**	0.024	−0.002	0.048	0.198**	–	−0.077	0.129*				
Age	−0.096	−0.092	−0.035	−0.077	016	−0.101	0.003	–	0.565**				
Education	032	0.112*	−0.096	−0.098	−0.078	0.050	0.061	0.429**	–				

Note h = subscales of the hope scale ** Correlation is significant at the 0.01 level (2-tailed)
* Correlation is significant at the 0.05 level (2-tailed)

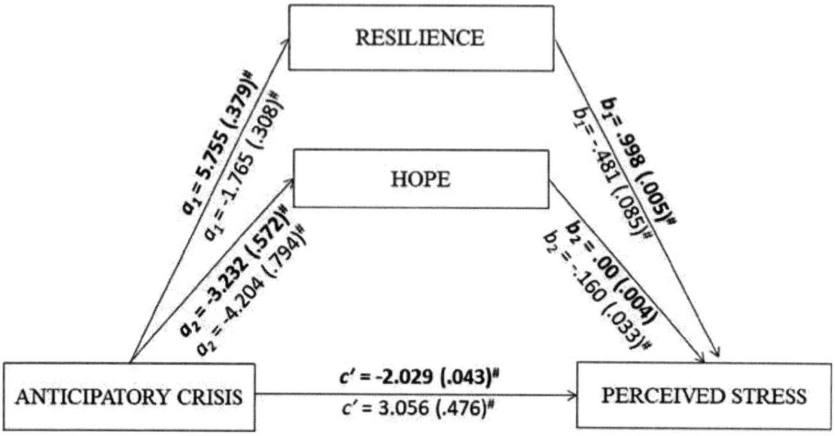

Fig. 29.2 The mediating effects of resilience and hope in the relationship between COVID-19 anticipatory crisis and perceived stress. $a_1, a_2, b_1, b_2, c' =$ path coefficient (unstandardized coefficient). a_1, a_2, b_1, b_2, c' (plain italics) are the values from the India-based sample. $\boldsymbol{a_1, a_2, b_1, b_2, c'}$ (boldface italics) are values from the Germany-based sample. $*p < 0.05$, $**p < 0.01$, $\#p < 0.001$

(1981) assert that a single variable (in this case two) would be explained entirely by a predictor and an outcome relation is often improbable.

An examination of the coefficients reveals that an increase in anticipatory crisis, when mediated by resilience, accounts for lowered perceived stress among respondents in Germany. Anticipatory crisis results in the increase in perceived stress through mediating effects of lowered resilience and hope. The individual effects of the two components of hope, agency ($b = -1.8075$, SE $= 0.4700$, 95% CI: $-2.7323, -0.8827$) and pathway ($b = -2.3965$, SE $= 0.4221$, 95% CI: $-3.2270, -1.5660$) were determined for the India-based sample as well.

We further investigated the conditional indirect effect of the country of residence such that the path between anticipatory crisis and resilience/hope is different for the two countries of residence, i.e., India-based and Germany-based. A heteroscedasticity consistent standard error and covariance matrix estimator was used for the analysis. The variables were mean centered prior to analysis to reduce multicollinearity in a regression model. The index of moderated mediation with resilience as the mediator is significant (4.8683, SE = 0.4482, 95% CI = 3.9554, 5.7358), as well as that with hope as the mediator (−0.6453, SE = 0.1862, 95% CI = −1.0407, −0.3047). Results show stark conditional direct effects of anticipatory crisis on perceived stress for the two nations with respondents in India reporting an increase in perceived stress corresponding with anticipatory crisis (b = 3.1550, SE = 0.5259, 95%CI = 2.1224, 4.1877), whereas an inverse relationship for Germany-based respondents (b = −1.9684, SE = 0.0821, 95%CI = −2.1296, −1.8071). The interaction terms of the anticipatory crisis and country of residence, based on the regression results, are statistically significant (b = 7.7347, SE = 0.4901, p < 0.001), indicating that the country of residence moderates the effect of anticipatory crisis on resilience. The conditional

Table 29.2 Conditional indirect effects on resilience and hope at different conditions of the moderator

	Resilience				Hope			
India	−1.814	0.313	0.00	−2.429, −1.199	−0.156	0.041	0.001	−0.236, −0.076
Germany	5.921	0.375	0.00	5.184, 6.657	−0.003	0.007	0.655	−0.017, 0.011

Note $n = 650$
Significance tests for the indirect effects were based on bias corrected confidence intervals derived from 5,000 bootstrapped samples

effects of anticipatory crisis on resilience at the two points of the moderator revealed that for the India-based respondents there was a negative effect (b = −1.8138, SE = 0.3132, p < 0.001) while that in the case of Germany was positive (b = 5.9208, SE = 0.3751, p < 0.001). This is indicative of an opposite interaction effect of the moderator. In the case of anticipatory crisis predicting hope, the analysis did not reveal any significant interaction with the moderator (b = 1.0485, SE = 0.9515, p < 0.271). In assessing the effect on perceived stress, country of residence was found to bear a significant interaction with anticipatory crisis (b = −5.1234, SE = 0.5304, p < 0.00), resilience (b = 1.4662, SE = 0.0932, p < 0.00), and hope (b = 0.1526, SE = 0.0416, p < 0.003). The conditional indirect effects of the moderator are summarized in Table 29.2. The pairwise contrasts between conditional indirect effects (b = −0.6453, SE = 0.1862, 95% CI = −1.0407, −0.3047) substantiates that the nature of mediation differs across the two groups.

Discussion

The onset and recurrence of the COVID-19 pandemic, public information, and risk communication have repeatedly exposed us to the adverse and distressing examples of its impact and a consequent vicarious experience of the crisis for many. Our investigation shows that COVID-19 has affected us by creating a sense of crisis, a fear of personal damage, and a threat to individual mental health even among those not physically harmed by the pandemic. Our findings are consistent with the previous studies that revealed fear, worry, anxiety, and psychological stress during this pandemic (Ahorsu et al., 2020; Grover et al., 2020). The probability of lagging behind in terms of expected career growth and employment serves as a major contributor to anticipating a crisis. However, anticipation, and not direct experiencing, leaves margin for planning and focus on relatively milder or positive instances, thereby alleviating the impact on perceived stress.

Confronting a crisis through direct or indirect experience is likely to increase awareness of one's vulnerabilities to its possible outcomes, elevating individual risk apprehension as well as preparedness (e.g. Terpstra, 2011). Resilience is associated with the belief that the benefits of personal actions will outweigh the hazards of the pandemic, leading to proactive crisis planning (Paton et al., 2008). On the contrary, negative beliefs like, "the impact of the pandemic is too great to be countered by individual initiatives," predispose one to remain in denial of one's competencies in effectively managing pandemic risks (health-related, academic, or professional), thus engendering perceived crisis and psychological distress. Our findings also reflect that apprehension of future crises among resilient people was associated with lower stress. When one's actions are appraised as instrumental in reducing vulnerability and preparing for the change or setback, it is likely to reduce distress and foster mental and physical wellbeing. The pandemic has compounded the stress that is usually associated with transitioning between life events like completing education and beginning a career. Adversities in the academic setting can be addressed by boosting resilience, particularly when people believe that resilience is a malleable individual capacity that can be developed (Yeager & Dweck, 2012). In the organizational context, resilience can facilitate performance and foster positive organizational behavior (Youssef & Luthans, 2007), and reduce burnout (West et al., 2020).

Hope has the potency to be a powerful motivator and make people believe that the future could be different. It can be estimated that despite being under the biggest lockdown in the world for a prolonged duration, people in India primarily adhered to the precautionary restrictions. As hope has a bearing upon the pandemic-induced stress in this study, it is likely that hope will generate positive emotions and capacitate evaluation of a stressful situation as an opportunity. However, mental health services and educational institutes need to exercise caution regarding the spiraling negative effects associated with hope, which accompanies failure. Though hope emerged to be negatively associated with stress in the India-based sample, the effects of anticipatory crisis on stress were not reverted singularly by hope. Cultural differences in hope between racial and ethnic groups provide insight into the variations in thinking patterns and actions. Chang and Banks (2007), in their study comparing hope in different ethnic groups in the US, showed that life satisfaction and avoidant style problem-solving predicted agency thinking, and positive affect predicted pathway-thinking among European Americans; while positive affect as well as negative affect and rational problem-solving predicted agency thinking, and positive affect and positive problem orientation predicted pathway thinking in Asian Americans. In other words, negative affect driven agency thinking may induce perceptions of inability to combat adversities. The role of the locus of hope may prove vital when addressing such crises.

Job loss concerns emerged as a major determinant of crisis anticipation during the pandemic. The World Economic Forum (2020) reported that among those currently employed, 57% in India and 26 percent in Germany anticipated losing their jobs in the ensuing 12 months. The proportion of those highly impacted by concerns of losing their employment, i.e., 25% in India and merely 45% in Germany, widens the gap between the two nations. This is in line with our findings that resilience is not a major contributor in mitigating stress among the participants in India, primarily due to the economic and social infrastructure and social security directives. The difference between resilience and hope becomes more prominent as we approach the two countries from the standpoint of their culture. Resilient people recognize the damaging impact of a crisis but at the same time allow themselves sufficient time and strength to transcend that efficiently. Unlike hope, resilience is not contingent upon the success or failure of one's initiatives. The inherent flexibility, adaptability, and preparedness for adverse and unknown conditions among resilient people (Youssef & Luthans, 2007) can aid in stress mitigation. This is reflective of Hofstede's cultural dimension of long-term orientation, by which people can pragmatically adapt to changed conditions, as is true in the case of Germany. Germany's socio-cultural orientation toward austerity and perseverance, social security policies, and infrastructure, facilitate the perception of the country as highly conducive to proactive initiatives by individuals, in terms of academic and career progress. India, on the other hand, also values pragmatism but at the same time is tolerant of ambiguous or uncertain futures, such that people are not usually driven by future securing initiatives and can adjust comfortably to what is being offered to them (Hofstede, 2011). As hope instills planning and the ability to perceive a problem as an opportunity, it seems reasonable to assume that hope is the most empowering aspect of approaching a crisis and dealing with stress among those living in India. As our study participants in the two countries are socio-culturally similar, future studies can provide more insight into the adoption of the cultural values of the country of residence and the consequent alteration in thought and behavior.

The present study highlights the need to build psychological resources to alleviate stress through promotion of resilience and hope by integrating counseling and stress management programs within the academic and workplace setups. Additionally, in conditions where hope is based on unrealistic outcomes or failure, mental health promoting programs based on resilience can prove to be more effective. As this pandemic has broadened the scope for community service in mental health promotion, the role of collective resilience (Drury et al., 2009) and collective hope (Snyder & Feldman, 2000) where people conjointly tackle a shared crisis, especially in contexts related to community health and survival, becomes more enhanced.

Limitations of the Study

In terms of generalizability, this study has a broader scope and will yield the best results when carried out in multiple cultural settings. In the present study India and Germany are contrasted due to their different socio-cultural orientation. The study had to be restricted to two countries due to the logistical difficulty in collecting data during the pandemic. Moreover, a probe into the duration of residence of people of Indian descent (expatriates) in Germany can provide additional insights into the subtle differences that might have developed over time in the socio-cultural patterns of thinking and preparedness to enlighten the uncertainty between the two groups.

As is usual with most cross-sectional studies and correlational nature of the data, findings from this study cannot assign a definitive causal relationship between predictors, moderators, mediators, and perceived stress during COVID-19 pandemic. In addition, through our study we cannot estimate temporal causality. Thus, we cannot rule out the possibility of a recursive relationship between anticipatory crisis and perceived stress, such that the degree of stress perceived could lead to crisis apprehension.

Conclusion

Amidst the unprecedented adversities that COVID-19 pandemic has inflicted, whether it is health, social, or economic, responding efficiently and preparing for a secure future emerges as the cardinal undertaking for societies, globally. Our study revealed that concerns about academic progress and employment have created a reasonable psychological burden among people who are not identified as vulnerable to being infected by the disease. However, those who are resilient have responded to stress more efficiently and enable reversing the effects of stress. Our study also revealed the differential mediation effects of hope between crisis apprehension and stress for the two groups. The study provides an understanding that individual response to the hazards of the pandemic can be mitigated through assertion of resilience competencies and expedient promotion of hope, and calls for community-based programs and effective public education for effective management of mental health burden.

References

Ahorsu, D. K., Lin, C. Y., Imani, V., Saffari, M., Griffiths, M. D., & Pakpour, A. H., (2020). The fear of COVID-19 scale: Development and initial validation. *International Journal of Mental Health and Addiction,* 1–9. Advance online publication. https://doi.org/10.1007/s11469-020-00270-8

Avey, J. B., Wernsing, T. S., & Luthans, F. (2008). Can positive employees help positive organizational change? Impact of psychological capital and emotions on relevant attitudes and behaviors. *The Journal of Applied Behavioral Science, 44*(1), 48–70.

Bäuerle, A., Steinbach, J., Schweda, A., Beckord, J., Hetkamp, M., Weismüller, B., & Skoda, E. M. (2020). Mental health burden of the COVID-19 outbreak in Germany: Predictors of mental health impairment. *Journal of Primary Care & Community Health, 11*, 2150132720953682. https://doi.org/10.1177/2150132720953682

Billings, R. S., Milburn, T. W., & Schaalman, M. L. (1980). A model of crisis perception: A theoretical and empirical analysis. *Administrative Science Quarterly, 25*(2), 300–316. https://doi:https://doi.org/10.2307/2392456

Brooks, S. K., Webster, R. K., Smith, L. E., Woodland, L., Wessely, S., Greenberg, N., & Rubin, G. J. (2020). The psychological impact of quarantine and how to reduce it: Rapid review of the evidence. *The Lancet, 395*(10227), 912–920. https://doi:https://doi.org/10.1016/S0140-6736(20)30460-8

Chang, E. C., & Banks, K. H. (2007). The color and texture of hope: Some preliminary findings and implications for hope theory and counseling among diverse racial/ethnic groups. *Cultural Diversity and Ethnic Minority Psychology, 13*(2), 94–103. https://doi.org/10.1037/1099-9809.13.2.94

Cohen, S., Kamarck, T., & Mermelstein, R. (1983). A global measure of perceived stress. *Journal of Health and Social Behavior, 24*, 386–396.
Crayne, M. P., & Medeiros, K. E. (2021). Making sense of crisis: Charismatic, ideological, and pragmatic leadership in response to COVID-19. *American Psychologist, 76*(3), 462–474. https://doi.org/10.1037/amp0000715
Dar, A. A., Deb, S., Thomas, S., Dhamodharan, M., Jahan, F., Sumaiya, B., & Gupta, S. (2021). Evidence and predictors of resilience among young adults exposed to traumatic events of the armed conflict in Kashmir. *Child and Youth Services, Online First.* https://doi.org/10.1080/0145935X.2021.1981133
Drury, J., Cocking, C., & Reicher, S. (2009). The nature of collective resilience: Survivor reactions to the 2005 London bombings. *International Journal of Mass Emergencies and Disasters, 27*(1), 66–95.
Duggal, D., Sacks-Zimmerman, A., & Liberta, T. (2016). The impact of hope and resilience on multiple factors in neurosurgical patients. *Cureus, 8*(10), e849. https://doi.org/10.7759/cureus.849
Folkman, S. (2010). Stress, health, and coping: synthesis, commentary, and future directions. The Oxford Handbook of Stress, Health, and Coping 453.
Grover, S., Sahoo, S., Mehra, A., Avasthi, A., Tripathi, A., Subramanyan, A., Pattojoshi, A., Rao, G. P., Saha, G., Mishra, K. K., Chakraborty, K., Rao, N. P., Vaishnav, M., Singh, O. P., Dalal, P. K., Chadda, R. K., Gupta, R., Gautam, S., Sarkar, S., ... Janardran Reddy, Y. C. (2020). Psychological impact of COVID-19 lockdown: An online survey from India. *Indian Journal of Psychiatry, 62*(4), 354–362. https://doi.org/10.4103/psychiatry.IndianJPsychiatry_427_20
Hayes, A. F. (2017). Introduction to mediation, moderation, and conditional process analysis: A regression-based approach. Guilford Publications.
Hofstede, G. (2011). Dimensionalizing cultures: The Hofstede model in context. *Online Readings in Psychology and Culture* 2(1). https://doi.org/10.9707/2307-0919.1014
Knolle, F., Ronan, L., & Murray, G. K. (2021). The impact of the COVID-19 pandemic on mental health in the general population: A comparison between Germany and the UK. *BMC Psychology, 9*(1), 1–17. https://doi.org/10.1186/s40359-021-00565-y
Lengacher, C. A., Johnson-Mallard, V., Barta, M., Fitzgerald, S., Moscoso, M. S., Post-White, J., & Kip, K. E. (2011). Feasibility of a mindfulness-based stress reduction program for early-stage breast cancer survivors. *Journal of Holistic Nursing, 29*(2), 107–117. https://doi.org/10.1177/0898010110385938
Lopez, S. J., Pedrotti, J. T., & Snyder, C. R. (2018). Positive psychology: The scientific and practical explorations of human strengths. Sage Publications.
Markovitz, G., 2020. World Economic Forum. At least half of people who have a job fear they'll lose it in the next 12 months. Retrieved on September 04, 2021 from https://www.weforum.org/agenda/2020/10/more-than-half-of-working-adults-fear-for-their-jobs/
Mimura, C., & Griffiths, P. (2008). A Japanese version of the Perceived Stress Scale: cross-cultural translation and equivalence assessment. *BMC Psychiatry*, *8*(1), 1–7. https://doi:https://doi.org/10.1186/1471-244X-8-85
Munoz, R. T., Hanks, H., & Hellman, C. M. (2020). Hope and resilience as distinct contributors to psychological flourishing among childhood trauma survivors. *Traumatology* 26(2) 177–184. https://doi:https://doi.org/10.1037/trm0000224
Paton, D., Parkes, B., Daly, M., & Smith, L., 2008.Fighting the flu: Developing sustained community resilience and preparedness. *Health Promotion Practice* 9(4_suppl) 45S-53S.
Petzold, M. B., Bendau, A., Plag, J., Pyrkosch, L., MascarellMaricic, L., Betzler, F., Rogoll, J., Große, J., & Ströhle, A. (2020). Risk, resilience, psychological distress, and anxiety at the beginning of the COVID-19 pandemic in Germany. *Brain and Behavior, 10*(9), e01745. https://doi.org/10.1002/brb3.1745
Qiu, J., Shen, B., Zhao, M., Wang, Z., Xie, B., & Xu, Y. (2020). A nationwide survey of psychological distress among Chinese people in the COVID-19 epidemic: Implications and policy

recommendations. *General Psychiatry, 33*(2), e100213. https://doi.org/10.1136/gpsych-2020-100213
Robert Koch Institut (2020). COVID-19: Fallzahlen in Deutschland und weltweit. Retrieved on September 06, 2021 from https://www.rki.de/DE/Content/InfAZ/N/Neuartiges_
Russo, S. J., Murrough, J. W., Han, M. H., Charney, D. S., & Nestler, E. J. (2012). Neurobiology of resilience. *Nature Neuroscience, 15*(11), 1475–1484. https://doi.org/10.1038/nn.3234
Schlichtiger, J., Brunner, S., Steffen, J., & Huber, B. C. (2020). Mental health impairment triggered by the COVID-19 pandemic in a sample population of German students. *Journal of Investigative Medicine, 68*(8), 1394–1396.
Smith, B. W., Dalen, J., Wiggins, K., Tooley, E., Christopher, P., & Bernard, J. (2008). The brief resilience scale: Assessing the ability to bounce back. *International Journal of Behavioral Medicine, 15*(3), 194–200.
Snyder, C. R., & Feldman, D. B. (2000). *Hope for the many: An empowering social agenda.* In Handbook of Hope, 389–412. Academic Press.
Snyder, C. R., Harris, C., Anderson, J. R., Holleran, S. A., Irving, L. M., Sigmon, S. T., & Harney, P. (1991). The will and the ways: Development and validation of an individual-differences measure of hope. *Journal of Personality and Social Psychology, 60*(4), 570–585. https://doi.org/10.1037/0022-3514.60.4.570
Tavakol, M., & Dennick, R. (2011). Making sense of Cronbach's alpha. *International Journal of Medical Education, 2*, 53–55. https://doi.org/10.5116/ijme.4dfb.8dfd
Terpstra, T. (2011). Emotions, trust, and perceived risk: Affective and cognitive routes to flood preparedness behavior. *Risk Analysis: An International Journal, 31*(10), 1658–1675.
Wang, C., Pan, R., Wan, X., Tan, Y., Xu, L., Ho, C. S., & Ho, R. C. (2020). Immediate psychological responses and associated factors during the initial stage of the 2019 coronavirus disease (COVID-19) Epidemic among the General Population in China. *International Journal of Environmental Research and Public Health, 17*(5), 1729. https://doi.org/10.3390/ijerph17051729
West, C. P., Dyrbye, L. N., Sinsky, C., Trockel, M., Tutty, M., Nedelec, L., Carlasare, L. E., & Shanafelt, T. D. (2020). Resilience and burnout among physicians and the general US working population. *JAMA Network Open, 3*(7), e209385. https://doi.org/10.1001/jamanetworkopen.2020.9385
World Health Organization. (2021). Coronavirus disease (COVID-19) pandemic. Retrieved on September 15, 2021 from https://www.who.int/emergencies/diseases/novel-coronavirus-2019
Yeager, D. S., & Dweck, C. S. (2012). Mindsets that promote resilience: When students believe that personal characteristics can be developed. *Educational Psychologist, 47*(4), 302–314.
Youssef, C. M., & Luthans, F. (2007). Positive organizational behavior in the workplace: The impact of hope, optimism, and resilience. *Journal of Management, 33*(5), 774–800.
Zhang, J., Lu, H., Zeng, H., Zhang, S., Du, Q., Jiang, T., & Du, B. (2020). The differential psychological distress of populations affected by the COVID-19 pandemic. *Brain, Behavior, and Immunity, 87* 49–50. https://doi:https://doi.org/10.1016/j.bbi.2020.04.031
Zhou, S. J., Zhang, L. G., Wang, L. L., Guo, Z. C., Wang, J. Q., Chen, J. C., Liu, M., Chen, X., & Chen, J. X. (2020). Prevalence and socio-demographic correlates of psychological health problems in Chinese adolescents during the outbreak of COVID-19. *European Child and Adolescent Psychiatry, 29*(6), 749–758. https://doi.org/10.1007/s00787-020-01541-4

Dr. Tusharika Mukherjee is an industrial and organizational psychologist working in the area of diversity, performance, and personality relationship and creating sustainable work organizations. She obtained her Ph.D. in Applied Psychology from the University of Calcutta and pursued her postdoctoral research in the area of situation contingent performance variability in the Department of Work and Organizational Psychology, Justus Liebig University Giessen, Germany. At present, she is associated with the Centre for International Development and Environmental Research at Justus Leibig University Giessen, Germany, as an independent lecturer and trainer. She has over thirteen years of experience in University teaching, research, conducting skill development workshops, and consultation. Her other academic and research experiences include intercultural communication competence, work-life integration, team and leadership development, and didactics

Prof. Sibnath Deb, Ph.D. & DSc is the Director of the Rajiv Gandhi National Institute of Youth Development, Ministry of Youth Affairs and Sports, Government of India. Prior to that, he was teaching in the Department of Applied Psychology, Pondicherry University (a central university), India as a full-time professor. Professor Deb was also acting as Director (I/C), Directorate of Distance Education, and Dean (I/C), School of Law, Pondicherry University. He also taught at the University of Calcutta. In 1994, Professor Deb did an intensive course on 'HIV/AIDS and Qualitative Research' from the University of Western Australia. From April 2009 to August 2009, Professor Deb visited the School of Public Health, Queensland University of Technology (QUT), Brisbane, Australia, as Visiting Faculty. Currently, he is also an Adjunct Professor at the School of Justice, QUT, Australia. During 2004–2008, he served the International Society for the Prevention of Child Abuse and Neglect (ISPCAN) as Council Member. In brief, he has 32 years of teaching, research and administrative experience and has produced 22 Ph.D.s in addition to publishing more than 100 research articles/book chapters in the leading national and international journals. Professor Deb has written nine books and edited 11 books. Some of his latest published books are (a) Child Safety, Welfare and Well-being: Issues and Challenges (2nd Edition, 2022, Springer Nature, Singapore); (b) School-based Family Counseling For Crisis and Disaster (Routledge, California, in press); (c) Health and Well-being: Challenges, Strategies and Future Trends (2022), Springer Nature, Singapore; (d) Youth Development in India: Future Generations in a Changing World (2021), New Delhi, Routledge. Professor Deb has received three national and three international awards in recognition of his contribution in the field of psychology including "Visitor's Award-2019" from the Hon'ble President of India Shri Ram Nath Kovind. His current areas of research interest include family dynamics, parenting styles, child safety, students' mental health, adolescent reproductive health and applied social psychology. ORCID ID:

Shayana Deb obtained M.Sc in Behavioral Science from the CHRIST (Deemed to be University), Bengaluru, India. She did her undergraduate with a triple major i.e., Biotechnology, Chemistry and Botany. She attended a number of online courses on different subjects based on her areas of academic interest. She has a special interest in child protection and youth development. On a voluntary basis, she worked in two research projects which created interest in her on child welfare and well-being issues and positive development of adolescence and youth. She has published three articles, eight book chapters and one conference proceedings as co-author. Recently one of her edited books on "Youth Development: Policies and Perspectives from India and Beyond" has been accepted by Springer Nature, Singapore.

Chapter 30
Doctoral Research by Youth: Analyzing the Role of Socio-Demographic Variables on Flourishing and Grit

Sibnath Deb, Aleena Maria Sunny, Shinto Thomas, Shayana Deb, Fathima G. Ashra, V. S. Sujith, and David Paul

Abstract The study examines the importance of socio-demographic variables like age, gender, family environment, and relationship with parents and friends in determining non-cognitive traits such as flourishing and grit, during the tenure of doctoral research. The cross-sectional correlational study comprises 400 Ph.D. scholars from a Central University in India, who were given a personal data sheet, the Flourishing Scale and the Grit Scale, for assessment. The results of the F-test showed that flourishing was significantly related to age, family environment and relationship with friends, and grit was significantly related to family environment and relationship with friends. Analysis using Pearson correlation found a weak correlation between flourishing and the three subscales of grit, namely ambition, consistency of interest, and perseverance of effort. Findings suggest that the socio-demographic variables are important contributors in the long-term goal-oriented behaviors and that flourishing and grit are two related but not correlated variables that influence completion and attrition of the doctoral research.

Keywords Academic achievement · Demographic variables · Doctoral attrition · Doctoral education · Flourishing · Grit

S. Deb (✉) · F. G. Ashra · V. S. Sujith · D. Paul
Department of Applied Psychology, Pondicherry University (A Central University), Puducherry, India
e-mail: sibnath23@gmail.com

A. M. Sunny
PGCE Teacher Trainee at, UCL Institute of Education, London, UK

S. Thomas
Teacher of Psychology, St. George's College, Weybrigde, UK

S. Deb
Department of Psychology, CHRIST (Deemed to be University), Bengaluru, India

S. Deb and S. Deb (eds.), *Handbook of Youth Development*,
https://doi.org/10.1007/978-981-99-4969-4_30

Introduction

Attrition and completion of doctoral research is a dynamic topic that deserves attention, but is often overlooked by academia. The dropout rate in doctoral research is consistently increasing and ranges between 30 and 50%, depending upon the discipline of study and the country (Gardner, 2008; Golde, 2005; MELS, 2013). It is found even among scholars who could secure prestigious fellowships (Wendler et al., 2012) and is a concern which requires pragmatic attention and scientific intervention. Most of the empirical efforts on studying doctoral attrition are often restricted to analysis based on the individual's academic capabilities and work environment. Besides, the influence of personal factors such as resilience (Castro et al., 2011), self-motivation (Ivankova & Stick, 2007) and personal goals, time and plan commitment (Martinsuo & Turkulainen, 2011) are also proven factors. However, Bair and Haworth (2004) considered the study of psychological variables that influences doctoral attrition to be a promising line of investigation. Now, measurement of non-cognitive traits is gaining prominence in education and positive psychology, in the explanation and prediction of achievement. Non-cognitive traits such as grit and flourishing were utilized to explain the consistent success of individuals with "lesser IQ" when compared to their "more intelligent" counterparts (Duckworth et al., 2007). Grit, as defined by Duckworth et al., is the "*perseverance and passion for long term goals, and involves working strenuously toward challenges, maintaining effort and interest over years despite failure, adversity, and plateaus in progress*" (2007, 1087–1088). This construct is understood in two dimensions: (a) "consistency of interests"—This is the ability to sustain interest for a long period of time and (b) "perseverance of effort"—This is the ability to exert effort in order to withstand failures and challenges (Duckworth et al., 2007). Similarly, flourishing, another non-cognitive trait, which Seligman stated to be the "gold standard of measuring wellbeing" (2018), is a "*dynamic optimal state of psychosocial functioning that arises from functioning well across multiple psychosocial domains*" (Butler & Kern, 2016, 2). The concept is synonymous with wellbeing, and Seligman hypothesized it to have five key elements viz., positive emotion, engagement, relationships, meaning, and accomplishment.

Expanded research concerning the construct of grit has repeatedly shown its significant influence upon academic achievement in various circumstances (Pate et al., 2017). Its proven association with academic motivation (Eskreis-Winkler et al., 2014), productivity and engagement (Hodge et al., 2018), performance (Kelly et al., 2014), and goal orientation (Muenks et al., 2017) further emphasizes the influential role of this construct in educational psychology. Grit was also found to take a different trajectory by exerting its impact on certain higher personal outcomes (Kannangara et al., 2018). Moreover, grit was found to be correlated to happiness (Singh & Jha, 2008), pursing engagement and pleasure in life (Von Culin et al., 2014), satisfaction and a sense of belonging (Bowman et al., 2015), sense of meaning in life (Von Culin et al., 2014), and higher accomplishment during one's life (Abuhassàn & Bates, 2015). These variables seem to be related to the five key elements of flourishing. On the whole, Vainio and Daukantaitė (2016) have found the positive association of grit with all three dimensions of wellbeing/flourishing: psychological wellbeing, satisfaction with life and harmony in life. Hence, existing literature provides an interesting lead in identifying flourishing as a potential non-cognitive trait in predicting academic success as well as doctoral attrition.

Several studies on these two constructs and their applications have found the existence of group differences and the expression of grit and flourishing. In other words, certain socio-demographic variables influence the development and expression of grit and flourishing among individuals (Kannangara et al., 2018). For instance, grit was found to be highly correlated with gender (Flaming & Granato, 2017) and age (Cupitt & Golshan, 2015). On the other hand, studies related to gender differences in flourishing have produced mixed results. Hence, the current study is correlational in nature and also explores the relationship between the socio-demographic variables of the participants and various non-cognitive traits, namely grit and flourishing among the Ph.D. scholars.

The Present Study and Hypotheses

The present study has a cross-sectional correlational design that intends to understand the role of socio-demographic variables such as age, gender, family environment, and relationship with family and friends in determining the development of grit and flourishing among Ph.D. scholars. On the basis of the links drawn between flourishing and grit from previous study findings, it was hypothesized that (i) there would be a significant difference in the mean scores of flourishing for different socio-demographic variables among Ph.D. scholars (H1); (ii) there would be a significant difference in the mean scores of grit for different socio-demographic variables among Ph.D. scholars (H2); and (iii) flourishing would be significantly associated with grit and its subscales viz. ambition, consistency of interest and perseverance of effort among Ph.D. scholars (H3).

Methodology

Participants

The participants were 400 Ph.D. scholars from Pondicherry University (A Central University). The sample included an equal number of men and women, who were aged 22 years and above.

Instruments

Structured Questionnaire

A specially designed structured questionnaire was used to collect background information about the study subjects. The information collected included gender, age, educational stream, semester performance, family type and size, relationship with family members, peer group members, and so on. Face validity of the questionnaire was ascertained by three experts.

Flourishing Scale

Flourishing scale, developed by Diener et al. (2010), consists of 8 questions which assess flourishing, as well as positive and negative feelings. It consists of items describing important aspects of human functioning, ranging from positive relationships, feelings of competence, to having meaning and purpose in life. The items were rated on a 7 points scale (1 = strongly disagree, 2 = disagree, 3 = slightly disagree, 4 = neither agree nor disagree, 5 = slightly agree, 6 = agree, 7 = strongly agree). The score ranges from 7 to 19. A high score indicates a person's emotional strength toward feeling of competence, thus having a more positive outlook and purpose in life and in developing positive relationships rapidly and successfully. The psychometric properties of the scale have been ascertained by several studies (Hone, Jarden, & Schofield 2014; Sumi, 2014; Silva & Caetano, 2013). Coefficient alpha in the current sample was 0.92.

Grit Scale

Grit Scale by Duckworth et al. (2007) consists of 17 questions which assess the perseverance and passion for long-term goals. The scale has three dimensions: (a) ambition, (b) consistency of interest, and (c) perseverance of effort. The items were rated on 5-point scale.

The first reverse score items 3, 5, 7, 9, 10, 13, and 16. Grit is calculated as the average score of items 2, 3, 5, 6, 7, 8, 9, 10, 11, 14, 16, and 17. The consistency of interest subscale is calculated as the average score for items 3, 5, 7, 9, 10, and 16. The perseverance of effort subscale is calculated as the average score for items 2, 6, 8, 11, 14, and 17. The brief grit scale score is calculated as the average score for items 3, 6, 7, 8, 9, 10, 11, and 17. Ambition is calculated as the average score for items 1, 4, 12, 13, and 15. The items were rated on 5 point scale (5 = very much like me, 4 = mostly like me, 3 = somewhat like me, 2 = not much like me, 1 = not like me at all). A number of previous studies ascertained the psychometric properties of Grit Scale and found it to be suitable (Duckworth & Quinn, 2009; Strayhorn, 2014). This scale was used by scholars and academics globally and they established its psychometric properties (Clark & Malecki, 2019; Rojas, Reser, Usher, & Toland, 2012; Duckworth & Quinn, 2009). The Cronbach's alpha of Grit Scale with the present sample was 0.91 and its three domains, i.e., Consistency of Interest (Domain 1), Perseverance of Efforts (Domain 2), and Ambition (Domain 3) with the present sample were 0.91, 0.89, and 0.90 respectively.

Procedure

Cluster sampling method was followed while selecting the Ph.D. scholars from the disciplines of humanities/social sciences, sciences, and commerce/management. After obtaining permission from the Heads of the Departments, a tentative time schedule was prepared for data collection and accordingly, the researchers contacted the Ph.D. scholars and explained the objective of the study. Informed consent forms, containing the details of the study, especially the benefits and consequences of the study, were given to all the study subjects. After getting familiarized with these details, interested participants were allowed to express their consent by signing the form. Informed consent was obtained from all the subjects. The investigator assured that the identity and details of the identity of the scholars and the information will not be revealed to any person and this will be used only for educational purposes. Date and time were decided as per the convenience of the study subjects. The participants were informed that they could withdraw from the study at their will and the benefits and risks of the study were explained to the participants.

Finally, based on voluntary consent, data were collected from 420 Ph.D. scholars by using a structured questionnaire, flourishing scale, and grit scale, in order to assess psychological wellbeing and perseverance for long-term goals. Self-administration method was followed for data collection. Approximately, 7 to 10 min were taken by participants for questionnaire completion.

Data Analysis

The data collected from the Ph.D. scholars were subjected to scrutiny. After scrutiny, 20 data sheets were found to be incomplete and they were rejected. Finally, complete data sheets of 400 students were fed to the system for analysis. The population distribution was found to be symmetric. F-test was used to compare the variances of subgroups under demographic variables such as age, gender, family environment, relationship with parents and friends, along with the scores obtained by the participants on flourishing scale and grit scale. Further, Pearson correlation was used to estimate the correlation between flourishing and grit as well as its subscales.

Results

To collate the data collected, descriptive and inferential statistics were used.

The characteristic of the sample population ($n = 400$) in terms of its distribution in subcategories of socio-demographic details, are demonstrated in Table 30.1 and is explained below. There is equal representation from both male and female gender subcategories. More than half of the population (59.3%) were aged between 25 and 26; half the population is from the discipline of commerce (51%), followed by humanities and social sciences (38.8%) followed by science (10.3%). Over 60.5% of the population belonged to nuclear families. Equal proportion of the sample population, that is 93.5%, have very good relationships with both parents and friends, and 89.5% of the population reported their family environment to be conducive. The population was found to be normally distributed.

Scores in flourishing were found to differ based on certain demographic variables of the study sample (Table 30.2). Three demographic variables, namely, age, family environment, and relationship with friends, have shown significant relationship with flourishing. Age was found to have a significant relationship with flourishing when compared across three age groups ($F = 5.01, p < 0.01$.). Participants aged between 25–26 (M = 48.14, SD = 6.27) were significantly more likely to score higher on flourishing, followed by those aged 27 and above (M = 47.38, SD = 6.00), followed by those aged between 23 and 24 (M = 44.89, SD = 11.37). Significant differences in flourishing were found between friendly and disturbed family environments ($F = 3.78$, $p < 0.01$). Participants hailing from a friendly family environment (M = 47.45, SD = 6.98) secured higher scores in flourishing as compared to those from disturbed family environments (M = 44.15, SD = 9.11). Analysis further revealed that participants who reported to have very good relationship with friends (M = 46.69, SD = 7.30) had significantly higher scores on flourishing in comparison to

Table 30.1 Socio-demographic characteristics of the sample

Socio-demographic variables		Number of participants (N)	Percentage of Sample (%)
Age	23–24	63	15.8
	25–26	237	59.3
	27 and above	100	25
Gender	Male	200	50
	Female	200	50
Family Environment	Friendly	358	89.5
	Disturbed	42	10.5
Relationship with parents	Very good	374	93.5
	Not so good	26	6.5
Relationship with friends	Very good	374	93.5
	Not so good	26	6.5

the ones who did not have a good relationship with their friends (M = 43.76, SD = 6.56), $F = 2.66, p < 0.01$. Other demographic variables, such as gender and family environment, did not show significance in their mean difference.

Data in Table 30.3 revealed two socio-demographic variables, such as family environment ($F = 2.59, p < 0.05$) and relationship with friends ($F = 2.56, p < 0.05$), to have significant relationship with grit. Table 30.3 showed a little difference in the mean of participants from friendly family environments (M = 20.15, SD = 3.29) and disturbed family environments (M = 20.69, SD = 3.64). Nevertheless, the family environment can be understood to have a significant relationship with grit among the participants. Finally, participants with "very good" relationships with friends (M = 47.67, SD = 7.30) were significantly grittier than the ones with "not so good" relationships with friends (M = 43.76, SD = 6.56). Variables such as age, gender, and relationship with parents did not show significant relationship with grit.

Further analysis of data between the three subscales of grit, viz. ambition, consistency of interest and perseverance of efforts, and the socio-demographic variables, yielded noteworthy findings. Ambition, the first subscale of grit, was found to be a significant factor regarding relationship with friends at $F = 2.53, p < 0.05$; wherein, participants who have "very good" (M = 9.38, SD = 1.64) relationship with friends were significantly more likely to be grittier as compared to those who do not have such equations with their peers (M = 8.30, SD = 2.12). The second subscale, consistency of interest, was found to have significant relationship with two socio-demographic variables, which are gender (F = 2.85, p < 0.01) and family environment (F = 2.46, p < 0.05). Notably, males (M = 9.62, SD = 2.47) scored significantly higher than females (M = 8.92, SD = 2.39) in this subscale and participants from "disturbed" family environments (M = 10.12, SD = 2.25) showed more consistency in interest

Table 30.2 Difference in the flourishing scores by socio-demographic variables

Socio-demographic variables		Total Flourishing Score (Mean and SD)	F value
Age	23–24	44.89(11.37)	5.01**
	25–26	48.14(6.27)	
	27 and above	47.38(6.00)	
Gender	Male	47.45(7.25)	
	Female	47.43(7.40)	
Family Environment	Friendly	47.84(6.98)	3.78**
	Disturbed	44.15(9.11)	
Relationship with parents	Very good	47.56(7.31)	
	Not so good	45.61(7.30)	
Relationship with friends	Very good	47.69(7.30)	2.66**
	Not so good	43.76(6.56)	

** *Significant at < 0.01*

Table 30.3 Difference in the grit score and its subscales by demographic variable

Socio-demographic variables		Total Grit Score (Mean & SD)	Ambition (Mean & SD)	Consistency of Interest (Mean & SD)	Perseverance of Efforts (Mean & SD)
Age	23–24	20.49(3.62)	9.53(2.08)	9.37(1.99)	11.12(2.70)
	25–26	20.09(3.32)	9.36(1.62)	9.21(2.47)	10.88(2.09)
	27 and above	20.29(3.21)	9.06(1.59)	9.35(2.69)	10.95(1.85)
Gender	Male	20.48(3.31)	9.21 (1.65)	9.62(2.47) 2.85**	10.86(1.90)
	Female	19.93(3.34)	9.41(1.75)	8.92(2.39)	11.01(2.36)
Family Environment	Friendly	20.15(3.29) 2.59*	9.33(1.67)	9.16(2.46)2.46*	10.98(2.10)
	Disturbed	20.69(3.64)	9.18(1.90	10.12(2.25)	10.56(2.46)
Relationship with parents	Very good	20.18(3.34)	9.30(1.70)	9.26(2.40)	10.92(2.15)
	Not so good	20.51(3.27)	9.48(1.65)	9.32(3.16)	11.19(2.03)
Relationship with friends	Very good	20.32(3.29) 2.56*	9.38(1.64) 2.53*	9.29(2.46)	11.02(2.09) 3.00**
	Not so good	18.59(3.56)	8.30(2.12)	8.87(2.33)	9.73(2.60)

* *Significant at < 0.05, ** Significant at < 0.01*

than those from "friendly" family environments (M = 9.16, SD = 2.46). Perseverance of effort was the third subscale in which only the variable "relationship with friends" showed significant relationship at $p < 0.01$ (F = 3.00). Here, participants who had "very good" relationships with friends (M = 11.02, SD = 2.09) had better scores than participants who reported "not so good" relationships with friends (M = 9.73, SD = 2.60).

Family relationships and relationships with friends were found to be significantly related to both flourishing and grit. Interestingly, analysis on the basis of gender showed little or no difference in the total means of both flourishing (Male = 47.45, Female = 47.43) and grit (Male = 20.48, Female = 19.93). However, gender as a variable did not prove to have a statistically significant relationship with either of these two variables, with the exception seen in the results of the grit subscale's "consistency of interest."

Table 30.4 displays the interrelation between the study variables, namely flourishing, grit, ambition, consistency of interest, and perseverance of effort, which were analyzed using Pearson correlation. Two interesting findings could be drawn from this data. Surprisingly, no significant association was found between flourishing and grit. However, significant but weak correlations were found between flourishing and all the three subscales of grit. Flourishing was significantly and positively associated with Ambition ($r = 0.198, p < 0.01$) and Perseverance of Effort ($r = 0.228, p < 0.01$), and significantly and negatively associated with Consistency of Interest ($r = -0.162$, $p < 0.01$). The correlation between grit and the sub-items of grit were positive as

Table 30.4 Correlation between flourishing, grit, and sub-items of grit

Variables	1	2	3	4
1. Flourishing				
2. Grit	0.027			
3. Ambition	0.198**	0.525**		
4. Consistency of Interest	-0.162**	0.767**	0.191**	
5. Perseverance of Effort	0.228**	0.678**	0.598**	0.048

* Significant at < 0.05, ** Significant at < 0.01

expected. Grit correlated highest with consistency of interest ($r = 0.767$, $p < 0.05$). Along with flourishing and grit, ambition was associated positively with consistency of interest ($r = 0.191$, $p < 0.01$) and perseverance of effort ($r = 0.598$, $p < 0.01$). However, no association was found between consistency of interest and perseverance of effort, which are two sub-items of grit.

Discussion

The present study produced a noteworthy relationship between flourishing and age, where it was found that people flourished with the advancement of age; it is in accordance with a pioneering study where age positively influenced flourishing and thereby, adult mental health (Keyes, 2002). Unlike this understanding, age did not have any impact on flourishing among older adults in a recent study by Momtaz et al. (2016). Similarly, grit and age were posited to be positively correlated by Duckworth et al. (2007) but, the present study didn't find age to be significantly impactful on grit and three of its subscales. This is a validation for one of the prominent findings of Hodges et al. (2013), that concerned age and other demographic variables, which cannot influence completion or attrition of higher education. Interesting findings by Cupitt and Golshan (2015), which goes along with that of Duckworth et al. (2007), found grit to be negatively associated with age, for students under 25, and found reduced consistency of interest and reduced persistence of effort during younger age. Research studies have provided mixed findings about age and its impact on flourishing and grit. The lack of clarity could probably be due to the involvement of both genetic and environmental factors. These findings indicate the existence of a pattern in age-related development of flourishing and grit, similar to what is found in the development of intelligence. Hence, investigating the role of age in development and maturation of non-cognitive variables would produce meaningful findings.

Similarly, the present analysis could not find any significance of gender differences in flourishing. Literature on the role of gender on flourishing and grit yields mixed findings. Little is known about the contribution of gender in an individual's pattern of flourishing (Csikszentmihalyi, 2014). This is a possible rationale why flourishing should be examined as a construct that includes various subdomains, which may behave differently with gender-related interests. Similarly, no gender difference was found in the overall grit score in the present study, as was previously found by Duckworth et al. (2007). But then, Flaming and Granato (2017) have found the correlation between grit and gender. Females were found to be grittier than males (Jaeger et al., 2010; Christensen & Knezek, 2014; Aswini & Deb, 2017). Unlike these findings, in the present study, males showed more consistency of interest, which is the second subscale of grit, as compared to females. Males in the age group of the present study could possibly be less curbed by external factors such as marriage and childbirth, unlike that of the female participants of the study, hence performing in a less taxing environment where consistency could be maintained. In addition to this, male participants may be under the pressure of being gainfully employed at the earliest and hence, they would be attempting to hasten their pursuit of doctoral research.

The present study gains support from several previous studies that have investigated the influence of social support on the development of both flourishing and grit in an individual. The study emphasizes upon the importance of social support, particularly from family and friends, in determining the levels of flourishing and grit and revealed the significant role played by the family environment among Ph.D. scholars as well. Individuals from friendly family environments were found to flourish better, as compared to their counterparts, probably implying the importance of nurturing family relationships while being involved in long-term tasks, which demand persistence and reassurance during setbacks. Indeed, previous research has identified the family to be a key motivator in ensuring success among students (Madhlangobe et al., 2014; Bethell et al., 2019). Similarly, while there are several studies that indicated positive influence of congenial families on grit, the present study found that individuals from disturbed family environments were grittier and showed more consistency of interest as compared to those from a friendly family environment. This could be explained by the increased likelihood of motivation for higher academic pursuit to arise out of the zeal to excel, achieve, and gain independence on their own. Particularly, in the accomplishment of long-term goals, the family environment may be perceived as burdening due to social pressure and high expectations of the family. The difficulty in predicting the direction of the influence of family on grit could possibly be due to these multiple factors that are individual-specific in nature. Considering the significance of family environment in predicting both flourishing and grit, this demographic variable may be considered as an area for future investigation in understanding the completion and attrition of doctoral education. The positive impact of social support on the development of both flourishing and grit, as explained by several previous investigations (Colbert et al., 2015; Wissing et al., 2019), was reinstated by the present study. This finding supports the idea that supportive friendships at workspaces offer a reciprocal and altruistic network that may motivate the individual to thrive till the target is achieved. Among the subscales of grit too, friendship was crucial in both ambition and perseverance of effort, adding to the overall impact on grit. However, this supportive ground may vary, depending on the nature, type, and distance of friendship and hence, open a direction for further examination.

Added investigation found flourishing to be correlated with all the subscales of grit, i.e., ambition, consistency of interest, and perseverance of effort, which are the core aspects of grit itself. Yet, no correlation was found between flourishing and grit, which could be the reason for the weakness of the correlation between flourishing and all the three subscales of grit. Explanation for this finding could be that grit and flourishing are two parallel concepts which predict related concepts such as wellbeing, resilience, or achievement-oriented behaviors, but they are not predictors of each other. They could be two related but not correlated variables, which are crucial in enduring tasks. The study offers a justification for exploring the two different yet related dynamics of flourishing and grit in understanding completion and attrition of long-term goal-oriented behaviors.

Conclusion

The study has provided substantial evidence on the prominence of demographic variables in determining the development of non-cognitive traits, thus enabling growth and achievement among students. The dynamics exhibited by the supportive and non-supportive social environment on the performance of participants were particularly interesting. It implied upon the need for further exploration into the varied functions of non-cognitive traits such as flourishing and grit. Much impact was created by healthy relationships with friends and hence, it was identified as one of most relevant understandings gained from the study. Current study findings were backed by existing literature on the related but not correlated relationship between flourishing and grit. Both these variables were understood to be crucial in long-term goal-directed behaviors.

Limitations and Future Study Directions

Although the present study provided evidence regarding the role of demographic variables as well as social support among Ph.D. scholars, it is important to understand its limitations as well. Apart from the typical drawbacks of a self-reported cross-sectional study, the paper has not gone beyond the preliminary examination of data. The collected sample was small in size and was restricted to only one university.

The study provided sufficient hints and directions for future research. Exclusive and in-depth investigation could be undertaken to examine the growth pattern of age in non-cognitive traits, particularly grit, which may resemble the one seen in cognitive abilities, such as intelligence. Further, studies could be undertaken to gain clarity upon the impact of gender on various non-cognitive traits, which may provide multi-faceted implications in identifying the correlates of an enabling environment, to be provided for students involved in long-term tasks. Detailed inferences could be drawn from the influence of both enabling and disabling family environment and social support on the completion and attrition of doctoral research.

Acknowledgements The authors wish to acknowledge the Heads of the departments for granting permission to meet the students for their participation in the study. The authors thank all the scholars of Pondicherry University for participating in the study voluntarily and providing data.

Ethical Approval Approval from the Institutional Ethics Committee of Pondicherry University (A Central University), Puducherry, India was obtained.

Disclosure of Potential Conflict of Interest The authors declare that there is no conflict of interest.

References

Abuhassàn, A., & Bates, T. C. (2015). Grit: Distinguishing Effortful Persistence from Conscientiousness. *Journal of Individual Differences, 36*(4), 205–214. https://doi.org/10.1027/1614-0001/a000175

Aswini, S., & Deb, A. (2017). Flourishing among postgraduate students: The role of resilience, meaningfulness and grit. *Indian Journal of Community Psychology, 13*(1), 24–38.

Bair, C. R., & Haworth, J. G. (2004). Doctoral student attrition and persistence: A meta-synthesis of research. In *Higher education: Handbook of theory and research* (pp. 481–534). Springer, Dordrecht.

Bethell, C. D., Gombojav, N., & Whitaker, R. C. (2019). Family resilience and connection promote flourishing among US children, even amid adversity. *Health Affairs, 38*(5), 729–737.

Bowman, N. A., Hill, P. L., Denson, N., & Bronkema, R. (2015). Keep on truckin' or stay the course? Exploring grit dimensions as differential predictors of educational achievement, satisfaction, and intentions. *Social Psychological and Personality Science, 6*(6), 639–645.

Butler, J., & Kern, M. L. (2016). The PERMA-Profiler: A brief multidimensional measure of flourishing. *International Journal of Wellbeing, 6*(3).

Castro, V., Garcia, E. E., Cavazos Vela, J., & Castro, A. (2011). The road to doctoral success and beyond. *International Journal of Doctoral Studies, 6*, 51.

Christensen, R., & Knezek, G. (2014). Comparative measures of grit, tenacity and perseverance. *International Journal of Learning, Teaching and Educational Research, 8*(1).

Colbert, A. E., Bono, J. E., & Purvanova, R. K. (2016). Flourishing via workplace relationships: Moving beyond instrumental support. *Academy of Management Journal, 59*(4), 1199–1223.

Csikszentmihalyi, M. (2014). Toward a psychology of optimal experience. In *Flow and the foundations of positive psychology* (pp. 209–226). Springer, Dordrecht.

Cupitt, C., & Golshan, N. (2015). Participation in higher education online: Demographics, motivators, and grit. In *STARS Conference* (pp. 1–4).

Diener, E., Wirtz, D., Tov, W., Kim-Prieto, C., Choi, D. W., Oishi, S., & Biswas-Diener, R. (2010). New well-being measures: Short scales to assess flourishing and positive and negative feelings. *Social Indicators Research, 97*(2), 143–156.

Duckworth, P. M., & Kelly,. (2007). Duckworth, AL, Peterson, C., Matthews, MD, & Kelly, DR (2007). *Grit: Perseverance and passion for long-term goals. Journal of Personality and Social Psychology, 92*, 1087–1101.

Larsson, M., Willander, J., Karlsson, K., & Arshamian, A. (2014). Olfactory LOVER: Behavioral and neural correlates of autobiographical odor memory. *Frontiers in Psychology, 5*, 312.

Flaming, N., & Granato, I. R. (2017). Personality and Gender: Grit Differences in Undergraduates. *Southwestern Psychological Association Conference. Oklahoma: Oklahoma City University.* https://doi.org/10.1080/00223890802634290

Gardner, S. K. (2008). 'What's Too Much and What's Too Little?': The Process of Becoming an Independent Researcher in Doctoral Education. *Journal of Higher Education, 79*(3), 326–350. https://doi.org/10.1353/jhe.0.0007

Golde, C. M. (2005). The Role of the Department and Discipline in Doctoral Student Attrition: Lessons from Four Departments. *The Journal of Higher Education, 76*(6), 669–700.

Hodge, B., Wright, B., & Bennett, P. (2018). The Role of Grit in Determining Engagement and Academic Outcomes for University Students. *Research in Higher Education* 59 (4). Springer Netherlands: 448–460. https://doi.org/10.1007/s11162-017-9474-y.

Hodges, B., Bedford, T., Hartley, J., Klinger, C., Murray, N., & O'Rourke, J. (2013). *and Neville Schofield*. Processes and Strategies for Improving Student Retention in University-Based Enabling Programs.

Ivankova, N. V., & Stick, S. L. (2007). Students' Persistence in a Distributed Doctoral Program in Educational Leadership in Higher Education: A Mixed Methods Study. *Research in Higher Education, 48*(1), 93–135. https://doi.org/10.1007/s11162-006-9025-4

Jaeger, B., Freeman, S., Whalen, R., & Payne, R. (2010). Successful Students : Smart or Tough?" *Proceedings of the 117th ASEE Annual Conference and Exposition*, AC 2010–1033.

Kannangara, C. S., Allen, R. E., Waugh, G., Nahar, N., Khan, S. Z. N., Rogerson, S., & Carson, J. (2018). All That Glitters Is Not Grit: Three Studies of Grit in University Students." *Frontiers in Psychology* 9 (AUG): 1–15. https://doi.org/10.3389/fpsyg.2018.01539.

Kelly, D. R., Matthews, M. D., & Bartone, P. T. (2014). Grit and Hardiness as Predictors of Performance among West Point Cadets. *Military Psychology, 26*, 327–342.

Keyes, C. L. (2002). The Mental Health Continuum : From Languishing to Flourishing in Life." *Journal of Health and Social Behaviour,* 43 (2): 207–222. https://www.jstor.org/stable/3090197?seq=1&cid=pdf-reference#references_tab_contents.

Madhlangobe, L., Chikasha, J., Mafa, O., & Kurasha, P. (2014). Persistence, Perseverance, And Success (Pps): A Case Study to Describe Motivational Factors That Encourage Zimbabwe Open University Odl Students to Enroll, Persist, And Graduate with Master's and Doctorate Credentials." *SAGE Open* 4 (3). https://doi.org/10.1177/2158244014544291.

Martinsuo, M., & Turkulainen, V. (2011). Personal Commitment, Support and Progress in Doctoral Studies. *Studies in Higher Education, 36*(1), 103–120. https://doi.org/10.1080/03075070903469598

MELS. (2013). "Education Indicators: 2012 Edition." *Ministry of Education, Leisure and Sports*. http://www.mels.gouv.qc.ca/sections/publications/publications/SICA/DRSI/Indicateurs_educ_2012_webP.p df.

Momtaz, Y. A., Hamid, T. A., Haron, S. A., & Bagat, M. F. (2016). Flourishing in Later Life." *Archives of Gerontology and Geriatrics* 63 (November). Elsevier Ireland Ltd: 85–91. https://doi.org/10.1016/j.archger.2015.11.001.

Muenks, K., Yang, J. S., & Wigfield, A. (2018). Associations between Grit, Motivation, and Achievement in High School Students. *Motivation Sciences* 4 (158–176). https://doi.org/10.1037/mot0000076.

Pate, A. N., Nalin Payakachat, T., Harrell, K., Pate, K. A., Caldwell, D. J., & Franks, A. M. (2017). Measurement of Grit and Correlation to Student Pharmacist Academic Performance. *American Journal of Pharmaceutical Education, 81*(6), 1–8. https://doi.org/10.5688/ajpe816105

Seligman, M. (2018). PERMA and the Building Blocks of Well-Being." *Journal of Positive Psychology* 13 (4). Routledge: 333–335. https://doi.org/10.1080/17439760.2018.1437466.

Singh, K., & Jha, S. D. (2008). Positive and Negative Affect, and Grit as Predictors of Happiness and Life Satisfaction. *Journal of the Indian Academy of Applied Psychology, 34*(April), 40–45. https://doi.org/10.1037/t06070-000

Vainio, M. M., & Daukantaitė, D. (2016). Grit and Different Aspects of Well-Being: Direct and Indirect Relationships via Sense of Coherence and Authenticity." *Journal of Happiness Studies* 17 (5). Springer Netherlands: 2119–2147. https://doi.org/10.1007/s10902-015-9688-7.

Culin, V., Katherine, R., Tsukayama, E., & Duckworth, A. L. (2014). Unpacking Grit: Motivational Correlates of Perseverance and Passion for Long-Term Goals. *Journal of Positive Psychology, 9*(4), 306–312. https://doi.org/10.1080/17439760.2014.898320

Wendler, C., Bridgeman, B., Markle, R., Cline, F., Bell, N., McAllister, P., & Kent, J. (2012). Pathways through Graduate School and into Careers. *Educational Testing Service*, 1–54. https://eric.ed.gov/?id=ED531249.

Wissing, M. P., Schutte, L., Liversage, C., Entwisle, B., Gericke, M., & Keyes, C. (2021). Important Goals, Meanings, and Relationships in Flourishing and Languishing States: Towards Patterns of Well-Being." *Applied Research in Quality of Life.* https://doi.org/10.1007/s11482-019-09771-8.